PEDIATRIC CARDIAC IMAGING

WILLIAM F. FRIEDMAN, M.D.

Professor and Chairman,
Department of Pediatrics, UCLA Medical Center;
J.H. Nicholson Professor of Pediatric Cardiology,
UCLA School of Medicine, Los Angeles

CHARLES B. HIGGINS, M.D.

Professor of Radiology and Chief,
Magnetic Resonance Imaging,
University of California, San Francisco

1984

W. B. SAUNDERS COMPANY

Philadelphia, London, Toronto, Mexico City, Rio de Janeiro, Sydney, Tokyo

W. B. Saunders Company: West Washington Square
Philadelphia, PA 19105

1 St. Anne's Road
Eastbourne, East Sussex BN21 3UN, England

1 Goldthorne Avenue
Toronto, Ontario M8Z 5T9, Canada

Apartado 26370—Cedro 512
Mexico 4, D.F., Mexico

Rua Coronel Cabrita, 8
Sao Cristovao Caixa Postal 21176
Rio de Janeiro, Brazil

9 Waltham Street
Artarmon, N.S.W. 2064, Australia

Ichibancho, Central Bldg., 22-1 Ichibancho
Chiyoda-Ku, Tokyo 102, Japan

Library of Congress Cataloging in Publication Data

Main entry under title:

Pediatric cardiac imaging.

1. Heart—Radiography. 2. Pediatric cardiology—Diagnosis. 3. Pediatric radiography. 4. Ultrasonic cardiography. 5. Radioisotopes in cardiography. I. Friedman, William F., 1936– II. Higgins, Charles B. [DNLM: 1. Angiocardiography—In infancy and childhood. 2. Echocardiography—In infancy and childhood. 3. Heart—Radiography. 4. Heart—Radionuclide imaging. 5. Heart diseases—Diagnosis. 6. Heart diseases—In infancy and childhood. 7. Nuclear magnetic resonance—In infancy and childhood. WS 290 P3707]

RJ423.5.R33P43 1984 618.92′6120757 84–1393

ISBN 0–7216–1287–3

Pediatric Cardiac Imaging ISBN 0-7216-1287-3

Last digit is the print number: 9 8 7 6 5 4 3 2 1

CONTRIBUTORS

LIONEL M. BARGERON, JR., M.D.
Professor of Pediatrics and Pediatric Cardiology, University of Alabama in Birmingham; Staff Physician, University Hospital, Birmingham, Alabama.
Angled Angiography

RICHARD L. BARON, M.D.
Clinical Assistant Professor of Radiology, University of Washington School of Medicine, Seattle; Staff Radiologist, Providence Hospital and The General Hospital of Everett, Everett, Washington.
Computed Tomographic Evaluation of the Great Arteries and Aortic Arch Malformations

LEE BENSON, M.D.
Assistant Professor of Pediatrics (Cardiology), UCLA School of Medicine, Los Angeles, California; Assistant Professor of Pediatrics (Cardiology) and Director of Pediatric Cardiac Catheterization Laboratory, Division of Cardiology, University of Toronto, Toronto, Ontario, Canada.
Positron Emission Tomography

THOMAS M. BIANCANIELLO, M.D.
Assistant Professor of Pediatrics, School of Medicine, SUNY at Stony Brook; Director, Division of Pediatric Cardiology, University Hospital, Stony Brook, New York.
Cardiac Imaging with Nuclear Magnetic Resonance

ELIAS H. BOTVINICK, M.D.
Associate Professor of Medicine and Radiology, University of California, San Francisco, California.
Cardiovascular Imaging with Nuclear Magnetic Resonance

EDWARD BUONOCORE, M.D.
Chairman, Department of Hospital Radiology, Cleveland Clinic, Cleveland, Ohio.
Digital Subtraction Angiography

JOACHIM H. BÜRSCH, M.D.
Professor of Pediatric Cardiology, University of Kiel; Attending Cardiologist, Departments of Pediatric Cardiology and Biomedical Engineering, Children's Hospital, University of Kiel, Kiel, West Germany.
Digital Angiocardiography for Assessment of Congenital Heart Disease

WESLEY COVITZ, M.D.
Associate Professor of Pediatrics, Medical College of Georgia, Augusta; Staff Pediatrician, Eugene Talmadge Memorial Hospital; Consultant in Pediatric Cardiology, Eugene Talmadge Memorial Hospital, University Hospital, Eisenhower Army Hospital, Augusta; Medical Center of Central

Georgia, Macon; Savannah Memorial Hospital, Savannah, Georgia; and Moncrief Army Hospital, Fort Jackson, South Carolina.
Radionuclide Studies of the Circulation

LAWRENCE E. CROOKS, Ph.D.
Associate Professor of Electrical Engineering; Assistant Director of Radiologic Imaging Laboratory, Department of Radiology and Radiologic Imaging Laboratory, University of California, San Francisco, California.
Cardiovascular Imaging with Nuclear Magnetic Resonance

THOMAS G. DiSESSA, M.D.
Assistant Professor of Pediatrics, UCLA School of Medicine; Director, Pediatric Echocardiography Laboratory, UCLA Hospital and Clinics, Los Angeles, California.
Echocardiographic Evaluation of Cardiac Performance

LARRY P. ELLIOTT, M.D.
Professor and Chairman, Department of Radiology, Georgetown University School of Medicine; Radiologist-in-Chief, Georgetown University Hospital, Washington, D.C.
Angled Angiography

CASIMIR EUBIG, Ph.D.
Associate Professor of Radiology, Medical College of Georgia, Augusta, Georgia.
Radionuclide Studies of the Circulation

ROBERT M. FREEDOM, M.D., F.R.C.P.(C.), F.A.C.C.
Professor of Pediatrics and Pathology, The University of Toronto School of Medicine; Senior Staff Physician, The Hospital for Sick Children, Toronto, Ontario, Canada.
Axial Angiocardiography in the Critically Ill Infant

WILLIAM F. FRIEDMAN, M.D.
J. H. Nicholson Professor of Pediatrics and Chairman, Department of Pediatrics, UCLA Medical Center, UCLA School of Medicine, Los Angeles, California.
Echocardiographic Evaluation of Cardiac Performance

MARK R. GOLDMAN, M.D.
Assistant Director of Cardiology, Newton-Wellesley Hospital, Newton; Clinical Associate in Medicine, Massachusetts General Hospital, Boston, Massachusetts.
Nuclear Magnetic Resonance Imaging

CURTIS E. GREEN, M.D.
Assistant Professor of Radiology, Georgetown University; Director, Section of Cardiac Radiology, Georgetown University Hospital, Washington, D.C.
Angled Angiography

FERNANDO R. GUTIERREZ, M.D.
Assistant Professor of Radiology, Mallinckrodt Institute of Radiology, Washington University School of Medicine, St. Louis, Missouri.
Computed Tomographic Evaluation of the Great Arteries and Aortic Arch Malformations

MARGERY A. HENEGHAN, M.D.
Assistant Professor of Radiology, School of Medicine, SUNY at Stony Brook; Director of Pediatric Radiology, University Hospital, Stony Brook, New York.
Cardiac Imaging with Nuclear Magnetic Resonance

ROBERT HERFKENS, M.D.
Assistant Professor of Radiology, Duke University Medical Center, Durham, North Carolina.
Cardiovascular Imaging with Nuclear Magnetic Resonance

CHARLES B. HIGGINS, M.D.
Professor of Radiology; Chief, Magnetic Resonance Imaging, Department of Radiology, University of California, San Francisco, California.
Digital Subtraction Angiography; Computed Tomography; Cardiovascular Imaging with Nuclear Magnetic Resonance

LEON KAUFMAN, Ph.D.
Professor of Physics; Director of Radiologic Imaging Laboratory, Department of Radiology and Radiologic Imaging Laboratory, University of California, San Francisco, California.
Cardiovascular Imaging with Nuclear Magentic Resonance

A. KURUC, B.S.
Research Associate, Division of Nuclear Medicine, Children's Hospital, Boston, Massachusetts.
Radionuclide Evaluation of Circulatory Shunts

PETER LANZER, M.D.
Clinical Affiliate Fellow in Cardiology and Thoracic Disease, Department of Medicine, University of California, San Francisco, California.
Cardiovascular Imaging with Nuclear Magnetic Resonance

MARTIN J. LIPTON, M.D.
Professor of Radiology and Medicine and Chief of Cardiovascular Imaging Section, University of California, San Francisco; Consultant, Veterans Administration Hospital, Palo Alto, and Letterman Army Hospital, San Francisco, California.
Computed Tomography; Cardiovascular Imaging with Nuclear Magnetic Resonance

ROBERT C. McKNIGHT, M.D.
Associate Professor of Radiology, Mallinckrodt Institute of Radiology, Washington University School of Medicine, St. Louis, Missouri.
Computed Tomographic Evaluation of the Great Arteries and Aortic Arch Malformations

JOSEPH PERLOFF, M.D.
Streisand Professor of Medicine and Pediatrics, UCLA School of Medicine, Los Angeles, California.
Positron Emission Tomography

GERALD M. POHOST, M.D.
Professor of Medicine and Director of Cardiology, University of Alabama Medical Center, Birmingham, Alabama.
Nuclear Magnetic Resonance Imaging

HEINRICH R. SCHELBERT, M.D.
Professor of Radiological Sciences, UCLA School of Medicine, Los Angeles, California.
Positron Emission Tomography

MARKUS SCHWAIGER, M.D.
Assistant Professor of Radiological Sciences, UCLA School of Medicine, Los Angeles, California.
Positron Emission Tomography

NORMAN H. SILVERMAN, M.D.

Associate Professor of Pediatrics and Radiology (Cardiology) and Director, Pediatric Echocardiography Laboratory, University of California, San Francisco, California.

An Ultrasonic Approach to the Diagnosis of Cardiac Situs, Connections, and Malpositions; Fetal Echocardiography

ROBERT A. SLUTSKY, M.D.

Associate Professor of Radiology and Radiologist, University of California, San Diego; Radiologist, Veterans Administration Hospital, La Jolla, California.

Radionuclide Evaluation of Cardiocirculatory Performance at Rest and with Exercise

INA LYNN DYER TONKIN, M.D.

Associate Professor of Radiology and Pediatrics, University of Tennessee Center for the Health Sciences; Attending Cardiovascular Radiologist, Director of Special Procedures Laboratory, and Co-Director of Cardiac Catheterization Laboratory, LeBonheur Children's Medical Center, Memphis, Tennessee.

The Definition of Cardiac Malpositions with Echocardiography and Computed Tomography

S. TREVES, M.D.

Associate Professor of Radiology (Nuclear Medicine), Harvard Medical School; Director, Division of Nuclear Medicine, Children's Hospital, Boston, Massachusetts.

Radionuclide Evaluation of Circulatory Shunts

PREFACE

The diagnosis of cardiovascular disease has become extremely precise. A major factor in this precision has been the depiction of cardiovascular anatomy in patients using several imaging techniques developed over the past three decades. Cardiac catheterization with angiography was the initial study that provided definitive diagnosis and subsequently fostered the amazing progress in the operative treatment of cardiovascular disease that has ensued over this time period. In the last decade we have experienced more progress in techniques for and change in concepts regarding cardiovascular imaging than in all preceding years combined. No longer does definitive anatomic diagnosis rely solely upon cardiac catheterization and angiography. Progress in cardiac diagnosis during the 1970's and continuing into the current decade has been characterized in a major way by the emergence of noninvasive and semi-invasive imaging techniques. These new techniques not only provide critical anatomic information but also assess global and regional myocardial function, blood flow and perfusion, and even *in vivo* myocardial metabolism.

The time seems appropriate to review the current status of cardiovascular imaging in pediatric cardiology. In general, there has been greater utilization and experience with the new cardiac imaging techniques in adult patients, and, indeed, some were initially developed for the assessment of ischemic myocardial disease. Most, if not all, of the new imaging techniques do have important applications in pediatric cardiology. Techniques such as angulated angiography have become established as critical for the preoperative evaluation of congenital cardiovascular abnormalities. Other modalities, such as computed tomography and magnetic resonance imaging, have infrequently been used for evaluating heart disease in children but may find considerable utility as greater experience accumulates.

In the past decade we have witnessed the introduction or rapid development of the following imaging modalities: sector scan echocardiography, radionuclide imaging, computed cardiac tomography, position emission tomography, and magnetic resonance imaging. Remarkable technical advances have supported these new and imaginative approaches to imaging the anatomy, physiology, and metabolism of the heart. Nonetheless, the complexity of cardiocirculatory disorders in the fetus, infant, and child still strains the capacities of these techniques in attaining precise diagnostic information.

Major aims of this volume were to review the latest experiences and refinements in the more familiar imaging modalities and to examine the capabilities and potential of the nascent imaging techniques for the diagnosis of heart disease in children. The latter aim should provide insight into future application of these new computer-based imaging techniques in pediatric cardiology.

The first portion of this volume gives an update on established methods of imaging the malformed heart. Thus, the sophisticated use of angulated views for cardiac angiography has received considerable attention. Angulated angiography and its applications are discussed in general and also in defining the frequently complex pathologic anatomy of the critically ill infant. Modern approaches to the evaluation of cardiocirculatory performance are detailed by using the non-invasive technique of radionuclide imaging and echocardiography. The use of echocardiography to help define abnormalities of situs and cardiac malpositions is described and serves as an example of how diagnostic accuracy can be improved beyond that achieved by even the traditional approach of cardiac catheterization.

The second portion of the book is intended to introduce and show the potential of several new cardiac imaging techniques. Not much experience is currently available with infants and children as the subjects for these new cardiovascular imaging techniques. The new techniques described in this volume include digital subtraction angiography and computed tomography for anatomic and physiologic imaging and positron emission tomography and magnetic resonance for the imaging of metabolic junctions. These later approaches, in particular, excite the imagination because they offer powerful tools for examining new dimensions of performance of the cardiovascular system. Positron emission tomography and magnetic resonance imaging will considerably expand our insights into the dynamic metabolic events associated with the transitional circulation, the responses of infants, children, and adolescents to diseases, alterations in the physical and chemical milieu associated with complex cyanotic heart disease, and the responses of the pediatric patient to cardioactive drugs.

The complexity of each imaging technique and the broad variety of imaging techniques currently extant make it unlikely that any single institution or person is any longer a pervasive authority on cardiovascular imaging. Consequently, the most practical approach to a volume that is intended to provide a truly updated view of this discipline is to gather a group of experts to review and discuss each of these many imaging modalities.

We express our appreciation to our splendid group of contributors for state-of-the-art presentations on cardiovascular imaging and for their pointing the way to exciting possibilities. We also thank Mrs. Linda Belfus at the Saunders Company for her advice and encouragement in the preparation of this volume

CHARLES B. HIGGINS
WILLIAM F. FRIEDMAN

CONTENTS

1

ANGLED ANGIOGRAPHY

General Approach and Findings

LARRY P. ELLIOTT, M.D., LIONEL M. BARGERON, JR., M.D.,
and CURTIS E. GREEN, M.D.

Advancements in cardiovascular surgical techniques have made feasible the repair of many complex congenital heart lesions that until recently had been considered inoperable. Because of this, it is untenable simply to make a generalized diagnosis of tetralogy of Fallot or ventricular septal defect from routine angiography. It is necessary to establish a "surgical diagnosis," which by definition, is one that demands more accuracy and refinement than that offered by conventional angiography or forward venous digital angiography (Fig. 1*A*). This accuracy and refinement can only be achieved with biplane cineangiographic systems (Fig. 1*B*).

This approach involves precise and consistent techniques in film exposure and development techniques that place the pathologic lesion at a right angle to the x-ray beam. The term that best describes these projection techniques is "axial" cineangiography.[2-6]

PRINCIPLES OF AXIAL CINEANGIOGRAPHY

Two basic patient (or equipment) maneuvers are involved: (1) the long axis of the heart is aligned perpendicular to the x-ray beam and (2) rotation of the patient results in the heart being radiographically sectioned at 30° angles. To accomplish this with fixed vertical and horizontal x-ray tubes, three positions were developed: (1) hepatoclavicular or four chamber, (2) long axial oblique, and (3) anteroposterior axial. The "sitting-up" projection, a fourth, will be discussed. The hepatoclavicular position profiles the posterior ventricular septum and atrial septum, separates the AV valves, places the four cardiac chambers en face, and clarifies mitral valve-semilunar valve and outflow tract relationships. The long axial oblique profiles the anterior ventricular septum, left ventricular outflow tract, and aortic valve-anterior mitral valve leaflet. The sitting-up view visualizes the bifurcation of the pulmonary trunk and separates true pulmonary arteries from systemic collaterals.

TECHNICAL CONSIDERATIONS OF THE FOUR-CHAMBER VIEW

Left Ventricle and Ventricular Septum. In the infant, raising the body 40 to 45° (or angling the tube 35 to 40° cranially in the adult) places the x-ray beam of the vertical image intensifier perpendicular to the long axis of the heart (Fig. 2). The 40 to 45° upward movement of the left shoulder or the combined left anterior oblique movement of the patient and image intensifier (adult) roughly aligns the atrial septum and the posterior part of the ventricular septum perpendicular to the x-ray beam. Therefore, in the initial phases of the ventriculogram, the posterior or inlet portion of the ventricular septum is first visualized. In addition, contrast medium fills the sinus, and the attachment of the posterior leaflet of the mitral valve is seen en face

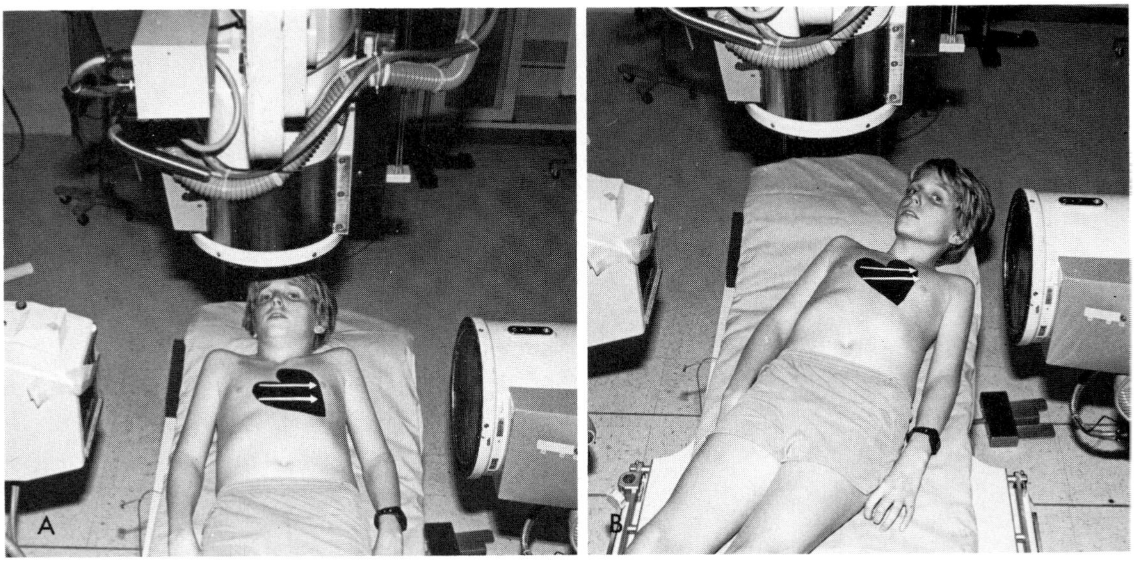

Figure 1. *A*, The relationship of the x-ray beam (white arrows) and the heart to the lateral x-ray tube, as seen with conventional angiography (fixed anteroposterior and lateral tubes). When the beam is not perpendicular to the long axis of the heart, there is always foreshortening of the ventricles, which obscures certain intracardiac structures, especially the left ventricular outflow tract and septum. *B*, The relationship of the lateral x-ray beam and heart to the lateral tube, as seen with axial alignment. One method of obtaining this angle is to slant the patient on the table in order to position the long axis of the heart perpendicular to the x-ray beam.

(Figs. 3 and 4). An anatomic landmark useful in proper positioning is the junction between the attachment of the anterior and posterior mitral valve leaflets and the junction of the left ventricular free wall and the posterior ventricular septum (see Figs. 3 and 4). During ventricular systole, the area of the free wall shows a slight localized bulge, characteristic of the projection (Fig. 4*B*). Distinctive ventricular septal defects (defects of the persistent arterioventricular

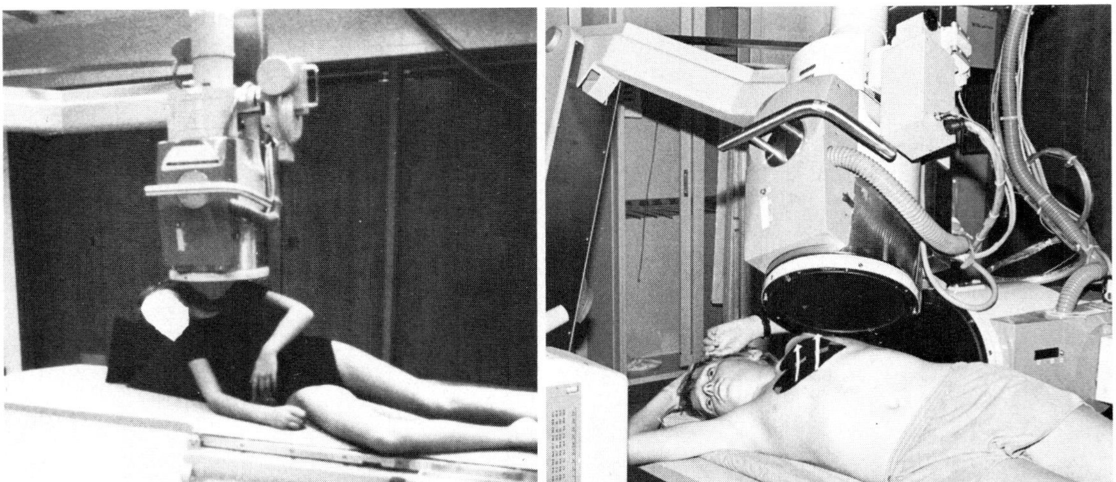

Figure 2. Two methods of obtaining the four-chamber view. *A*, The fixed tube system with the vertical image tube serving as the source of the four-chamber view. The patient sits at a 35 to 45° angle and the left shoulder is elevated 35 to 45°. For axial alignment with the lateral image tube (complementary right anterior oblique view), the patient is slanted 20 to 25° in relation to the table. *B*, The mobile anteroposterior tube (Philips parallelogram). The patient is rotated 20 to 25° in the left anterior oblique position, and the anteroposterior image is moved leftward 20 to 25°, with cranial movement of 30 to 40°.

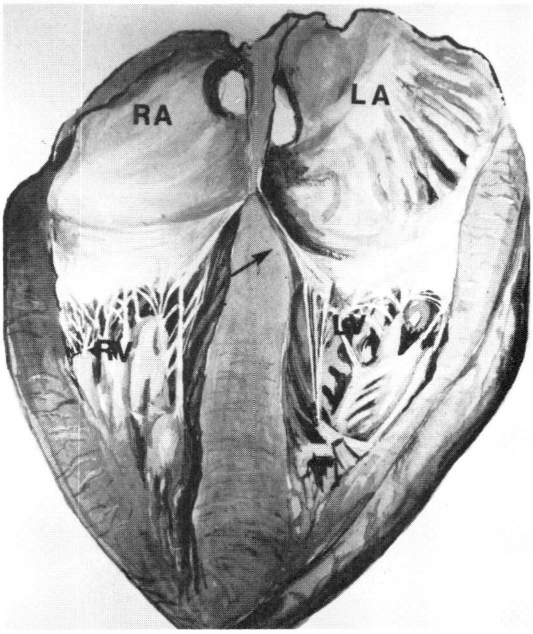

Figure 3. Drawing of an actual heart specimen as it would be seen by the vertical image intensifier in the four-chamber view. This shows the relationship of the two atrioventricular valves, the atrial septum, and the posterior ventricular septum. The arrow points to the junction of the posterior ventricular septum with the free wall of the septum and the junction of the posterior mitral valve commissure. This region is crucial and is seen best in the first few frames of the cine before opacification of the left ventricular outflow tract. RA: right atrium, LA: left atrium, RV: right ventricle, and LV: left ventricle.

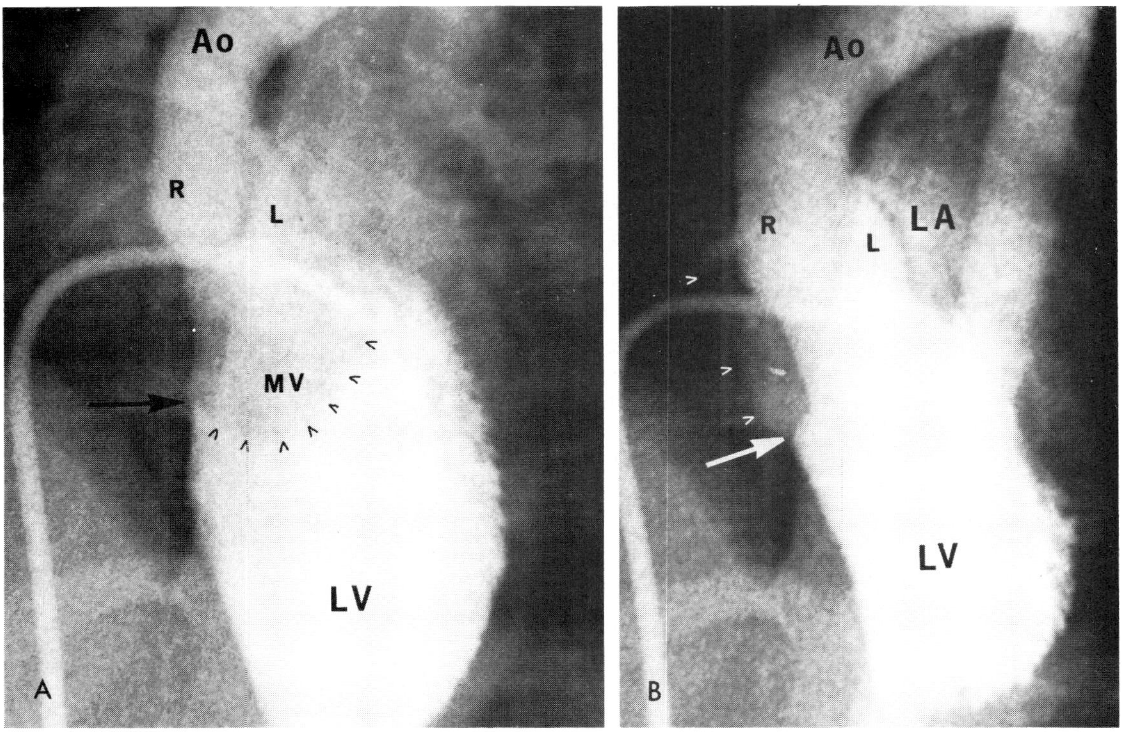

Figure 4. Normal left ventricle (LV) in a four-chamber view. *A*, Diastole. The arrow shows the crucial junction of the posterior mitral valve and the anterior mitral valve commissure with the posterior and free wall of the ventricular septum. The arrowheads depict the posterior mitral valve attachment. The left ventricular outflow tract is opacified and is seen between the mitral valve (MV) and the aortic valve (Ao). The left atrium is opacified because of catheter-induced incompetence of the mitral valve. However, note how the left atrium is completely separated from the right atrium. This is of great help in diagnosing mitral valve incompetence and shunting between the left ventricle and the right atrium. *B*, Systole. The junction of the mitral valve, posterior ventricle, and free wall septum (arrow) is usually characterized by a localized bulge during systole. The entire length of the muscular septum is also well visualized. The arrowheads show the relationship of the atrial septum ot the ventricular septum. LA: left atrium, R: right cusp, and L: left cusp.

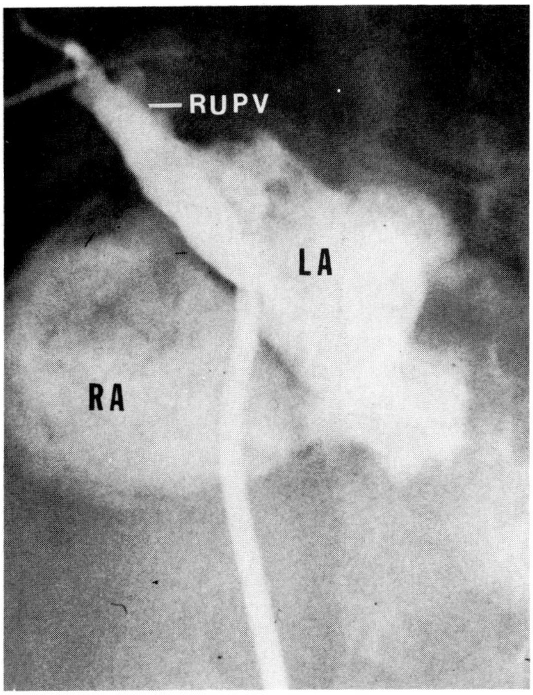

Figure 5. Analysis of the atrial septum. The patient is in the four-chamber view, and the catheter tip is in the right upper pulmonary vein (RUPV). The atrial septum is in profile. The right atrium (RA) opacifies via a defect in the ostium primum in the most inferior aspect of the atrial septum. LA: left atrium.

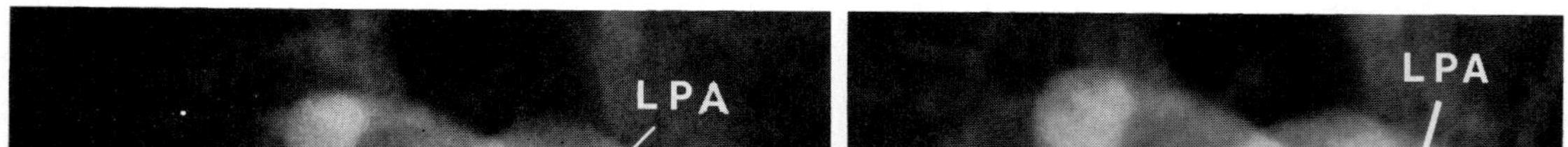

Figure 6. Normal right ventricle (RV) in the four-chamber view. *A*, Ventricular diastole. This view gives a clear visualization of the entire tricuspid valve ring (arrowheads), the pulmonary valve, pulmonary trunk (P), the bifurcation and course of the left pulmonary artery (LPA). *B*, Ventricular systole. This view also depicts accurately the location and size of the ventricular septal defect in conditions involving systemic pressures in the right ventricle, especially in the transposition and double outlet right ventricle complexes.

canal type) occur in this area and can be localized best in this projection.

Atrial Septum. The septum is best visualized by injecting through the tip of the catheter into the proximal portion of the right upper pulmonary vein (Fig. 5). Defects occurring anywhere along the septum are then visualized, since contrast material streams along the septum in order to reach the mitral valve (see Fig. 5).

Additional Left-Sided Structures and Relationships. A number of other structures are usually well visualized in this projection. Mitral valve incompetence and shunting between the left ventricle and the right atrium can usually be distinguished and is especially helpful in the diagnosis of the persistent common atrioventricular canal spectrum of the lesion.

Relationships between the mitral valve and semilunar valve are distinctly visualized in conditions marked by a double-outlet right ventricle or bilateral infundibula.

Abnormal attachments of the mitral valve to the left ventricular outflow tract or subaortic diaphragms can be seen to best advantage in this projection.

In transposition complexes, the pulmonary valve, pulmonary trunk, and the origin of the left pulmonary artery from the pulmonary trunk are best outlined with the same injection.

The transverse aortic arch and ductus region are opened up so that a patent ductus arteriosus can be distinguished easily from the pulmonary artery of the upper lobe crossing the ductal region, a phenomenon that may cause confusion after conventional left ventriculography in patients with a large ventricular septal defect.

Right Ventricle and Pulmonary Trunk. From the side of the right ventricle, the ventricular septum is seen in profile (Fig. 6). The tricuspid valve ring is well visualized, and this view is extremely valuable in detecting the phenomenon of "straddling" valve. With straddling, the valve ring would be deviated further to the left. The inflow portion of the ventricle is seen to the right of the septum and is not superimposed over the left ventricle (see Fig. 6*A*).

COMPLEMENTARY AXIAL RIGHT ANTERIOR OBLIQUE VIEW WITH FOUR-CHAMBER VIEW

This view is approximately 70 to 80° from that obtained with the vertical tube and the patient in this same position. It is not always needed but often gives much additional information. The slanting of the body 10 to 15° away from the horizontal image intensifier places the long axis of the heart perpendicular to the x-ray beam. The 45° sitting position and the 45° upward rotation of the left shoulder allows the horizontal image intensifier to view the heart in an elongated and tilted right anterior oblique view.

Left Ventricle. Left ventriculography yields a tilted right anterior oblique view with excellent visualization of the mitral valve, posterior papillary muscle, left ventricular outflow tract, and a number of cusps of the aortic valve. This projection is also the best for visualizing the supracristal ventricular septal defect (see Fig. 16*A*).

Right Ventricle and Pulmonary Trunk. The horizontal tube produces an excellent view of the ostium of the right ventricular infundibulum, the musculature comprising the posterior wall of the infundibulum itself (this musculature between the two semilunar valves is usually termed the body of the crista supraventricularis in normal hearts and infundibular septum in abnormal ones), as well as the sinus and inflow portions of the right ventricle (Fig. 7).

LONG AXIAL OBLIQUE VIEW

Method of Positioning. In infants and most children, the technique of positioning involves the following maneuvers (Fig. 8). The entire torso or long axis of the patient's body is slanted 30° away from the horizontal image intensifier, or in some instances the child is positioned with the feet to the right side of the table, and the right shoulder is elevated 15 to 20° (see Fig. 8*A*).

In large children and adults, the patient is rotated into a 30 to 35° left anterior oblique position, and the anteroposterior image intensifier of the parallelogram is rotated 35 to 40° to the left and angled cranially 25 to 30° (see Fig. 8*B*). A third method is shown in Figure 8*C*. So much of the angulation depends on the position of the heart in the thorax. A heart horizontally positioned will require more angulation of the patient or the cranial tube than a heart vertically positioned. This is not a cookbook technique.

Angiocardiographic Aspects of the Long Axial Oblique View. Of the two planes of viewing in the infant and small child, the horizontal tube is usually the most useful. Slanting the body on the table places the long axis of the heart perpendicular to the x-ray beam (see Fig. 8*A*). The second maneuver, rotation of the right shoulder, places the anterior portion of the ventricular septum and the left ventricular outflow tract in profile (Figs. 9 and 10). The lateral tube is essentially viewing the ventricular sep-

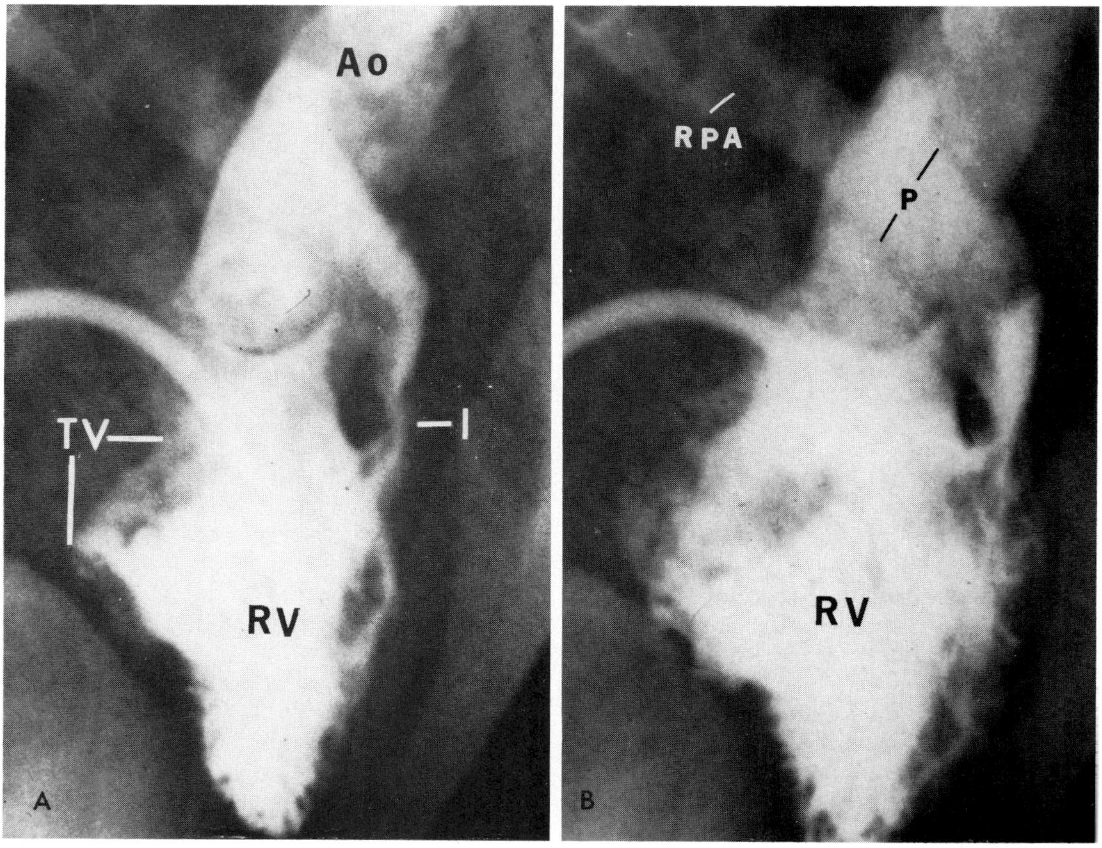

Figure 7. Right ventricular cineangiogram with the four-chamber view in tetralogy of Fallot. *A*, Ventricular systole. The tricuspid valve (TV) is in profile, and the sinus and inflow portions are well visualized. The infundibular stenosis (I), created by the anteriorly deviated infundibular septum or body of the crista supraventricularis, is vividly demonstrated. *B*, Ventricular diastole. The pulmonary valve, annulus, trunk (P), and origin and full length of the pulmonary artery (RPA) are well visualized. Ao: aorta.

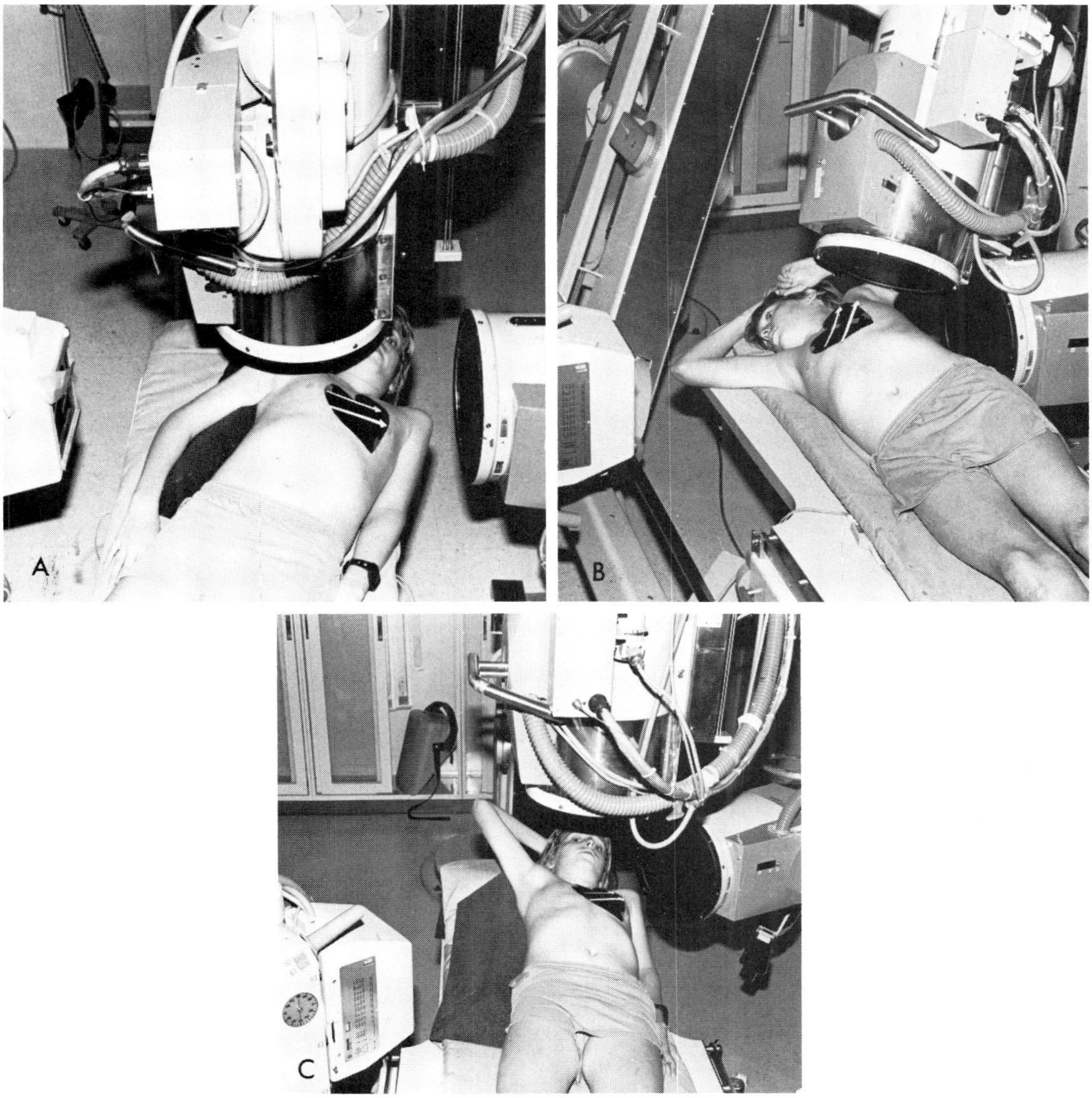

Figure 8. Three techniques of obtaining the long axial oblique view. *A*, The fixed tube system with the lateral tube used as the source of the axial oblique view. The left shoulder is elevated 15 to 20°, and the patient is slanted 25 to 30° in relation to the table. *B*, Mobile anteroposterior tube (Philips parallelogram) serves as the source of view. The patient is rotated in the left anterior oblique position 30 to 35° on a sponge wedge with leftward movement of the anteroposterior image tube 35 to 40°, and cranial angulation 20 to 25°. *C*, When both tubes are mobile, the lateral image tube is the primary source of view. The left shoulder of the patient is elevated 15 to 20°; the lateral image is cranially angulated 25 to 30°. A complementary right anterior oblique view is obtained by moving the anteroposterior tube 30 to 45° to the right (not shown).

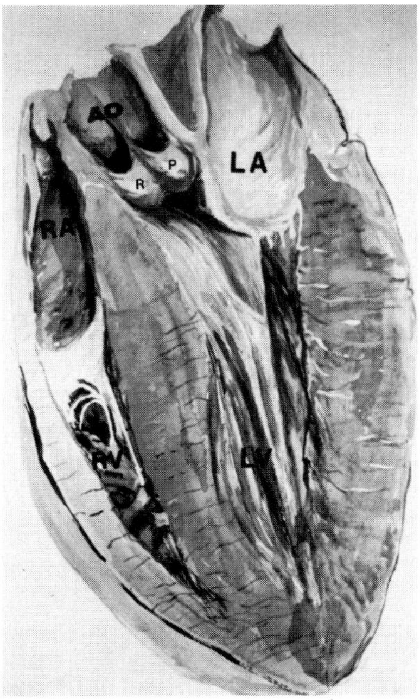

Figure 9. An artist's rendition of a necropsy specimen as seen on a cineangiogram in the long axial oblique view. The left ventricular outflow tract, anterior leaflet of the mitral valve, and the anterior aspect of the entire muscular septum are in profile. RA: right atrium, LA: left atrium, Ao: aorta, R: right aortic valve cusp, P: Posterior aortic valve cusp, RV: right ventricle, LV: left ventricle.

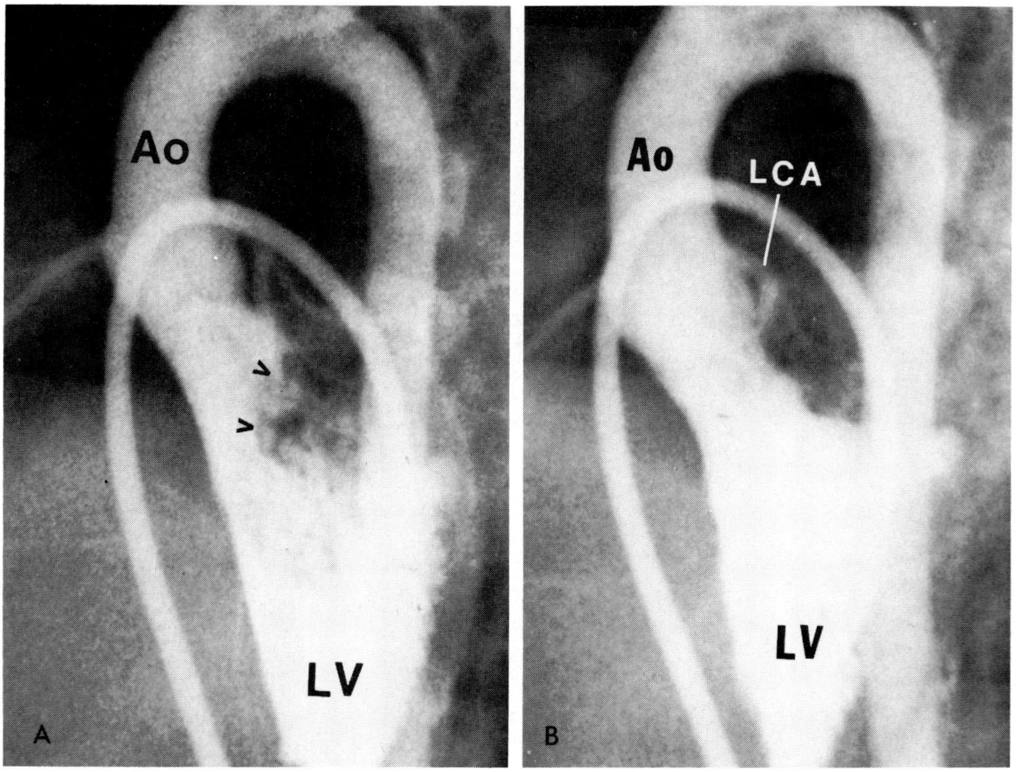

Figure 10. Normal left ventricular cineangiogram utilizing the long axial oblique view. Both phases (A and B) vividly depict the anterior portion of the ventricular septum, the left ventricular outflow tract, and the entire muscular septum below. *A*, Ventricular diastole. This left ventriculogram can be considered a virtual cast of the left ventricle (LV) shown in Figure 9. Arrowheads designate the anterior leaflet of the mitral valve. *B*, Ventricular systole. The left coronary artery (LCA) and its bifurcation are well visualized. Ao: aorta.

tum as a steep 65 to 70° left anterior oblique view with the long axis of the heart perpendicular to the x-ray beam.

In the adult, the anteroposterior tube is the primary source of information, hence the movement of both the patient and tube to ultimately create a steep 60 to 70° left anterior oblique projection (see Fig. 8*B*). The cranial movement of the image intensifier places the ventricular septum and outflow tract in profile, which is analogous to the 30° slanting movement of the infant on the table (see Fig. 8*A*).

When the long axial oblique view is compared with the four-chamber view, a left anterior oblique view of the ventricular septum 20 to 30° steeper is obtained with the long axial oblique projection (compare Figs. 3 and 4 with Figs. 9 and 10). This results in the anterior and outflow tract septa being viewed in profile, rather than the posterior ventricular septum.

Figure 9 shows an artist's rendition of an actual necropsy specimen as seen angiocardiographically in this view. Note how the left ventricular outflow tract and the region of the subaortic valve are emphasized. The free edge of the anterior leaflet of the mitral valve is also seen in profile. This area is well demonstrated because the left outer shoulder of the left ventricle has been displaced inferiorly and no longer overlies the outflow area as in the conventional left anterior oblique view.

Figure 10 shows a left ventriculogram in the long axial oblique view. It is strikingly similar to the drawing in Figure 9. In diastole (see Fig. 10*A*), the anterior leaflet of the mitral valve is seen in profile. The left ventriculogram vividly depicts the anterior portion of the ventricular septum in the area of the left ventricular outflow tract and the muscular septum below this. The relationship of the mitral valve to the left ventricular outflow tract itself can also be fully appreciated. This is a particularly informative view in patients with hypertrophic obstructive cardiomyopathy[7] (asymmetric septal hypertrophy) as well as in patients with prolapse of the anterior leaflet of the mitral valve.[5] The left main, anterior descending, and proximal circumflex coronary arteries are well delineated.

COMPLEMENTARY AXIAL RIGHT ANTERIOR OBLIQUE VIEW WITH LONG AXIAL OBLIQUE VIEW

With the vertical image intensifier in the infant or child (see Fig. 8*A* and *C*) and the horizontal image intensifier in the adult (Fig. 8*B*), the right and left ventricles are placed in a right anterior oblique view of approximately 45°. The 45° right anterior oblique projection offers an advantage over the conventional, single plane, right anterior oblique views of 30° by lessening the degree of foreshortening of the ventricle.[5] This is especially valuable in adult patients with ventricular asynergy.[5]

Left Ventricle and Thoracic Aorta. The atrioventricular part of the cardiac septum (Fig. 11) is well delineated in this projection. Since this structure is usually absent or appears "bitten out" in persistent common atrioventricular canal lesions (see Fig. 11*C*), this projection is of particular value in determining whether a given case falls within this spectrum of lesions. When correlated with the findings derived from the long axial oblique view, this view depicts well the variations in mitral valve movement and often demonstrates the site of mitral valve incompetence.

Relationship of the Mitral Valve to the Left Atrium. When correlated with the findings of the long axial view, this view yields considerable information about which leaflets are involved in the various forms of mitral valve disease, especially in the prolapsing mitral valve.[5]

With the long axial oblique technique in tetralogy of Fallot, right ventriculography yields about the same information as the right ventricular injection in the anteroposterior projection. This is an excellent projection with which to view the trabecula septa marginalis region of the right ventricle.

ANTEROPOSTERIOR AXIAL TECHNIQUE

This is a biplane mode of filming in which both shoulders are elevated approximately 10 to 15°, and the patient is slanted 15 to 20° on the table. It closely approximates the position used in the conventional anteroposterior and lateral projections. Both of these maneuvers place the ventricles and their outflow tracts in better profile.

We use this positioning for an initial injection when the chamber position is unknown or when the case is complex and the diagnosis uncertain.

SITTING-UP VIEW

This view was designed to visualize better the pulmonary trunk and its bifurcation.[8] The same results can be obtained if the patient's body is (1) in the supine position with cranial

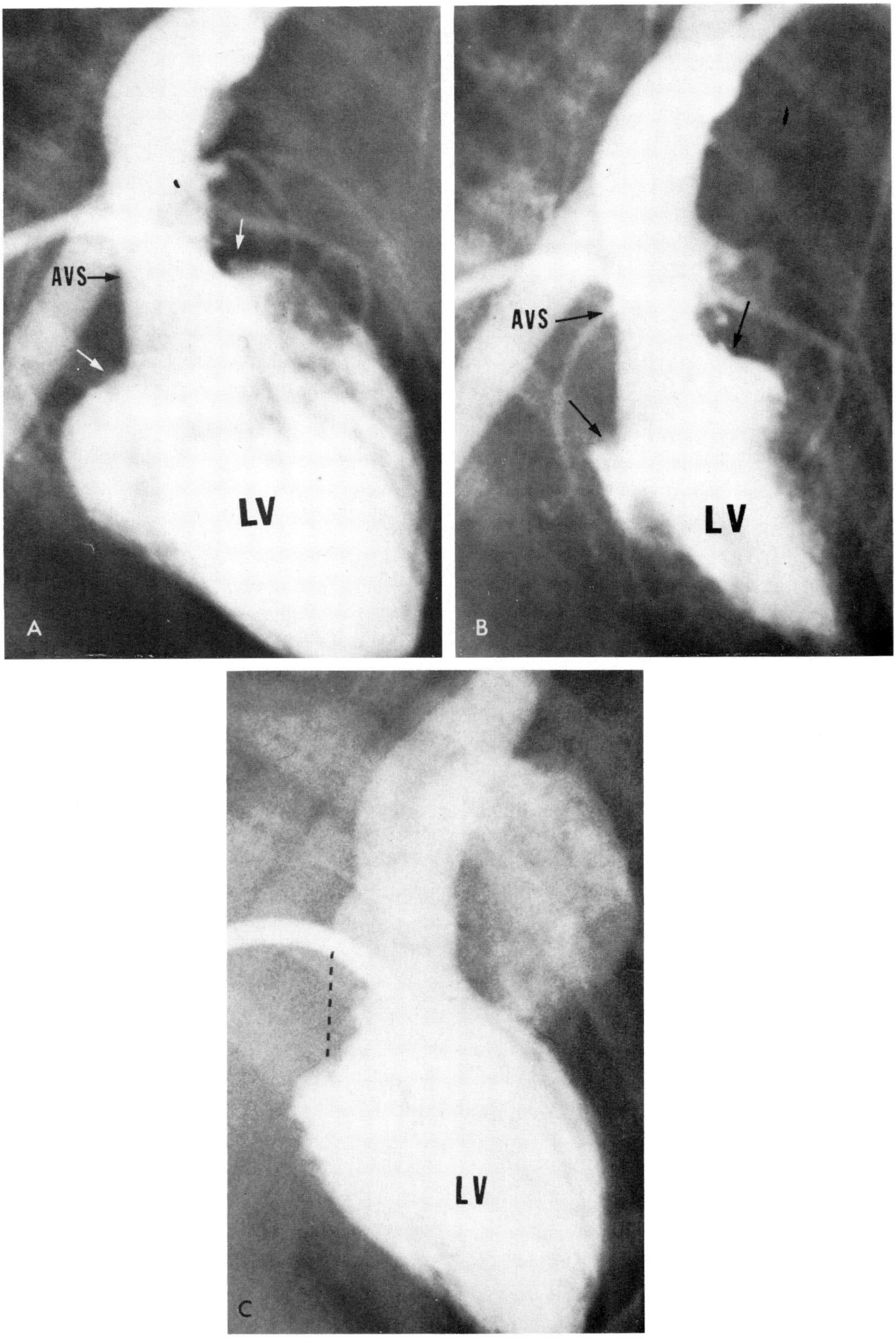

Figure 11. Normal left ventricular cineangiogram (right anterior oblique view) from the x-ray beam perpendicular to the long axial oblique view. *A*, Ventricular diastole. The balck arrows show the region of the atrioventricular septum (AVS); the white arrows show the mitral valve commissure. This view is especially useful in patients with either the supracristal form of ventricular septal defect or a defect in the atrioventricular septum, which is fundamental to all lesions classified as persistent, common lesions of the atrioventricular canal. *B*, Ventricular systole. *C*, A right anterior oblique view shows a large defect in the atrioventricular septum.

angulation of the image intensifier (Fig. 12*A*); (2) elevated with cranial angulation of the image intensifier (Fig. 12*B*); or (3) elevated 45 to 60° in a straight sitting-up position (Fig. 12*C*).

This view is optimal for visualization of the bifurcation of the right and left pulmonary arteries, the pulmonary valve, annulus, and pulmonary trunk (Fig. 12*D*). The sitting maneuver places the pulmonary trunk and its bifurcation in a position almost perpendicular to the x-ray beam. With conventional angiocardiographic techniques, the pulmonary trunk is foreshortened and is superimposed over the bifurcation of the pulmonary trunk. This view or a modification of it is always used in performing angiography in patients with tetralogy of Fallot or pulmonary atresia with a common arterial trunk (usually a tetralogy with pulmonary atresia). In lesions involving a common arterial trunk, this view is especially important since it allows accurate detection and separation of systemic collateral or bronchial arteries from true central pulmonary arteries.

The sitting maneuver projects the true pul-

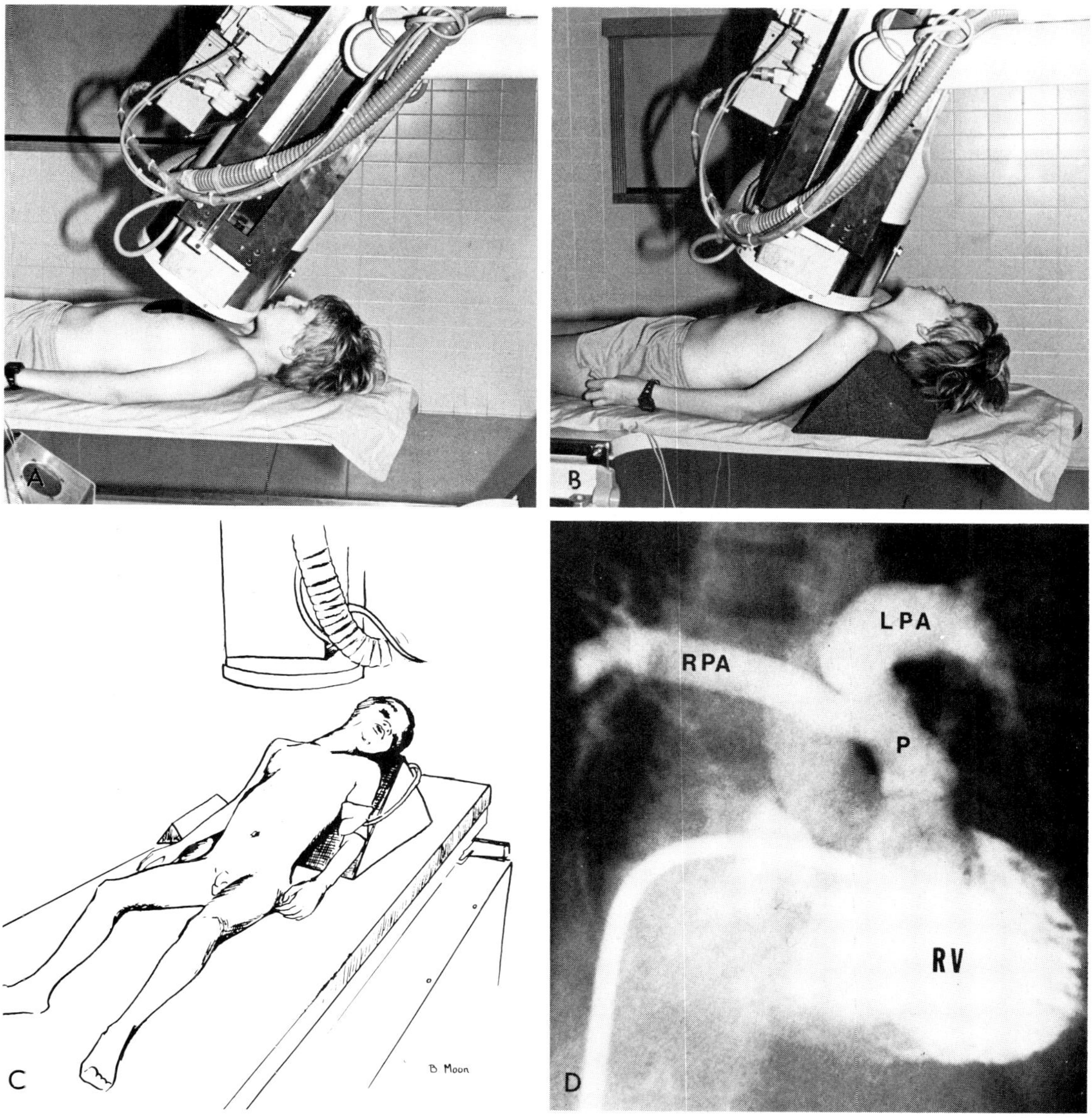

Figure 12. Three techniques in obtaining the sitting-up view, as shown in relation to the vertical image intensifier. *A*, Patient is supine with the image intensifier moved cranially 50°. *B*, Combination of propping the patient and cranial movement of the x-ray tube. *C*, Patient is in a 45° sitting position. Fixed anteroposterior tube alone. *D*, Right cineventriculogram, sitting position, in a patient with tetralogy of Fallot. This particular view yields superb visualization of the bifurcation of the pulmonary trunk (P) and the pulmonary valve and its annulus. LPA: left pulmonary artery, RPA: right pulmonary artery, RV: right ventricle.

monary arteries inferior to the labyrinth of systemic collateral or bronchial arteries and serves as an effective substitute for subtraction techniques.

SPECIFIC LESIONS

Ventricular Septal Defects. The location of the ventricular septal defect must be identified, including its site of entry and exit, as seen from both the left and right ventricular sides. With precise knowledge of the location of the ventricular septal defect, the surgeon can make a more informed decision about the optimal surgical approach.

The long axial oblique view is almost invariably used as the initial injection. The rationale for this is that most defects are located in the left ventricular outflow tract or muscular septum, areas that are profiled by the long axial oblique view.

An exception is the ventricular septal defect located in the posterior or inlet septum. Since this defect tends to show left axis deviation on electrocardiography, patients with clinical evidence of a ventricular septal defect and left axis deviation should undergo a four-chamber view as the initial examination.

Perimembranous Ventricular Septal Defect. Two forms of perimembranous ventricular septal defects are shown in Figure 13. In case 1 (Fig. 13*A*) a small defect is shown, and in case 2 (Fig. 13*B*), a large defect is demonstrated. In both, the origin of the perimembranous ventricular septal defect is depicted arising in the center of the left ventricular outflow tract at the junction of the right and posterior cusps (see Fig. 13*A*). In Figure 13*B*, the perimembranous location is indicated by its adjacent position to the aortic valve, and, more important, by the fact that the anterior wall of the outflow tract septum is intact and the trabeculated muscular and posterior (inlet) septum are well visualized and reveal no additional defects.

Ventricular Septal Defect of the Anterior Outflow Tract Septum. In case 3, a large ventricular septal defect confined to the most anterior aspect of the outflow tract septum is shown (Fig. 14). As with the perimembranous

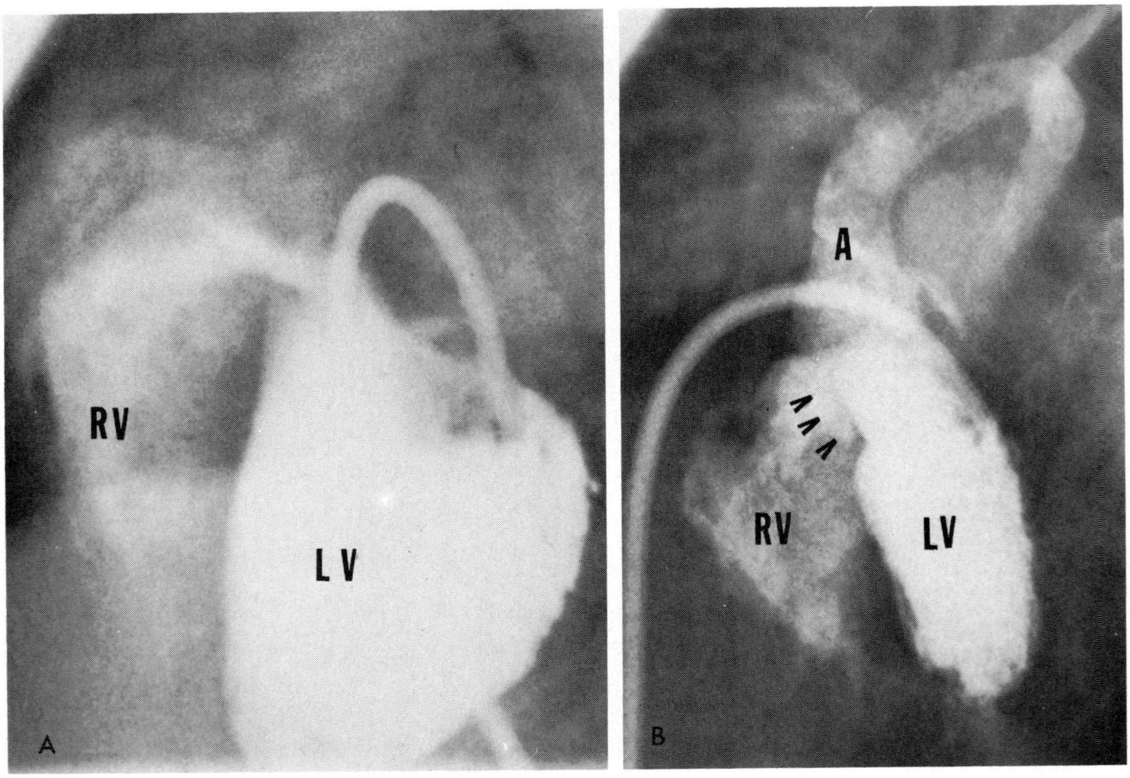

Figure 13. Two cases of ventricular septal defect are studied using the long axial oblique view. *A*, The defect in the outflow tract of the septum is nearly confined to the membranous septum. *B*, A large defect involves the membranous septum and surrounding muscle (perimembranous). Arrows designate the continuation of the anterior outflow tract area through the defect. LV: left ventricle, RV: right ventricle.

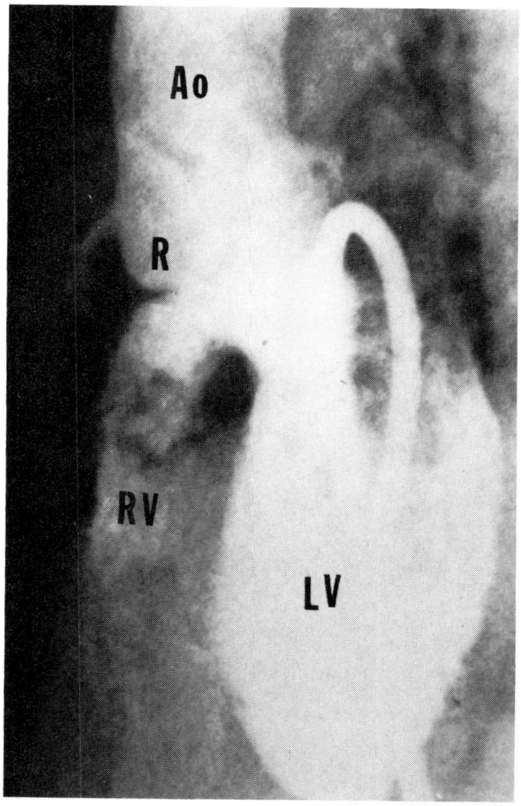

Figure 14. A large ventricular septal defect involves the most anterior aspect of the outflow tract of the left ventricle (LV). The right aortic valve cusp (R) forms the superior margin of the defect, and the anterior wall of the outflow tract septum is silhouetted by the defect itself. RV: right ventricle, Ao: Aorta.

ventricular septal defect, this defect resides immediately beneath an aortic valve cusp. In contradistinction to the perimembranous ventricular septal defect, there is a break or discontinuity in the anterior wall of the outflow tract septum, indicating that the defect is anterior to the perimembranous region. Moreover, the subaortic location is confined to the right cusp. This type of ventricular septal defect is often observed in patients with a deviated or hypoplastic body of the crista supraventricularis or infundibular septum.[1]

Muscular Ventricular Septal Defect. In Figure 15 (case 4), a ventricular septal defect is seen in two axial projections. Conventional anteroposterior and lateral cineangiograms failed to demonstrate adequate anatomic detail, but a biplane long axial oblique view showed the defect to be in the mid portion of the muscular septum (see Fig. 15*A*). The mid septal wall, which in this view is the anterior portion of the septum, forms a continuous linear density through the defect, indicating that the ventricular septal defect is more posterior. To locate the lesion more precisely, a four-chamber view (30° less than the long axial oblique view) was performed (see Fig. 15*B*). The continuity of the mid portion of the muscular septal wall was interrupted, indicating that the ventricular septal defect was in the posterior aspect of the muscular ventricular septum. Because of the unusual location of this lesion, the surgeon chose to approach it through the left ventricle. A right atrial or a right ventricular approach would probably have resulted in a serious problem of identification.

Supracristal Ventricular Septal Defect. This defect is one in which the axial right anterior oblique view is optimal for determining the location of the defect. As shown in Figure 16, the right anterior oblique view shows a wide jet emanating from the left ventricle and coursing immediately into the pulmonary trunk. The body of the crista supraventricularis (infundibular septum) is obscured or not apparent. In the other defects involving the outflow tract septum, the body of the crista supraventricularis forms a pillar of muscle between the aortic valve and contrast column (see Fig. 7). The companion left anterior oblique view suggests the presence of this type of ventricular septal defect by virtue of the more vertical course of the contrast column as well as the decreased opacification of the sinus portion of the right ventricle.

Persistent Common Atrioventricular Canal.

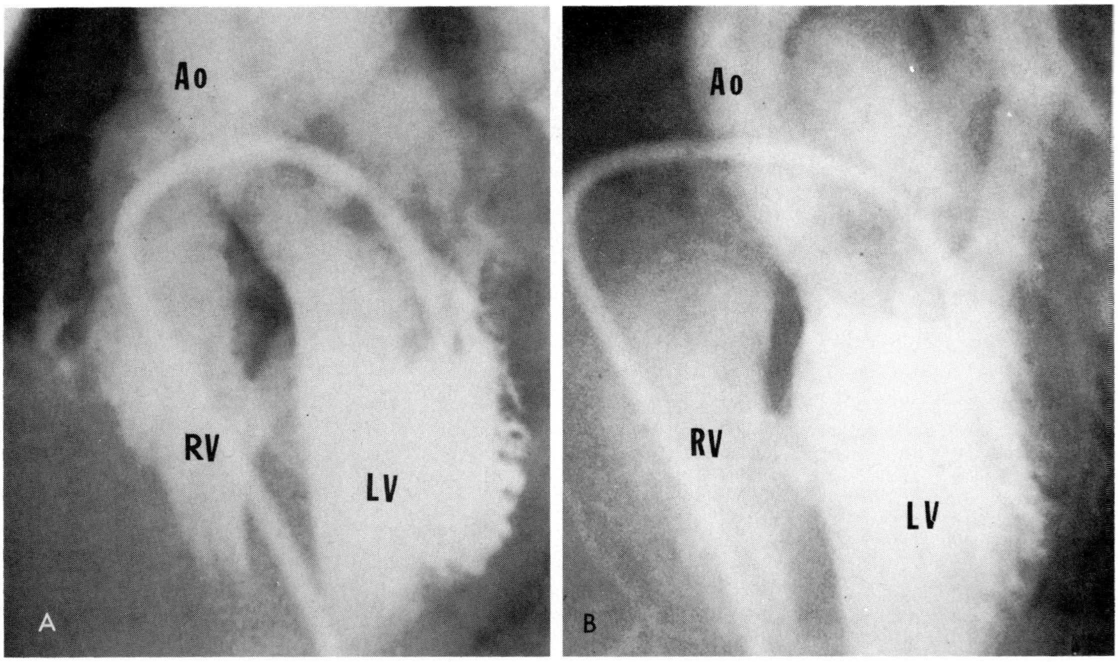

Figure 15. Large posterior, muscular ventricular septal defect. Left ventriculography was performed by using both the long axial oblique view (A) and the four-chamber view (B). To locate the ventricular septal defect precisely, cineangiographic sectioning with these two techniques was performed. The anterior septum is profiled in *A*; the posterior septum is visualized in *B*. LV: left ventricle, RV: right ventricle, and Ao: aorta.

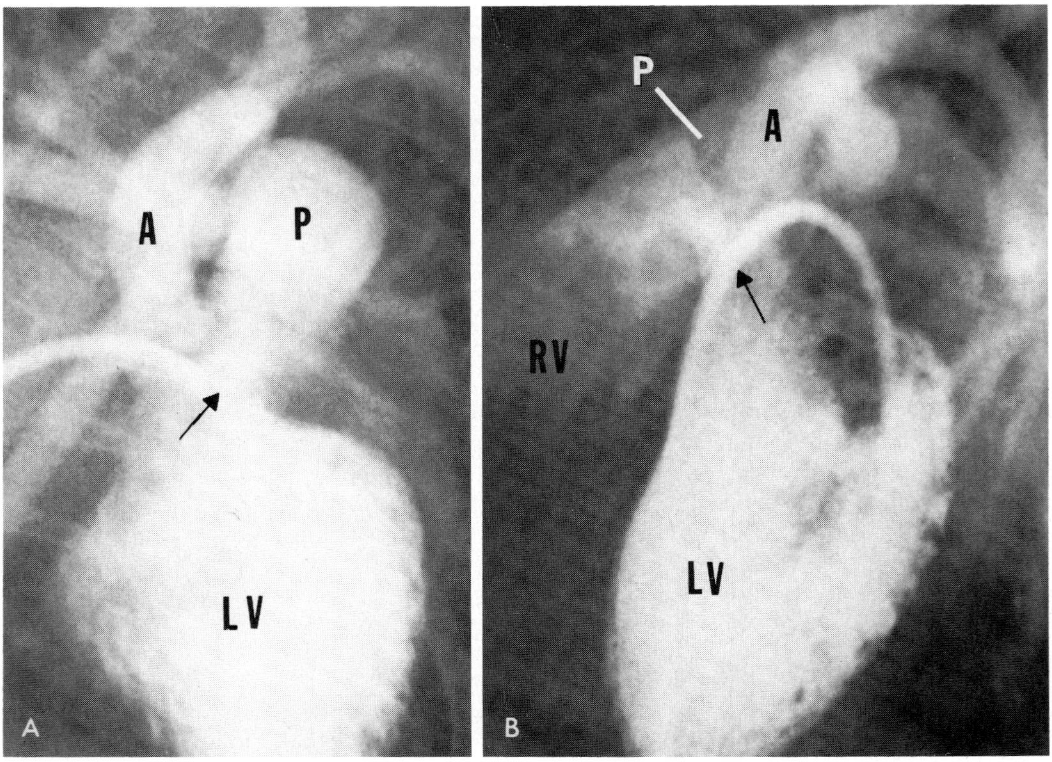

Figure 16. Supracristal type of ventricular septal defect. *A*, Axial right anterior oblique view 90° to the long axial oblique view. There is a wide jet coursing directly from the left ventricle (LV) into the pulmonary trunk (P). In this ventricular septal defect, the body of the crista supraventricularis is obliterated. In a perimembranous defect, it would be seen as muscle bundle between the two semilunar valves. *B*, Long axial oblique view (90° to A). The jet leaving the left ventricle (LV) barely opacifies the upper aspect of the right ventricle (RV) and is angled upward into the pulmonary trunk (P). A: atrium.

The technique of axial cineangiography allows the diagnostician to view persistent, common arterioventricular canal lesions much more accurately than in the past. Fundamentally, the lesions that form the spectrum of persistent common atrioventricular canals can be divided into three major types:

1. The complete type involves a common atrioventricular (AV) valve with a large interventricular communication and an ostium primum defect (the latter not necessarily a large defect).

2. The intermediate or transitional type is essentially a complete type, differentiated only by a piece of valve tissue that forms a bridge between the anterior and posterior leaflets of the common AV valve.

3. The partial type is characterized by two distinctly formed AV valves: a separation of the anterior leaflet of the mitral valve into a superior and inferior component, and an ostium primum defect. The two-component anterior mitral leaflet essentially closes the interventricular communication by its anomalous attachment onto the concave crest of the deficient ventricular septum. The separation or cleft in the anterior leaflet is necessary to valve function and is therefore a compensatory mechanism to promote normal valve function.

Our angiocardiographic examination of persistent common atrioventricular canal lesions is preceded by the following protocol of questions:

1. What is the status of the ventricular septum, including the atrioventricular septum, the posterior or inlet septum, and the outflow tract septum?

2. What type of atrioventricular valve is involved? Is it a common AV valve? If so, does the valve override into the right or left ventricle? Is it free-floating or nonfree-floating? Is there bridging tissue between the anterior and posterior leaflets, placing the AV canal within the intermediate or transitional type, rather than the complete type? Or are there two formed AV valves, in which the anterior leaflet of the mitral valve reveals a variably sized cleft?

3. Regardless of the anatomic configuration of the AV valve, is the valve competent or incompetent? And if incompetent, what is the direction and location of the regurgitant jet?

4. The least important—what is the status of the atrial septum?

Status of the Ventricular Septum. Varying degrees of absence of the AV component of the muscular septum are characteristic of all three forms of persistent common AV canal. Angiographically, this is seen in the axial right anterior oblique view (obtained as the complementary view with either the four-chamber or long axial oblique views) as an irregular notch or bite in the atrioventricular part of the left ventricular outflow tract (see Fig. 11*C*).

The three basic configurations of the posterior or inlet septum most commonly seen in persistent common AV canal lesions are shown in Figure 17. In Figure 17*A*, there is a large defect

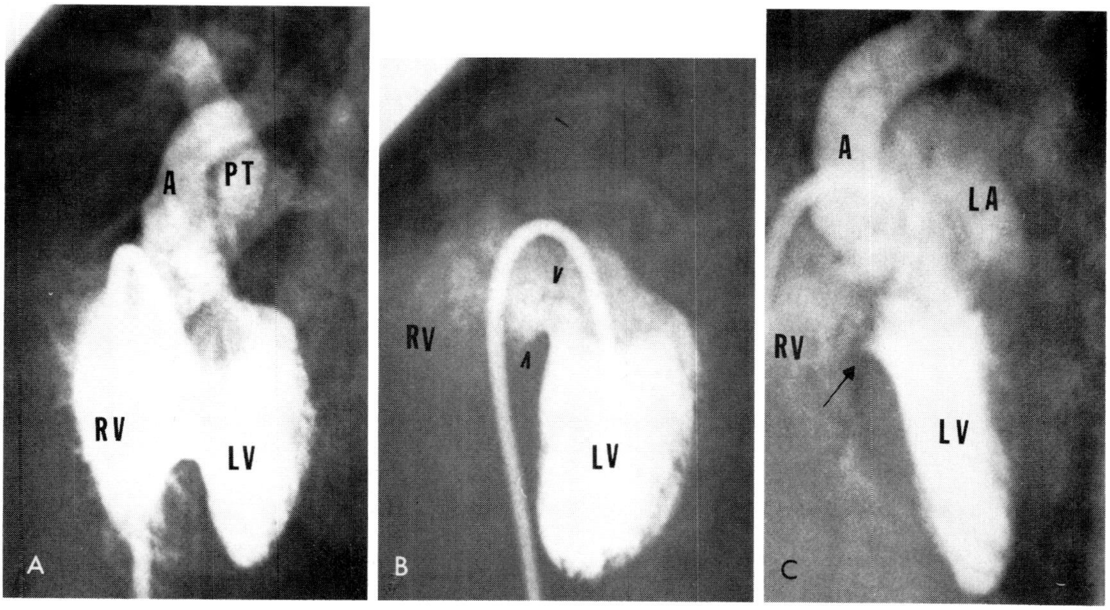

Figure 17. Variations in the posterior septum in three examples of the complete form of persistent common atrioventricular canal as seen in the four-chamber view. *A*, Extremely large posterior ventricular septal defect. *B*, Posterior ventricular septal defects of a small to moderate size (between arrowheads). *C*, Intact posterior ventricular septum (arrow). RV: right ventricle, LV: left ventricle, A: atrium, and LA: left atrium.

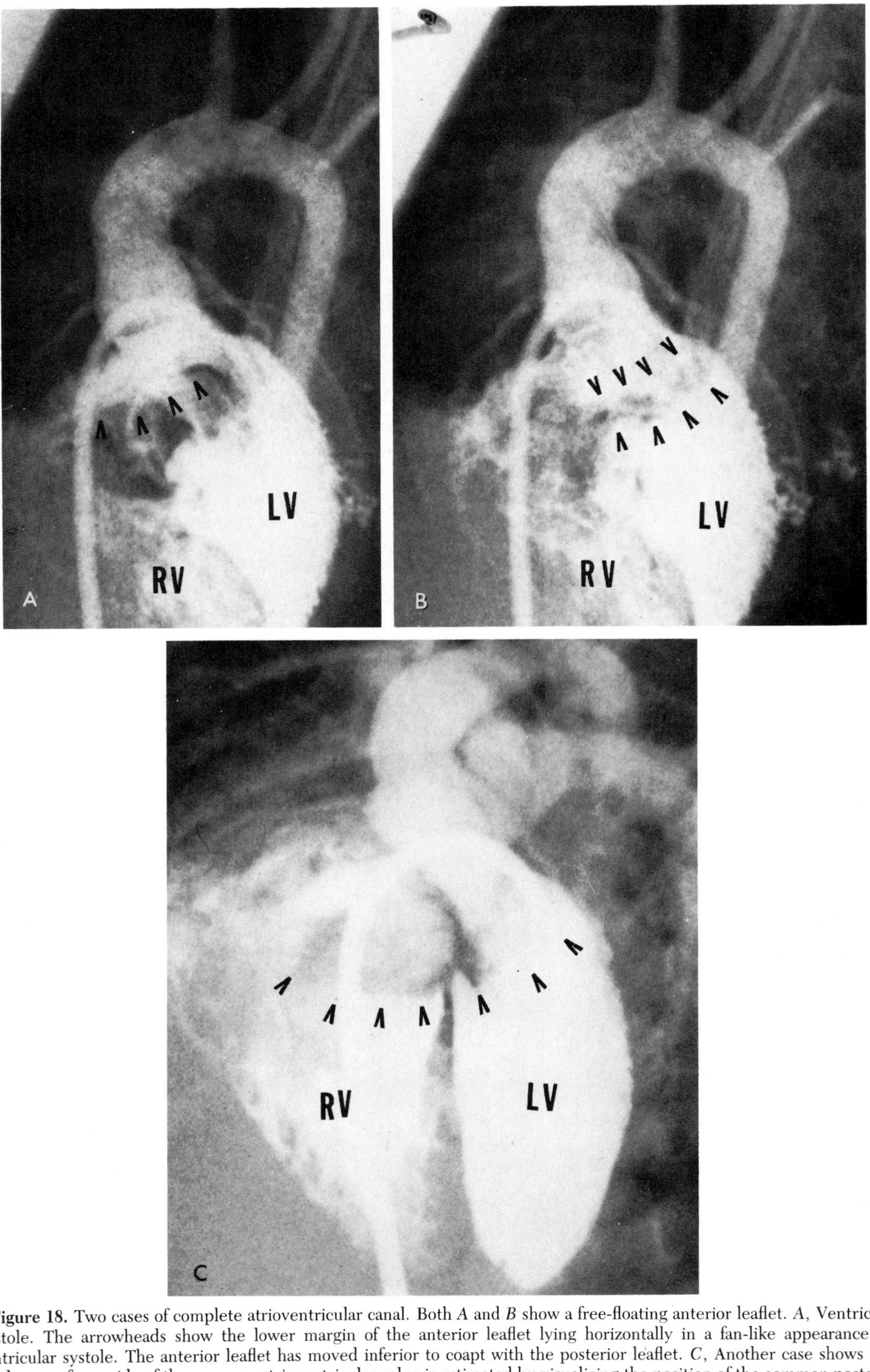

Figure 18. Two cases of complete atrioventricular canal. Both *A* and *B* show a free-floating anterior leaflet. *A*, Ventricular diastole. The arrowheads show the lower margin of the anterior leaflet lying horizontally in a fan-like appearance. *B*, Ventricular systole. The anterior leaflet has moved inferior to coapt with the posterior leaflet. *C*, Another case shows how the degree of override of the common atrioventricular valve is estimated by visualizing the position of the common posterior leaflet attachment or annulus in relationship to the ventricular septum. Moderate override is present into the right ventricle (RV). LV: left ventricle.

in the posterior or inlet ventricular septum. In Figure 17*B*, a moderately sized defect is demonstrated, and in Figure 17*C*, the posterior ventricular septum is intact. When the interventricular communication is as large as that shown in Figure 17 (*A* and *B*), the lesions almost always fall within the category of complete or intermediate forms of persistent common AV canal. With the intact posterior septum (see Fig. 17*C*), a partial or complete form of persistent common AV canal may be present.

Status of the AV Valves. There are three basic types of AV valves: (1) the common AV valve, (2) two formed AV valves with a variably sized cleft separating the anterior leaflet of the mitral valve into a superior and inferior component (partial type), and (3) a common AV valve with bridging tissue from the anterior leaflet to the posterior one (intermediate type).

In the four-chamber view, common AV valves are characterized by a continuation of the posterior valve annulus as a common or continuous line across the top of the ventricular septum (Fig. 18*A* and *C*). The valve may show an equal degree of override (Fig. 18*B*) or displacement, most commonly to the right (see Fig. 18*C*) but sometimes to the left. The degree of override of the common AV valve can thus be determined.

A formed yet cleft anterior mitral leaflet has both a superior and an inferior component (Fig. 19). These two components displace the column of contrast material during diastole, creating an elongated left ventricular outflow tract (see Fig. 18*A*). They can then be seen to coapt together during systole (see Fig. 18*B* and *C*). These findings are the hallmark of the partial form of persistent common AV canal. Almost invariably, there is some jetting of contrast medium across the incompetent mitral valve into the right atrium, left atrium, or both simultaneously. On occasion, contrast material will also jet into the right ventricle. An interventricular shunt, therefore, does not rule out a partial canal.

The common AV valve with bridging tissue (intermediate type) is characterized by the formation of a pseudoannulus (Fig. 20). This is created by contrast medium trapped beneath the bridging tissue and caught up in the short chordae that usually insert into a crest of the deficient ventricular septum. The size of the ventricular septal defect is usually as large as that of the complete type, but the interventricular shunt may be reduced because of partial closure of the ventricular septal defect by chordal attachments onto the septum.

In patients with a common AV valve, the status of the anterior leaflet is also determined by whether it is free-floating or bound by chordae tendineae (nonfree-floating). In most cases, a free-floating leaflet is characterized during diastole as a continuous crescent or fan-like structure beneath the aortic valve (see Fig. 18*A*). It usually overrides the ventricular septum and shows considerable excursion during systole as it traverses inferiorly and coapts with

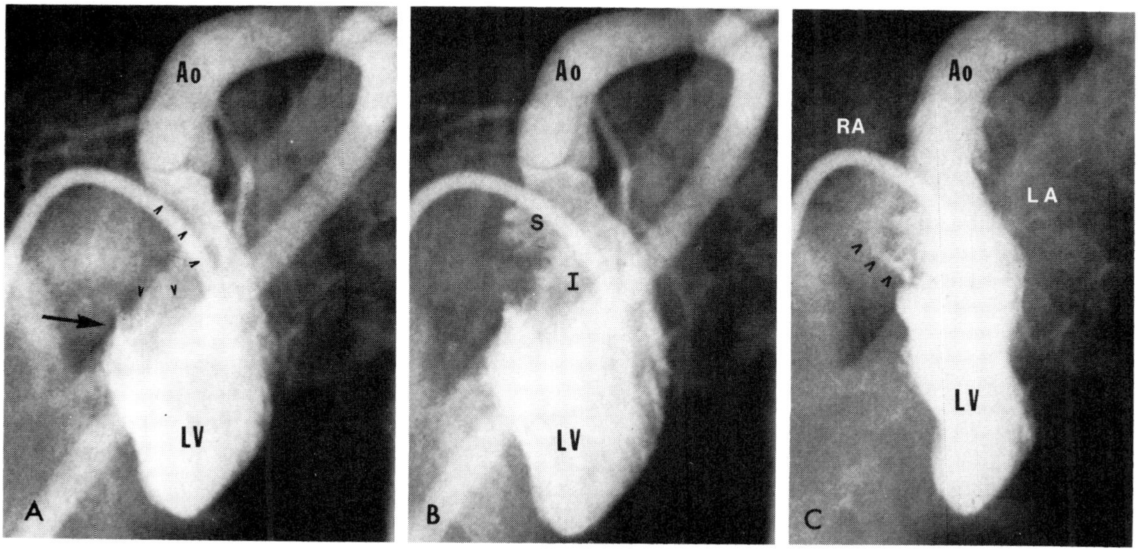

Figure 19. A four-chamber view of the partial form of atrioventricular canal. Left cineventriculogram. *A*, Diastole. Arrowheads show elongated and narrow outflow tract. A posterior ventricular septum (arrow) is intact at the attachment of the normally formed posterior mitral valve. *B*, Early systole. S: superior component, I: inferior component of the divided or cleft anterior mitral leaflet. *C*, Mid systole. Arrowheads depict a jet to the right atrium (RA). The left atrium (LA) shows minimal opacification as well. Note the clear-cut separation of the two atrial chambers. LV: left ventricle, Ao: Aorta.

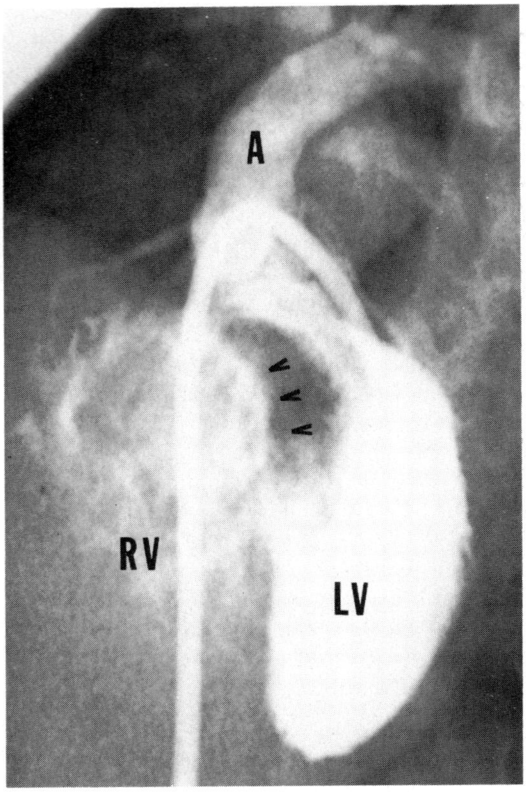

Figure 20. Left cineventriculogram. Four-chamber view of an intermediate form of persistent common atrioventricular canal. There is a defect of moderate size in the posterior ventricular septum. The arrows outline a vertical, thin, linear, opaque line that gives the impression of a valve ring. This represents momentarily trapped contrast media underneath the chordae, which attaches the thin bridging tissue to the crest of the ventricular septum. RV: right ventricle, LV: left ventricle, A: atrium.

the posterior leaflet (see Fig. 18*B*). On cine studies, this has an oval or fish-mouth-like movement.

With the leaflet that is not free-floating, the anterior leaflet has a restricted degree of motion. It may produce a well-demarcated left ventricular outflow tract and reduce the size of the interventricular communication in the left ventricular outflow tract (Fig. 21).

Determination of the degree of competence of the AV valves is important, surgically. The four-chamber view separates the atria from the ventricles. Jets of contrast medium, attributable to valvular incompetence and passing from the left ventricle to the right atrium, from the left ventricle to the left atrium (see Fig. 21*B*), or from both ventricles to both atria simultaneously, can easily be differentiated.

Status of the Outflow Tract Septum. This area of the ventricular septum is not profiled in the four-chamber view. However, defects, which in persistent common AV canal lesions are usually located beneath the anterior common leaflet, are apparent in this area (see Fig. 21). In most cases, this injection is omitted.

Status of the Atrial Septum. The atrial septum is best analyzed with a right upper lobe pulmonary vein injection, provided it connects normally to the left atrium (see Fig. 5). This is best performed in the four-chamber view also.

Atrial Septal Defect. Atrial septal defects are demonstrated with unusual clarity when contrast medium is injected into the right upper pulmonary vein (provided it connects normally to the left atrium) and is filmed in the four-chamber view.

Ostium Secundum Defect. The right upper pulmonary vein cineangiogram outlines nicely the septum secundum and allows an accurate estimate of its size (see Fig. 7*A*).

Sinus Venous Defect. These defects must be visualized with a left atrial injection because of the 90 per cent incidence of anomalous connection of the right upper pulmonary vein to the superior vena cava. The catheter tip should be positioned as close as possible to the right upper corner of the left atrium. The superior vena cava will appear to override the atrial septum.

Tetralogy of Fallot with Pulmonary Atresia (Pseudotruncus Arteriosus). In tetralogy of Fallot, the major extracardiac problem with pulmonary valve atresia is the differentiation of the true central pulmonary arteries from the systemic collateral or aortopulmonary arteries (Fig. 22). This decision has life and death significance for the patient and cannot be compromised.

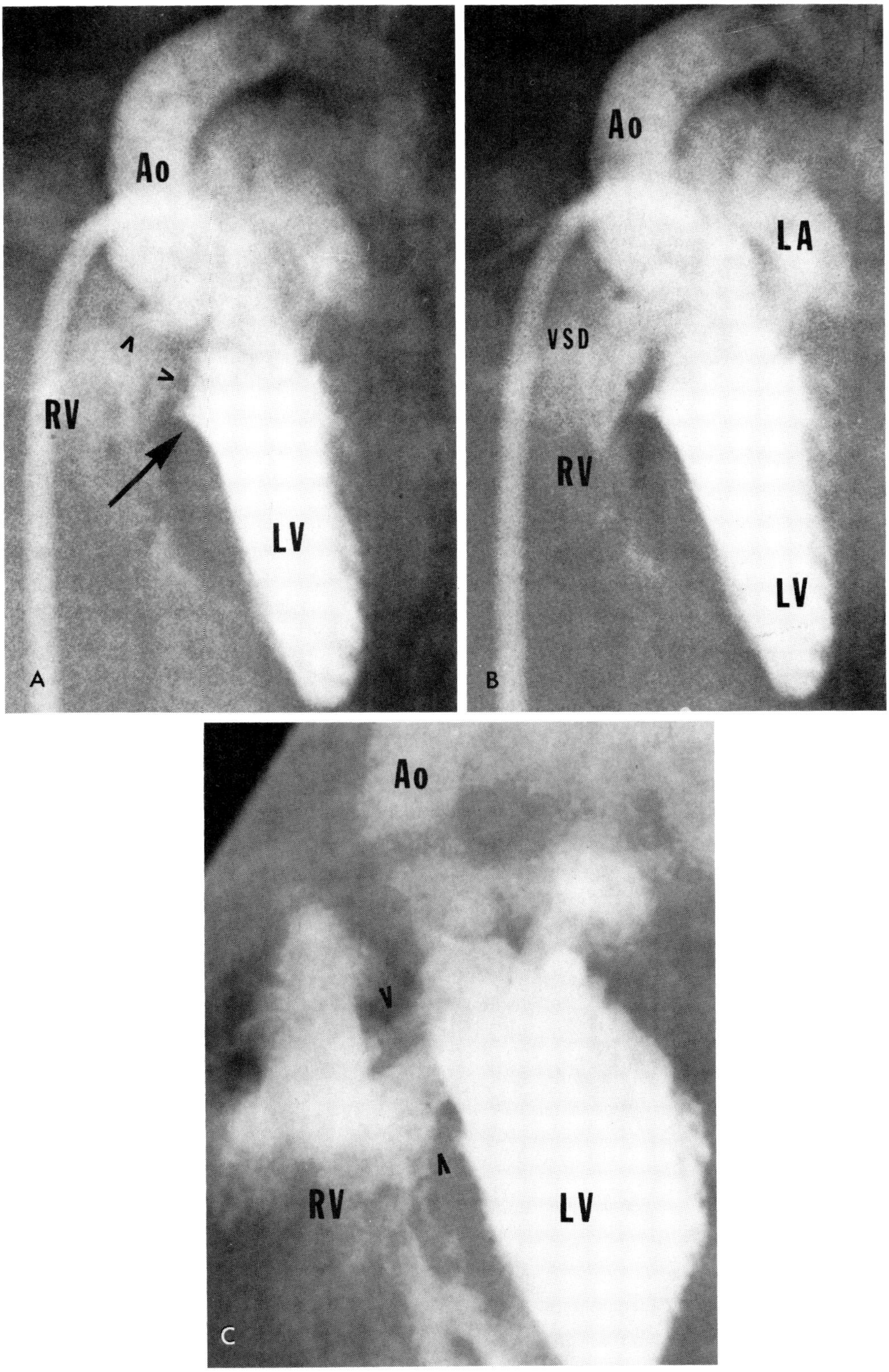

Figure 21. Left cineventriculogram. Four-chamber view of a complete form of atrioventricular canal. *A* and *B*, The posterior ventricular septum underneath the posterior leaflet is intact, but there is evidence of a large interventricular communication as shown by opacification of the right ventricle (RV). The arrowheads in *A* depict the superior and inferior leaflets that showed relatively poor mobility and were consistent with leaflets that were not free-floating. The left atrium (LA) opacifies because of common atrioventricular valve incompetence. *C*, By placing the defect (arrowheads) in profile, a long axial oblique view of the same case shows that the ventricular septal defect (VSD) is located in the outflow tract of the septum, underneath the anterior leaflet. LV: left ventricle, Ao: Aorta.

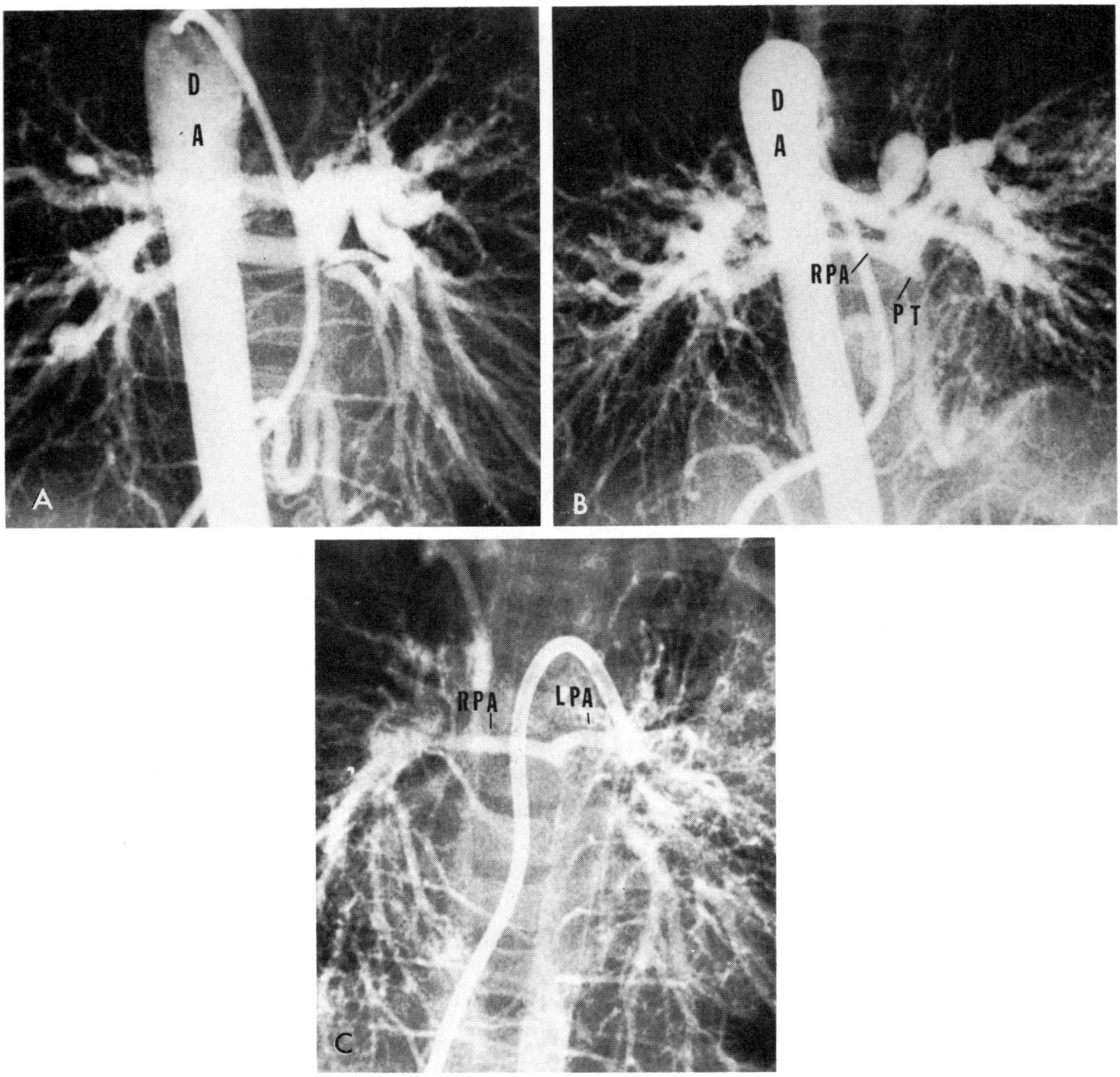

Figure 22. Two cases of tetralogy of Fallot with pulmonary atresia (pseudotruncus arteriosus). *A*, Upper descending thoracic aortogram (DA) in the straight anteroposterior view. Large systemic collateral or bronchial arteries are noted to fill bilaterally. These communicate in the hilar region with true intrapulmonary arteries. A central true pulmonary arterial tree is not visualized. *B*, Descending thoracic aortogram (DA) performed with the patient in a sitting position. (Same patient as in *A*.) A true central pulmonary arterial tree and nubbin like pulmonary trunk (PT) are visualized. The very proximal left pulmonary artery is present but was interrupted from the intrapulmonary component. RPA: right pulmonary artery. *C*, A view in another patient in a sitting position shows the "sea-gull"-like configuration of a true pulmonary arterial tree. Cineangiography can show true pulmonary artery trees much smaller than this and is more sensitive than seriographic filming. RPA; right pulmonary artery, LPA; left pulmonary artery.

In conventional anteroposterior angiograms, the central pulmonary arteries are superimposed on the labyrinth of systemic collateral arteries (see Fig. 22*A*). Neither are necessary since the collateral and true pulmonary arteries can be differentiated by positioning the patient in an upright sitting position or angling the x-ray image intensifier in a cranial direction (toward the feet) (see Fig. 22*B* and *C*). With cranial angulation, the true pulmonary arteries show a distinctive shape and motion.

Case 1: Inoperable Pulmonary Atresia-Ventricular Septal Defect without Central Pulmonary Arteries. Conventional anteroposterior thoracic aortography (see Fig. 22*A*) may show numerous systemic collateral arteries arising from the upper descending aorta, as well as a large patent ductus arteriosus. When such a maze of vessels exists, differentiating a true pulmonary arterial system from the systemic arteries may often be difficult or impossible.

The sitting-up view (see Fig. 22*B*) shows

complete separation of the true pulmonary arteries from the systemic collateral or bronchial arteries. The pulmonary trunk fills in a retrograde manner from the patent ductus, and there is discontinuity of the main and left pulmonary artery. A later frame showed a large left pulmonary artery filling from the systemic collateral or bronchial collaterals.

Case 2: Tetralogy of Fallot with Pulmonary Atresia. Figure 22*C* shows a late arterial phase of an upper descending thoracic aortogram. The true pulmonary arteries, together with the pulmonary trunk, show a characteristic V-shaped configuration. When viewed in a cineangiographic projector, this confluence shows a characteristic movement, the "sea gull sign."[3, 4] We are convinced that high quality cine studies, with their inherent ability to show movement, are superior to seriographic filming.

Case 3. This case demonstrates the importance of refusing to accept, even after multiple thoracic aortograms, angiographic data that indicate that true and confluent pulmonary arteries are not present. When this occurs, wedge pulmonary venous angiography should be performed.

Large systemic collateral arteries opacifying intrapulmonary arteries in both lungs are shown in Figure 23*A*. A central confluent true pulmonary arterial tree is not apparent. A second

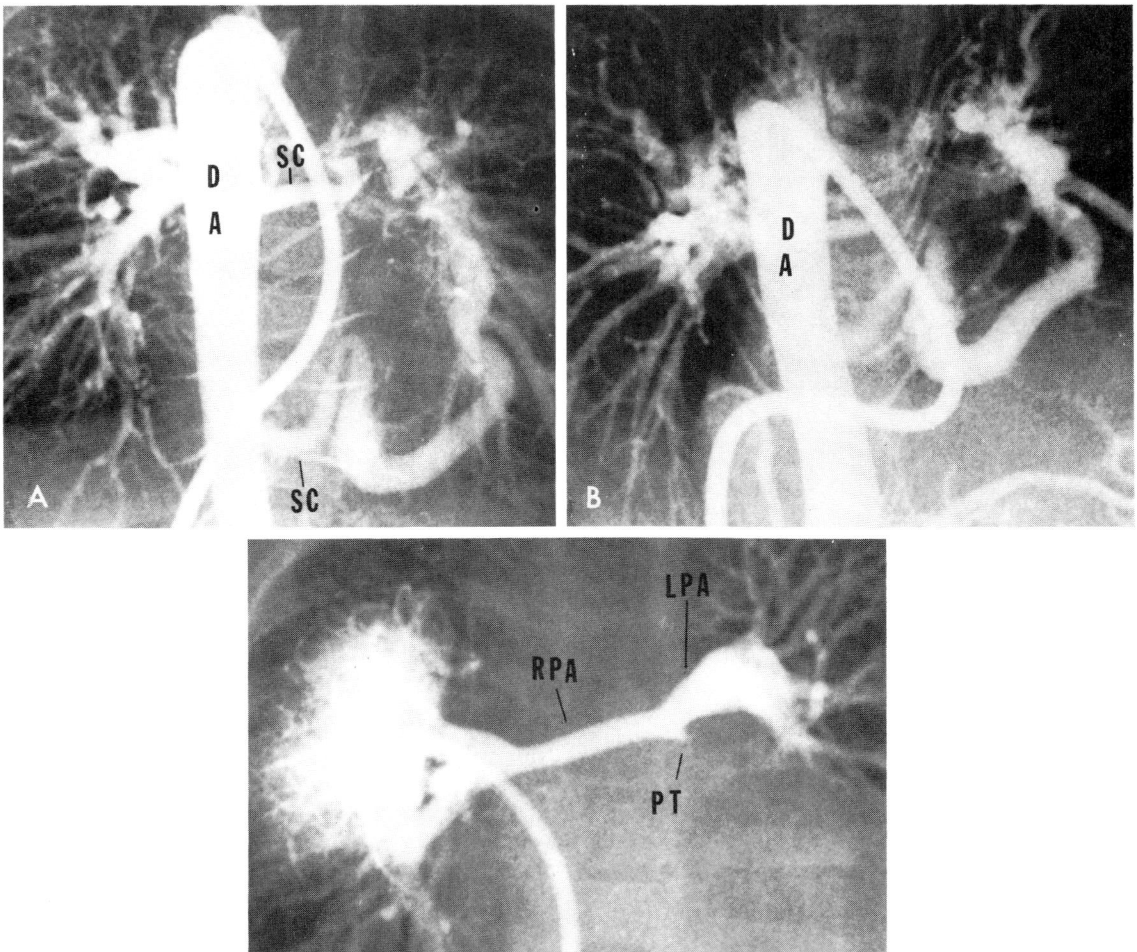

Figure 23. Tetralogy of Fallot with pulmonury atresia. *A*, Straight anteroposterior view. The upper descending thoracic aortogram (DA) shows large collateral arteries (SC) bilaterally. A true central pulmonary arterial tree was not visualized. *B*, Identical injection to *A* (sitting-up view). Again, a true central pulmonary arterial tree was not visualized. *C*, A pulmonary venous angiogram of the right upper pulmonary lung wedge. Contrast material flows retrograde into a true right and left pulmonary arterial tree. An inoperable type 4 truncus had been diagnosed at another institution.

injection in a sitting-up view, which again does not reveal a true pulmonary arterial tree, is shown in Figure 23*B*. A right pulmonary venous wedge cineangiogram was performed (Fig. 23*C*). This study shows retrograde filling of a true and confluent pulmonary arterial tree without stenosis of the major arterial origins.

Tetralogy of Fallot. Although tetralogy of Fallot is one of the most common forms of congenital heart disease amenable to repair, our experience with axial cineangiography indicates that many surgically significant lesions are not apparent on conventional filming techniques, including the much ballyhooed venous forms of digital subtraction angiography. These lesions include stenosis of the origin of the pulmonary arteries (especially the left pulmonary artery), additional ventricular septal defects, the complete form of the persistent common AV canal, and coronary artery anomalies.

In our approach to tetralogy, we now insist upon demonstrating (1) the entire pulmonary artery from the supravalvar area to and past its bifurcation (Figs. 24*A* and 25), (2) the entire ventricular septum (Fig. 26), (3) the size of both ventricles and their relationship to their respective AV valves, (4) the position and type of AV valves, and (5) the anatomic configuration of the coronary artery.

Usually, the initial injection is a biplane right ventriculogram with the four-chamber technique (see Fig. 24*A*). If possible, the second injection should be a four-chamber left ventriculogram, and the third, a sitting-up right ventriculogram in case the pulmonary trunk, its origin, and the central pulmonary arteries are not opacified.

Complete Transposition of the Great Arteries. The long axial oblique view best demonstrates the various forms of subpulmonary stenosis and location of the ventricular septal defects seen in complete transposition.

With regard to right ventriculography, it is essentially a "fielder's choice" as to which axial view is used for the right ventriculogram. At the present time, we use the four-chamber view primarily.

There are basically five variations of left ventricular outflow tract obstruction:[9] (1) pulmonary valve stenosis, (2) subpulmonary fibrous

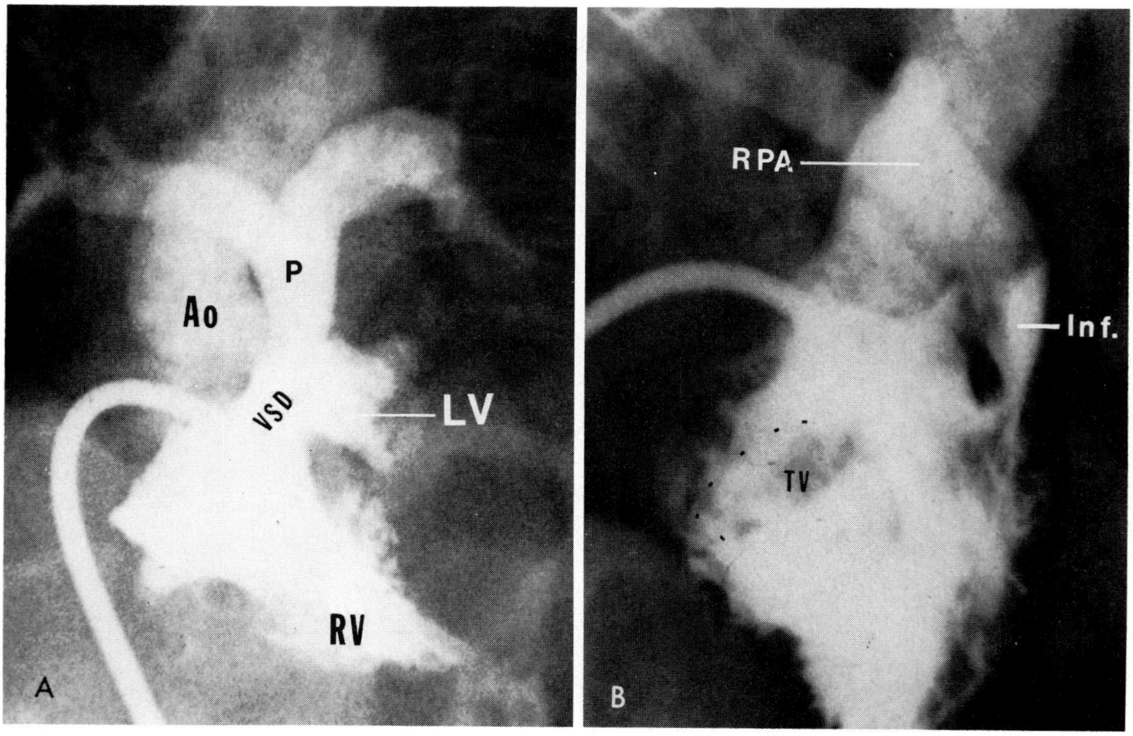

Figure 24. Tetralogy of Fallot. *A*, Four-chamber view. The subaortic ventricular septal defect (VSD) and remaining septum are brought into profile, and the bifurcation of the pulmonary trunk (P) is clearly seen. The right ventricular infundibulum is not well visualized in this view. *B*, Right anterior oblique view, companion to the four-chamber view. The infundibulum (Inf.) is brought into profile. Note the anteriorly deviated body of the crista supraventricularis or infundibular septum. Ao: aorta, RV: right ventricle, LV: left ventricle, RPA: right pulmonary artery, hash marks: tricuspid valve (TV) ring.

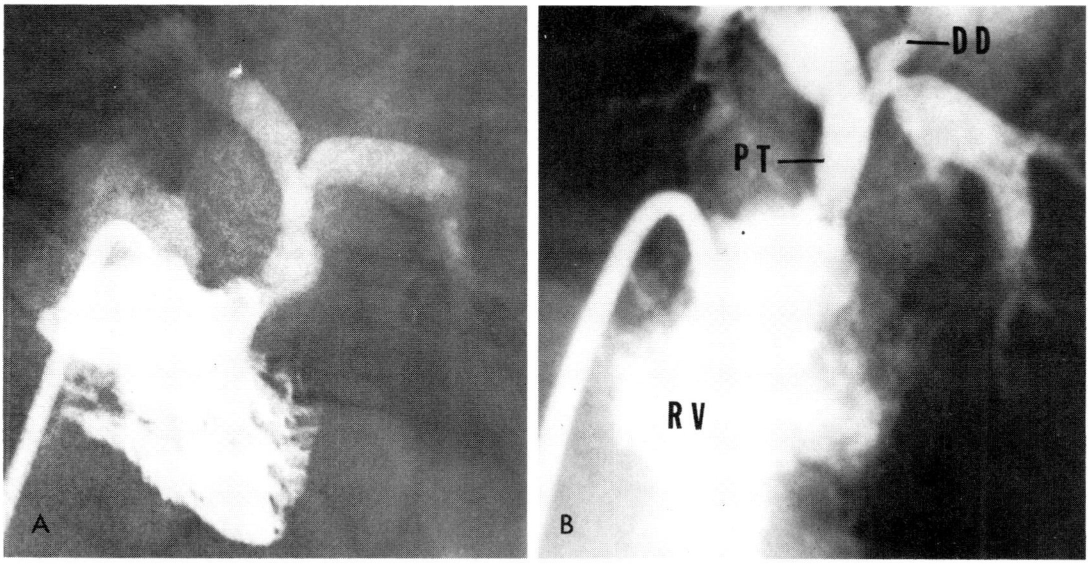

Figure 25. Tetralogy of Fallot with stenosis of the bifurcation of the pulmonary trunk. Right cineventriculograms were performed in both cases in a sitting-up position with some elevation of the right shoulder and slanting of the patient on the table. *A*, This ventriculogram profiles one of the most hazardous forms of pulmonary truncus. The pulmonary valve annulus, pulmonary trunk, and the origin of both pulmonary arteries show significant stenosis. *B*, Right cineventriculogram in the same view. In this case, not only is the pulmonary trunk (PT) profiled, but the severe stenosis of the origin of the left pulmonary artery at the site of the insertion of the ductus diverticulum (DD) is also vsiualized. RV: right ventricle.

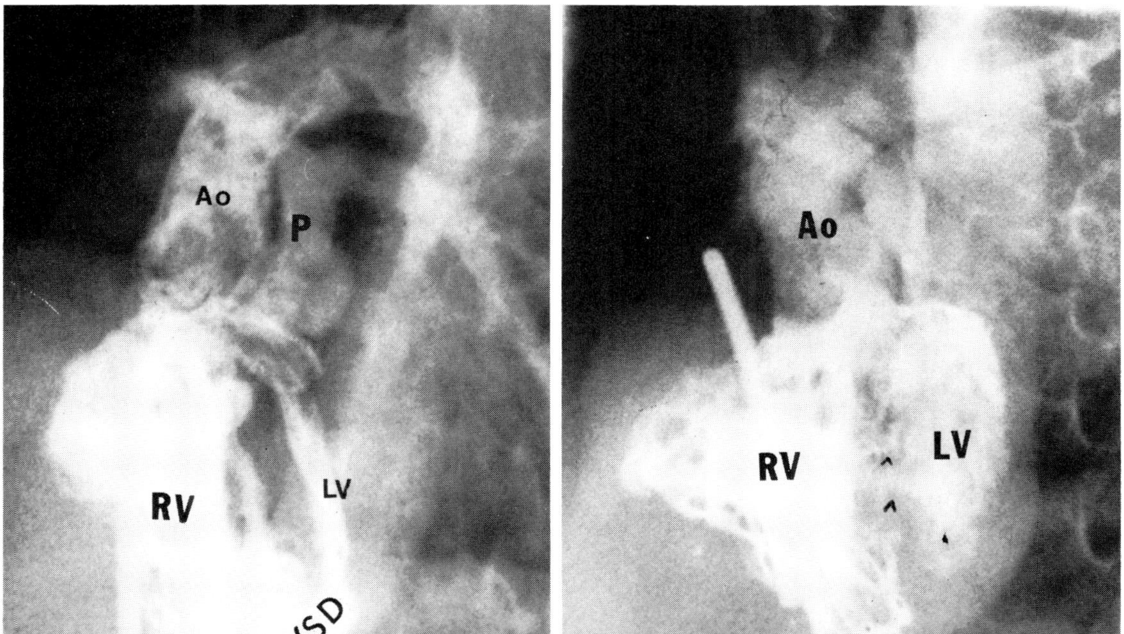

Figure 26. Two case of tetralogy of Fallot with additional complication of muscular ventricular septal defects. Four-chamber view. *A*, A right cineventriculogram shows a high, classic, subaortic ventricular septal defect (VSD), with the additional finding of a large muscular ventricular septal defect in the apex. *B*, A right cineventriculogram shows a large, typical, subaortic ventricular septal defect in profile, but numerous small muscular defects (arrowheads) are present, creating a so-called "Swiss cheese" septum. Ao: aorta, LV: left ventricle, RV: right ventricle, P: pulmonary trunk.

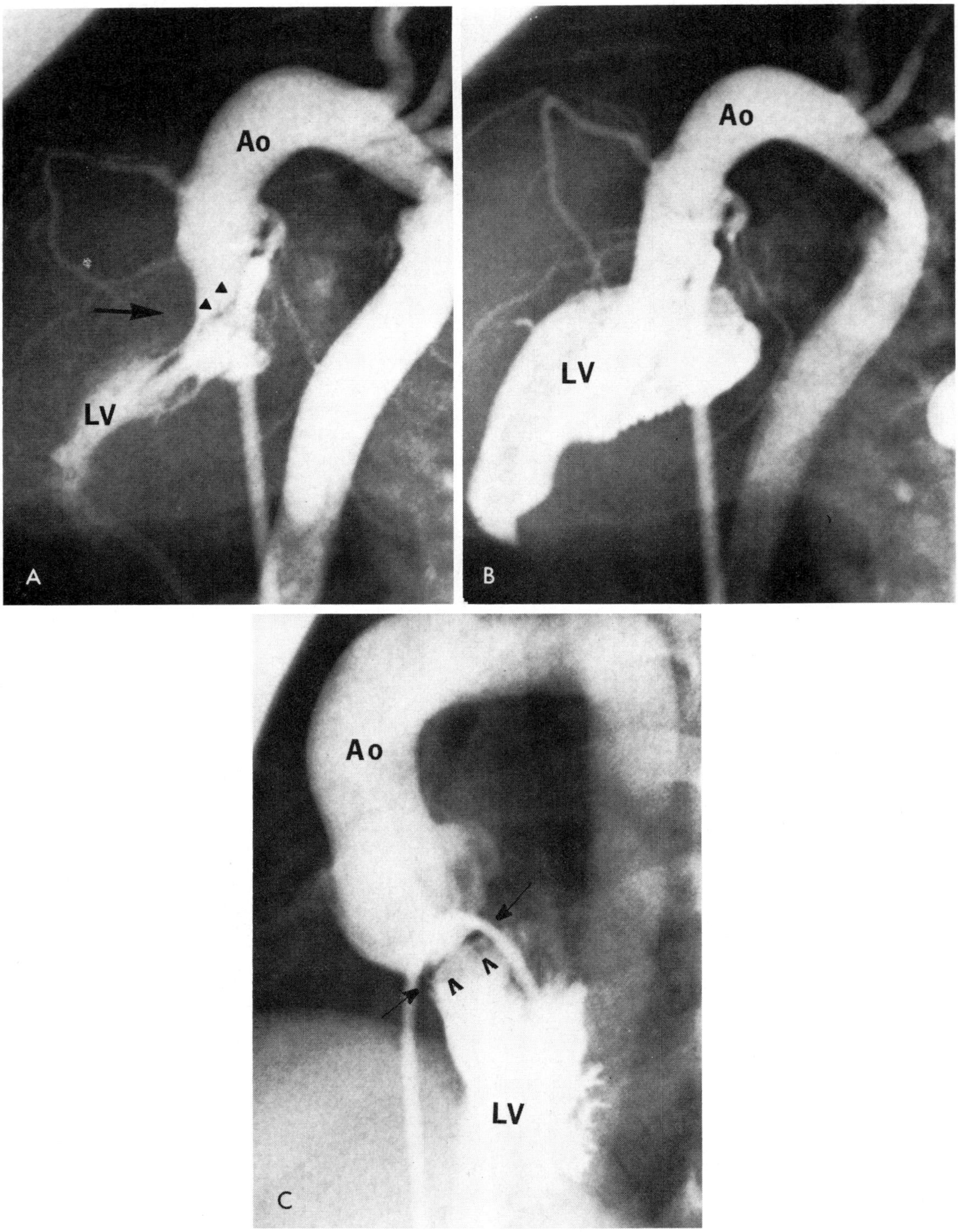

Figure 27. Two forms of subaortic stenosis. Equal hypertrophic obstructive cardiomyopathy is evident in both *A* and *B*. Left ventriculograms were performed in the long axial oblique view. *A*, Ventricular systole. The extremely thickened ventricular septum is depicted (arrow), as is the abnormal apposition of the systolic mitral valve (arrowheads). *B*, Ventricular diastole showing left ventricular hypertrophy and the return of the anterior leaflet to a normal position. *C*, Discrete subaortic stenosis demonstrated on a left ventriculogram performed from the long axial oblique view. Outside cineventriculograms suggested hypertrophic obstructive cardiomyopathy. The discrete subaortic valve diaphragm is shown in profile (arrows). Ao: aorta, LV: left ventricle.

diaphragm, (3) subpulmonary fibromuscular tunnel, (4) a dynamic form, characterized by a septal bulge with mitral valve apposition, and (5) an uncommon form involving an aneurysm of the membranous portion of the ventricular septum. Approximately 50 per cent of patients with left ventricular outflow tract obstruction will have an associated ventricular septal defect, which may be either isolated or multiple.

Subaortic Stenosis. The last two lesions to be discussed are relatively common ones that create various degrees of subaortic stenoses. They may cause either discrete subaortic stenoses or hypertrophic obstructive cardiomyopathy, often termed "asymmetric septal hypertrophy" or "idiopathic hypertrophic subaortic stenosis."

Axial left ventriculography has made an outstanding contribution to the delineation of the abnormality in the left ventricular outflow tract.[7] The long axial oblique view is the preferred one and is so definitive as to circumvent biventricular angiography in cases of hypertrophic obstructive cardiomyopathy.[7]

An infant with hypertrophic obstructive cardiomyopathy underwent radiographic study. The long axial oblique view can be seen to profile satisfactorily the anterior leaflet of the mitral valve and the septal bulging of the ventricular septum. In Figure 27*A*, thickening of the anterior leaflet of the mitral valve with abnormal anterior restriction is apparent. This, together with the septal bulge, created subaortic stenosis. A diastolic frame of the same case is shown in Figure 27*B*. Note how clearly the papillary muscles and the coronary artery anatomy are delineated.

Discrete subaortic stenosis (Fig. 27*C*) was demonstrated in a child who was referred to our institution with the diagnosis of hypertrophic obstructive cardiomyopathy, based upon excellent anteroposterior and lateral cineangiograms. The biplane long axial oblique study showed a discrete subaortic diaphragm. A superior septal bulge as well as abnormal systolic motion of the mitral valve was absent. The subaortic diaphragm was simply not seen on the anteroposterior and lateral left ventriculogram.

REFERENCES

1. Anderson RH, Becker AE, Van Mierop LHS: What should we call the "crista"? Br Heart J, *89*:856, 1977.
2. Bargeron LM Jr, Elliott LP, Soto B, et al: Axial cineangiography in congenital heart disease. I. Concept, technician and anatomic considerations. Circulation, *2*:1075, 1977.
3. Elliott LP, Bargeron LM Jr, Bream PR, et al: Axial cineangiography in congenital heart disease. II. Specific lesions. Circulation, *56*:1084, 1977.
4. Elliott LP, Bargeron LM Jr, Soto B, et al: Axial cineangiography in congenital heart disease. Radiol Clin North Am, *18*:515, 1980.
5. Elliott LP, Green CE, Rogers WJ, et al: Advantages of the caudocranial left anterior oblique left ventriculogram in adult heart disease. Am J Cardiol *49*:369, 1982.
6. Fellows KE, Keane JF, Freed MO: Angled views in cineangiography of congenital heart disease. Circulation, *56*:485, 1977.
7. Green CE, Elliott LP, Coghlan CH: Improved cineangiographic evaluation of hypertrophic cardiomyopathy by caudocranial left anterior oblique view. Am Heart J, *102*:1015, 1981.
8. Kattan KR: Angled view in pulmonary angiography. A new roentgen approach. Radiology, *94*:79, 1970.
9. Sansa M, Tonkin IL, Bargeron LM Jr, et al: Left ventricular outflow tract obstruction in transposition of the great arteries: An angiographic study of 74 cases. Am J Cardiol *44*:88, 1979.

2

AXIAL ANGIOCARDIOGRAPHY IN THE CRITICALLY ILL INFANT

Indications and Contraindications

ROBERT M. FREEDOM, M.D., F.R.C.P.(C.), F.A.C.C.

The application of axial angiocardiography has provided a new sophistication to the invasive study of the patient with structural heart disease. Although axial projections have been used in patients with acquired heart disease (usually coronary arteriography or hypertrophic cardiomyopathy),[48] its widest application is for the patient with congenital heart disease. After the reports of Elliott and Bargeron and their colleagues in 1977 (although there were earlier reports[49, 60]), some form of axial angiography has probably been adopted by most catheterization laboratories, attesting to its acceptance as well as its relevance.[12, 20, 21, 31] Axial angiography has been applied to the normal heart[8, 9, 16] and to patients with tetralogy of Fallot,[74] atrioventricular septal defect,[71] posterior ventricular septal defect,[47] vascular ring,[78] obstruction of the left ventricular outflow tract in isolation[52] or complicating transposition of the great arteries,[67, 79] and univentricular heart.[73, 75] Many of the patients subjected to axial angiography had likely undergone a previous catheter study using the classic angiographic projections of anteroposterior, lateral, and right and left anterior oblique views. These previous investigations provided the framework for application of axial techniques. A legacy of classic angiocardiography can be found in other studies.[14, 19, 50, 68] Indeed, often these earlier studies provided the basic information about the atrial situs, atrioventricular and ventriculoarterial connections, and the spatial relationships between the ventricles and great arteries. More recently, cross-sectional echocardiography has provided the same type of information. What then is the role of axial angiography in the critically ill infant in whom contrast material must be judiciously used? The first article of this symposium has defined the general approach to axial angiography. This article will explore some of those conditions in critically ill infants, when axial angiography is desirable, and when such techniques may prove confusing.

AXIAL ANGIOGRAPHY IN THE CONTEXT OF SEGMENTAL APPROACH TO CONGENITAL HEART DISEASE

The medical and surgical management of the neonate with congenital heart disease mandates a thorough knowledge of the atrial situs and atrioventricular and ventriculoarterial connections and a precise assessment of associated intracardiac and extracardiac anomalies. What must be also integrated is the appreciation of the spatial relationships between the ventricles and the internal organization of the ventricle.[4, 23, 38, 83] It has become increasingly evident that the spatial relationship between the two cardiac ventricles, the internal organization of the ventricle (its inlet-outlet axis),[83] and the type of atrioventricular connection convey important but fundamentally different aspects of the congenitally malformed heart.[38] Nowhere are these concepts better exemplified than in patients with so-called superoinferior ventricles.[34, 38, 83]

When selective ventricular angiography is performed by using axial projections, one assumes a "normal" spatial relationship between the cardiac ventricles and the normal curvilinear topography of the ventricular septum. Thus, assuming the normal topography of the ventricular septum, it is relatively straightforward to define a posterior muscular or inlet ventricular septal defect by using the hepatoclavicular four-chamber projection or to detect the perimembranous defect with the left long axial oblique projection. But if the ventricular mass is aligned about a horizontal ventricular septum or a vertically disposed septum,[6, 7] then axial angiography will possibly not define the position of the ventricular septal defect to advantage.[6, 23, 34, 58] As a guideline, then, axial angiography should be provided as the initial procedure when one is reasonably confident (from cross-sectional dimensional echocardiographic examinations or limited spot-injections of small amounts of contrast material) of the normal curvilinear contour of the ventricular septum.

CONTRAINDICATIONS TO AXIAL VENTRICULAR ANGIOGRAPHY

Among certain congenital heart malformations, distortions of the "usual" spatial relationships between ventricles may contraindicate axial ventricular angiography as the initial approach. This is particularly true when the ventricular septum is best profiled in the frontal projection.[6, 7, 34, 38] The ventricular septum is best profiled in the frontal plane in hearts with so-called superoinferior or upstairs-downstairs ventricles. This spatial relationship between the ventricles is characterized by an abnormal disposition of the ventricles about a horizontal ventricular septum (Fig. 1).

A significant departure from selective frontal ventriculography would result in overlapping of the cardiac ventricles. One of the more consistent features of hearts with superoinferior ventricles is that the ventricular septal defect will also be best profiled in the frontal projection. Yet this unusual spatial disposition of the cardiac ventricles is predictive neither of the internal organization of the ventricle nor of the type of atrioventricular connection.[23, 34, 38, 83] For most patients with superoinferior ventricles, the atrioventricular connections are either concordant or discordant, or there is concordance or discordance of one atrioventricular valve and straddling of the other. Usually, selective atriography must be performed in these patients to determine both the type of atrioventricular connection and the internal organization of the ventricle. Selective angiography is best performed in the hepatoclavicular projection so that the crux of the heart is profiled. Furthermore, this projection is ideal for demonstrating straddling of the atrioventricular valve.

The ventricles are usually disposed about a vertical axis in patients with congenitally cor-

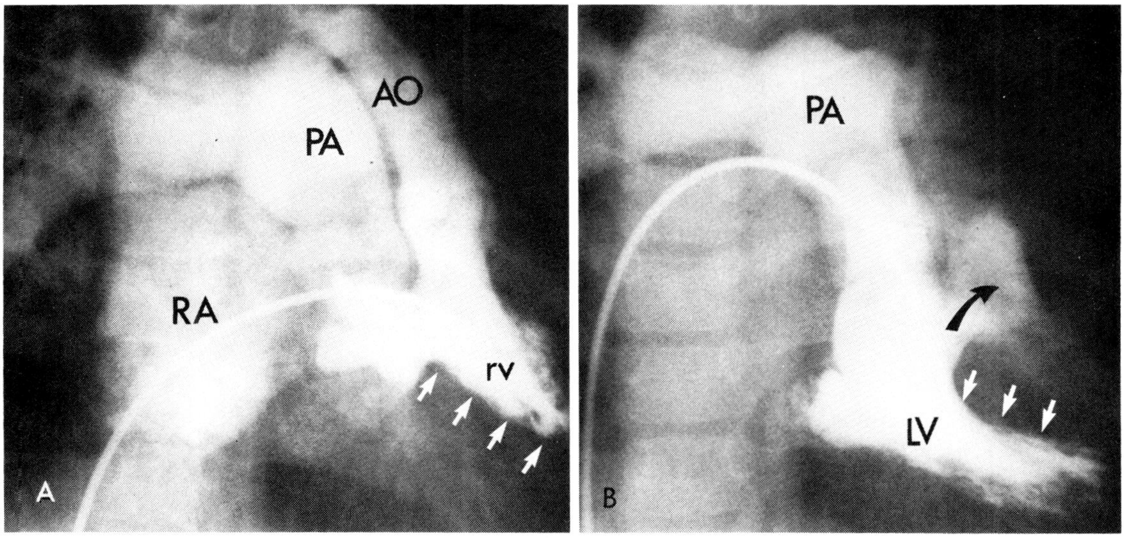

Figure 1. A horizontal ventricular septum (white arrows) with a superoinferior ventricular relationship. *A*, frontal injection in the superiorly positioned right ventricle (rv) with opacification of a levopositioned aorta (AO) and medially positioned pulmonary artery (PA), with some regurgitation of contrast material into the right atrium (RA). *B*, This frontal left ventriculogram (LV) shows the horizontal disposition of the ventricular septum, and the ventricular septal defect (black arrows) is profiled.

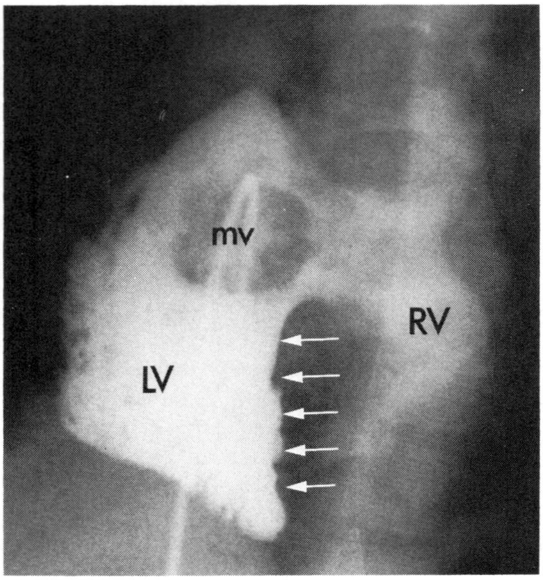

Figure 2. The ventricular septum has a vertical disposition (white arrows) in patients with atrioventricular discordance as demonstrated by this left ventriculogram (LV). mv: mitral valve, RV: morphologic right ventricle.

rected transposition of the great arteries (atrioventricular and ventriculoarterial discordance) (Fig. 2).[7, 31] Thus, as in the patient with superoinferior ventricles, the ventricular septum is best profiled in the frontal projection. This projection should demonstrate to advantage the ventriculoarterial connection, the subpulmonary infundibulum, and the dimension of the ventricular septal defect. Obviously, if the ventricular septal defect is not clearly profiled in the frontal projection, then perhaps some axial angulation or a four-chamber projection will be necessary. This is particularly true if the ventricular septal defect involves the posterior or inlet portion of the septum. Once the position of the ventricular septum is defined, right or left long axial oblique ventriculography may be necessary to define further the morphology of the arterial outflow tracts.[7, 31]

The necessity of defining precisely the type of atrioventricular and ventriculoarterial connections is demonstrated in the next series of figures (Fig. 3). Does this baby require balloon septostomy? From Figures 3*A* and 3*B*, the ventricles are apparently in an inverted relationship, and for the individual with atrial situs solitus, this would suggest the presence of atrioventricular discordance. But despite this angiographic evidence of an "inverted" ventricular relationship, the atrioventricular connections are concordant as shown by selective right atriography (Fig. 3*C*), and the ventriculoarterial connections are discordant. Thus, this patient has "transposition" physiology and anatomy, and balloon atrioseptostomy is indicated.

Cardiac malpositions, especially dextrocardia, may contraindicate axial angiography, unless from the noninvasive assessment, one is fairly certain of the disposition of the ventricular septum, the atrioventricular connections, and the size of the ventricles. The majority of ill neonates with dextrocardia requiring cardiac catheterization will have either (1) severe fixed obstruction to pulmonary blood flow (duct-dependent pulmonary blood flow) or (2) unobstructed pulmonary blood flow. Usually in the first group, the immediate surgical management necessitates definition of the (1) caliber and origin of the pulmonary arteries; (2) the laterality of the aortic arch and disposition of the brachiocephalic arteries; (3) the nature of the pulmonary venous connections;[41] and (4) the functional status of the systemic atrioventricular valve and the atrial septum. With rare exception, the morphology of the ventricles and the exact position of the ventricular septal defect(s) do not influence the type of palliative surgery. Ventricular angiography is necessary, but at the first catheter study, we would usually perform the first ventricular injection in the frontal and lateral projections if there were reservations about the disposition of the ventricular septum.

The assessment of the neonate with dextrocardia and increased pulmonary blood flow may require axial angiography, especially if the ventricular anatomy conforms to that of univentricular heart and an outlet chamber. It might be necessary to define the caliber of the outlet chamber and the size of the outlet foramen, especially when the ventriculoarterial connec-

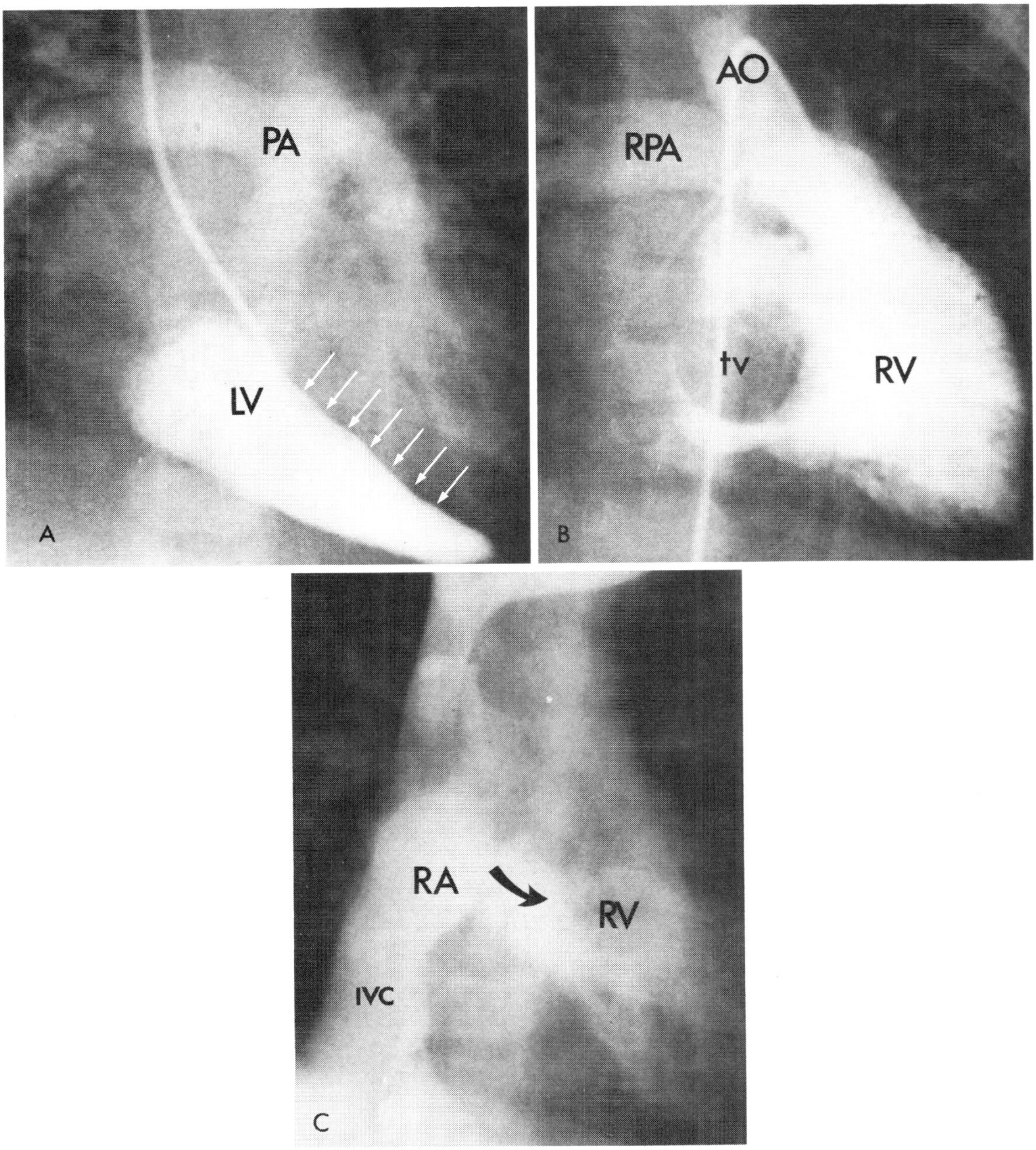

Figure 3. These two ventriculograms suggest atrioventricular and ventriculoarterial discordance, but selective atriography clearly demonstrates that the arterioventricular connections are discordant. *A*, Selective left ventriculogram (LV) in the frontal plane reveals this ventricle to be right-sided, and the position of the ventricular septum (arrows) is abnormal. The morphologic left ventricle (LV) supports the pulmonary artery (PA). *B*, The morphologic right ventricle appears to be to the left of the morphologic left ventricle and supports the discordantly connected aorta. *C*, Yet selective injection of contrast material in the right atrium (RA) demonstrates opacification of the right ventricular inlet, not the left ventricular inlet. IVC: inferior vena cava.

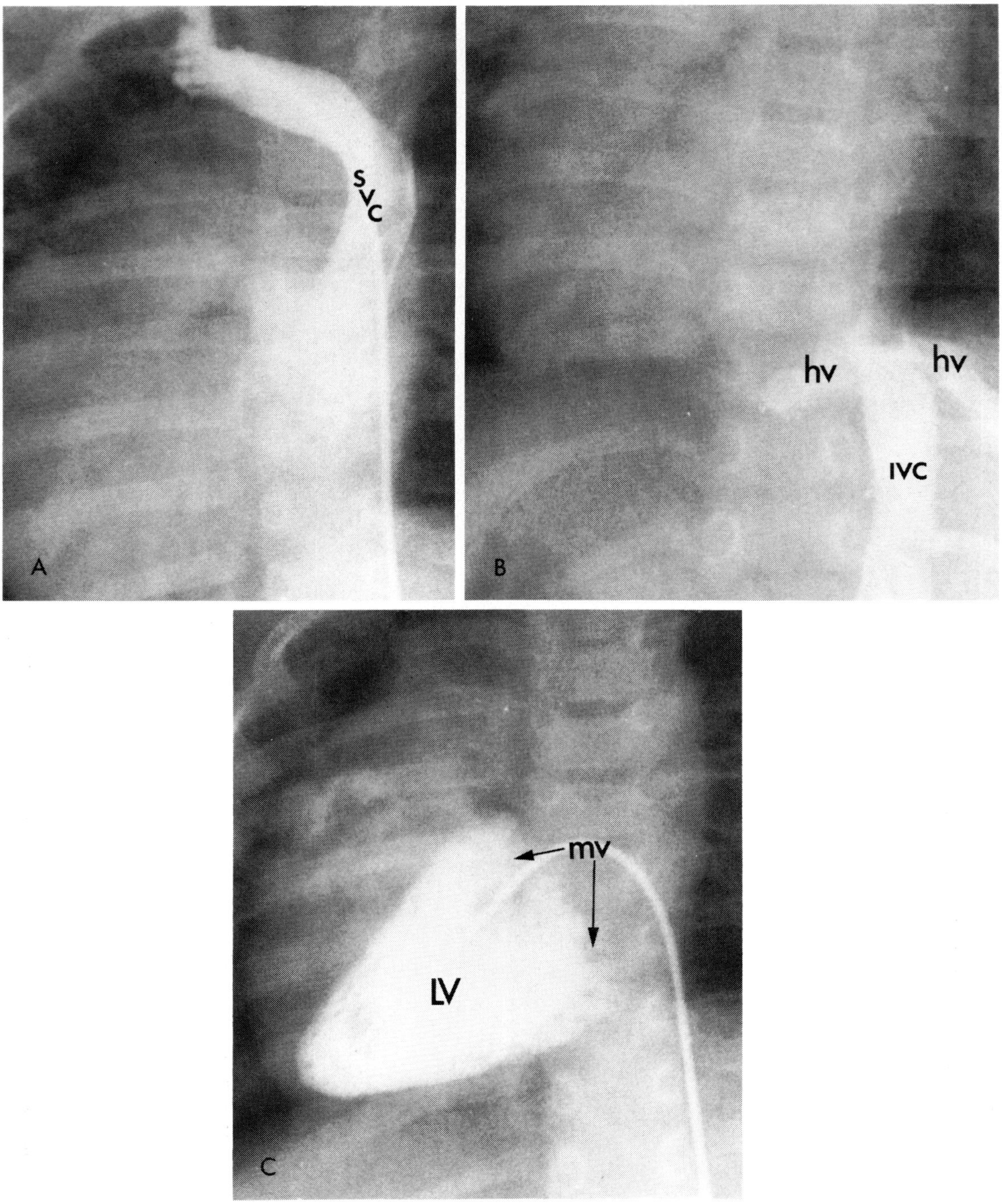

Figure 4. An infant with complex congenital heart disease associated with dextrocardia. *A*, Injection of contrast material in the right brachiocephalic vein in the frontal plane shows a left-sided superior vena cava (svc). *B*, Injection in the left-sided inferior vena cava (ivc) shows normal hepatic veins (hv), and thus the systemic venous return is to the left-sided right atrium. *C*, Injection of the left-sided ventricle in the frontal plane via the mitral valve reveals typical left ventricular (LV) morphology.

Illustration continued on opposite page.

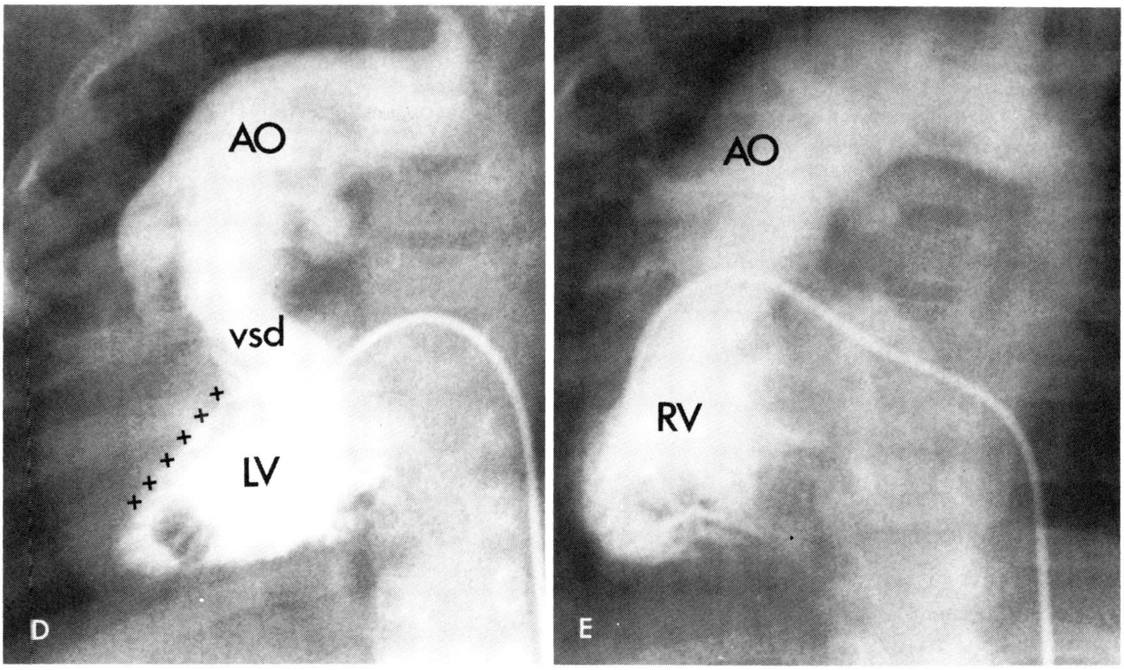

Figure 4 *(Continued). D,* Slightly later in this injection, the ascending aorta (AO) opacifies via a ventricular septal defect (VSD), which is nicely profiled. The ventricular septum (x) is more vertically disposed than normal. *E,* The right-sided morphologically right ventricle (RV) supports the aorta (AO). Thus, this patient with dextrocardia has atrial situs inversus and atrioventricular discordance with the right ventricle having a right-hand pattern of internal organization. The aorta originates from the right ventricle. There is also pulmonary atresia.

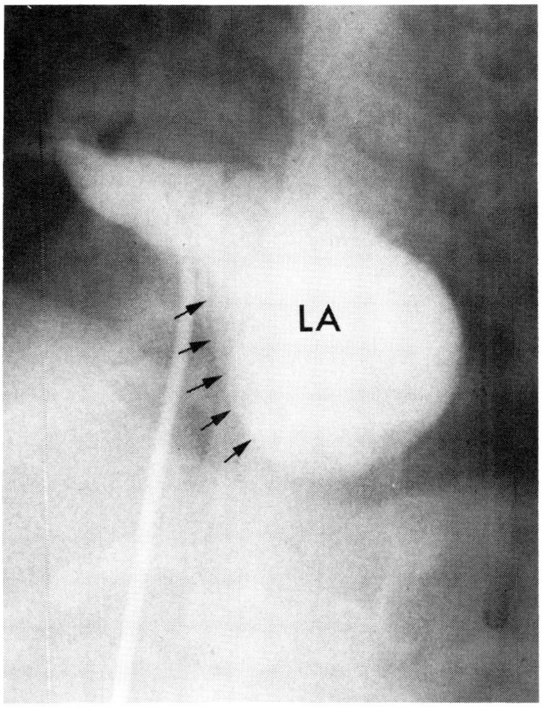

Figure 5. Left atriogram (LA) filmed in the hepatoclavicular four-chamber projection with injection of contrast material in the right superior pulmonary vein. The atrial septum (arrows) is clearly seen.

tion is discordant. However, in the sick neonate, it is possible by the judicious use of contrast material to define fully the type of atrioventricular, ventriculoarterial, and systemic venous connections (Fig. 4).

THE ATRIAL SEPTUM

The atrial septum is ideally profiled in the hepatoclavicular or four-chamber projection (Fig. 5). This projection demonstrates to advantage the alignment or malalignment of the atrial septum with the ventricular septum, and when necessary, the size of an atrial septal defect(s) can be shown with clarity (Fig. 6).

Among patients with atresia or severe stenosis of the right or left atrioventricular orifice, a restrictive interatrial communication can profoundly influence the hemodynamics and clinical course (Figs. 5 and 7). A severely restrictive interatrial communication with formation of aneurysm can be readily diagnosed by cross-sectional echocardiographic techniques and by standard anteroposterior and lateral selective right or left atriography.[27, 62, 66] This use of the hepatoclavicular projection clearly shows the plane of the atrial septum, and in the patient

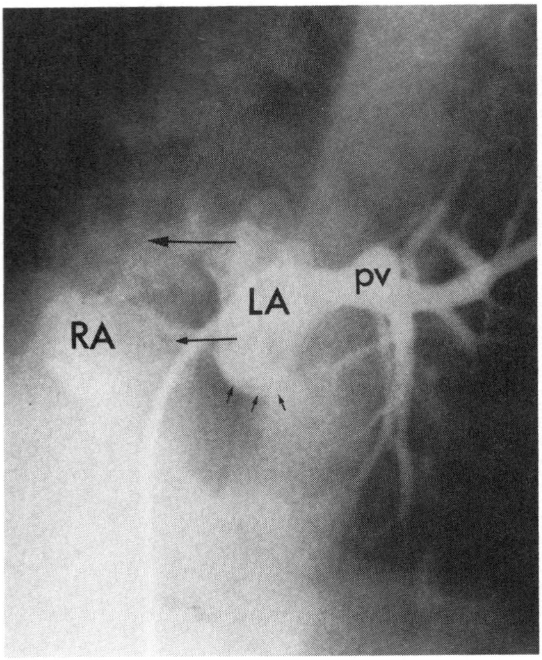

Figure 6. Diminutive left atrium (LA) in a patient with complex congenital heart disease and atresia (small black arrows) of the systemic atrioventricular valve. Left atriogram demonstrates atresia of the atrioventricular valve and two small interatrial communications (black arrows), with opacification of the right atrium (RA). The pulmonary veins (pv) are distended. Four-chamber projection.

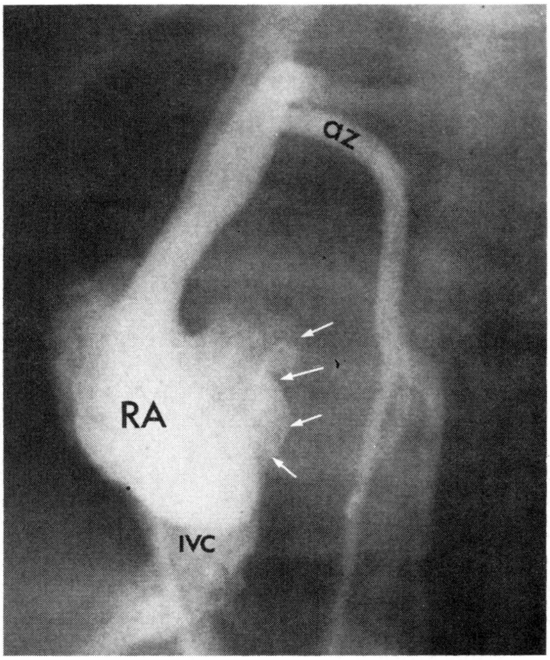

Figure 7. Aneurysm of atrial septum (white arrows) in a neonate with tricuspid atresia shown by right atriogram (RA) performed in hepatoclavicular projection. There is substantial reflux into the azygous vein (az) and inferior vena cava (ivc). The mean right atrial pressure was 18 mmHg; left atrial mean pressure was 4.0 mmHg.

with classic tricuspid atresia, aneurysmal herniation of the septum primum can be unequivocally demonstrated (Fig. 7).

THE ATRIOVENTRICULAR SEPTAL DEFECT

An extensive literature is now devoted to the angiocardiography of the atrioventricular septal defect, but most of these observations have relied on the classic angiographic projections (frontal, lateral, and right and left anterior oblique projections) (see references 31 and 80 for recent summaries). More recently, however, axial angiography has been applied to patients with this form of congenitally malformed heart.[31, 71]

The hepatoclavicular or four-chamber projection demonstrates to advantage the inlet portion of the ventricular septum, the disposition of the common atrioventricular orifice relative to the ventricular septum, and the size of the ventricular component of the atrioventricular septal defect. The advantage of the axial approach to angiography is clearly illustrated in the angiograms from a patient with the complete form of atrioventricular septal defect (Fig. 8). The standard lateral or left anterior oblique left ventriculogram clearly demonstrates a left-to-right shunt at ventricular level, but the size of the ventricular septal defect and its localization within the ventricular septum are not defined (see Fig. 8*A*). Yet using the hepatoclavicular projection in the same patient (Figs. 8*B* and *C*), the left ventriculogram indicates that the common atrioventricular orifice is equally disposed over the ventricular septum.[15] It unequivocally demonstrates the size of the ventricular septal defect and shows that the remainder of the muscular septum is intact. Because defects in other portions of the ventricular septum can coexist (however uncommon) with the atrioventricular septal defect, right and left long axial oblique left ventriculograms may also be necessary.

That subaortic stenosis and obstructive anomalies of the aortic arch can complicate the atrioventricular septal defect is clear.[24, 30, 31, 36, 39, 59] The mechanisms responsible for the subaortic

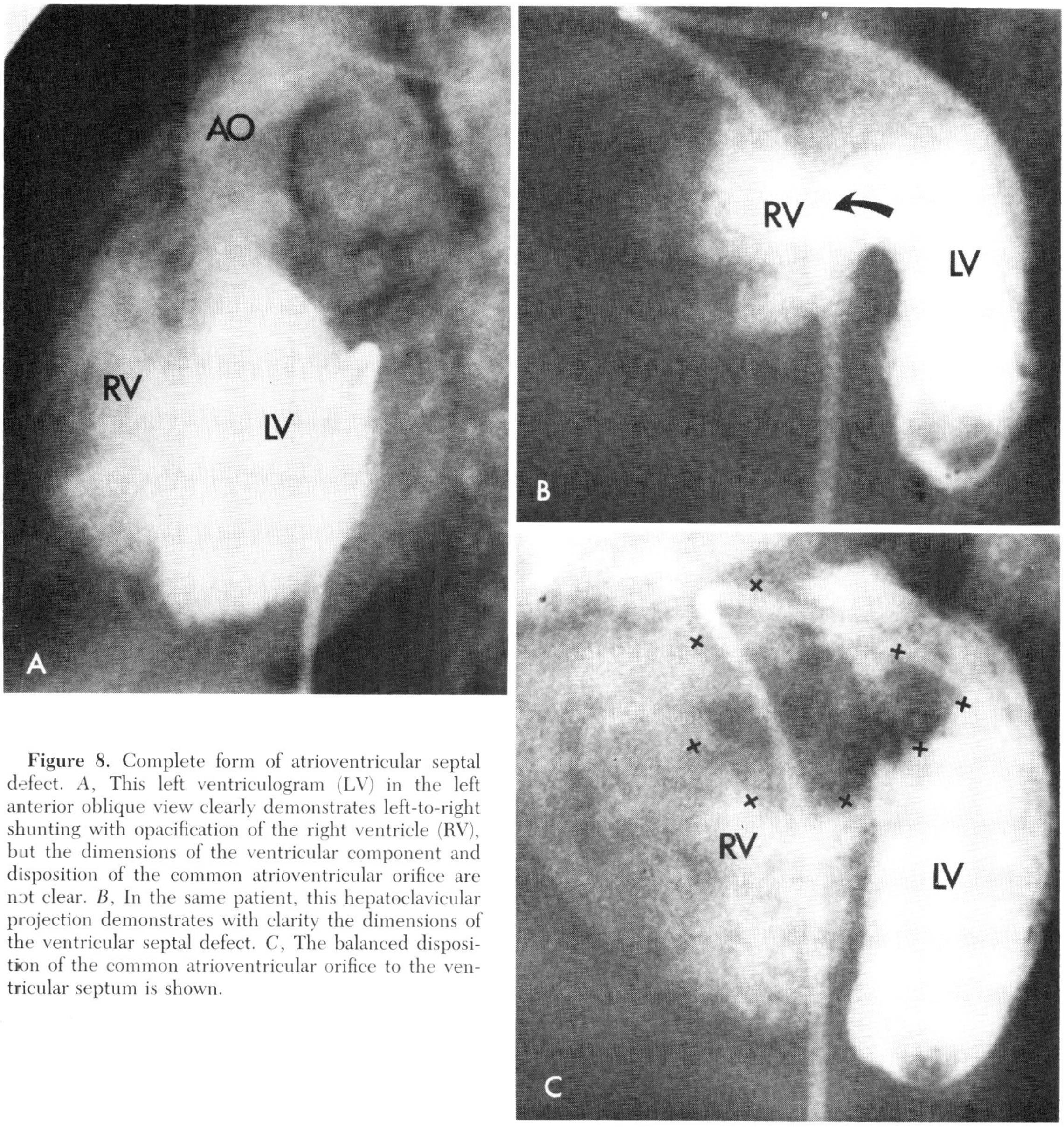

Figure 8. Complete form of atrioventricular septal defect. *A*, This left ventriculogram (LV) in the left anterior oblique view clearly demonstrates left-to-right shunting with opacification of the right ventricle (RV), but the dimensions of the ventricular component and disposition of the common atrioventricular orifice are not clear. *B*, In the same patient, this hepatoclavicular projection demonstrates with clarity the dimensions of the ventricular septal defect. *C*, The balanced disposition of the common atrioventricular orifice to the ventricular septum is shown.

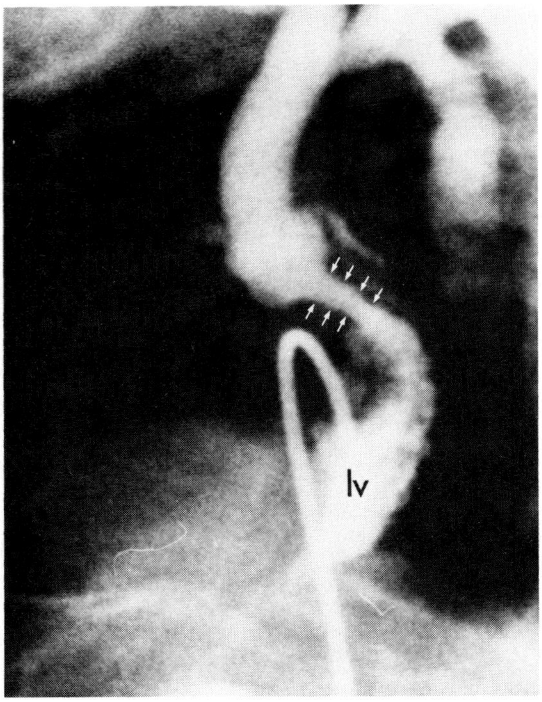

Figure 9. Subaortic stenosis (white arrows) in a neonate with a dominant right form of an atrioventricular septal defect demonstrated by a four-chamber left ventriculogram (lv).

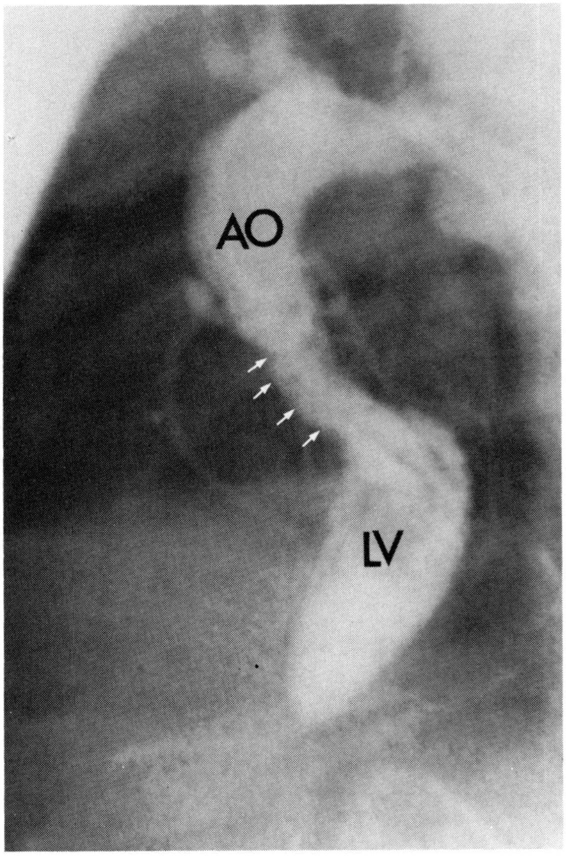

Figure 10. A neonate with a tunnel form of subaortic stenosis complicating left atrial isomerism, an ostium primum atrial septal defect, and multiple, small, muscular ventricular septal defects. The subaortic stenosis probably results both from a maladherent mitral valve and from persistence of the left ventriculoinfundibular fold. This left long axial oblique ventriculogram (LV) shows the elongated (white arrows) left ventricular outflow tract. The ascending aorta (AO) exhibits mild dilatation.

stenosis include a maladherent anterior "mitral" leaflet, accessory tissue tags, or a fibrous diaphragm. Not infrequently, some combination of these mechanisms can result in obstruction of the subaortic vestibule. Subaortic stenosis can complicate the primum atrial septal defect or the complete form of atrioventricular septal defect. When the complete form of the defect is complicated by subaortic stenosis, the common atrioventricular orifice may be equally disposed to both ventricles (so-called balanced form),[15] or the common atrioventricular orifice may be disposed primarily to the morphologic right ventricle (so-called dominant right form) (Figs. 9 to 11).[15, 30]

The definition of functional subaortic stenosis and its anatomic basis may require left ventriculography filmed in several projections (see Figs. 8 to 11). The four-chamber projection (see Fig. 8) may not profile the subaortic area to advantage, and the right and left long axial oblique projections may be required to profile the subaortic area (see Fig. 11).

ATRIOVENTRICULAR JUNCTION

Anomalies of the atrioventricular junction are perhaps best defined by cross-sectional echocardiographic techniques. Although almost any significant structural anomaly can be defined by a combination of atrial and ventricular angiography, these invasive procedures should be used to complement or augment the echocardiographic examination.

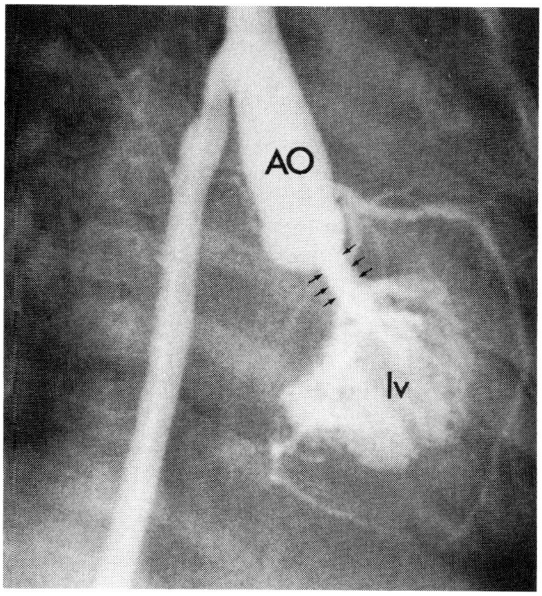

Figure 11. Another infant with severe subaortic stenosis complicating a dominant right form of atrioventricular septal defect. This baby had severe congestive heart failure after repair of a thoracic coarctation. This left ventriculogram (LV) in the elongated right axial projection shows a "fixed," tunnel-like subaortic obstruction, resulting in large part from a maladherent mitral valve.

Selective right atriography performed in the hepatoclavicular four-chamber projection in the patient with tricuspid atresia will demonstrate the blind floor of the right atrium. Usually, selective right atriography will not distinguish between the tricuspid atresia resulting from an absent or atretic orifice and that resulting from an imperforate connection. The exception to the generalization is, of course, the imperforate variant of Ebstein's anomaly.[5, 39, 61] The displacement of the posterior and septal aspects of the tricuspid valve from its normal position and the failure to opacify the trabecular zone of the right ventricle from right atrial or "ventricular" angiography are diagnostic of this condition.[31, 39, 45] The right atriogram filmed in the four-chamber projection will also demonstrate the abnormal right venous valves that subdivide the right atrium and reveal an aneurysm of the atrial septum. The straddling right or left atrioventricular valve can also be demonstrated by right or left atriography (Fig. 12) filmed in the four-chamber projection, and a stenotic atrioventricular valve can be readily imaged as well.[11]

PULMONARY ARTERIES

Craniocaudal angulation is ideally suited for profiling the main pulmonary artery and the origins of the branch pulmonary arteries.[16, 26, 31, 49, 74] This gives the perspective of "looking down" on the bifurcation of the main pulmonary artery into its right and left branches. Ideally, one would like to perform a selective pulmonary arteriogram by using this radiologic projection (Fig. 13), but in the critically ill neonate with severe obstruction to pulmonary blood flow in concert with other intracardiac anomalies, it may be difficult to probe the pulmonary artery without compromising the patient's condition (Figs. 14 and 15). Fortunately, selective right or left ventriculography (depending on which ventricle supports the pulmonary artery) with a craniocaudal angulation will often suffice. At times either the right or left shoulder may have to be elevated in order to define most clearly the anatomy of the caliber of the pulmonary arteries.

VENTRICULAR SEPTAL DEFECT

Data from the New England Regional Infant Cardiac Program and clinical experience of most

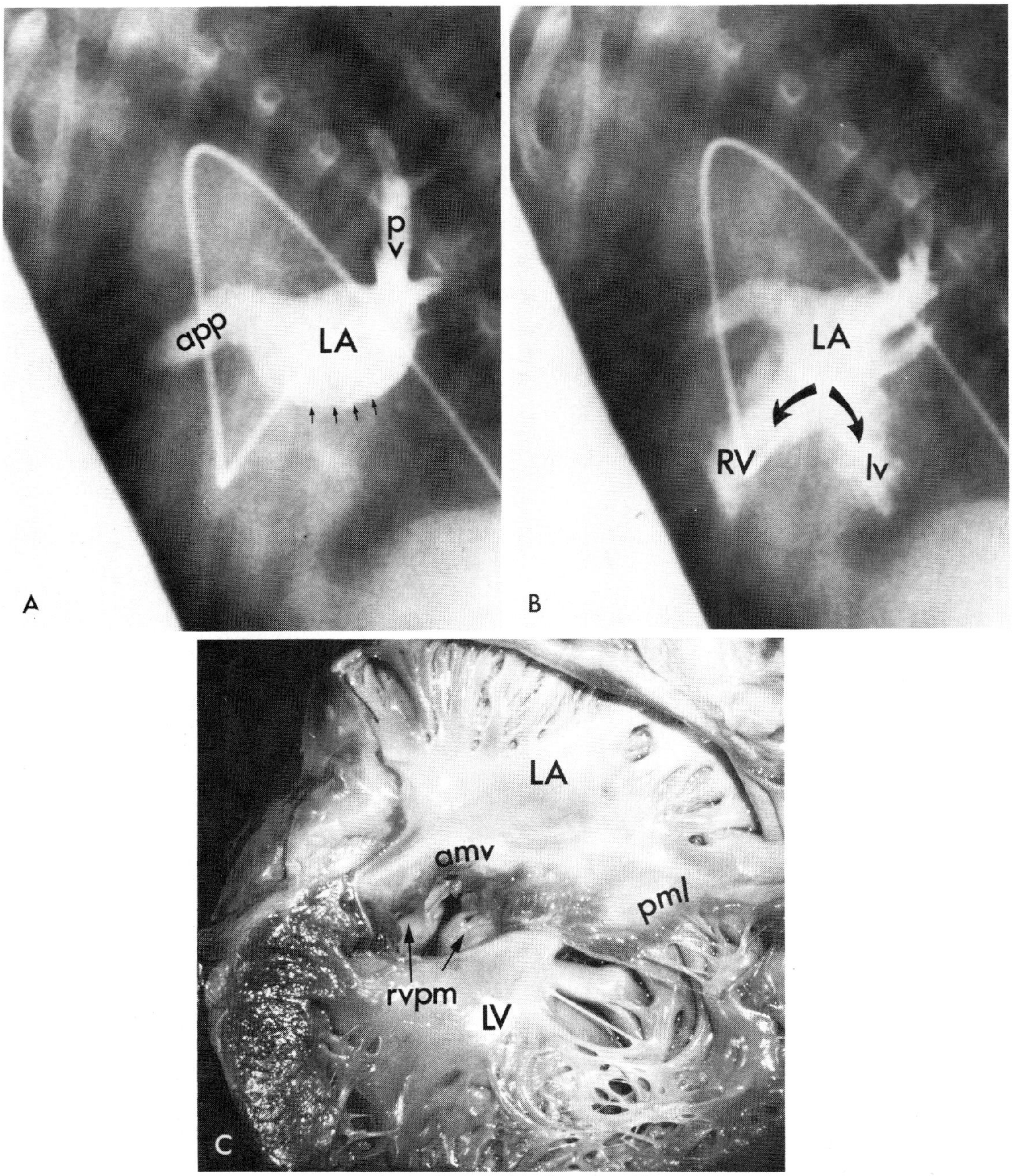

Figure 12. A straddling mitral valve in an infant with Taussig-Bing double-outlet right ventricle, small left ventricle, and intact atrial septum. *A*, Retrograde left atriogram (LA) in four-chamber projection before atrial systole. The closed mitral valve is seen (arrows). app: left atrial appendate, pv: pulmonary vein. *B*, Straddling of the mitral valve (curved arrows) is evident. *C*, This internal view of the left atrium (LA) and left ventricle (LV) shows insertion of the anterior mitral valve (amv) into the right ventricular papillary muscles (rvpm). pml: posterior mitral leaflet.

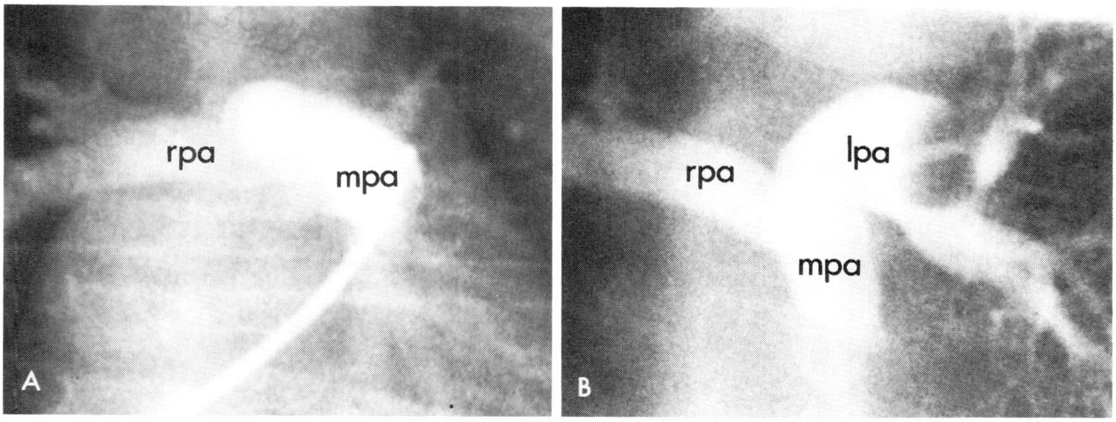

Figure 13. The pulmonary arteries in an infant with tetralogy of Fallot. *A*, In this frontal, main pulmonary arteriogram (mpa), the origin of the right pulmonary artery (rpa) is seen fairly well, but the origin of the left pulmonary artery is not demonstrated. *B*, The same patient with craniocaudal angulation clearly shows the origins of both branch pulmonary arteries.

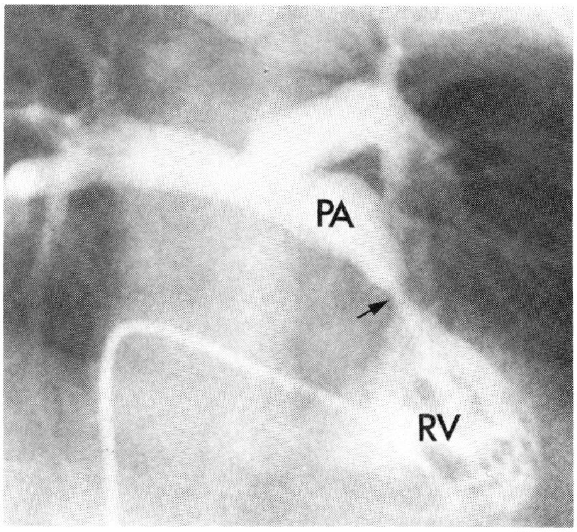

Figure 14. Isolated infundibular pulmonary stenosis (arrow) in an infant with hypoxia. Suprasystemic right ventricular pressures is shown in this right ventriculogram (RV) filmed with craniocaudal angulation. The caliber and bifurcation of the pulmonary arteries are clearly demonstrated.

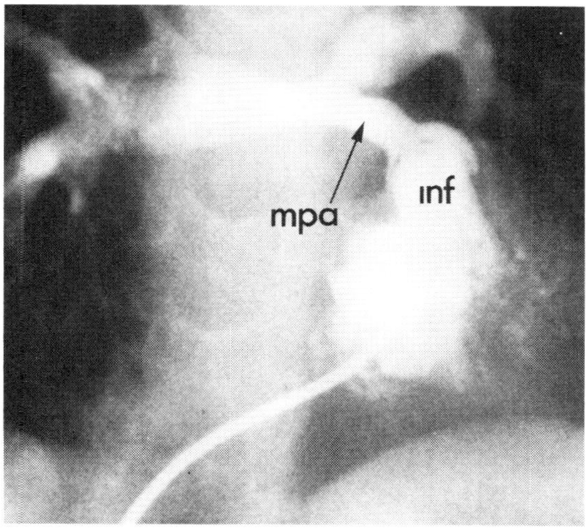

Figure 15. Severe hypoplasia of the main pulmonary artery is demonstrated by craniocaudal angulation of this right ventriculogram performed with injection of contrast material in the infundibulum (inf).

pediatric cardiology centers suggest that the ventricular septal defect is the most common cardiac anomaly in the first year of life.[44] Although the majority of such isolated defects are small to moderate in size, with many of these either spontaneously closing or becoming smaller during the first five years of life, some babies will require surgical intervention in the first year of life. The direction in most surgical centers of primary intracardiac repair (rather than palliative pulmonary artery banding) necessitates accurate preoperative diagnosis of the number of such defects, their size relative to the aortic root,[64] and the positions(s) of such defects within the ventricular septum.

Because the ventricular septum is curvilinear, conventional angiocardiographic projections will not invariably profile the ventricular septal defect to advantage (despite claims to the contrary[79]). The application of axial angiographic techniques allows one to distinguish between those defects involving primarily the inlet (or posterior muscular) septum from those involving the perimembranous septum, that is, the trabecular or infundibular (or outlet) septum.[46, 86] Because a defect involving primarily one portion or zone of the ventricular septum may extend to and become confluent with a defect involving a contiguous portion of the ventricular septum,[72] more than one axial projection may be required to characterize the defect(s) fully (Figs. 16 to 19).[47]

In addition to providing the surgeon with important information about how he or she might approach the ventricular septal defect (through the right atrium, right ventricle, apex of left ventricle, aorta, or pulmonary artery), the position of the ventricular septal defect can provide information about other associated intracardiac anomalies.[87] The recognition that the ventricular septal defect is posterior, muscular, and involving the inlet septum mandates that one exclude straddling or overriding of the tricuspid valve.[53] When one recognizes that the ventricular septal defect involves the infundibular septum, it is necessary to define whether such a defect represents isolated deficiency (so-called supracristal defect) of the infundibular septum, or whether the defect results from malalignment of the infundibular septum from the trabecula septomarginalis.[29] Thus, a "malalignment" defect with posterior and caudal extension of the infundibular septum provides the potential for subaortic stenosis, and one would think that pulmonary artery banding, which might accelerate the subaortic stenosis, would be contraindicated.[22, 65] Conversely, if the defect results from malalignment, but malalignment of the tetralogy type, then one might consider deferring surgery, hoping for increasing obstruction to pulmonary blood flow.

Finally, although a large number of studies have been addressed to the natural history of ventricular septal defect in isolation,[25] such assessments (with rare exception)[1, 2, 43] have tended not to differentiate between the various anatomic types of the defect.[25, 51, 85] As summarized by Freedom, these studies would be better served if natural history phenomena were interpreted in the context of the specific anatomic type of ventricular septal defect.[25]

TETRALOGY OF FALLOT

An extensive literature is devoted to the morphology of tetralogy of Fallot and to the angiocardiography of this lesion. (See reference 31 for a thorough review of the angiography of Fallot's tetralogy and variants.) With rare exceptions, however, the literature on angiography has relied on standard frontal, lateral, and right and left anterior oblique projections.[14, 19, 50, 68] Soto in collaboration with Bargeron has recently published a beautiful angiographic-pathologic correlative study of tetralogy of Fallot that used axial angiography.[74]

The essence of the tetralogy complex is malalignment between the infundibular septum and the trabecula septomarginalis.[13] The maligned infundibular septum is deviated anteriorly and superiorly, thus narrowing the right ventricular outflow tract. Hypertrophy of the septal band of the right ventricle (so-called trabecula septomarginalis) and muscle bundles intrinsic to the anterior wall of the right ventricle may also contribute significantly to obstruction of the right ventricular outflow tract in tetralogy of Fallot. Pulmonary valve stenosis and obstructive pulmonary annulus are common in the more severe forms of tetralogy (Fig. 20). The caliber and distortions of the pulmonary arteries must also be unequivocally shown as well (see Figs. 13 to 15).

The previous comments have focused on the infundibular anatomy, but rotational anomalies of the ventricles, right or left ventricular hypoplasia, straddling atrioventricular valves (either tricuspid or mitral), atrioventricular septal defect, subaortic stenosis, and so on can complicate the infundibular anomaly characteristic of tetralogy of Fallot. Such complicating features must be defined before intracardiac repair, but their recognition assumes lesser importance if only palliative surgery is contem-

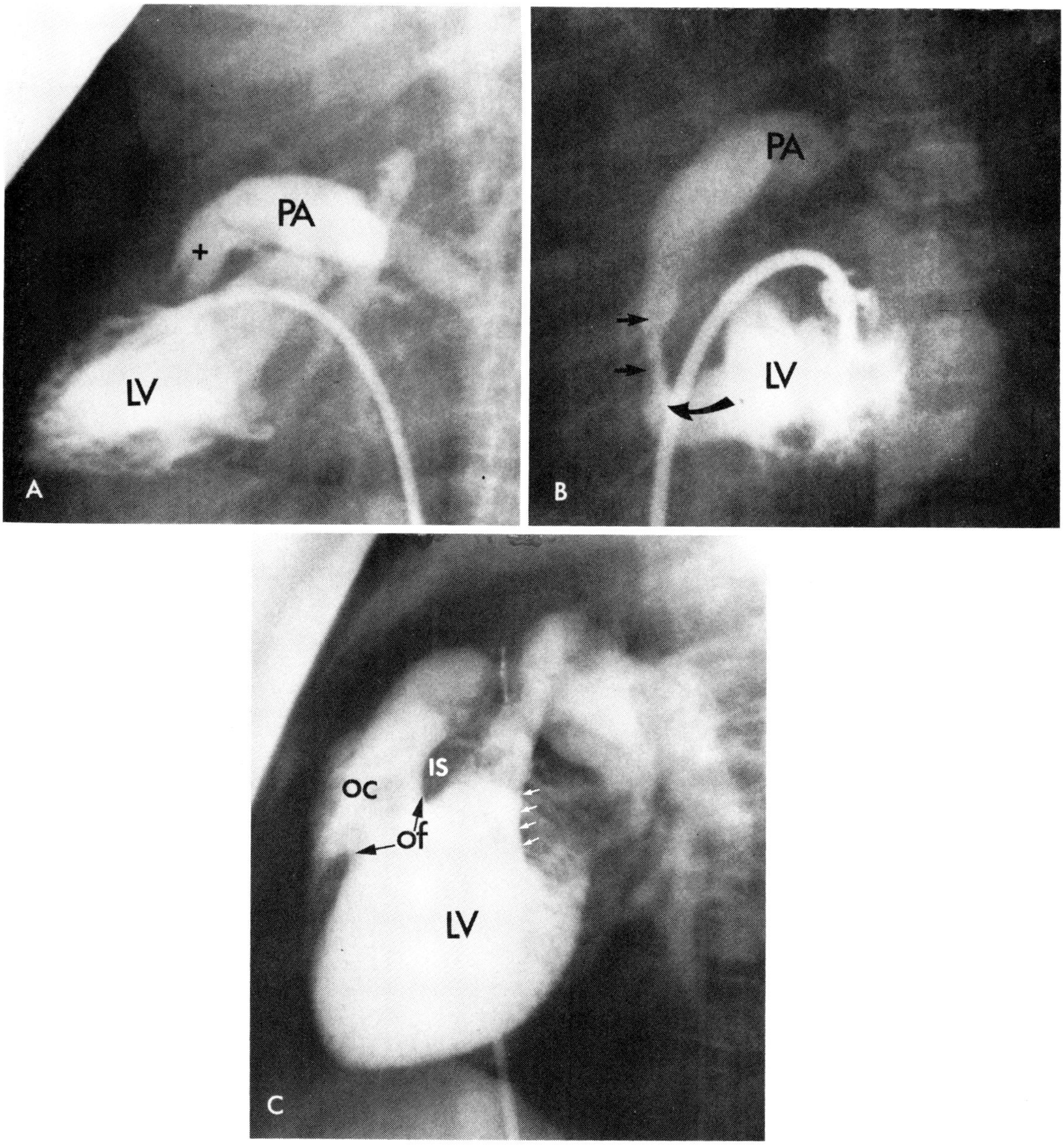

Figure 16. An infant with tricuspid atresia, ventricular septal defect, and pulmonary stenosis. *A*, This lateral left ventriculogram (LV) shows opacification of the distal infundibulum (x) and the pulmonary artery (PA), but the position and size of the outlet foramen (ventricular septal defect) and the nature of the subpulmonary stenosis are not clearly shown. *B*, The same patient with the left ventriculogram filmed in the left long axial oblique view has a large muscular ventricular septal defect (curved arrow) and diffuse hypoplasia (black arrows) of a subpulmonary trabecular zone and proximal infundibulum. *C*, A different patient with tricuspid atresia, normal ventriculoarterial connections, and banded pulmonary artery in whom this long axial oblique left ventriculogram demonstrates the dimension of the outlet foramen (of), and the plane of the left atrioventricular valve (white arrows) is clearly shown.

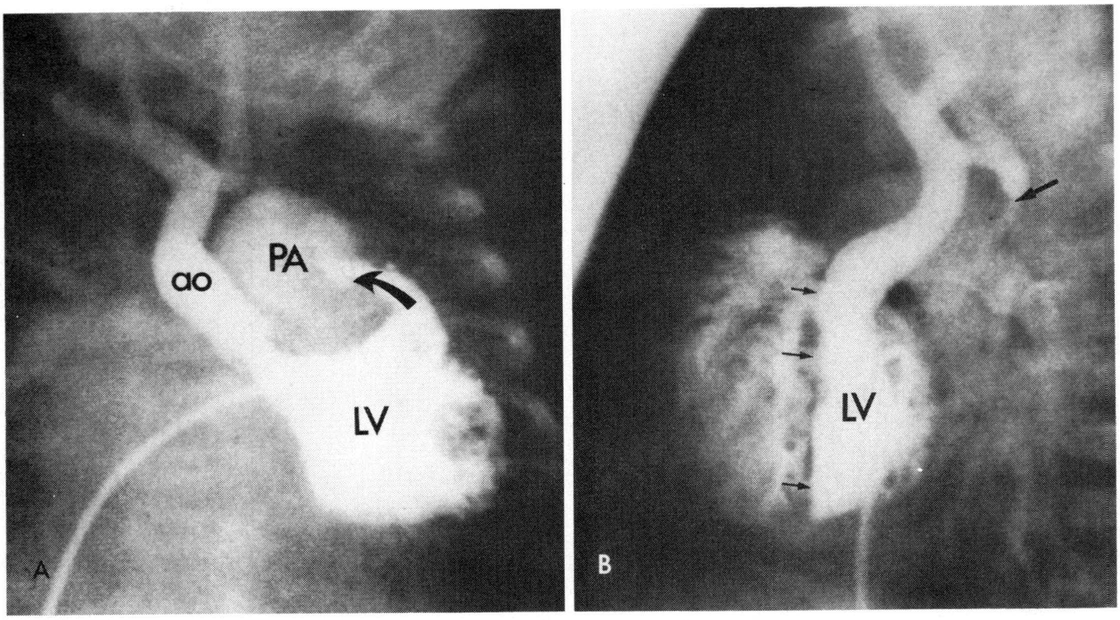

Figure 17. Coarctation syndrome in a neonate. *A*, Frontal left ventriculogram (LV) demonstrates opacification (arrow) of a very large pulmonary artery (PA) relative to a considerably smaller aorta (ao). *B*, The left long axial oblique left ventriculogram reveals a "swiss-cheese" ventricular septum (small black arrows) and a severe thoracic coarctation (arrow).

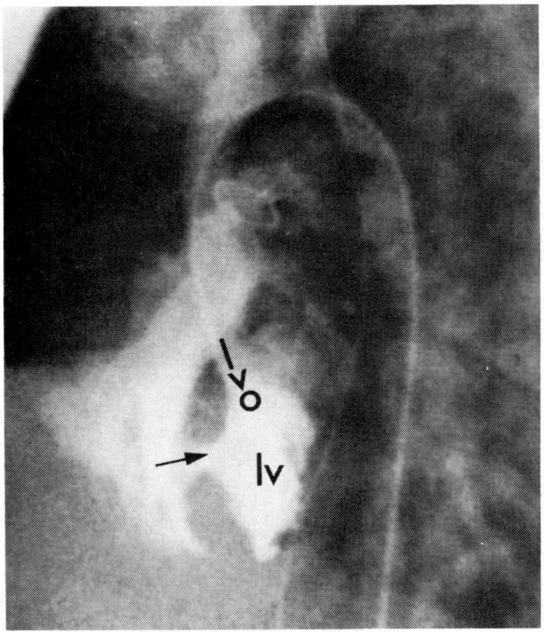

Figure 18. A muscular ventricular septal defect with mild subaortic stenosis,[54] previously repaired thoracic coarctation, and banded pulmonary artery in a neonate weighing 2.0 kg. This left long axial oblique left ventriculogram (LV) clearly shows the ventricular septal defect (arrow), but the aortic area is not clearly defined (lvo).

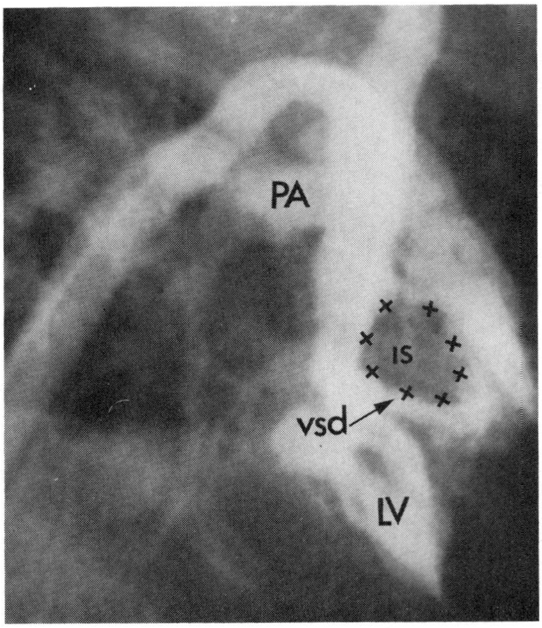

Figure 19. Subaortic stenosis resulting in part from a hypertrophied infundibular septum (is) in an infant with ventricular septal defect. The left ventriculogram (LV) in right long axial oblique projection demonstrates significant hypertrophy of the infundibular septum (x). The left ventricular outflow tract is narrowed. The ventricular septal defect (vsd) is relatively small.

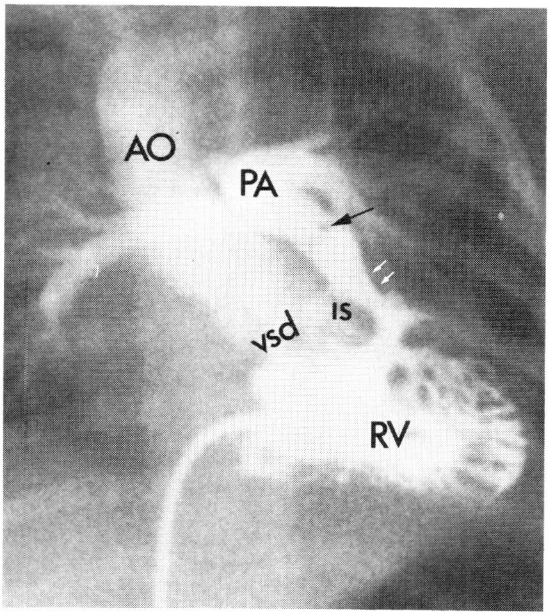

Figure 20. Tetralogy of Fallot in an infant weighing 2.6 kg. This right ventriculogram filmed with craniocaudal angulation demonstrates hypertrophy of the right ventricle (RV) and severe infundibular stenosis from the malaligned infundibular septum (is) and from contributions of free wall muscle bundles (small white arrows). The pulmonary arteries (PA) are reasonably well profiled, as is the stenotic pulmonary valve. The ascending aorta (AO) is opacified via the ventricular septal defect.

plated. However, "silent" lesions (cor triatriatum, supravalvar mitral ring, and so on), which could be unmasked by construction of a shunt, must be fully defined before palliation.[31]

For the critically ill, hypoxic infant with Fallot's tetralogy, a right ventriculogram in the elongated right axial oblique projection (about 30° right anterior oblique projection with 30° craniocaudal angulation) will provide information about (1) the size of the right ventricle, (2) the nature of the infundibular anatomy and contributions from the anterior muscular wall and the trabecula septomarginalis, (3) the functional status of the pulmonary valve and the pulmonary annulus, and (4) the caliber and distribution of the pulmonary arteries (see Fig. 20). The lateral view to this projection should provide information about the ventricular septal defect and the degree of aortic override. Aortography will be necessary to define the origin and epicardial distribution of the coronary arteries. Selective left ventriculography in various projections may be necessary to exclude (1) obstruction of left ventricular outflow tract, (2) atrioventricular septal defect, (3) other ventricular septal defects (involving the trabecular or inlet septum) and so forth.

LEFT VENTRICULAR OUTFLOW TRACT IN TRANSPOSITION OF THE GREAT ARTERIES

Obstruction of the left ventricular outflow tract in patients with complete transposition of the great arteries may be fixed or dynamic.[10, 67, 79] In most neonates with more than trivial subpulmonary obstruction, the obstruction is fixed and may become progressively severe. A number of pathologic mechanisms can be responsible for obstruction of the left ventricular outflow tract. For optimum medical and surgical management, these precise mechanism(s) for the obstruction of the left ventricular outflow tract and their severity must be identified.

Selective left ventricular cineangiography is best performed in the right and left long axial oblique projections (Figs. 21 to 23). This projection is achieved by elevating the right shoulder 15 to 20° with a sponge wedge and then slanting the body 25 to 30° across the table. These maneuvers serve to elongate the left ventricular outflow tract and to prevent the "shoulder" of the left ventricle from obscuring the left ventricular outflow tract (Fig. 21A). With the long axial oblique projections, it should be relatively easy to identify the pathologic mechanism responsible for the obstruction of the left ventricular outflow tract (see Figs. 22 and 23).

SUBAORTIC STENOSIS IN INFANTS WITH VENTRICULAR SEPTAL DEFECT AND OBSTRUCTIVE ANOMALIES OF THE AORTIC ARCH (NORMAL ATRIOVENTRICULAR AND VENTRICULOARTERIAL CONNECTIONS)

The relatively discrete forms of subaortic stenosis are rarely diagnosed in the critically ill infant with concordant atrioventricular and ventriculoarterial connections. Certainly, muscular subaortic stenosis (hypertrophic obstructive cardiomyopathy) and fibrous diaphragms have been identified in the neonate and infant, but subaortic stenosis is more commonly diagnosed, superimposed on a substrate of anomalies of the systemic atrioventricular junction, muscular abnormalities of the left ventricle, and defects of the ventricular septum.[33, 36] That obstructive anomalies of the aortic arch should complicate such cardiac anomalies is not surprising.[82] Because of the considerable heterogeneity of those mechanisms capable of producing subaortic ste-

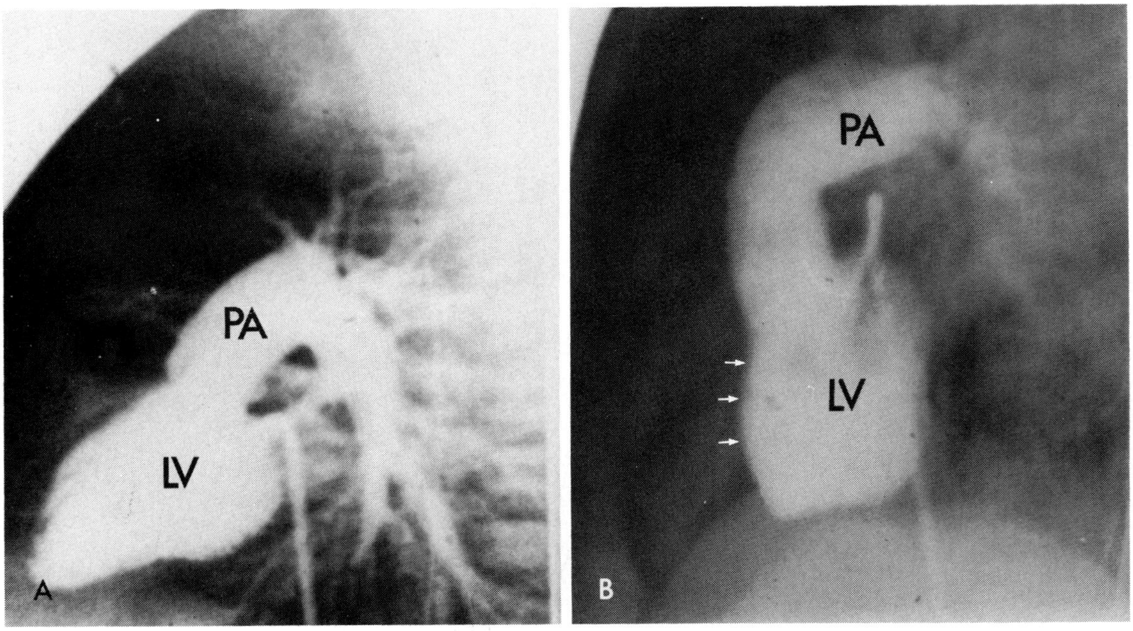

Figure 21. A normal left ventricular outflow tract in complete transposition of the great arteries and intact ventricular septum. *A*, Classic left ventriculogram (LV) in lateral projection shows that this ventricle supports the pulmonary artery. The plane of the ventricular septum is not profiled, nor is the left ventricular outflow tract. *B*, The same patient in an elongated left axial oblique projection.

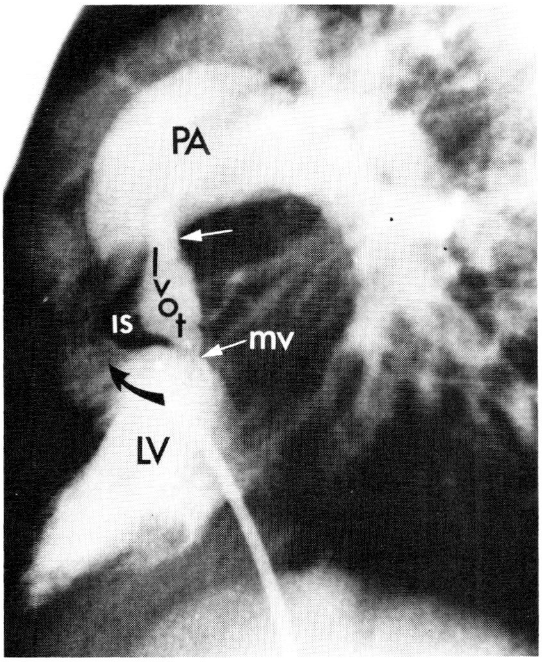

Figure 22. Multiple mechanisms are responsible for left ventricular outflow tract stenosis in this patient with transposition of the great arteries and ventricular septal defect. This elongated left axial oblique ventriculogram (LV) demonstrates severe left ventricular outflow tract stenosis (lvot) resulting from (1) malaligned infundibular septum (is), (2) persistence of the left-sided ventriculoinfundibular fold, producing mitral valve (mv)-pulmonary valve (white arrow) discontinuity, and (3) pulmonary valve stenosis. The ventricular septal defect (curved arrow) is inferior to the malaligned infundibular septum.

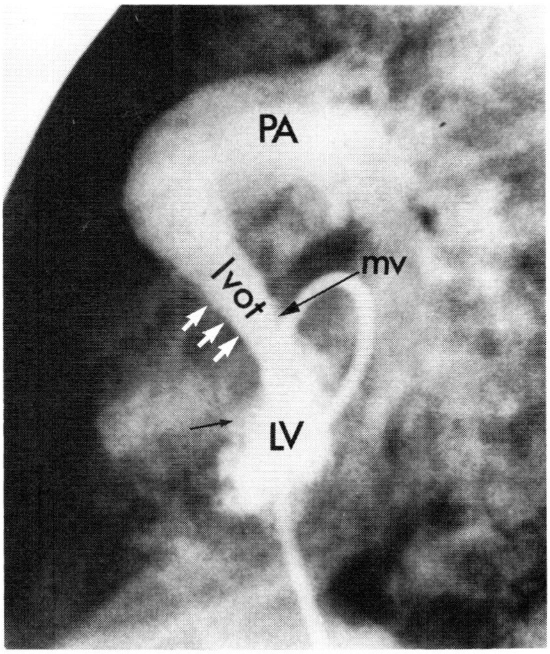

Figure 23. Severe tunnel form of obstruction of the left ventricular outflow tract (lvot), complicating complete transposition of the great arteries, a small left ventricle (LV), and a restrictive, muscular ventricular septal defect (arrow). The pulmonary artery (PA) is dilated. There is discontinuity between mitral valve (mv) and pulmonary valve.

nosis, the topography of the left ventricular outflow tract must be understood.

Walmsley characterizes the left ventricular outflow tract as the left ventricular region that lies between the ventricular septum and the anterior leaflet of the mitral valve. The anterior wall of the left ventricular outflow tract is thus anteromedial, and the muscular and membranous portions of the ventricular septum compose the anterior wall.[84] The membranous septum is partly atrioventricular, with the right face of the membranous septum having attachments both with the medial wall of the right atrium and with a small part of the septal leaflet of the tricuspid valve. Superiorly, the membranous septum is continuous with the right lateral wall of the root of the aorta. The posterior aspect of the left ventricular outflow tract is formed by the anterior mitral leaflet and partly by the fusion of the anterior and posterior mitral leaflets. Furthermore, there is a contribution to the posterior wall of the left ventricular outflow tract from the so-called intervalvar septum. This intervalvar septum is a fibrous lamina that originates from the region of the left and noncoronary aortic sinuses and extends inferiorly and joins the upper muscular wall of the left atrium, becoming continuous with the lamina fibrosa of the anterior leaflet of the mitral valve.

Superiorly, the anterior mitral leaflet is in fibrous continuity with the adjacent left and noncoronary sinuses of the aortic valve. Rosenquist et al. have defined the normal spectrum of aortic and mitral valve discontinuity and have suggested that the width of the fibrous (and muscular band) varied from 0.0 to 7.0 mm.[63] It has been suggested that this spectrum of aortic-mitral separation results from varying degrees of resorption of musculature having its origin along the inner curvature of the heart tube. This inner curvature of the heart tube has been termed "bulboauricular" or "conoventricular flange" or the "ventriculoinfundibular fold."[3] There is increased mitral aortic separation in patients with discrete subaortic stenosis,[63] and this lack of resorption or persistence of the ventriculoinfundibular fold is frequently accompanied by hypoplasia of the aortic valve can-

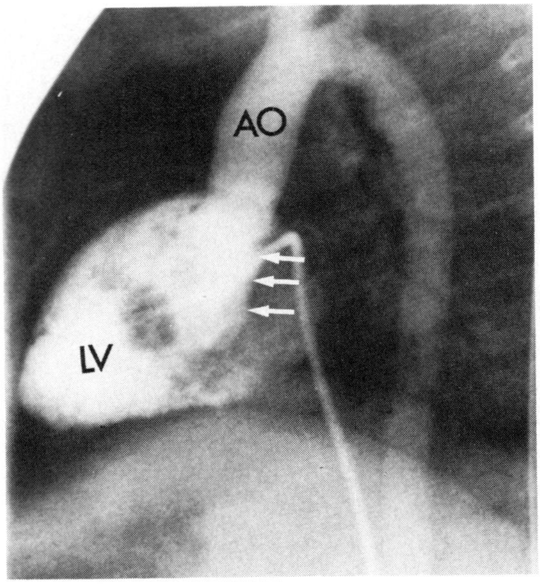

Figure 24. "Classical" left ventriculogram (LV) filmed in the lateral projection demonstrates (arrows) mitral valve-aortic valve continuity, but the left ventricular outflow tract is obscured by the shoulder of the left ventricle.

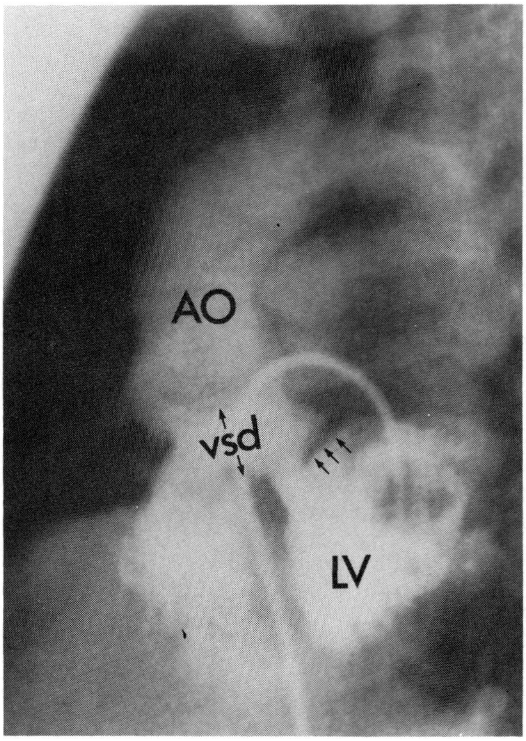

Figure 25. Subaortic stenosis below the level of a ventricular septal defect in an infant with severe congestive heart failure and clinical findings of a hypertensive ventricular septal defect. This left ventriculogram (LV) filmed in the left long axial oblique projection shows the large ventricular septal defect (vsd), an intact muscular ventricular septum, and a fibrous membrane (arrows) attached to the anterior leaflet of the mitral valve. AO: aorta.

nulas. Moulaert and Oppenheimer-Dekker have shown that persistence of the left extremity of the bulboatrioventricular flange results in a muscular type of subaortic stenosis.[55-57] They have termed this muscular remnant the "anterolateral muscle bundle" of the left ventricle, and its position between the left coronary aortic leaflet and the anterior mitral leaflet indicates its origin from the unresolved inner curvature of the heart tube.

A ventricular septal defect can occur in patients with subaortic stenosis, and not infrequently, the two defects have an intimate, if not causal, relation (See Figs. 18, 19, 24 and 25). From the studies of Van Praagh, Moulaert, and Freedom and their respective colleagues,[29, 55-57, 82] the caudal malalignment of the infundibular septum (that portion of the ventricular septum separating the arterial outlets) from the anterior and posterior limbs of the trabecula septomarginalis will clearly result in a type of muscular subaortic stenosis *above* the ventricular septal defect. This infundibular malalignment type of ventricular septal defect is common in patients with interruption of the aortic arch and in those patients with aortic atresia, ventricular septal defect, and normal left ventricle.[29, 32, 35] It has been suggested elsewhere that occlusion of the subaortic vestibule (resulting in subaortic atresia, ventricular septal defect, and normal left ventricle) could result from fusion of the caudal extension of the infundibular septum and the ventriculoinfundibular fold (Fig. 26).[32, 35]

Moene et al. have described a particular relationship between aortic arch hypoplasia of variable severity and central muscular defects (see Fig. 18).[54] Of particular concern are the associated left ventricular anomalies including the so-called anterolateral muscle bundle, the posteromedial muscle, and the anteroseptal twist. This appears to be a genuine association, and the morphologic bases for subaortic stenosis are *superior* to the ventricular septal defect. Among patients with central muscular ventricular septal defect and obstructive anomalies of the aortic arch, there appears to be a consistent association of left ventricular muscular anomalies with anatomic and functional disturbances of the mitral and aortic valves.

Obstruction of the left ventricular outflow tract can occur below the ventricular septal defect,[17] and this can be muscular (see Figs. 18 and 19), fibrous (see Fig. 25), or related to an accessory tissue tag.[24, 29, 31, 33, 36, 37]

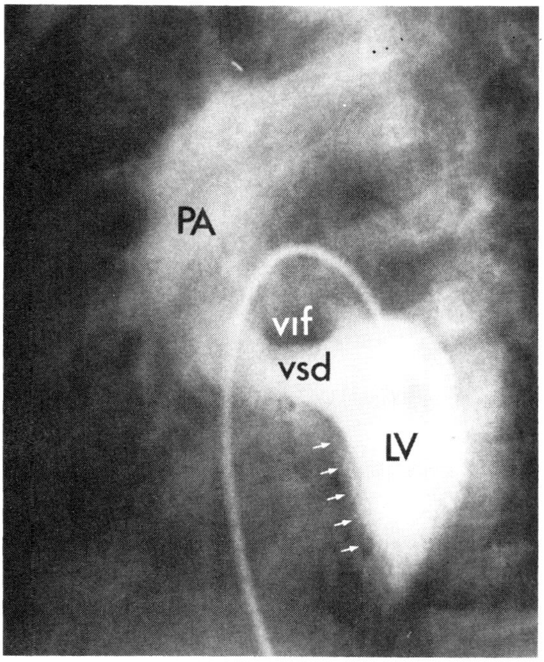

Figure 26. Left ventriculogram (LV) in left long axial oblique view in a patient with aortic atresia, ventricular septal defect (vsd), and normal left ventricle. The muscular ventricular septum is intact (white arrows). The left ventricle empties through a moderately large ventricular septal defect (vsd), which lies beneath a muscular bar that has virtually occluded the subaortic vestibule. This muscular bar probably represents fusion of a malaligned infundibular septum with the ventriculoinfundibular fold (vif).

UNIVENTRICULAR HEART AND SUBAORTIC STENOSIS

The morphologic bases of subaortic stenosis in patients with univentricular heart have received considerable attention.[18, 24, 28, 40, 69] The most common form of univentricular heart in which subaortic stenosis may be found is characterized by a single left ventricle, a well-formed outlet chamber, and discordantly connected, transposed great arteries. The transposed aorta originates above the outlet chamber, and the unobstructed and usually larger pulmonary artery is supported by the main left ventricular chamber. Subaortic obstruction usually results from alterations in or about the outlet foramen, the foramen between the single left ventricle and the infundibular outlet chamber. This outlet foramen may be actually obstructive at birth, or rarely it may be sealed.[36] Furthermore, a marginal outlet foramen may become obstructive, and there is now considerable evidence to suggest that palliative pulmonary artery banding may potentiate obstruction at the outlet foramen.[40, 42, 69, 70] When an obstructive anomaly of the aortic arch complicates a single left ventricle, a well-defined infundibular outlet chamber, and transposed great arteries, it is likely that the outlet foramen is actually or potentially obstructive even in utero, thus favoring pulmonary blood flow at the expense of the aortic blood flow. Even when the outlet foramen is severely obstructive in the critically ill neonate, it is unusual to record a pressure gradient across it. Thus, it becomes important to profile the outlet foramen during cardiac angiography. This outlet foramen is usually elliptical, and the septum between the infundibular chamber and the main left ventricular cavity can be profiled either by selective injection in the outlet chamber or by selective injection in the main left ventricular chamber (Fig. 27).

When the outlet chamber is relatively right-sided and anterior (as in the patient with the usual type of tricuspid atresia), the left long axial oblique projection will usually profile the outlet foramen to advantage (see Figs. 16*C* and 27). Conversely, if the outlet chamber is leftward, superior, and posterior, injection of contrast material in the frontal plane will usually suffice. There is, however, considerable variation in the topography of the outlet chamber, and several, small injections of contrast material by hand may be necessary to define the most precise axial projection.[28]

DOUBLE-OUTLET RIGHT VENTRICLE

Double-outlet right ventricle characterizes an abnormal ventriculoarterial connection. In the purest sense, both great arteries originate completely from the morphologic right ventricle. When the ventricular septum is intact, this determination poses little difficulty. But most patients with this abnormal ventriculoarterial connection have a ventricular septal defect, and thus one or both semilunar roots may override the ventricular septal defect. Thus the dilemma. There is not unanimity of opinion about how much of each great artery must originate morphologically from the right ventricle to satisfy the definition of the abnormal ventriculoarterial connection. We have adopted the convention of Tynan and his colleagues that double-outlet right ventricle is that condition in which more than half of each great artery originates morphologically from the right ventricle.[81]

The management of the neonate with this abnormal ventriculoarterial connection neces-

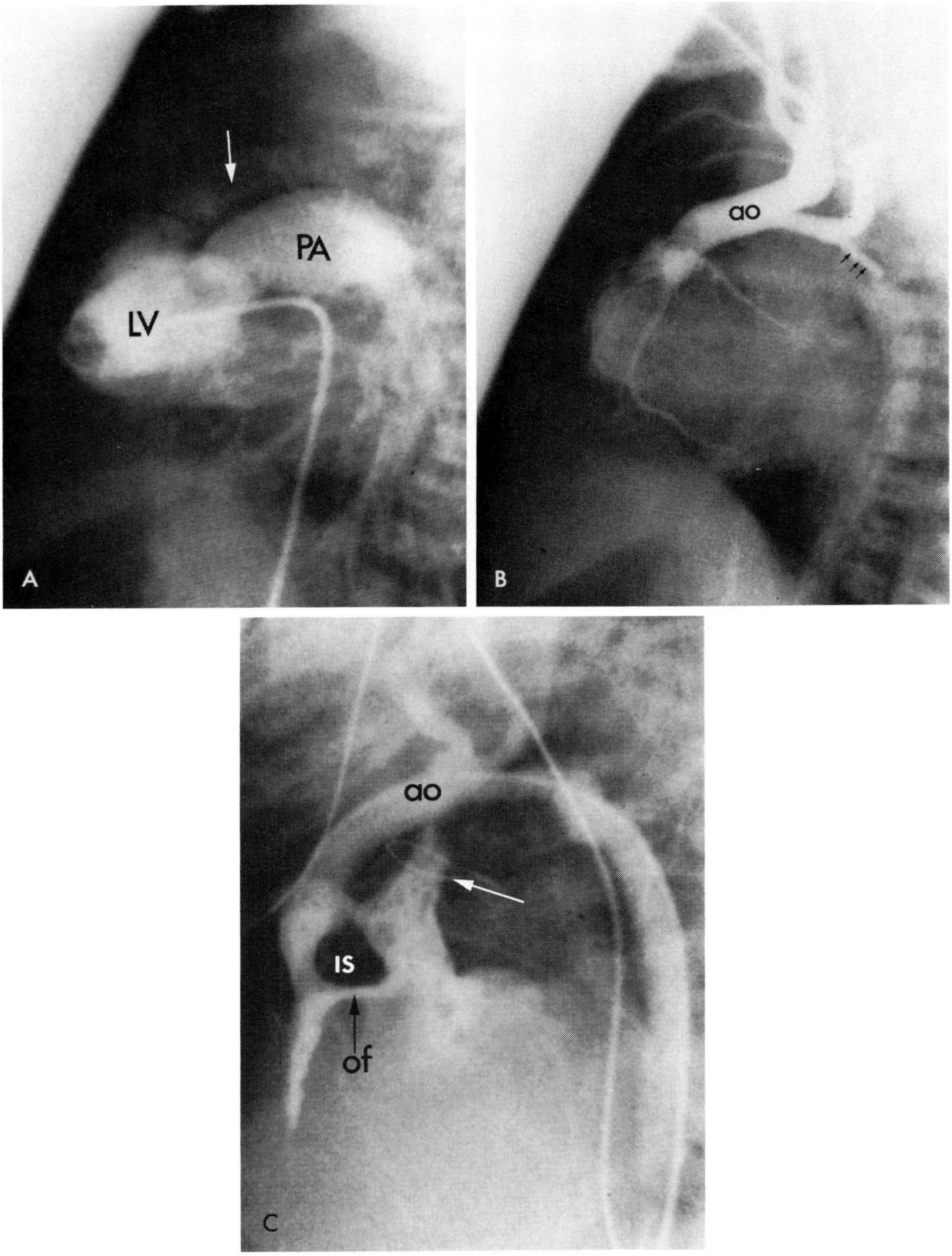

Figure 27. Severe coarctation of the aorta in a neonate with tricuspid atresia and discordant ventriculoarterial connections. *A*, This lateral left ventriculogram (LV) shows a very large posteriorly positioned pulmonary artery (PA) and a faintly opacified anterior aorta (white arrow). The outlet foramen is not profiled but certainly could be restrictive. *B*, The retrograde aortogram via the right axillary artery shows a small ascending aorta (ao) and extreme isthmic hypoplasia (black arrows). *C*, Several weeks after repair of the coarctation and pulmonary artery banding (white arrow), this selective injection in the outlet chamber demonstrates a markedly restrictive outlet foramen (of) and a hypertrophied infundibular septum (is).

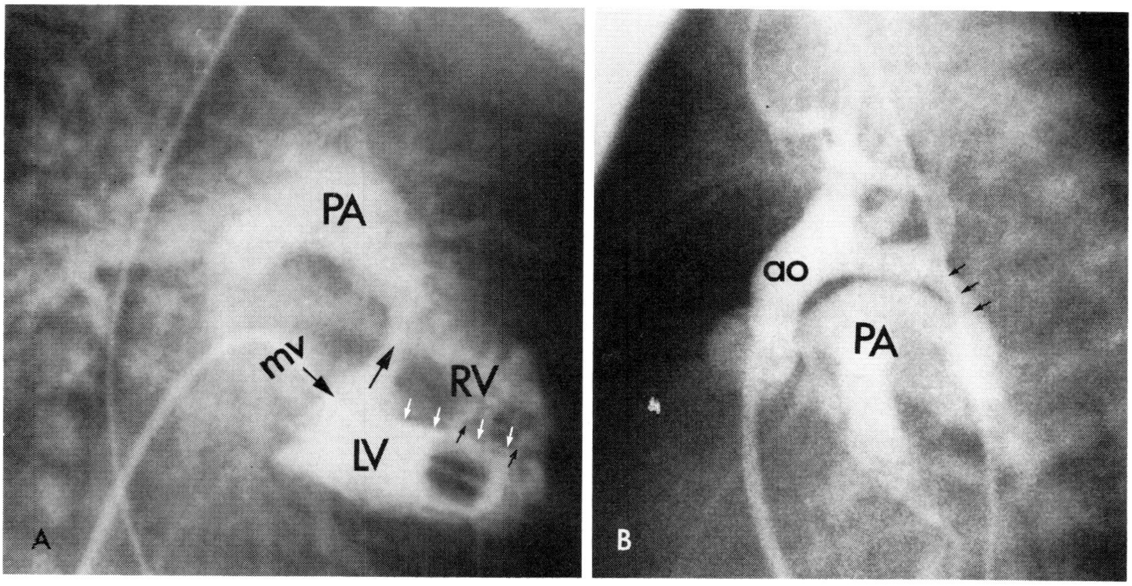

Figure 28. Taussig-Bing type of double-outlet right ventricle with both subpulmonary ventricular septal defect and multiple muscular ventricular septal defect and complicated by a severe obstructive anomaly of the aortic arch. *A*, Right long axial oblique left ventriculogram (LV) performed via the mitral valve (mv) shows the larger subpulmonary ventricular septal defect (larger black arrow) and multiple small muscular defects (small black arrows). The plane of the ventricular septum is shown reasonably well in this projection (white arrows). *B*, Selective aortogram (ao) in this patient shows the diffusely hypoplastic aortic isthmus with opacification of the larger pulmonary artery (PA) via a patent ductus arteriosus.

sitates the definition of the size and position of the ventricular septal defect, the presence or absence of pulmonary or (less commonly) obstruction of the aortic outflow tract, and the status of the mitral valve (Fig. 28).[76] When the ventricular septal defect is subpulmonary, the circulation is similar to that of the patient with complete transposition of the great arteries and a large ventricular septal defect (Fig. 29). There is preferential opacification of the larger pulmonary artery. The subaortic ventricular septal defect is also profiled in this projection, but in

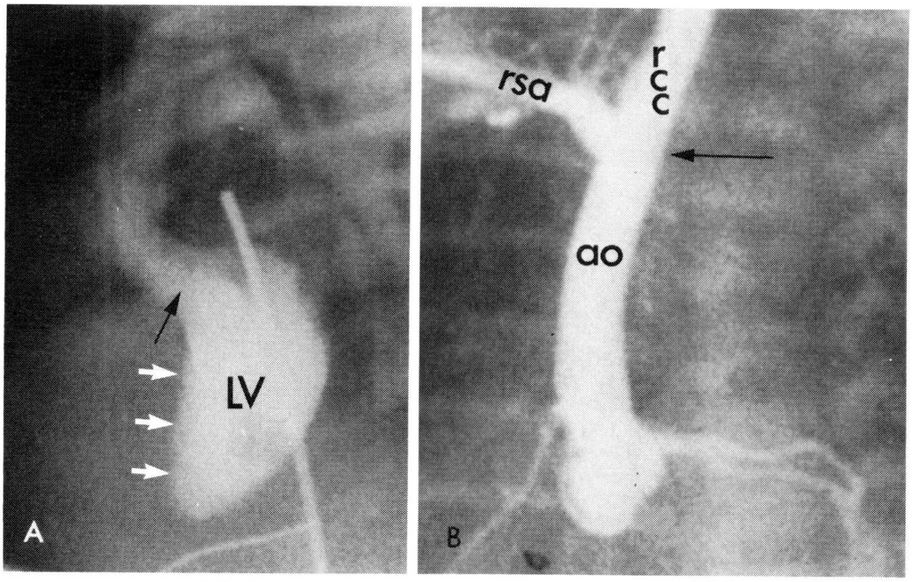

Figure 29. Taussig-Bing type of double-outlet right ventricle and type C interruption of aortic arch. *A*, Left long axial oblique left ventriculogram (LV) shows an intact muscular septum (white arrows) and an anteriorly positioned ventricular septal defect. *B*, The frontal aortogram performed via the right axillary artery shows interruption of the aortic arch (arrow) distal to the innominate artery. rcc: right common carotid artery, rsa: right subclavian artery.

this situation, left ventricular angiography preferentially opacifies the aorta.

CONCLUSIONS

That axial projections provide a new and important dimension to cardiac angiography is beyond question, and the application of these projections is usually mandatory if medical or surgical intervention is to be optimized. Yet there are caveats to the blind application of these techniques. The presence of an abnormal disposition of the ventricles about a horizontal or vertical ventricular septum may contraindicate the use of these projections at the initial catheter investigation. Judicious use of cross-sectional echocardiographic examination before invasive studies and small test doses of contrast material should facilitate the optimum angiographic projection without unduly jeopardizing the patient's condition.

REFERENCES

1. Alpert BS, Cook DH, Varghese PJ, et al: Spontaneous closure of small ventricular septal defect: Ten-year follow-up. Pediatrics, *63*:204, 1979.
2. Alpert BS, Mellits ED, Rowe RD: Spontaneous closure of small ventricular septal defects. Probability notes in the first five years of life. Am J Dis Child, *125*:194, 1973.
3. Anderson RH, Becker AE, Van Mierop LHS: What should we call the 'crista'? Br Heart J, *39*:856, 1977.
4. Anderson RH, Shinebourne EA, Gerlis LM: Criss-cross atrioventricular relationships producing paradoxical atrioventricular concordance or discordance. Their significance to nomenclature of congenital heart disease. Circulation, *50*:176, 1974.
5. Anderson RH, Wilkinson JL, Becker AE: The bulbus cordis—a misunderstood region of the developing human heart: Its significance to the classification of congenital cardiac malformations. *In* Rosenquist GC, Bergsma D (eds): Morphogenesis and malformation of the cardiovascular system. The National Foundation—March of Dimes. Birth Defects: Original Article Series. Vol 14, No. 7, p. 1, 1978.
6. Attie, F, Munoz-Castellanos L, Ovseyevitz, J, et al: Crossed atrioventricular connections. Am Heart J, *99*:163, 1980.
7. Attie F, Soni J, Oveseyevitz J, et al: Angiographic studies of atrioventricular discordance. Circulation, *62*:407, 1980.
8. Bargeron LM Jr: Angiographic recognition of specific anatomic structures. *In* Becker AE, Losekoot G, Marcelletti C, et al (eds): Paediatric Cardiology, vol 3. Edinburgh, Churchill Livingstone, 1981, pp. 33–47.
9. Bargeron LM Jr: Axial angiography. *In* Becker AE, Losekoot G, Marcelletti C, et al (eds): Paediatric Cardiology, vol 3. Edinburgh, Churchill Livingstone, 1981, pp. 65–87.
10. Bargeron LM Jr: Angiography relevant to complicating features. *In* Becker AE, Losekoot G, Marcelletti C, et al (eds): Paediatric Cardiology, vol 3. Edinburgh, Churchill Livingstone, 1981, pp. 179–184.
11. Bargeron LM Jr: Straddling valves. *In* Becker AE, Losekoot G, Marcelletti C, et al (eds): Paediatric Cardiology, vol 3. Edinburgh, Churchill Livingstone, 1981, pp. 426–430.
12. Bargeron LM Jr, Elliott LP, Soto B, et al: Axial cineangiography in congenital heart disease. I. Concept, technical and anatomic consideration. Circulation, *56*:1075–1083, 1977.
13. Becker E, Connor M, Anderson RH: Tetralogy of Fallot. A morphometric and geometric study. Am J Cardiol, *35*:402, 1975.
14. Beuren AJ: Die angiokardiographische darstellung kongenitaler Herzenfeher. Ein Atlas. Berlin, Watter De Gruyter Co., 1966, p. 182.
15. Bharati S, Lev M: The spectrum of common atrioventricular orifice. Am Heart J, *86*:553, 1973.
16. Ceballos R, Soto B, Bargeron LM Jr: Angiographic anatomy of the normal heart through axial angiography. Circulation, *64*:351, 1981.
17. Dirksen TH, Moulaert AJ, Buis-Liem TN, et al: Ventricular septal defect associated with left ventricular outflow tract obstruction below the defect. J Thorac Cardiovasc Surg, *75*:688, 1978.
18. Doty DB, Marvin WJ Jr, Lauer RM: Single ventricle with aortic outflow obstruction. Operative repair by creation of double outlet to the aorta and application of the Fontan principle. J Thorac Cardiovasc Surg, *81*:636, 1981.
19. Edwards JE, Carey LS, Neufeld HN, et al: Congenital Heart Disease. Correlation of Pathologic Anatomy and Angiocardiography. Philadelphia, W. B. Saunders Co., 1965.
20. Elliott LP, Bargeron LM Jr, Bream PR, et al: Axial cine-angiography in congenital heart disease. II. Specific lesions. Circulation, *56*:1084, 1977.
21. Fellows KE, Keane JF, Freed MD: Angled views in cineangiocardiography of congenital heart disease. Circulation, *56*:485, 1977.
22. Freed MD, Rosenthal A, Plauth WH Jr, et al: Development of subaortic stenosis after pulmonary artery banding. Circulation (Suppl), *47*:3, 7, 1973.
23. Freedom RM: The supero-inferior ventricle and criss-cross atrioventricular connections: An analysis of the myth and mystery. Mod Probl pediatr, *22*:48, 1983.
24. Freedom RM: The morphologic and therapeutic implications of an obstructive anomaly of the aortic arch in infants with complex congenital heart disease (univentricular heart, dominant right for of AV defect). *In* Parenzan L, Crupi G, Graham G (eds): Congenital Heart Disease in the First Three Months of Life. Medical and Surgical Aspects. Bologna, Patron Editore, 1981, p. 341.
25. Freedom RM: The natural history of ventricular septal defect, with morphologic considerations. *In* Moss AJ (ed): Paediatric Updates. New York, Elsevier, 1979, p. 251.
26. Freedom RM, Olley PM: Pulmonary arteriography in congenital heart disease. Cathet Cardiovasc Diagn, *2*:309, 1976.
27. Freedom RM, Rose RD: Aneurysm of the atrial septum in tricuspid atresia. Diagnosis during life and therapy. Am J Cardiol, *38*:265, 1976.
28. Freedom RM, Rowe RD: Morphological and topographical variations of the outlet chamber in complex congenital heart disease: An angiocardiographic study. Cathet Cardiovasc Diagn, *4*:345, 1978.

29. Freedom RM, Bain H, Esplugas E, et al: The ventricular septal defect in interruption of the aortic arch. Am J Cardiol, *39*:572, 1977.
30. Freedom RM, Bini M, Rowe RD: Endocardial cushion defect and significant hypoplasia of the left ventricle: A distinct clinical and pathological entity. Eur J Cardiol, *7*:263, 1978.
31. Freedom RM, Culham JAG, Moes CAF: The angiocardiography of congenital heart disease. New York, MacMillan and Co., in press, 1982.
32. Freedom RM, Culham JAG, Rowe RD: Aortic atresia with normal left ventricle: Distinctive angiocardiographic findings. Cathet Cardiovasc Diagn, *3*:283, 1977.
33. Freedom RM, Culham JAG, Rowe RD: Angiocardiography of subaortic obstruction in infancy. Am J Roentgenol, *129*:813, 1977.
34. Freedom RM, Culham JAG, Rowe RD: The criss-cross and superoinferior ventricular heart: An angiocardiographic study. Am J Cardiol, *42*:620, 1978.
35. Freedom RM, Dische MR, Rowe RD: Conal anatomy in aortic atresia, ventricular septal defect, and normally developed left ventricle. Am Heart J, *94*:689, 1977.
36. Freedom RM, Dische RD, Rowe RD: The pathologic anatomy of subaortic stenosis and atresia in the first year of life. Am J Cardiol, *39*:1035, 1977.
37. Freedom RM, Fowler RS, Duncan WJ: Rapid evolution from "normal" left ventricular outflow tract to fatal subaortic stenosis in infancy. Br Heart J, *45*:605, 1981.
38. Freedom RM, Gingell RL, Rowe RD: The superoinferior ventricle and "criss-cross" atrioventricular connection: An angiographic analysis of the important differences between abnormal spatial relationships between ventricles, the internal organization of the ventricle, and the type of atrioventricular connection. Submitted for publication.
39. Freedom RM, Harder J, Culham JAG, et al: Ventricular hypoplasia: Angiocardiographic features with surgical applications. *In* Godman MJ (ed): Paediatric Cardiology, vol 4. Edinburgh, Churchill Livingstone, 1981, p. 117.
40. Freedom RM, Hirose M, Patel RG, et al: The morphologic basis of subaortic stenosis in single ventricle with angiocardiographic and therapeutic considerations. Pediatr Cardiol, in press.
41. Freedom RM, Olley PM, Coceani T, et al: The prostaglandin challenge: Test to unmask obstructed total anomalous pulmonary venous connections in asplenia syndrome. Br Heart J, *40*:91, 1978.
42. Freedom RM, Sondheimer H, Dische MR, et al: Development of subaortic stenosis after pulmonary artery banding in common ventricle. Am J Cardiol, *39*:78, 1977.
43. Freedom RM, White RD, Pieroni DR, et al: The natural history of the so-called aneurysm of the membranous ventricular septum in childhood. Circulation, *49*:375, 1974.
44. Fyler DC: Report of the New England Regional infant cardiac program. Pediatrics (Suppl), *65*:388, 1980.
45. Gerlis LM, Anderson RH: Cor triatriatum dexter with imperforate Ebstein's anomaly. Br Heart J, *38*:108, 1976.
46. Goor DA, Lillehei CW, Rees R, et al: Isolated ventricular septal defect. Developmental basis for various types and presentation of classification. Chest, *58*:468, 1970.
47. Green CE, Elliott LP, Bargeron LM Jr: Axial cineangiographic evaluation of the posterior ventricular septal defect. Am J Cardiol, *48*:331, 1981.
48. Green CE, Elliott LP, Coghlan HC: Improved cineangiographic evaluation of hypertrophic cardiomyopathy by caudocranial left anterior oblique view. Am Heart J, *102*:1015, 1981.
49. Kattan KR: Angled views in pulmonary angiography. A new roentgen approach. Radiology, *94*:74, 1970.
50. Kjellberg SR, Mannheimer E, Rudhe U, et al: Diagnosis of congenital heart disease. Chicago, Year Book Publishers, 1959, p. 338.
51. Hoffman JIE: Natural history of congenital heart disease. Problems in its assessment with special reference to ventricular septal defects. Circulation, *37*:97, 1968.
52. Kelley MJ, Higgins CB, Kirkpatrick SE: Axial left ventriculography in discrete subaortic stenosis. Radiology, *135*:77, 1980.
53. Milo S, Yenho S, Macartney FJ, et al: Straddling and overriding atrioventricular valves. Morphology and Classification. Am J Cardiol, *44*:1122, 1979.
54. Moene RJ, Oppenheimer-Dekker A, Wenink ACG: Relation between aortic arch hypoplasia of variable severity and central muscular ventricular septal defects. Emphasis on an associated left ventricular abnormalities. Am J Cardiol, *48*:111, 1981.
55. Moulaert AJ, Bruins CC, Oppenheimer-Dekker A: Anomalies of the aortic arch and ventricular septal defects. Circulation, *53*:1011, 1976.
56. Houlaert AJ, Oppenheimer-Dekker A: Anterolateral muscle bundle of the left ventricle, bulboventricular flange and subaortic stenosis. Am J Cardiol, *37*:78, 1976.
57. Oppenheimer-Dekker A, Gittenberger-De Groot AC, Roozendaal H: The ductus arteriosus and associated cardiac anomalies in interruption of aortic arch. Pediatr Cardiol, *2*:185, 1982.
58. Otero Coto E, Quero Jiminez M, Cabrera A, Deverall PB, et al: Aortic levopositions without ventricular inversion. Eur J Cardiol *8*:523, 1978.
59. Piccoli GP, Yen Ho S, Wilkinson JL, et al: Left-sided obstructive lesions in atrioventricular septal defects. J Thorac Cardiovasc Surg, *83*:453, 1982.
60. Puyau FA, Burko H: The tilted left anterior oblique position in the study of congenital cardiac anomalies. Radiology, *87*:1069, 1966.
61. Rao PS, Jue KL, Isabel-Jones J, et al: Ebstein's malformation of the tricuspid valve with atresia. Differentiation from isolated tricuspid atresia. Am J Cardiol, *32*:104, 1973.
62. Reder RF, Hsu-Cmong Y, Steinfeld L: Aneurysm of the interatrial septum causing pulmonary venous obstruction in an infant with tricuspid atresia. Am Heart J, *102*:786, 1981.
63. Rosenquist GC, Clark EB, McAllister HA, et al: Increased mitral-aortic separation in discrete subaortic stenosis. Circulation, *60*:70, 1979.
64. Rowe RD: Angiocardiography in the prognosis for young infants in congestive failure with ventricular septal defect: The value of the defect ascending aorta diameter ratio. *In* Barratt-Boyes BG, Neutze JM, Harris EA, et al (eds): Heart Disease in Infancy. Diagnosis and Surgical Treatment. Edinburgh, Churchill Livingstone, 1973, p. 119.
65. Rosenthal A, Freed MD, Fyler DC, et al: Observations on the development of subaortic stenosis following pulmonary artery banding. Chest, *65*:420, 1974.
66. Sahn DJ, Allen HD, Anderson R, et al: Echocardiographic diagnosis of atrial septal aneurysm in an infant with hypoplastic right heart syndrome. Chest, *73*:227, 1978.
67. Sansa M, Tonkin IL, Bargeron LM Jr, et al: Left ventricular outflow tract obstruction in transposition

of the great arteries: An angiographic study of 74 cases. Am J Cardiol, *44*:88, 1979.
68. Schumacher G, Buhlmeyer K: Diagnostic augeborener Herzfehler. Band 2. Systematik der angeborensen Herzfehler. Germany, Verlagsgellschaft mbH, 1980, p. 413.
69. Somerville J: Changing form and function in one ventricle hearts. Herz, *4*:206, 1979.
70. Somerville J, Becu L, Ross D: Common ventricle with acquired subaortic obstruction. Am J Cardiol, *34*:206, 1974.
71. Soto B, Bargeron LM Jr, Pacifico AD, et al: Angiography of atrioventricular defects. Am J Cardiol, *48*:492, 1981.
72. Soto B, Becker AE, Moulaert AJ, et al: Classification of venttricular septal defects. Br Heart J, *43*:332, 1980.
73. Soto B, Bertranou EG, Bream PR, et al: Angiographic study of univentricular heart of ventricular type. Circulation, *60*:1325, 1979.
74. Soto B, Pacifico AD, Ceballos R, et al: Tetralogy of Fallot: An angiographic pathologic correlative study. Circulation, *64*:558, 1981.
75. Soto B, Pacifico AD, Di Scascio G: Univentricular heart: An angiographic study. Am J Cardiol, *49*:787, 1982.
76. Sriadaromont S, Ritter DG, Felkdt RH, et al: Double outlet right ventricle: Anatomic and angiographic correlations. Mayo Clin Proc, *53*:555, 1978.
77. Taylor JFN, Chrispin A: Interventricular septal defects shown by left ventricular cineangiography. Br Heart J, *33*:285, 1971.
78. Tonkin IL, Elliott LP, Bargeron LM Jr: Concomitant axial cineangiography and barium esophagography in the evaluation of vascular rings. Radiology, *135*:69, 1980.
79. Tonkin IL, Sansa M, Elliott LP, et al: Recognition by developing left ventricular outflow tract obstruction in complete transposition of the great arteries. Radiology, *134*:53, 1980.
80. Towbin R, Schwartz D: Endocardial cushion defects: Embryology, anatomy, and angiography. A.J.R., *136*:157, 1981.
81. Tynan M, Becker AE, Freedom RM, et al: Analysis of the ventriculo-arterial junction—connexions, infundibulum morphology and arterial relationships. *In* Godman MJ (ed): Paediatric Cardiology, vol 4. Edinburgh, Churchill Livingstone, 1981, p. 182.
82. Van Praagh R, Bernhard WF, Rosenthal A, et al: Interrupted aortic arch: Surgical treatment. Am J Cardiol, *27*:200, 1971.
83. Van Praagh S, LaCorte M, Fellows KE, et al: Superoinferior ventricles. Anatomic and angiocardiographic findings in ten postmortem cases. *In* Van Praagh R, Takao A (eds): Etiology and Morphogenesis of Congenital Heart Disease. New York, Futura Publishing Co.. 1980, p. 317.
84. Walmsley R: Anatomy of left ventricular outflow tract., Br Heart J, *41*:263, 1979.
85. Weidmann WH, Blount SG Jr, Dushane JW, et al: Clinical course in ventricular septal defect. Circulation (Suppl), *56*:56, 1977.
86. Wenmink ACG: Embryology of the ventricular septum. Separate origin of its components. Virch Arch (Pathol Anat), *390*:71, 1981.
87. Wenink ACG, Oppenheimer-Dekker A, Moulaert AJ: Muscular ventricular septal defects: A reappraisal of the anatomy. Am J Cardiol, *43*:259, 1979.

3

DIGITAL SUBTRACTION ANGIOGRAPHY

Techniques and Applications for Evaluating Cardiac Anatomy and Function

CHARLES B. HIGGINS, M.D., and EDWARD BUONOCORE, M.D.

Central cardiovascular dynamics can be studied without cardiac catheterization by digital processing of fluoroscopic images of the heart obtained after central intravenous injection of contrast media. Although digital subtraction angiography has been used for studying peripheral vasculature during the past few years,[4, 11, 14] this technique has only been recently applied toward assessing cardiac morphology and physiology. The conversion of fluoroscopic x-ray data into a digital form has an added advantage for the study of the central cardiovascular system since it not only permits contrast enhancement of the images but also facilitates quantitative and functional analysis of the x-ray data. The several applications described in this article suggest that digital subtraction angiography (DSA) will prove to be a powerful tool for studying cardiovascular physiology in animals and for evaluating heart disease in patients.

FLUOROSCOPIC DATA ACQUISITION AND PROCESSING

In digital subtraction angiography, detected x-ray information is converted into digital form, and in this form, contrast enhancement and quantitative analysis of the images can be performed. Ideally, the video signals are directly digitized and immediately processed, so that the images are not degraded by the introduction of noise.[5, 15] However, adequate images of the relatively large ventricular chambers have been obtained by recording the video signal initially on videotape and later digitizing and processing the images with the computer. This technique of post processing, although introducing some noise, has proven to be adequate for assessing left ventricular function because the left ventricle is a relatively large structure with predictable, nonrandom, periodic motion enabling effective frequency filtering of random noise during processing of the images. On the other hand, high-resolution visualization of the much smaller and relatively stationary peripheral arteries may critically depend on direct digitization of the amplified video signal.

Briefly, the process can be described in the following way: either the direct video image from the television or an image intermediately stored on videotape or videodisc is converted into digital form by an analog to digital converter (Fig. 1). After computer processing (subtraction, filtering, and so on), the digital data can then be reversed by a digital to analog converter into an analog (video) form for display on a video monitor or in a film format.

An electrocardiographic signal is obtained along with the video data in order to identify and subtract end-diastolic and end-systolic images or to permit digitization of a single heart beat at a rapid framing rate. We have used a

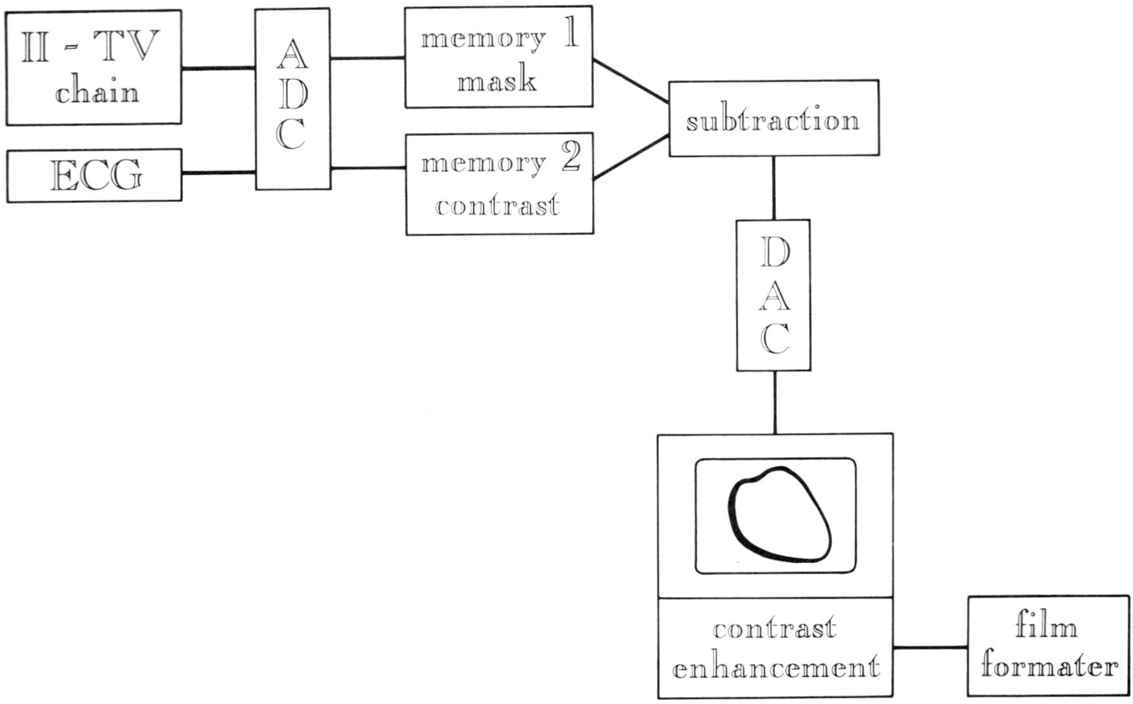

Figure 1. Diagram of digital fluoroscopic system for cardiac functional studies. ECG signal is recorded along with video data.

technique in which the operator visually identifies the heart beat in which the left ventricle is maximally opacified and digitizes this single heart beat at the rate of 30 frames (60 t.v. fields) per second. Simultaneous recording of the electrocardiogram ensures that the recording extends from one R wave to the succeeding R wave.

CONTRAST ENHANCEMENT

The contrast between structures containing contrast media and overlying noncardiovascular structures is improved several fold by density windowing and by various forms of filtering and subtraction (or division). Density "windowing" spreads densities within the area of interest over the entire grey scale level. This technique of density "windowing" is analogous to the technique used in computed tomography, in which only those structures having attenuation values within the operator-selected window are displayed.

Although the data are acquired with 256 levels of grey, not all of these levels correspond to intensities of interest. For example, regions over the lung fields have minimum x-ray attenuation, or maximum x-ray transmission. Since these values are not of interest in cardiac studies, they are not displayed, and the attenuation values corresponding to the ventricle and its surrounding structures are spread out over the entire grey scale.

FILTERING

In some of our studies, temporal frequency filtering is performed on the video data as the initial step in improving image quality. Dynamic studies of the cardiovascular system are particularly well suited to this technique. Since the motion of the heart is relatively smooth and undulatory, the individual time-varying frames comprising the study should also be expected to change smoothly and continuously. Any abrupt, stepwise changes occurring from one frame to the next are therefore most likely attributable to random statistical noise. Such rapid, abrupt changes are characterized by high temporal frequencies; the smooth periodic motion of the heart and great vessels contains predominantly very low temporal frequencies.

By frequency filtering in the time domain (temporal frequency filtering), medium and high frequency noise is eliminated while retaining the important low frequencies that contain the image data. For our studies, temporal frequency filtering is performed by using a truncated convolution operator so that processing time is minimized.

Recursive filtering has recently been introduced as an "on-line," real-time process for noise reduction.[17] This technique reduces the constraints on the digitizer, TV system, and x-ray equipment. Important for cardiac studies, image degradation due to subject motion is reduced by recursive filtering.

SUBTRACTION METHODS

Several different types of subtraction techniques have been used for cardiac studies. In mask mode subtraction, the digitized data from peak opacified frames are subtracted from multiple averaged frames of the same area recorded before the arrival of the contrast medium (Fig. 2). Theoretically, overlying nonvascular structures that do not contain contrast material at the instant when the cardiac structure is maximally opacified are erased from the image. Mask mode subtraction considerably improves the visibility of faintly opacified vascular structures.

Another form of subtraction is time interval difference subtraction (TID). In TID, the sets of frames subtracted from each other all contain contrast medium but are separated slightly in time. Conseqently, the resultant substracted image (TID image) is a display of the difference in contrast levels between the two sets of frames. Thus, the TID image indicates instantaneous changes in contrast levels throughout the ventricle during the cardiac cycle.

An important type of subtraction used to evaluate left ventricular contraction is functional subtraction.[7] We have accomplished functional subtraction by taking the mask mode image at end diastole and end systole and subtracting one from the other (Fig. 3). The end-diastolic and end-systolic images can be selected by reference to a computer-generated transmission vs. time curve. An ejection shell image was

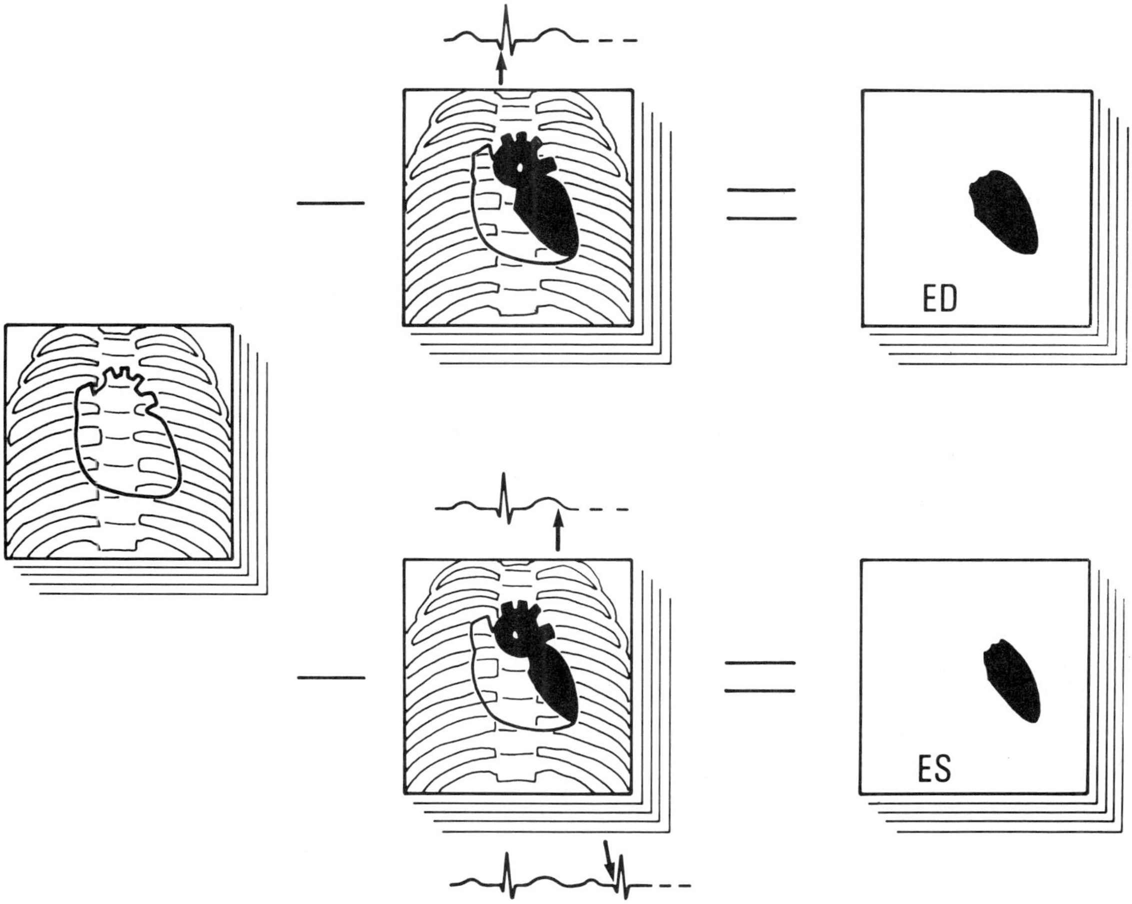

Figure 2. Diagram depicting the technique of mask mode subtraction in reference to the ECG. This procedure provides mask mode images at end diastole and end systole.

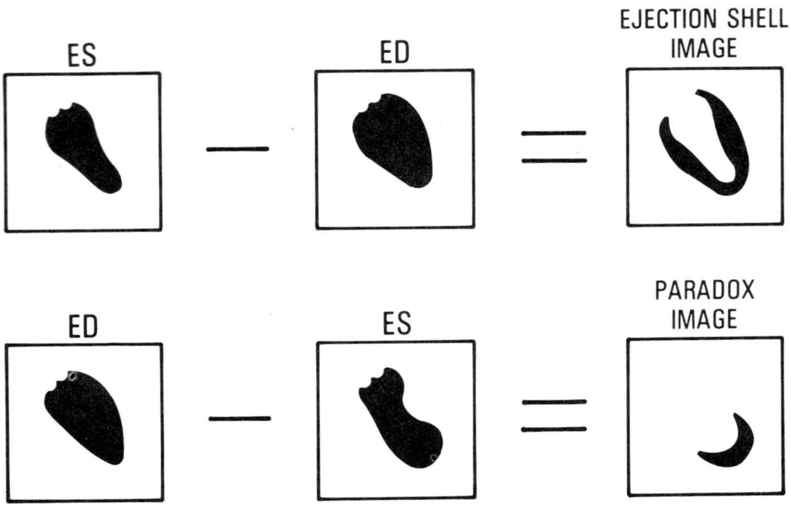

Figure 3. Conceptual diagram of the technique of functional subtraction. In this process, mask mode end-diastolic (ED) and end-diastolic (ES) images are subtracted from each other.

created by subtracting the end-systolic from the end-diastolic image and a functional paradox image created by subtracting the end-diastolic from the end-systolic image (Fig. 3).

SYSTEM SPECIFICATIONS FOR CARDIAC IMAGING

The capabilities of the image processing computer necessary for evaluating cardiac function are different from those considered optimal for evaluating vascular morphology by digital subtraction studies. Compared with peripheral vessels, the left ventricle is a large structure, so that spatial resolution is less critical. Spatial resolution is determined to a major extent by the pixel size or matrix density. On the other hand, temporal resolution (frame rate) needs to be considerably greater for evaluation of cardiac function compared with that necessary for depicting vascular morphology. At normal heart rate, the frequency response needed to evaluate left ventricular wall motion must exceed 10 to 15 cycles (frames) per second. At higher heart rates, such as engendered by exercise, the framing rate must increase accordingly. Consequently, we have used a temporal resolution of 30 frames per second and have been less concerned with spatial resolution.

Lower framing rates are usually adequate for merely evaluating the anatomy of the heart and great vessels. Depiction of thoracic aortic abnormalities has been accomplished with a framing rate of one per second, but a framing rate of two to four per second is preferable in children. Considering the high heart rates and rapid circulation times encountered in infants, the rate of four per second may be essential. The framing rate necessary for the diagnosis of intracardiac anomalies should be equal to or greater than four frames per second and preferably eight or more frames per second.

LEFT VENTRICULAR DIMENSIONS

In an experimental animal model in which left ventricular major and minor axis dimensions, left ventricular wall thickness, and myocardial segment length were continuously measured with multiple pairs of sonic dimension crystals, left ventricular volumetric and functional data derived from DSA could be verified by these independent measurements.[7, 22, 23] Volumes were calculated from mask mode DSA images by using standard single-plane techniques. From the filtered, contrast-enhanced left ventricle image, an approximate end-diastolic region of interest was defined by the operator and an x-ray transmission vs. time curve for the digitized heart beats was generated by the computer. The end-diastolic image was defined as the image with minimum x-ray transmision (maximum left ventricular volume). Left ventricular volumes determined from DSA images correlated closely with those obtained from sonocardiometry ($r = 0.91$) (Fig. 4).

Since the pair of sonomicrometer crystals measure the long axis and only one short axis of the left ventricle, it must be considered that the correlation between this measurement and volumes derived from DSA images might be

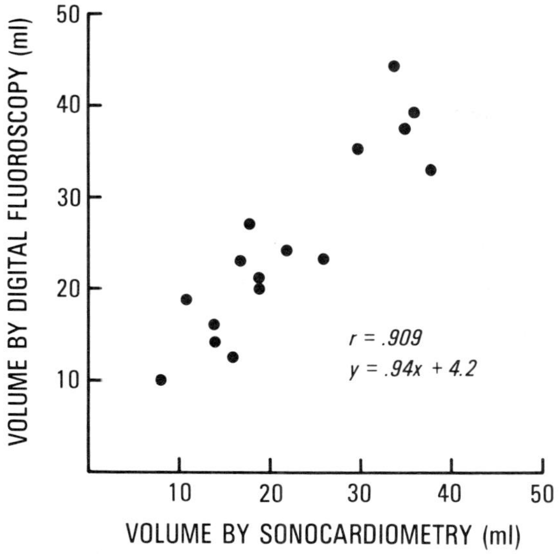

Figure 4. End-systolic and end-diastolic volumes measured from digital intravenous fluoroscopic images are plotted against volumes calculated from sonocardiometer measurements.

decreased in the presence of regional abnormalities in contraction.

Measurement of thickening of the free wall of the left ventricle during the cardiac cycle from DSA images closely approximated sonocardiometric measurements (r = 0.98).[23] Cardiac output calculated from DSA images (ejection fraction × heart rate) correlated with and closely approximated cardiac output determined by simultaneously recorded thermodilution measurements (Fig. 5).[1]

Mask mode images in patients were used to measure end-diastolic, end-systolic, and stroke volumes and ejection fraction (Figs. 6 and 7). In patients, left ventriclar volumes and ejection fraction calculated from the mask mode DSA images closely approximated those measured on direct left ventriculograms (Fig. 7). When end-diastolic and end-systolic volumes measured from mask mode DSA images were plotted against those determined from direct left ventriculograms, the correlation coefficient was 0.96.[18] There was no significant difference in volumes and ejection fractions calculated by the two methods. Similar correlatons between DSA and direct left ventriculography have been shown by other groups[21, 26] using geometric measurements. In addition, a videodensitometric method for calculating ejection fraction from DSA images has shown an adequate correlaton with ejection fractions measured from direct left ventriculography.[24]

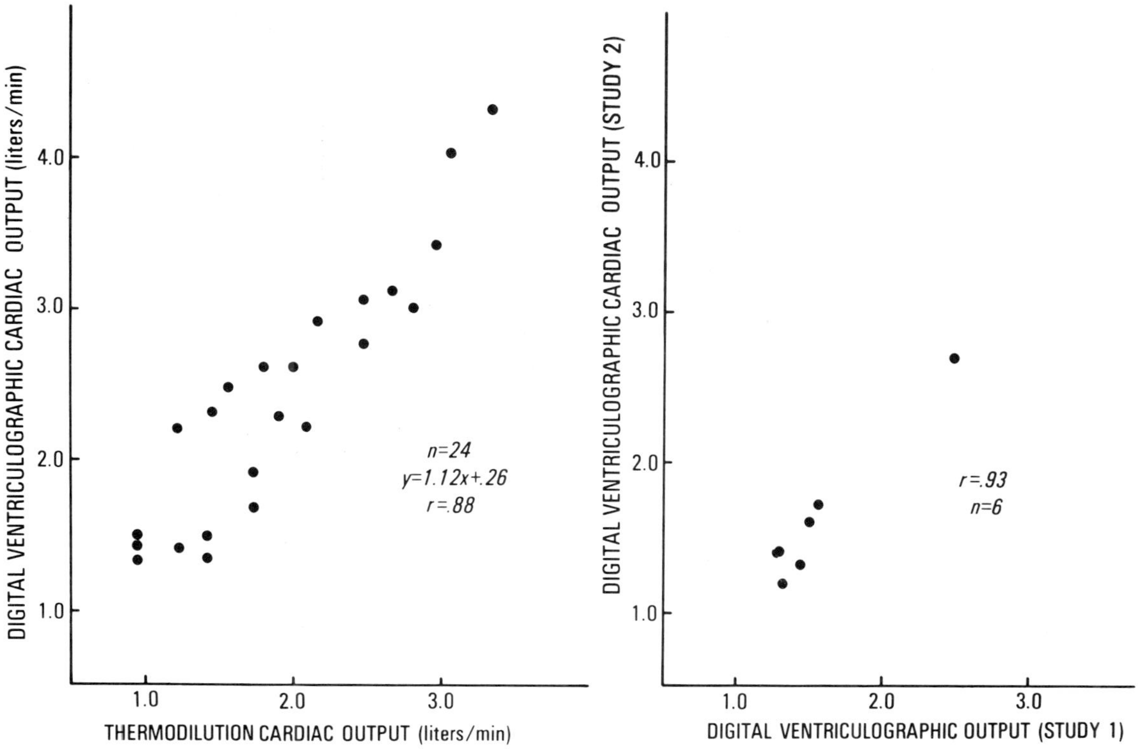

Figure 5. Cardiac output determined by digital intravenous ventriculography is plotted against thermodilution cardiac output (left). The reproducibility of the digital estimate of cardiac output is shown in the right panel (where the first and second measurements are plotted against each other).

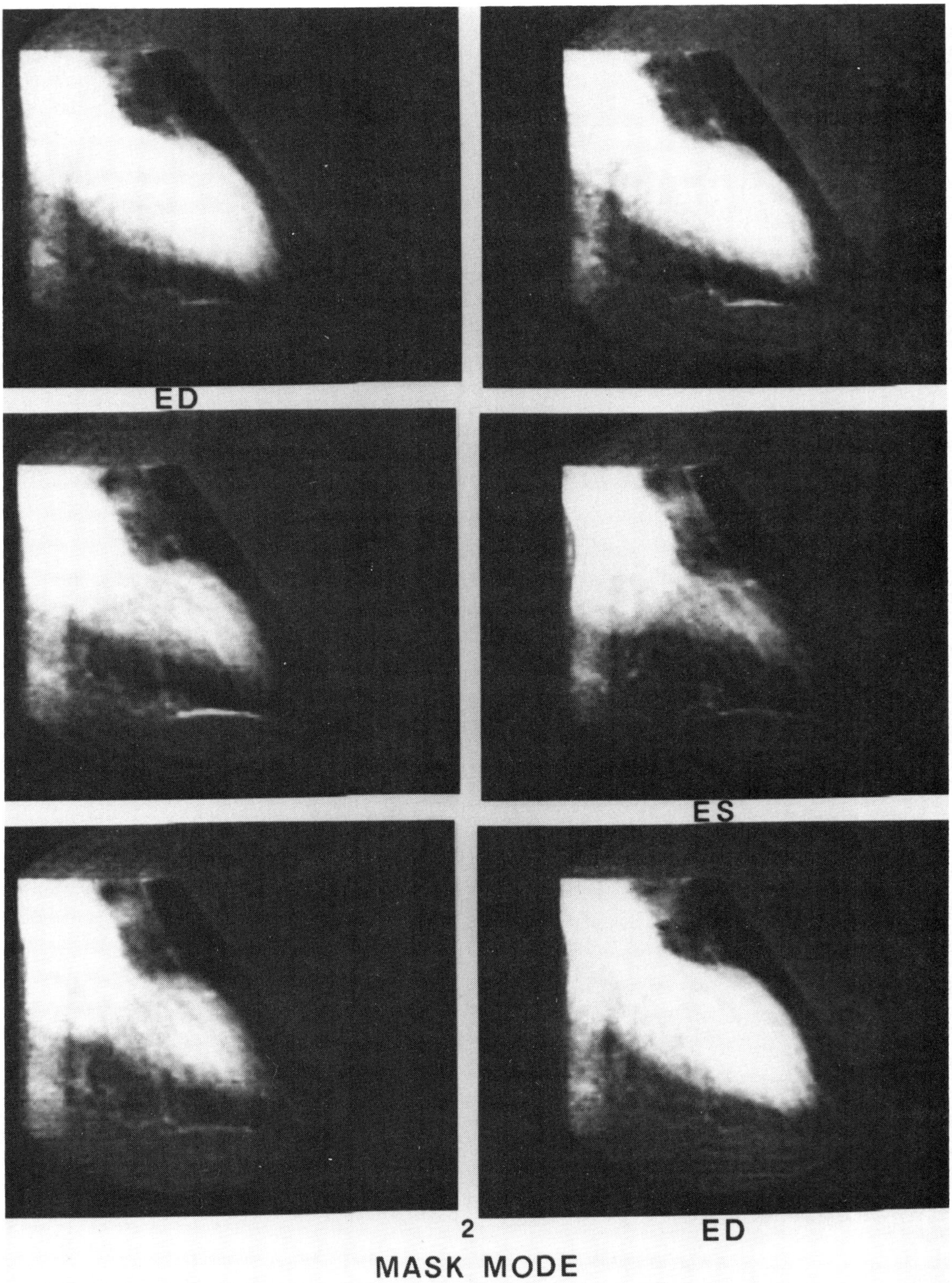

Figure 6. A series of mask mode images obtained from a patient with occlusion of the left anterior descending artery. The study was obtained after central intravenous injection of 40 ml of Renografin 76. These mask mode images in the right anterior oblique projection reveal hypokinesis of the anterolateral wall.

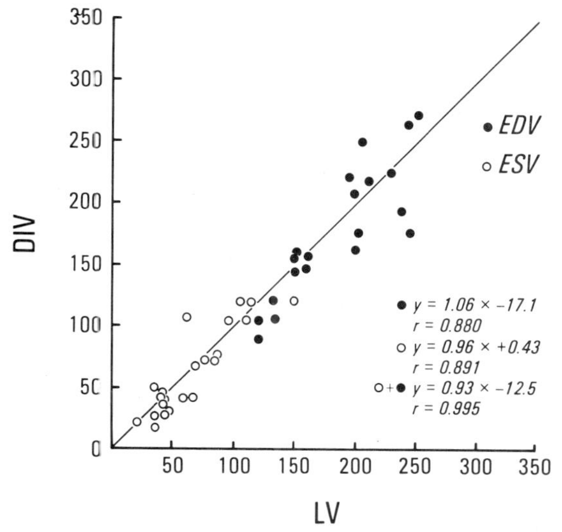

Figure 7. Left ventricular volumes in patients as determined by digital intravenous fluoroscopy (DIV) are plotted against the volumes determined by direct left ventriculography (LV).

LEFT VENTRICULAR FUNCTIONS

An advantage of DSA for assessing cardiac physiology is that the video data is converted into a digital form. This conversion facilitates quantitative analysis of the images and through-computer processing and production of parametric images.[9] Analysis of segmental function from DSA images using the radial shortening method has correlated well with similar analysis using direct line left ventriculography.[13] Additionally, we have created three different types of functional or parametric images:

1. Ejection shell images and paradox images are functional images that provide a display of left ventricular segmental contraction (Fig. 8).
2. Amplitude images display the amplitude of contraction of each pixel from a region of interest surrounding the left ventricle. This is derived from the first harmonic of the Fourier analysis of the volume curve for each pixel.
3. Phase analysis image displays the time of contraction of each pixel (from the region of interest around the left ventricule) relative to the QRS complex.[19] This parametric image provides a measure of the synchrony of the left ventricular contraction and demonstrates regions of tardokinesis.

An ejection shell image is created by subtracting the end-diastolic from the end-systolic image, and a functional paradox image is created by subtracting the end-systolic from the end-diastolic image (Fig. 8). In the functional images, all negative pixels (algebraic sign opposite that arbitrarily set as positive) are set to zero. Because all negative pixels in the functional images are set to zero, an image for motion of a left ventricular segment is observed on the ejection shell only when that segment is larger on the end-diastolic image compared with the end-systolic image. Likewise, if a segment is larger on the end-systolic image compared with the end-diastolic image, then an image of this difference is contained on the paradox image. A stroke volume image is derived as the difference between maximum and minimum density of each pixel within the area of interest at any time during the cardiac cycle. Thus, this stroke volume image would result if all segments contracted with complete synchrony.

CONGENITAL CARDIOVASCUALR ANOMALIES

Digital subtraction angiography was found early to provide excellent demonstration of coarctation of the aorta (Fig. 9) and other thoracic aortic abnormalities.[3, 4, 14, 16] For this purpose, DSA has been considered comparable to direct aortography.[3, 16] The technique has been useful for the exclusion of a vascular anomaly as the cause of a mediastinal mass.[3, 16] Vascular rings such as double aortic arch and right aortic arch have been diagnosed with DSA.[3] Patency of surgically created systemic to pulmonary shunt is well demonstrated by DSA, but because of the overlapping of opacified structure, the anastomosis of the shunt may not be visible (Fig. 10). It has also been comparable to aortography for the evaluation of surgical repairs of coarctation of the aorta. A postoperative DSA study in a patient with a hypoplastic descending aorta is shown in Figure 11. The graft from the left subclavian artery to the descending aorta is demonstrated along with the hypoplastic aorta.

The DSA technique after the intravenous injection of contrast medium has also detected obstructive lesions of both the right and left heart, a variety of intra- and extracardiac shunts,[27] and transposition of the great vessels.[2] Early and late frames from a DSA study after intravenous injection of contrast medium in a child with tricuspid atresia are shown in Figure 12. The early frame demonstrates densely opacified right and left atria and early opacification of the left ventricle. These relationships are vividly displayed because of the nearly complete erasure of noncontrast-containing mediastinal structures, bones, diaphragm, and liver. The later frame shows complete opacification of the left-sided chambers, thoracic aorta, and its branches but almost no opacification of pulmonary vessels. This image depicts the disparity between systemic and pulmonary blood flows.

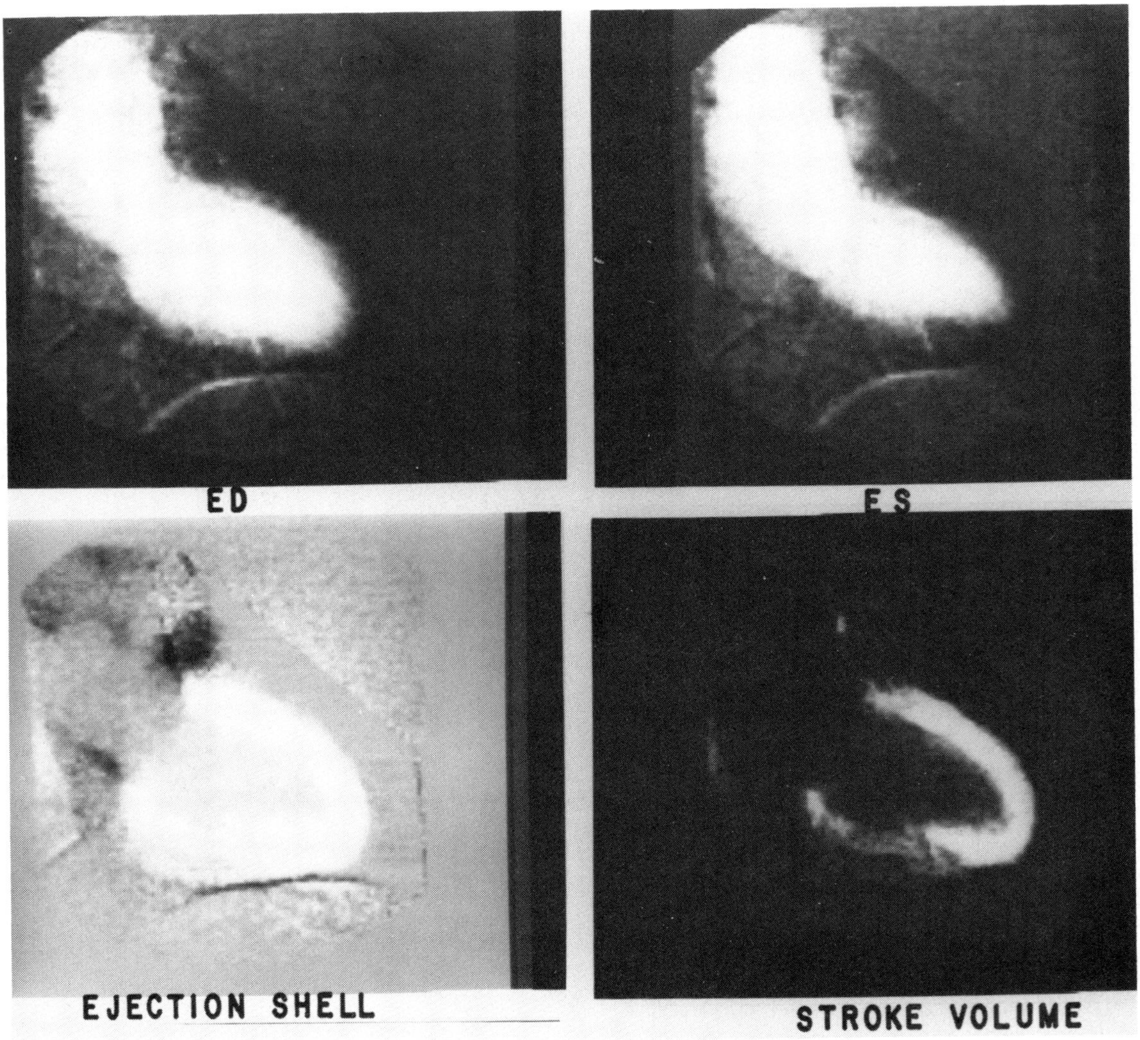

Figure 8. Functional subtraction and mask mode images at end diastole and end systole in the right anterior oblique projection in a patient with occlusion of the right coronary artery. Stroke volume and ejection shell images show hypokinesis of the diaphragmatic segment compared with normal contraction of the apical and anterolateral segments.

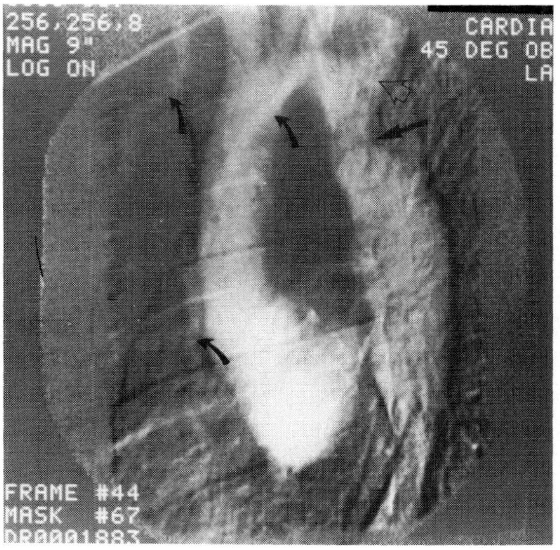

Figure 9. Mild coarctation (arrow) of the aorta demonstrated on DSA study after intravenous injection of contrast medium. Dilated left subclavian artery (open arrow) and internal mammary arteries (curved arrows) are also shown.

Dense opacification of the right-sided cardiac chambers and pulmonary vessels is shown in a child with rhabdomyoma of the right ventricle (Fig. 13). The subtraction technique has removed the nonopacified mediastinal structures and bony strctures. The infundibular stenosis due to the tumor is clearly demonstrated. The obstruction of the right ventricular outflow tract is demonstrated as well on the DSA study as that usually achieved with selective right ventriculography.

DETECTION AND QUANTIFICATION OF SHUNTS

After intravenous injection of contrast medium, early opacification of left-sided cardiac chamber has permitted the diagnosis of right-to-left shunts (see Fig. 12). On the other hand, reopacification of right-sided chambers during the levo phase indicates an intracardiac left-to-right shunt. Reopacification of the right atrium during the levo phase of an intravenous DSA study is demonstrated in Figure 14. Again, visualization of contrast medium in the right-sided cardiac chamber is facilitated by the subtraction of extraneous densities such as mediastinal soft tissues and skeletal structures. A left anterior oblique view of the levo phase of intravenous DSA is shown in Figure 15. There is shunting of contrast medium into the right ventricle across an outflow type of ventricular septal defect.

Left-to-right shunts have been quantified on DSA studies by placing a videodensitometric cursor on the pulmonary artery and plotting x-ray density vs. time curves.[27] A gamma variate fit of the curve is used to separate the activity caused by the first pulmonary transit from that of early recirculation due to the shunt. The technique for calculation $\dot{Q}p/\dot{Q}s$ from the DSA

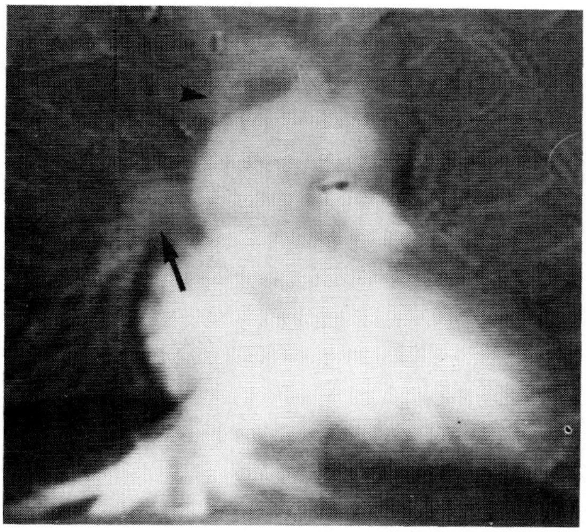

Figure 10. Patent Blalock-Taussig shunt is demonstrated on DSA study (arrowhead). The distal anastomosis is not visualized because of overlapping opacified vascular structures. Contrast medium has opacified the pulmonary arteries (arrow).

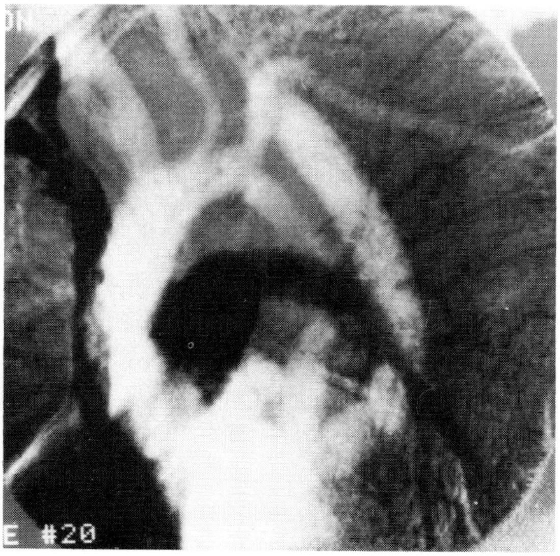

Figure 11. DSA study shows graft between left subclavian artery and descending aorta in a patient with a hypoplastic descending aorta.

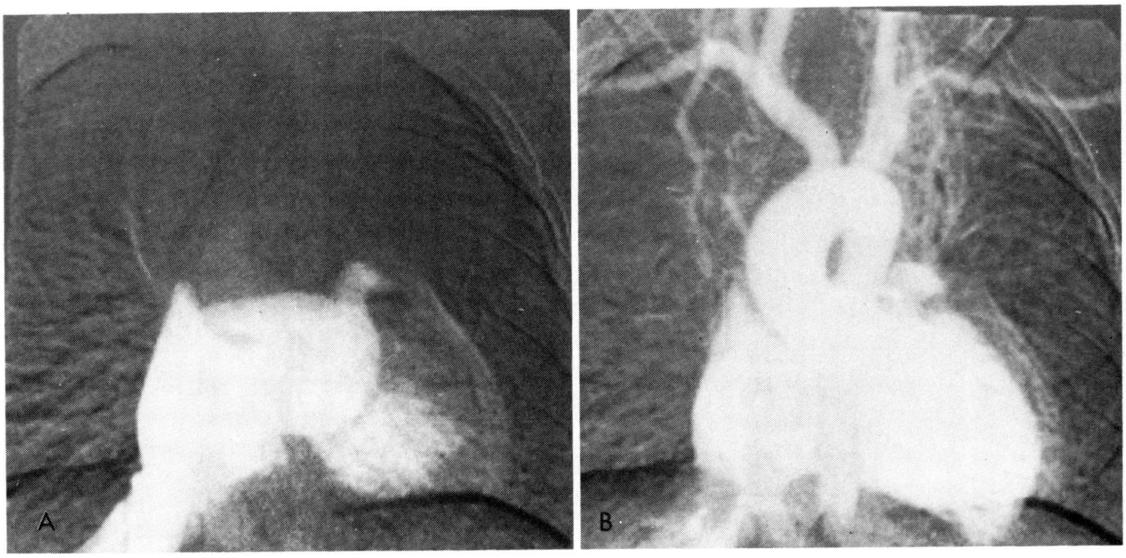

Figure 12. *A*, Early and, *B*, late frames of a DSA study after intravenous injection of contrast medium in a patient with tricuspid atresia. Note, on the early frame, the direct shunting of contrast medium from the right to the left atrium and the contrast void in the area of the right ventricle.

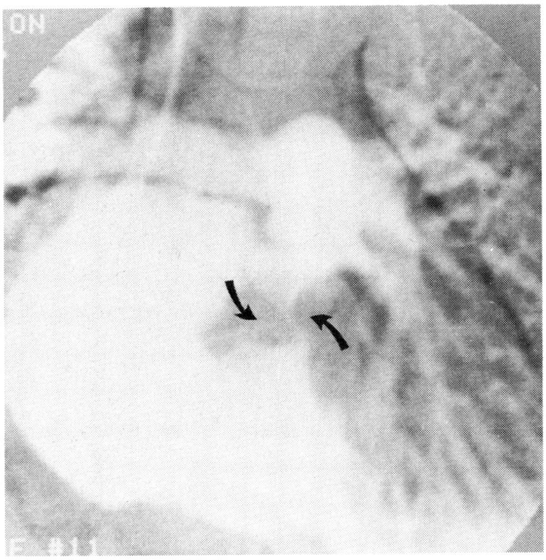

Figure 13. DSA study in a patient with rhabdomyoma of the right ventricle causing obstruction of the right ventricular outflow tract (curved arrows).

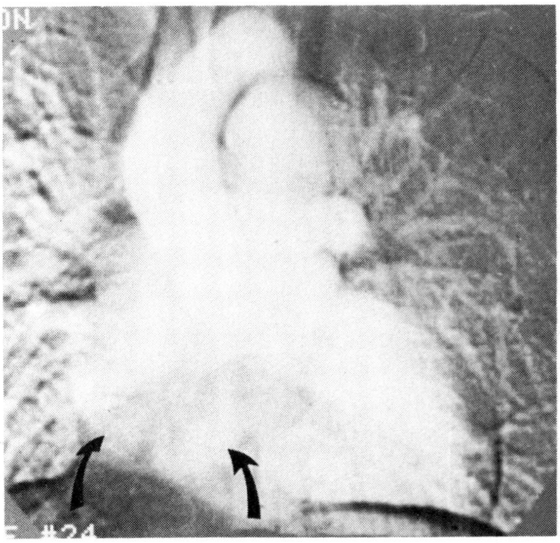

Figure 14. Levo phase of DSA study after intravenous injection of contrast medium shows reopacification of the right atrium (curved arrows) in a patient with an atrial septal defect.

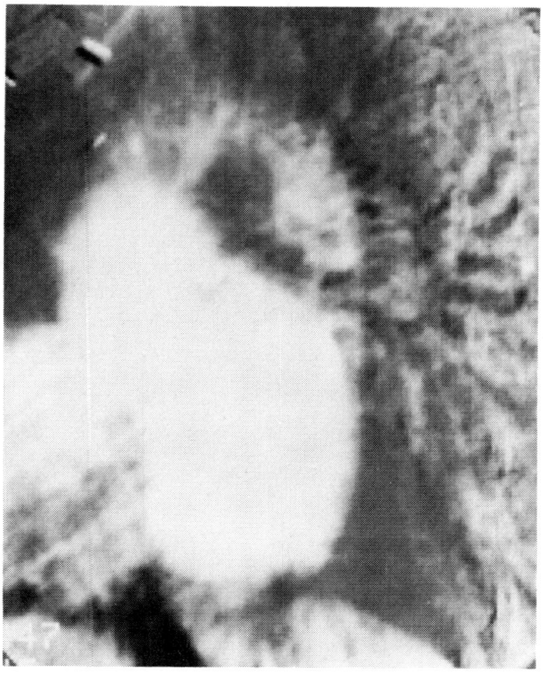

Figure 15. Levo phase of DSA study in a patient with an outflow type of ventricular septal defect.

study is similar to that applied to radionuclide studies.[25] Comparison of Q̇p/Q̇s determined at cardiac catheterization has indicated a good correlaton between the measurements (r = 0.91) (Fig. 16). Calculation of Q̇p/Q̇s from DSA studies after surgical repair of the shunts revealed a Q̇p/Q̇s value of less than 1.2 in ten patients evaluated postoperatively.[27] Calculation of the Q̇p/Q̇s from DSA studies was also compared with similar estimates obtained from the radionuclide angiogram. The correlation between the DSA and the radionuclide estimate of Q̇p/Q̇s was also very good (r = 0.89) (Fig. 17).

LIMITATION OF DSA AND COMPARISON TO OTHER CARDIAC IMAGING MODALITIES

Some potential limitatons and inaccuracies are inherent in the quantitative analysis of segmented left ventricular functions with DSA. With digital subtraction techniques, subject movement and respiratory motion degrade the subtraction image and introduce inaccuracies into the quantitation of segment motion. An additional inaccuracy inherent in analysis of left ventricular wall motion is the complx cardiac motion during systole involving translation and rotary motion of the left ventricular segments, but errors from this factor are considered to be negligible.[10]

Although several methods of reorientation of the major axis of the left ventricle from systole to diastole have been employed for wall motion analysis of cineventriculograms, this reorientation may be ambiguous in the presence of regional abnormalities of wall motion, since phase variations in the amplitude of motion of left ventricular segments occur in ischemia.[12] These variations cannot be completely resolved even by reorientation of the left ventricular major axis. This limitation applies to a radio-

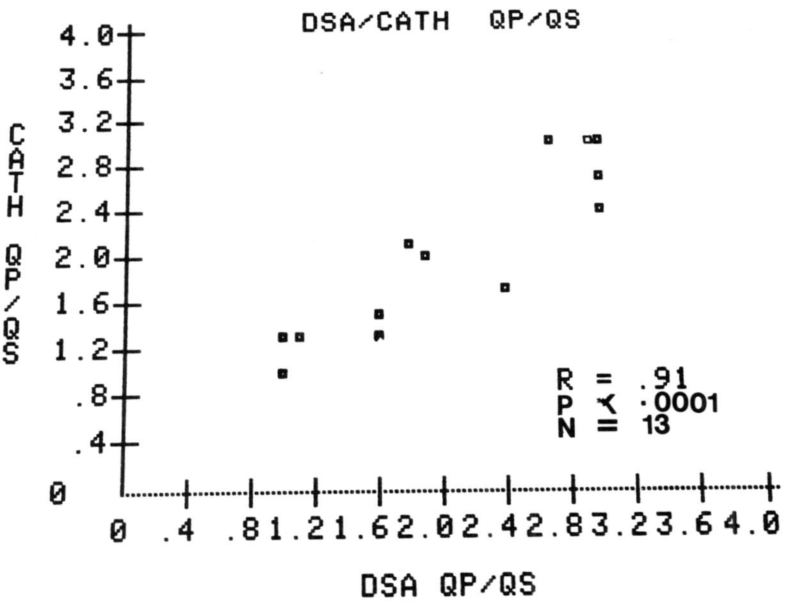

Figure 16. The Q̇p/Q̇s calculated from oximetry data obtained at cardiac catheterization is plotted against the Q̇p/Q̇s estimated by videodensitometric time curves obtained from the DSA study in 13 patients.

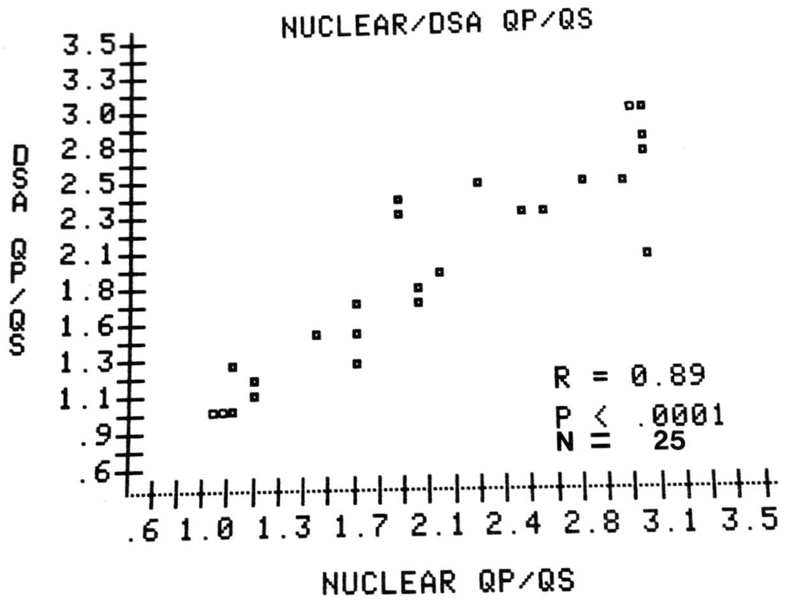

Figure 17. The $\dot{Q}p/\dot{Q}s$ calculated from the DSA study is plotted against the Qp/Qs determined from radionuclide angiogram.

graphic method using geometric (area-length) measurements but can be averted by using videodensitometric measurements if proper corrections are made for the nonhomogeneity of the image system. The stroke volume images derived from DSA images, as shown in this article, are not subject to the possible inaccuracies of measuring amplitude of regional wall motion at any instance as a result of phase variations. The stroke volume image is derived as the difference image between the maximum and minimum density value for each pixel within the area of interest at any time during the cardiac cycle.

An additional consideration is that the intravenous administration of ionic contrast medium causes hemodynamic alterations including changes in left ventricular loading factors and myocardial contractility.[8] This factor may be minimized by a new nonionic contrast medium, which induces smaller hemodynamic changes and does not depress myocardial contractility.[6]

It is natural to compare a new imaging modality with other accepted modalities. Direct contrast left ventriculography is conventionally accepted as the "gold standard" by which other techniques are compared. Although the degree of ventricular opacification is not as dense using central venous contrast injection, our preliminary experience and that of others[11, 14, 20] have shown that satisfactory definition of edge is obtained. Arrhythmias induced by catheter recoil during direct ventriculography are not encountered with DSA, and opacification of the left ventricle is more uniform with DSA than compared with that for direct ventriculography. These latter two considerations have in our initial experience produced an advantage for DSA in evaluating left ventricular function.

Many of the data manipulation techniques that we use with digital intravenous ventriculography are similar to those used with radionuclide ventriculography. If DSA is compared with nuclear techniques, the most obvious advantage is the superior spatial resolution of DSA, allowing visualization of anatomic detail usually not apparent on scintigraphic images. The latter consideraton and the results of the current study suggest that DSA may be a better technique for evaluating segmental left ventricular contractile function since it provides distinct visualization of the endocardial edge of left ventricular segments. Moreover, radionuclide studies are usually acquired over many beats and therefore provide a mean sample of left ventricular dimensions and function. In some situations, the single beat analysis produced by DSA may be advantageous, particularly when evaluating the effects of acute intervention. However, the greater ease of performing rest-exercise radionuclide ventriculographic and myocardial perfusion studies will likely cause these techniques to be retained for the routine evaluation of many patients.

Two-dimensional (2D) sector scan echocardiography is another noninvasive modality that might be compared with DSA. Although 2D echocardography is less invasive than DSA, echograms provide tomographic slices of the heart rather than the global visualization provided by DSA. The tomographic images obtained with echocardiography have inherent advantages for anatomic visualization of values, pericardial fluid, and even wall thickness in those patients in whom technically satisfactory studies may be obtained. Digital fluoroscopy, on the other hand, will probably be more useful for assessing global and regional wall motion, ejection fraction, and ventricular volumes with unambiguous edge definition of the entire ventricle and easily interpretable images.

REFERENCES

1. Carey PH, Slutsky RA, Ashburn WL, et al: The validation of cardiac output by digital intravenous ventriculography in dogs: Correlation with thermodilution estimates. Radiology, *143*:623–626, 1982.
2. Chung KJ, Hesselink JR, Chernoff HL, et al: Digital subtraction angiography in patients with transposition of great arteries after surgical repair. Circulation (Suppl), *66*:II-104, 1982.
3. Crummy AB: Digital subtraction arterography of the thoracic vasculature. *In* Mistretta CA, et al.: (eds): Digital Subtraction Angiography Chicago: Year Book Publishers, 1982.
4. Crummy AB, Strother CM, Sackett JF, et al: Computerized fluoroscopy: Digital subtraction for intravenous angiocardiography and arteriography. AJR, *135*:1131–1140, 1980.
5. Frost MM, Fisher HD, Nudelman S, et al: A digital video acquisition system for extraction of subvisual information in diagnostic medical imaging. IV. Optical instrumentation in medicine. Proc Soc Photo Opt Eng, *127*:208, 1977.
6. Gerber KH, Higgins CB, Yuh YS, et al: Regional myocardial hemodynamic and metabolic effects of ionic and nonionic contrast media in the normal and ischemic state. Circulation, *65*:1307–1314, 1982.
7. Gerber KH, Slutsky RA, Ashburn WL, et al: Detection and assessment of severity of regional ischemic left ventricular dysfunction by digital fluoroscopy. Am. Heart J, *104*:27–35, 1982.
8. Higgins CB, Gerber KH, Mattrey RF, et al: Evaluation of hemodynamic effects of intravenous administration of ionic and nonionic contrast materials. Implications for deriving physiologic measurement from CT and digital cardiovascular imaging. Radiology, *142*:681–686, 1982.
9. Higgins CB, Norris SL, Gerber KH, et al: Quantitation of left ventricular dimensions and function by digital video subtraction angiography. Radiology, *144*:461–469, 1982.
10. Ingels NB, Daughters GT II, Stinson EB, et al: Measurement of mid-wall myocardial dynamic in intact man by radiography of surgically implanted markers. Circulation, *52*:859–867, 1975.
11. Kruger RA, Mistretta CA, Houck TL, et al: Computerized fluoroscopic techniques for intravenous study of cardiac chamber dynamics. Invest Radiol, *14*:279–287, 1979.
12. Leighton RF, Pollack MEM, Welch TG: Abnormal left ventricular wall motion at mid-ejection in patients with coronary heart disease. Circulation, *52*:238–244, 1975.
13. Mancini GBJ, Einsidler E, Norris SL, et al: Quantitative assessment of segmental wall motion abnormalities at rest and after atrial pacing using digital intravenous ventriculography. (Abstr.). Circulation (Suppl), *91*:II–8, 1982.
14. Meaney TF, Weinstein MA, Buonocore E, et al: Digital subtraction angiography of the human cardiovascular system. AJR, *135*:1153–1160, 1980.
15. Mistretta CA: The use of general description of the radiological transmission image for categorizing image enhancement procedures. Opt Eng, *13*:134, 1974.
16. Moodie DS, Yiannikas J, Gill CC, et al: Intravenous digital subtraction angiography in the evaluation of congenital abnormalities of the aorta and aortic arch. Circulation (Suppl), *66*:II–104, 1982.
17. Nelson JA, Miller FJ Jr, Kruger RA, et al: Digital subtraction angiography using a temporal band pass filter: Initial clinical results. Radiology, *145*:309, 1982.
18. Norris SL, Mancini GBJ, Slutsky, RA, et al: Comparison of digital intravenous ventriculography with conventional ventriculography for quantitative left ventricular volume and ejection fraction. Am J Cardiol, *51*:1399–1403, 1983.
19. Norris SL, Widmann TF, Mancini GBJ, et al: Assessment of wall motion by regional phase analysis of digital intravenous ventriculograms. (Abstr.). Circulation (Suppl), *91*:II–190, 1982.
20. Ovitt TW, Christenson PC, Fisher HD, et al: Intravenous angiography using digital video subtraction: X-ray imaging system. AJR, *135*:1141–1144, 1980.
21. Sasayama S, Nonogi H, Kawai C, et al: Automated method for left ventricular volume measurement by cine ventriculography with minimal doses of contrast medium. Am J Cardiol, *48*:746–53, 1981.
22. Slutsky RA, Carey PH, Higgins CB: The effect of acute incremental volume overload on cardiac chamber size, function and the pulmonary circulation: Analysis by digital intravenous ventriculography. Am Heart J, *104*:254, 1982.
23. Slutsky RA, Gerber KH, Higgins CB: Digital intravenous ventriculography: Analysis and validation of wall thickness changes during ischemia and inotropic stimulation of dogs. Am J Cardiol, *50*:874–880, 1983.
24. Tobis J, Nalcioglu O, Seibert JA, et al: Comparison of videodensitometry and area-length methods for computing left ventricular ejection fraction from digital intravenous ventriculograms. (Abstr.). Am J Cardiol, *49*:964, 1982.
25. Treves, S, Parker JA: Detection and quantification of intracardiac shunts. *In* Strauss HW, Pitt B (eds): Cardiovascular Nuclear Medicine. St. Louis, C. V. Mosby Co., 1979, p. 148.
26. Vas R, Diamond GA, Forrester JS, et al: Computer enhancement of direct and venous injected left ventricular contrast angiography. Am Heart J, *102*:719, 1982.
27. Yiannikas J, Moodie DS, Gill CC, et al: Pre- and postoperative assessment of patients with left to right shunts using digital subtraction angiography. Circulation (Suppl), *66*II–104, 1982.

4

DIGITAL ANGIOCARDIOGRAPHY FOR ASSESSMENT OF CONGENITAL HEART DISEASE

JOACHIM H. BÜRSCH, M.D.

Computerized image processing has been applied increasingly in recent years to various diagnostic aspects of cardiovascular radiology. Its widespread use since 1980 can be attributed to the invention of digital intravenous arteriography, which affords simple venous cannulation rather than arterial catheterization procedures, for the evaluation of arterial disease.[18, 19] The great number of adult patients potentially taking advantage of intravenous examinations and the reliability of digital subtraction techniques indicates clearly the usefulness and efficacy of this new diagnostic approach. Likewise, imaging of the heart has been performed for the assessment of left ventricular function.[9, 10, 20] Therefore, subtraction angiography is now regarded as an alternative modality to conventional angiocardiography with the specific advantage of being a less invasive procedure.

Moreover, when the technique is applied to pediatric patients, improved safety can be expected with digital subtraction angiography not only for intravenous contrast studies but also for conventional angiography using central circulatory injections.[5, 13, 14] It is also possible to decrease the amount of contrast medium injected and the radiation dosage. This feature is particularly important for studies of critically ill children with complex cardiac malformations who need to undergo repeated angiographic examinations. Furthermore, image enhancement permits visualization of circulatory structures that are usually only faintly opacified, such as the capillary perfusion phase of organs (lung).

Finally, by application of indicator dilution principles, digital processing provides data on the flow of the contrast bolus throughout the vasculature on a quantitative basis.[2, 15, 17] This approach appears specifically promising for blood flow studies in children with vascular malformations and shunting at the arterial level.

It is the purpose of this chapter to survey recent developments in digital angiocardiography and to outline the potential value of this technique for the diagnosis of congenital heart disease.

ACQUISITION OF IMAGES

Computerized processing of angiograms is based on the scanning of video images in a raster fashion. The number of lines greatly defines the spatial resolution of the imaging system. Accordingly, the same number of picture elements is used to resolve the spatial information along each video line. Our experience is that an image matrix with 256 × 256 picture elements is adequate for most of the problems under study in pediatric cardiology, since these studies require visualization of relative large vascular structures, i.e., the heart and great vessels. Quantitation of grey-scale intensities with a resolution of 256 discrete values (per picture element) is adequate for these studies.

There are basically two modalities for the acquisition of images: real-time digital processing and off-line processing from video tape or video disk. Digital imaging has some restrictions if real-time processing is used. Owing to limitations of digital computers in handling data flow rates in real time, a maximum rate of four images per second can be acquired with most of the conventionally available systems. Therefore, direct computer processing has the disadvantage of a low image acquisition rate. If no more than two digitized images have to be processed at a time, this can be readily handled by digital equipment without using computers. However, the latter system permits only simple arithmetic operations, such as continuous mask image subtraction.

On the contrary, off-line processing of angiograms provides the greatest versatility with respect to the rate and sequence of image selection as well as to the algorithms that can be applied for data processing.[3] For these reasons most of our pediatric examinations have been performed by video tape processing, and this approach will possibly continue unless immediate digital storage of several hundred images becomes feasible. Very recently a special purpose processor has been designed that differs from the current systems in that real-time access to a large digital memory is available and a dedicated hardware and software configuration provides real-time processing with a rate of about 50 images per second.[6]

Processing of tape recordings is achieved by operating the video tape in a shuttle mode, thereby providing digitization in a stroboscopic manner.[4] Electrocardiogram (ECG)-gated images or even the whole image series (e.g., 50 images/sec) can be digitized. Identification of images and automatic selection are provided by numerical coding of the images during the time course of tape recording. In addition, digitally readable parameters such as ECG and pressure data are used for further analysis. Postprocessing enables selection of video images of comparable cardiac phases (end-diastolic and end-systolic phases) and respiratory phases (position of diaphragm). The latter may even be performed automatically by calculating the cross-correlation of grey levels from selected parts of the image (measure of similarity).[5] If quantitative studies are considered on the basis of roentgen density measurements, adequate filtering of the incident radiation beam with 0.2 mm copper is necessary, as well as fixed settings of the x-ray tube voltage and current.

PROCESSING OF IMAGES

Two different principles have been applied to digital processing of pediatric angiograms. The first aims at image enhancement for optimal visualization of the cardiovascular structures. The second utilizes functional parameter extraction for studies of circulatory dynamics (Fig. 1). Image enhancement is based on the elimination of nonopacified background structures (mask mode subtraction). An ECG-gated mask image is selected from the preinjection period and subtracted from corresponding images during opacification. Optimal angiographic contrast is achieved by individual rescaling of grey levels, possibly using statistical methods and spatial filtering of images. In addition, it is our experience that the angiographic contrast can be significantly enhanced by integration of several images from both the preinjection and the contrast phases (Fig. 1, left panel). Integration and averaging of regional image values contribute to an optimal image quality by noise reduction. As an alternative to mask mode subtraction, the difference in images between a set of frames following one another within short time intervals (time interval difference) during the opacification phase has also been tested for studies of the cardiac chambers and the great arteries.

Functional parameter extraction from angiograms is based on the quantitative analysis of temporal changes in roentgen densities of each picture element (pixel). In order to establish

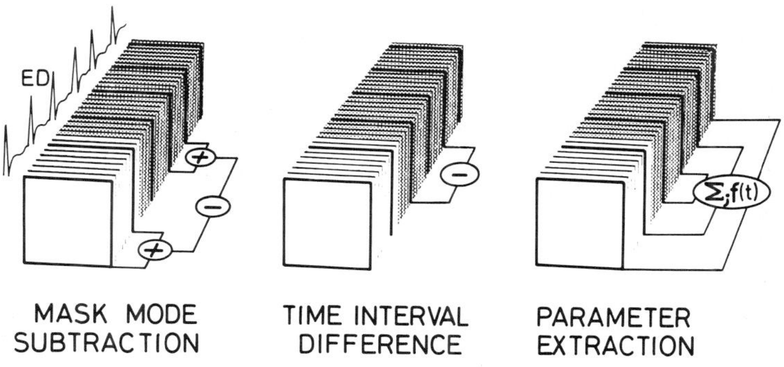

Figure 1. Illustration of the three processing modes that have been applied to digital imaging in pediatric cardiology. The temporal sequence of images is indicated by the ECG (upper left), and the time course of contrast opacification is symbolized by grey shading images. The selection of end-diastolic images and mathematical operations is indicated. Mask subtraction and the time interval difference are two modalities of subtraction angiography. Parameter extraction is utilized for functional imaging studies.

radiopaque dilution curves, the continuous sequence of images throughout the angiogram has to be digitized. For studies of blood flow at the central arteries, which are of primary interest to the pediatric cardiologist, data analysis is mostly restricted to images of identical cardiac phases in order to account for phasic motion and variations in thickness of these vessels. Parameters of regional time, and vascular volume were utilized to calculate regional blood flow and flow distribution data.

SUBTRACTION ANGIOGRAPHY

Improved safety is considered an important advantage of digital subtraction techniques for angiographic examinations. The ability to enhance significantly the contrast qualities of opacified structures has promoted the use of digital techniques for intravenous angiography. We have delivered the contrast medium by peripheral venous injections rather than by using catheters for high-volume flow injections into central veins. Radiation exposure is low in studies employing fluoroscopic radiation levels (80 kV, 2 mA, continuous radiation).

Besides peripheral venous studies, contrast enhancement has proved useful in conventional selective angiographic examinations. Angiograms may be recorded synchronously with the cinefilm (50 or 100 images/sec) using high-energy radiation pulses (80 kV, 250 mA, 2 msec). Subtraction angiography has improved angiographic diagnostic qualities in cases with low-contrast opacification or overlap of cardiovascular structures or both. Thereby, extended catheterization maneuvers applying multiple selective injections can be avoided for the most part.

Peripheral Venous Injections

When contrast medium is injected into a peripheral vein, such as the antecubital or jugular vein, satisfactory opacification of the right side of the heart is usually obtained in accordance with the relatively high concentration and bolus integrity during the early phase of circulatory contrast flow.[12] The injected bolus of contrast material into a peripheral vein is flushed with a comparable volume of saline or dextrose. This approach has been successful in newborns for studying the arterial-ventricular relationship, especially as a screening procedure in suspected transposition of the great arteries (Fig. 2). In general, cardiac malformations with right-to-left shunting can be adequately studied by this technique. Usually 3 ml of Urografin-76% are injected in infants and flushed with 3 ml of saline. In children up to the age of four years, about 0.75 ml/kg body weight is "hand-injected." Continuous fluoroscopic recording over about a 15-sec period (5 sec before and 10 sec after the onset of contrast injection) was utilized to select corresponding ECG-gated images from the preinjection period and from the opacification phase. Optimal matching of the image background structures can be achieved by selecting images from the end-expiratory phases, as determined by the position of the diaphragm. Suspended respiration is not required in children but in general has been attempted in those older than five years of age.

The excellent quality with which the right cardiac chambers can be visualized by intravenous angiocardiography has permitted right ventricular dimension and volume measurements. Contrast enhancement in these studies is preferably based on the subtraction of images from two different phases of cardiac opacification. Instead of mask mode subtraction, the difference between maximal right atrial and right ventricular contrasts is calculated, thereby yielding different grey intensities in the two cavities (Fig. 3). The separation of the atrial from the ventricular chamber facilitates ventricular contour detection. Ventricular volume determination from biplane roentgen projection images may be performed.

Visualization of the left side of the heart is another perspective of digital subtraction angiography. Delivery of "tight" bolus of contrast material is a prerequisite for minimizing the dilution of contrast medium after pulmonary vascular perfusion. Delivery of volumes of more than 20 ml within 3 sec is usually not feasible by hand injection. The use of a power syringe is therefore essential in children over the age of four years. Figure 4 depicts schematically an injection device used for flushing of the contrast medium. In order to promote safety using the peripheral vein approach (Abbocath—T20 × 1¼), a test injection of saline is usually performed before angiography with the actual flow rate (less than 10 ml/sec) in order to ensure adequate positioning of the small venous catheter. During injection the device must be manually kept in position to prevent any displacement from recoil. Visualization of the left chambers of the heart and the aorta can be readily achieved with contrast volumes of 0.75 ml/kg body weight. An example from a post-

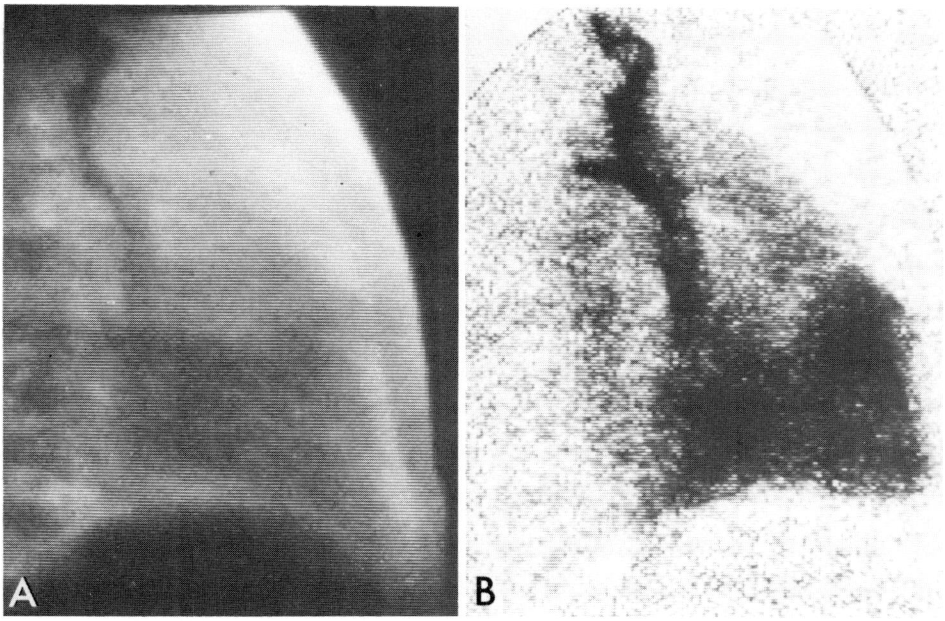

Figure 2. TV monitor picture for comparison of the angiographic contrast before and after digital processing. The nonprocessed image *(A)* is taken from the time period of maximal contrast accumulation in the right side of the heart. Substantially improved anatomic information is obtained after mask subtraction *(B)* is performed to document the origin of the aorta from the right ventricle in a newborn with transposed great arteries. Three ml of Urografin-76% had been injected into the jugular vein. This early example of clinical application was presented by Heintzen et al. at the 3rd International Symposium on Coronary Heart Disease in Frankfurt, February, 1978.

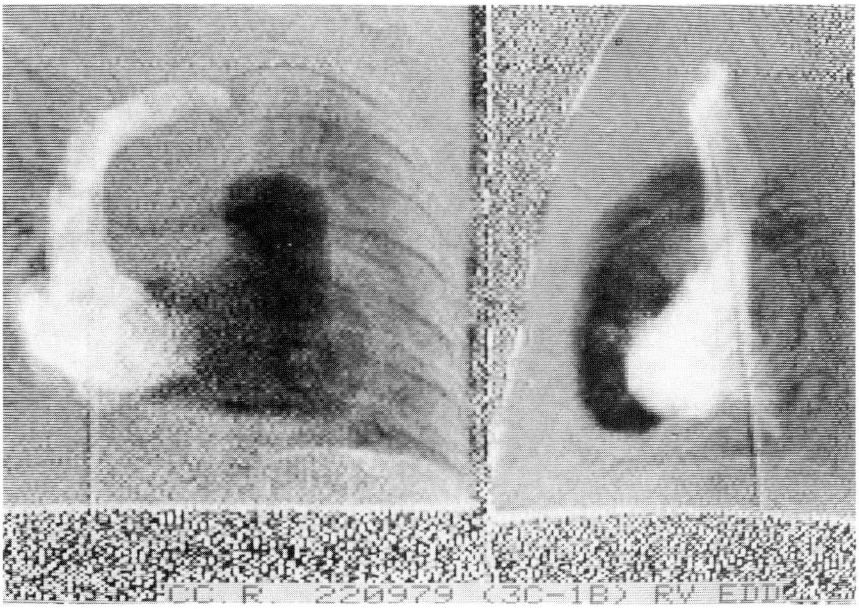

Figure 3. TV monitor picture in the biplane roentgen projection mode of the right side of the heart in a child after intravenous injection of contrast medium. End-diastolic images were selected for processing (time interval: two cardiac cycles). The different grey intensities of the right atrium and the right ventricle help to separate these two cardiac chambers from each other for outlining contours and subsequent right ventricular volume determination.

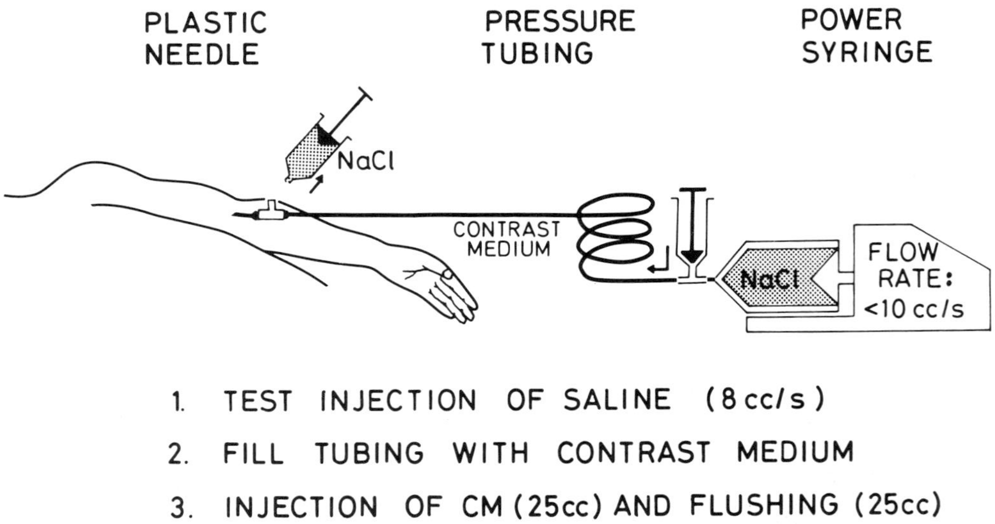

Figure 4. Schematic drawing of the procedure for peripheral vein injections of contrast medium. Volume and flow data are representative for a patient of about 30 kg of body weight.

operative study is illustrated in Figure 5. The effectiveness of image enhancement based on subtraction angiography is apparent by comparison with nonprocessed images at the time of maximal opacification of the cardiac chambers. The enhancement factor is estimated to be in the range of 2 to 4. Time interval difference subtraction has also been used by subtracting the end-systolic from end-diastolic images. Because contrast differences between these two cardiac phases are small compared with mask mode subtraction, visualization especially of the end-systolic contour has not been found to be reliable. This approach is probably not particularly useful in studies of congenital heart disease.

Contrast in the right side of the heart was usually completely cleared before maximal opacification of the left ventricle occurred. The normal separation of right- and left-sided opacification has served as the basis for the detection of left-to-right shunting in septal defects and aorticopulmonary anastomoses. A systematic experimental study has been used to demonstrate the feasibility of intravenous angiography in such lesions.[1, 7] With the hepatoclavicular view, ventricular septal defects and patent ductus arteriosus have been directly visualized, whereas atrial septal defects were indicated by shunting from the left to the right atrium (Fig. 6). Peripheral venous angiography has been used clinically for postoperative follow-up as well as outpatient examinations.

Central Circulatory Injections

If digital equipments meets the requirements for video tape processing, contrast enhancement studies may be applied as an additional option to the cineangiograms. There are two major clinical indications for contrast enhancement techniques. First, these techniques may be used when opacification of vascular structures is inadequate owing to unfavorable contrast flow conditions. Second, they may be employed when combined with small volume injections in order to minimize the total amount of contrast medium used in a study, e.g., in critically sick children.

Our experience gained from a large number of cases has indicated some specific fields of interest for additional digital imaging in conventional angiocardiography:

1. The group of children who have undergone catheterization of the right side of the heart only can have a more adequate angiographic visualization of the left chambers of the heart than is usually obtained with the standard levophase angiograms. Unexpected lesions as well as left ventricular function can be analyzed, thereby providing a complete angiographic examination.

2. There is another group of patients with congenital heart disease and concomitant reduced blood flow. Low-contrast opacification due to subnormal blood flow through small and stenotic vessels can be overcome by contrast enhancement. Typically of interest are newborns with aortic arch anomalies (coarctation), in whom selective aortography may be difficult to perform.

3. In patients with pulmonary atresia and other lesions restricting pulmonary blood flow, contrast enhancement may help to elucidate aorticopulmonary collaterals as well as the mor-

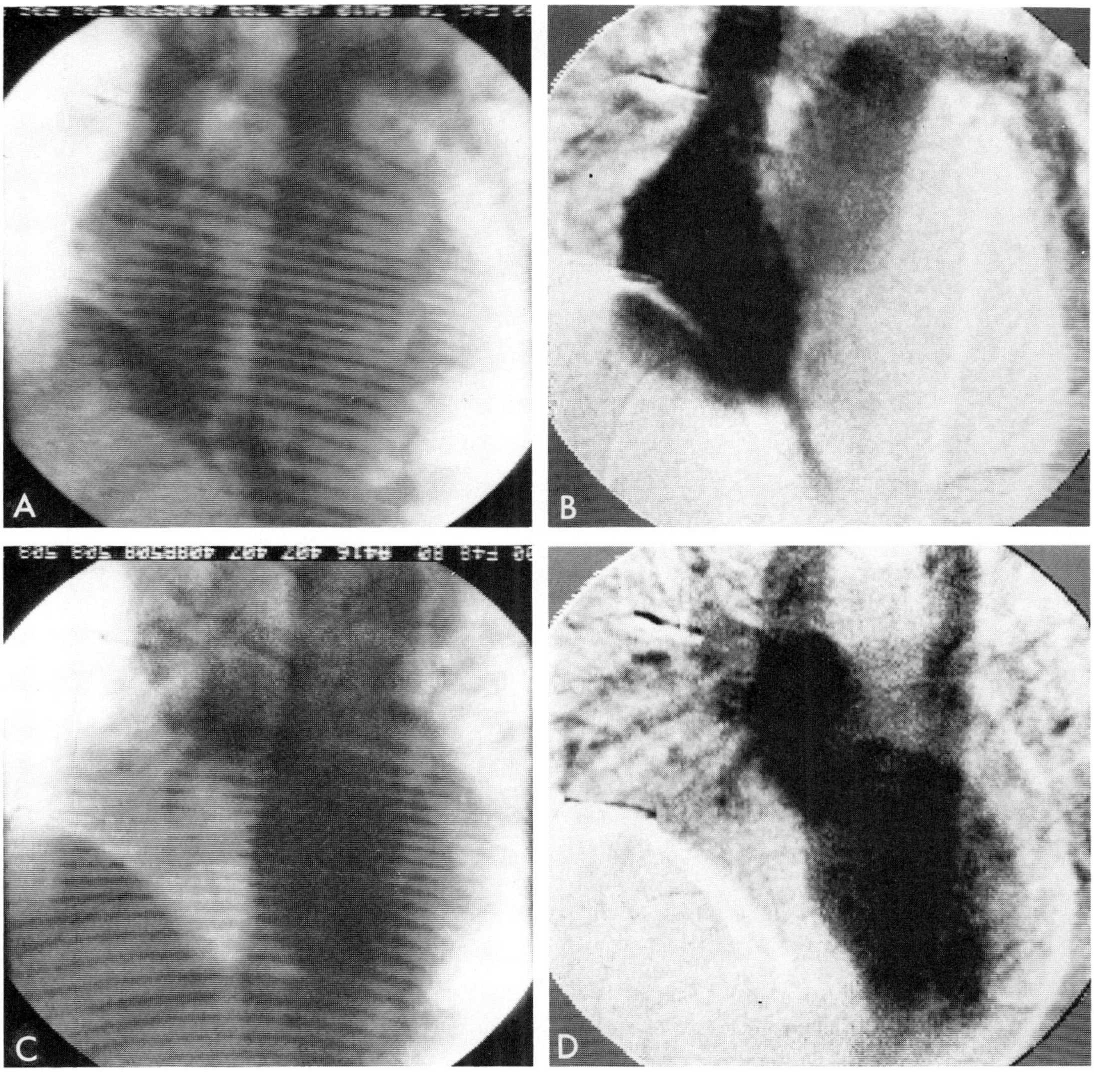

Figure 5. Comparison of angiograms (hepatoclavicular view) by peripheral vein injections before *(A)* and after *(C)* mask mode subtraction. The dextrogram *(B)* shows slight pulmonary enlargement. The levogram *(D)* appears normal. Case after surgical closure of a ventricular septal defect.

phology of central pulmonary arteries. An example of a sequence of processed images is illustrated in Figure 7, which shows contrast flow to the left lung via a small vessel and a hypoplastic central pulmonary artery.

4. Anomalous pulmonary venous drainage constitutes a wide range of abnormal connections. Conventional pulmonary artery injection often fails to demonstrate clearly the morphology of the pulmonary veins, particularly if narrowing of the vascular lumen is under question. The pulmonary veins may be partly obscured by residual contrast in the pulmonary arteries. Digital contrast enhancement can considerably improve angiographic quality during the late pulmonary vein perfusion phase (Fig. 8).

5. Finally, selective contrast injections, using low concentrations and small volumes, may be applied to study ventricular dynamics without significant alterations in cardiac function. The advantage and usefulness of this approach are currently being tested for ventricular volume determinations and may be of relevance for repeated sequential studies of the functional status of the heart and circulation.

FUNCTIONAL ANGIOGRAPHY

The extraction of functional parameters from an image sequence provides quantitative information on the cardiac and blood flow dynamics.[11] Computerized processing has been used to study objectively the degree and temporal

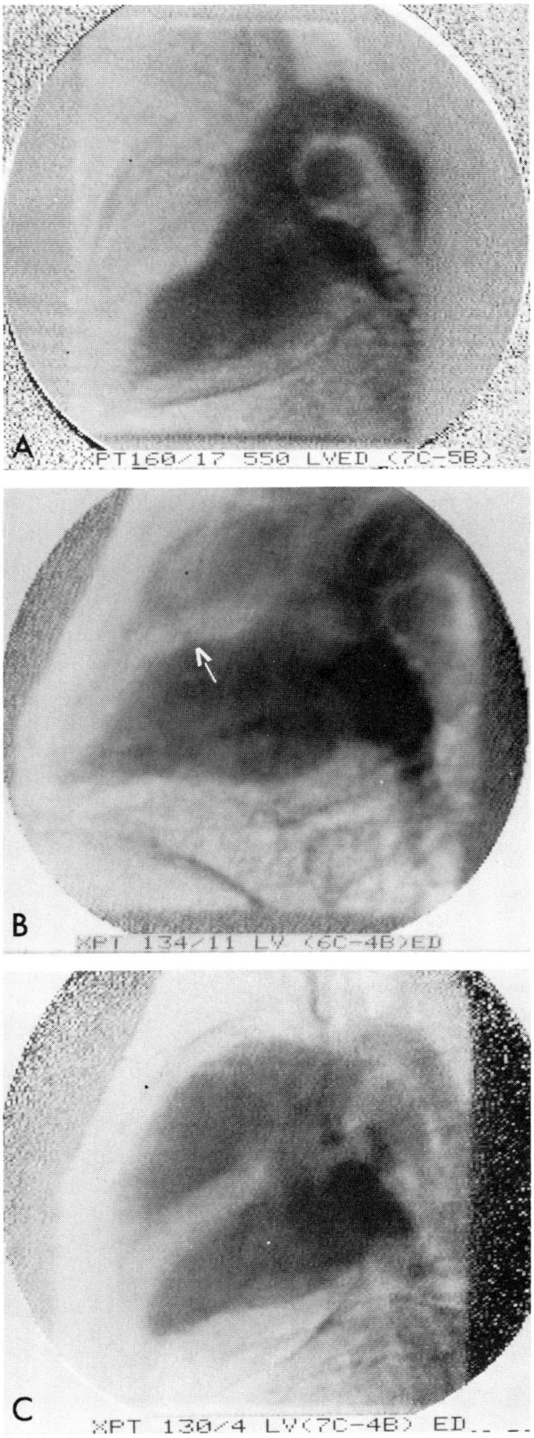

Figure 6. Contrast-enhanced angiocardiograms in experimental left-to-right shunting in pigs. Mask subtraction using end-diastolic images was applied in all cases. *A*, Aorticopulmonary anastomosis. *B*, Small ventricular septal defect (arrow). *C*, Large atrial septal defect.

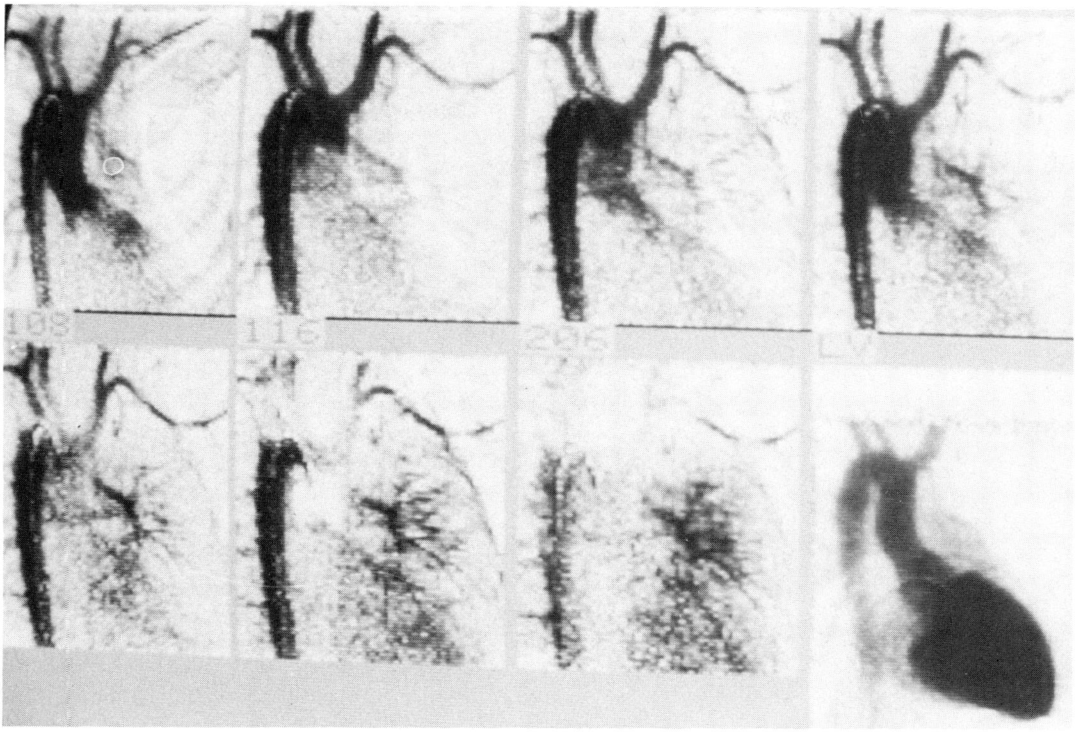

Figure 7. Serial images (from left to right) after digital processing by mask subtraction after aortic root injection. Perfusion of a small central pulmonary vessel, as well as of the pulmonary parenchyma, is recognized. The lower right image shows a separate left ventricular injection for comparison.

sequence of the roentgen absorption by contrast material flowing through the circulation. Flow parameters are extracted from the angiographic image series by utilizing indicator dilution principles.[8] Each picture element (pixel) constitutes a minute sampling area for the detection of temporal changes in image brightness by analyzing consecutively the total image sequence. On the basis of the exponential attenuation of roentgen absorption in relation to the amount of x-ray transmission (Lambert-Beer's law), the regional brightness values are logarithmically converted. As a result, mass-time curves of the contrast medium bolus are obtained (densograms). According to the 256 × 256 image matrix, up to 65,000 densograms can be obtained from one angiogram.

Each pixel densogram is used to calculate a time parameter. By a method similar to analytic procedures in indicator dilution studies, a representative time value may be derived from the forward triangle of each curve (indicator front) or from the entire curve (mean circulation time). If this time information is pictorially displayed on the video monitor by different grey intensities or colors, the progressive passage of the contrast bolus through the vasculature can be viewed. As depicted in Figure 9,

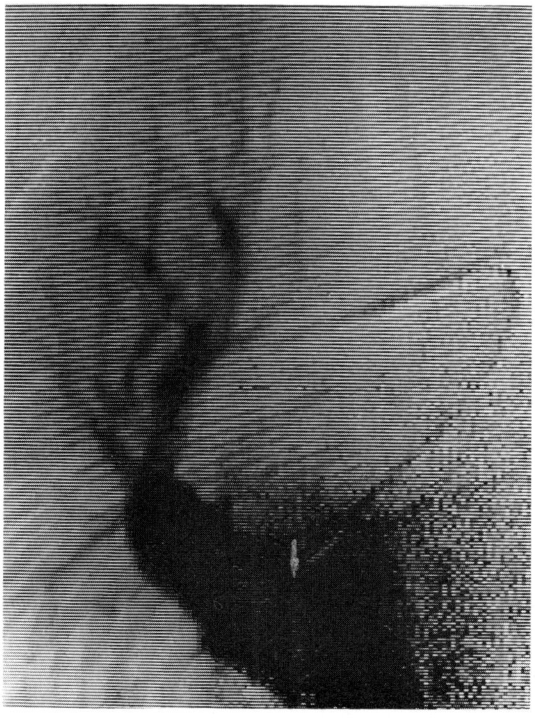

Figure 8. Mask mode subtraction image of the right pulmonary veins in a patient with abnormal pulmonary venous drainage to the right atrium. Contrast material had been injected into the right pulmonary artery.

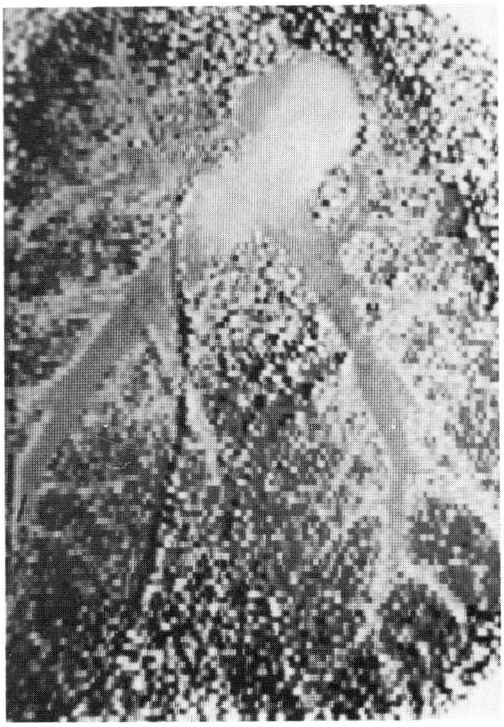

Figure 9. Time parameter image of the pulmonary vasculature in a pig. Increasing grey intensities are indicative of the temporal delay of contrast flow from the pulmonary trunk (light) to the peripheral arteries and the tissue (dark).

the increase in grey intensities illustrates the propagation of contrast medium from the central to the peripheral circulatory segments of the pulmonary circulation. Even though these time parameters are obtained from a three-dimensional object and are displayed in a two-dimensional projection image, they provide new quantitative information on blood flow dynamics.

Time parameters have been utilized to study organ perfusion semiquantitatively.[16] With respect to problems in pediatric cardiology, it may be useful for comparative studies of blood flow in the left and the right lung as well as for interventional studies. e.g., examination of vasodilator effects. Time parameter extraction is also the basis for flow distribution measurements in the great arteries.[8] If time values are grouped in accordance with the elapsed time after contrast injection, identical time increments can be calculated. The assignment of time data to specific vascular regions provides an indication of vascular segments that have been perfused within identical time intervals. These time-dependent vascular segments are pictorially displayed and provide regional (segmental) volume flow calculations in all vessel segments. Volume flow data are determined from the indicator mass absorption within each segment. This determination is achieved by calculating the area under each pixel densogram. Because the curve areas are linearly related to vascular thickness (volume element), a relative measure of the segmental vascular volume is obtained by summing up all area data from each segment. Both the volume and the time parameters may be used to calculate relative volume flow in each vascular segment.

Functional imaging is illustrated for flow distribution studies at the aorta (Fig. 10). The density information and the time parameters are depicted in a child with a Blalock-Taussig anastomosis. Contrast medium in these studies is usually injected into the left ventricle. ECG-gated imaging accounts for cardiac phase-dependent motion and diameter variations of the aortic arch. From more than 20 end-diastolic images, the time-density information is analyzed at each picture element and time and volume parameters are calculated. Because a rather low temporal resolution of data sampling (ECG-gated) is utilized in these studies, the segmentation was based on rather large time increments relative to the interval of one cardiac cycle. Accordingly, the vascular segments confine the propagation of blood within one cardiac cycle in each of the vessels (Fig. 11). The ratio of segmental volumes to time intervals reveals regional flow data as a percentage of the maximum flow rate. The example illustrates a 14 per cent aorticopulmonary flow through the anastomosis as related to the total left ventricular output (100 per cent).

The described method for functional parameter extraction based on densitometric analyses affords strict motionlessness of image background structures. Therefore, it has been applied only in patients who were able to cooperate and suspend respiration over an adequate period of time (15 sec).

The assessment of circulatory parameters by digital angiography is practical in relation to the present developmental stage of this new diagnostic imaging technique. It is believed that other new uses will continue to be devised and may possibly lead to an extended quantitative analysis of patient angiograms in the future.

ACKNOWLEDGMENTS

The techniques described were developed and studied in the Department of Pediatric Cardiology and Biomedical Engineering at the University of Kiel, West Germany. The author is indebted to

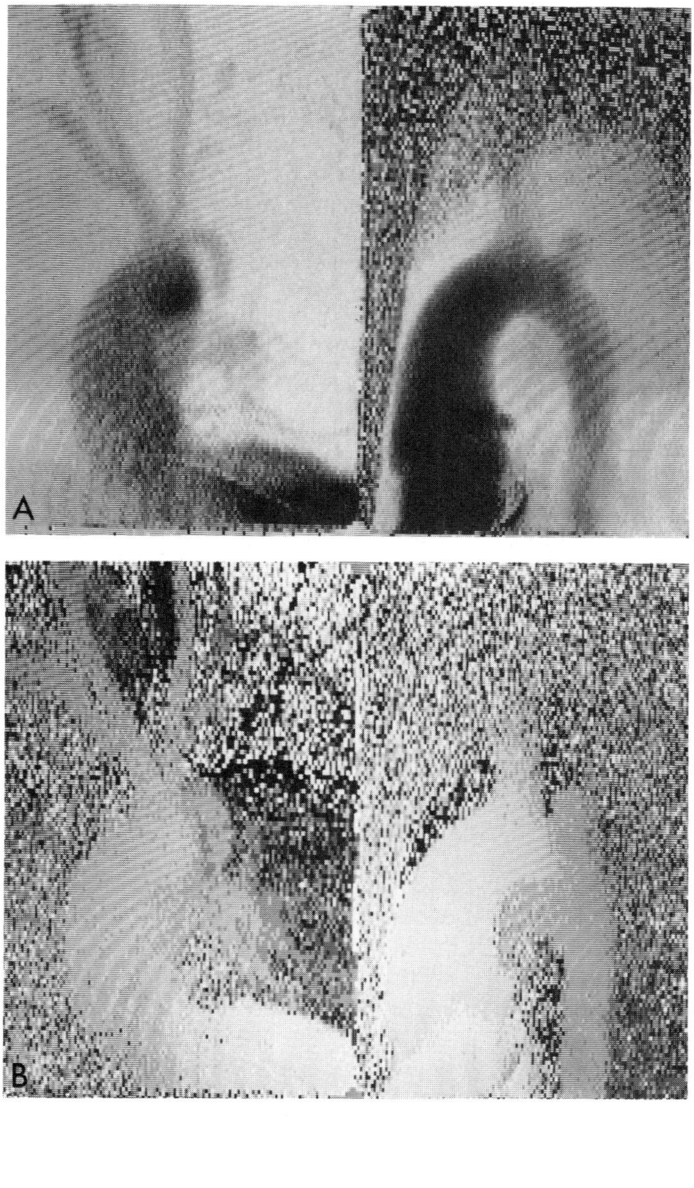

Figure 10. Parameter images of the aorta in a patient with a Blalock-Taussig anastomosis as viewed in the biplane projection mode (anteroposterior [ap] and lateral). Contrast medium had been injected into the left ventricle. *A*, Depth parameter image indicating the regional thickness of vessels by grey intensities. *B*, Time parameter image indicating the temporal sequence of contrast flow by increasing grey intensities.

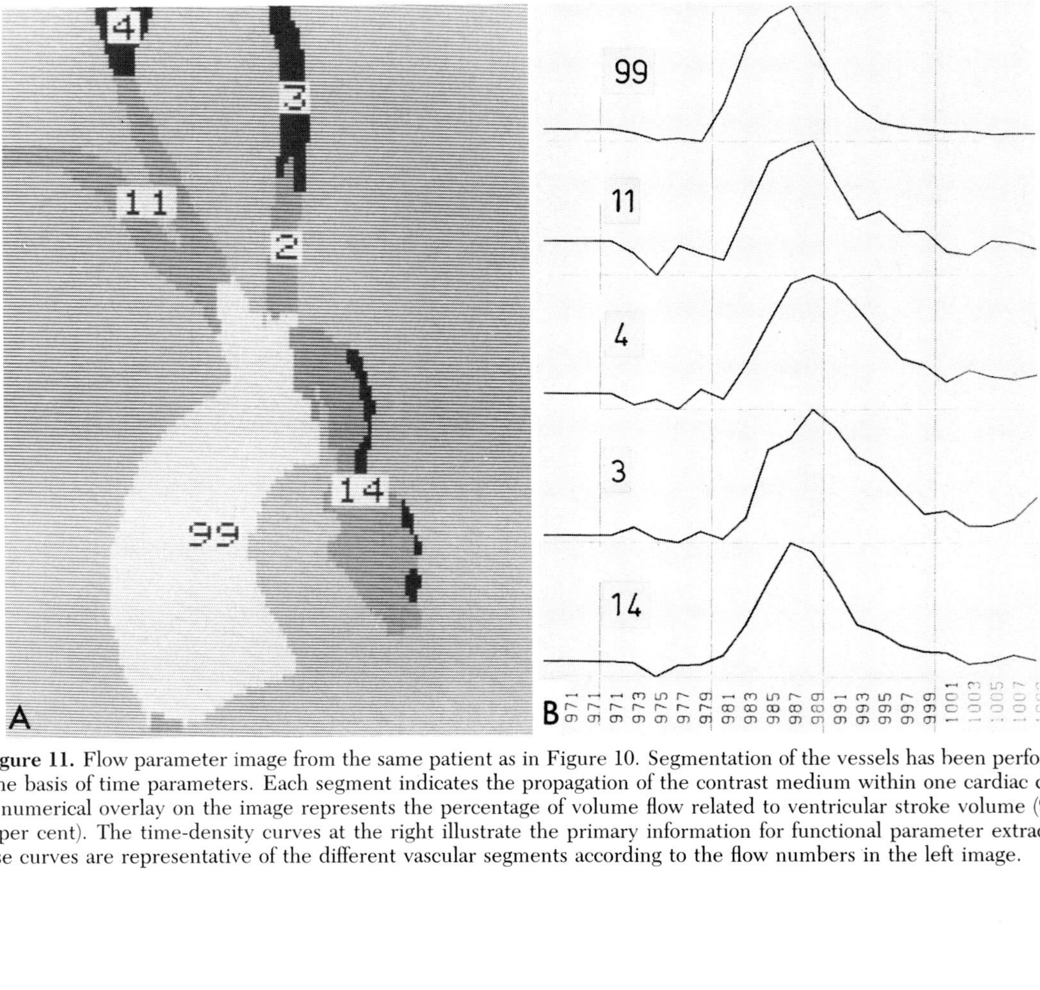

Figure 11. Flow parameter image from the same patient as in Figure 10. Segmentation of the vessels has been performed on the basis of time parameters. Each segment indicates the propagation of the contrast medium within one cardiac cycle. The numerical overlay on the image represents the percentage of volume flow related to ventricular stroke volume (99 = 100 per cent). The time-density curves at the right illustrate the primary information for functional parameter extraction. These curves are representative of the different vascular segments according to the flow numbers in the left image.

Professor Heintzen and his collaborators, especially Drs. Brennecke, Hahne, and Radtke, whose work and thinking have contributed greatly to the contents of this chapter.

REFERENCES

1. Bogren, HG, Bürsch JH, Brennecke R, et al: Intravenous angiocardiography using digital imaging processing: Experience with axial projections in normal pigs and in pigs with experimentally generated left-to-right shunts. SPIE, *314*:287–292, 1981.
2. Böhm M, Höhne KH: The processing and analysis of radiographic image sequences. *In* Höhne KH (ed): Digital Image Processing in Medicine. Berlin, Springer, 1981, pp. 42–92.
3. Brennecke R, Brown TK, Bürsch JH, et al: Digital processing of videoangiographic image series using a minicomputer. Proc. Comp. Cardiol. Long Beach, CA, IEEE Computer Society, 1976, pp. 255–260.
4. Brennecke R, Brown TK, Bürsch JH, et al: A digital system for roentgen video image processing. *In* Heintzen PH, Bürsch JH (eds): Roentgen-Video-Techniques. Stuttgart, G. Thieme, 1978, pp. 150–157.
5. Brennecke R, Bürsch JH, Bogren HG, et al: Digital intravenous imaging techniques in pediatric cardiology. *In* Mistretta CA, Crummy AB, Strother CM, et al (eds): Digital Subtraction Arteriography: An Application of Computerized Fluoroscopy. Chicago, Year Book Medical Publishers, 1982, pp. 133–141.
6. Brennecke R, Hahne HJ, Moldenhauer K, et al: A special purpose processor for digital angiocardiography. Design and applications. Proc Comp Cardiol. Long Beach, CA, IEEE Computer Society, 1979, pp. 343–346.
7. Bürsch JH, Bogren HG, Radtke W, et al: Cardiac imaging by digitized intravenous angiocardiography. Proc Comp Cardiol. Long Beach, CA, IEEE Computer Society, 1982, pp. 321–324.
8. Bürsch JH, Hahne HJ, Brennecke R, et al: Assessment of arterial blood flow measurements by digital angiography. Radiology, *14*:39–47, 1981.
9. Crummy AB: Digital subtraction arteriography of the thoracic vasculature. *In* Mistretta CA, Crummy AB, Strother CM, et al (eds): Digital Subtraction Arteriography: An Application of Computerized Fluoroscopy. Chicago, Year Book Medical Publishers, 1982, pp. 83–86.
10. Engels PHC, Ludwig JW: Digital subtraction arteriography of the left ventricle using time interval difference mode. *In* Mistretta CA, Crummy AB, Strother CM et al (eds): Digital Subtraction Arteriography: An Application of Computerized Fluoroscopy. Chicago, Year Book Medical Publishers, 1982, pp. 123–124.
11. Heintzen PH, Bürsch JH (eds): Roentgen video techniques for dynamic studies of structure and function of the heart and circulation. Stuttgart, G. Thieme, 1978.
12. Heintzen PH, Brennecke R, Bürsch JH: Computerized videoangiocardiography. *In* Kaltenbach M, Lichtlen P (eds): Coronary Heart Disease. Stuttgart, G. Thieme, 1978, pp. 116–121.
13. Heintzen PH, Brennecke R, Bürsch JH: Digital cardiovascular radiology. *In* Höhne KH (ed): Digital Image Processing in Medicine: Lecture Notes in Medical Informatics. Berlin, Springer, 1981, pp. 1–14.
14. Heintzen PH, Brennecke R, Bürsch JH: Improved safety by computerized video-angiocardiography. Ann Radiol, *22*:349–350, 1979.
15. Heintzen PH, Brennecke R, Bürsch JH, et al: Quantitative analysis of structure and function of the cardiovascular system by roentgen-video-computer techniques. Mayo Clin Proc. 57(Suppl):78–91, 1982.
16. Höhne KH, Böhm M, Erbe W, et al: Computer angiography: A new tool for x-ray functional diagnostics. Med Progr Technol, *6*:23, 1978.
17. Höhne KH, Böhm M, Erbe W, et al: Die Messung und differenzierte bildliche Darstellung der Nierendurchblutung mit der Computerangiographie. Fortschr Röntgenstr, *129*:667–672, 1978.
18. Meaney TF, Weinstein MA, Buonocore E, et al: Digital subtraction angiography of the human cardiovascular system. AJR, *135*:1153–1160, 1980.
19. Mistretta CA, Crummy AB, Strother CM, et al: Digital Subtraction Arteriography: An Application of Computerized Fluoroscopy. Chicago, Year Book Medical Publishers, 1982.
20. Vas R, Diamond GA, Forrester JS, et al: Computer enhancement of direct and venous-injected left ventricular contrast angiography. Am Heart J, *102*:719–725, 1981.

5

RADIONUCLIDE EVALUATION OF CIRCULATORY SHUNTS

S. TREVES, M.D., and A. KURUC, B. S.

Major advances in cardiac surgery combined with the advent of short-lived radionuclides and practical gamma scintillation cameras have provided much of the impetus for the development of noninvasive techniques to diagnose intracardiac shunts. With first-pass radionuclide angiography, the heart, great vessels, and lungs are evaluated after intravenous injection of a small bolus of radionuclide solution. During the initial part of the study, most of the radionuclide is concentrated in one or two heart chambers at a time. First-pass radionuclide angiography uses this temporal separation to provide sequential visualization of the cardiovascular structures. In addition, it is possible to obtain computer-generated time versus activity curves for regions of interest over these structures. Analysis of these curves permit the detection, localization, and quantitation of intracardiac shunts and shunts between the great arteries.

PROCEDURE

Radionuclide angiography is a reasonably simple procedure that can be performed on outpatients. There is no patient preparation. Because the study itself can be completed in less than 30 sec, it is usually unnecessary to sedate the patient.

The procedure requires the use of a gamma camera, a digital computer system, and the appropriate radionuclide. The anterior projection is adequate for the detection and quantitation of shunts. Since the calculation of shunt flow presupposes no complicating malformations, such as valvular incompetence or large bronchial collateral circulation, the angiocardiogram is carefully analyzed to evaluate the cardiovascular anatomy. The presence of left-to-right or right-to-left shunting is then determined, and the shunt flow calculated.

Qualitative and quantitative analysis of first-pass radionuclide angiography is greatly simplified if the radionuclide is delivered to the cardiopulmonary system as a compact bolus. The procedure used for this study is designed to achieve this effect. The patient is placed supine, and a vein is entered with a 23 or 21 gauge butterfly needle set. A disposable injector with a one-way valve (Paramedical Disposables, Inc., Watertown, MA) is used for the simultaneous rapid injection of the bolus of radionuclide and a saline flush.

The sites of injection, in order of preference, are an external jugular vein, an antecubital vein via a 12 in intracath, and antecubital veins without catheters. In our clinic, more than 95 per cent of the studies are performed with a butterfly needle in an external jugular vein. For small infants whose venous access is more difficult, an antecubital vein is frequently used. Since the bolus travels only a short distance, and there is low intrathoracic resistance in these infants, a compact bolus is most often produced. Satisfactory results can be obtained even in premature infants.

The patient should be relaxed during the injection; crying or a Valsalva maneuver, which increases the intrathoracic pressure, may cause fragmentation of the bolus and thus prejudice the results. If the child is irritable and uncooperative, a mixture of meperidine hydrochloride, 25 mg/ml; chlorpromazine hydrochloride, 6.25 mg/ml; and promethazine hydrochloride, 6.25 mg/ml, may be administered intramuscularly. The recommended dose is 1.0 ml in children with a body weight over 15 kg with a maximum of 2.0 ml. This mixture should not be used in children less than one year old.

A series of images are recorded on the computer at two to four frames per sec for 25 sec. The images are examined visually to assess the cardiac anatomy and flow patterns. Time-activity curves are then analyzed to quantify shunts. The duration and shape of the injected bolus is assessed from a time-activity curve recorded over the superior vena cava, with care taken to exclude the overlying lung activity. Ideally, the bolus should be 3 sec or less in duration from the initial appearance of activity in the superior vena cava to about 10 to 15 per cent of the peak activity on the downslope. If a poor injection has occurred, a second dose 50 per cent greater than the first can be used in a second attempt. Data recording is begun a few seconds before the second injection, so that the computer can subtract the relatively stable background activity from the previous injection. If the second attempt fails, the study should be rescheduled for another day.

QUANTITATIVE ANALYSIS

Linear Time-Invariant System Models for Vascular Beds. Shunt quantitation by radionucleide angiocardiography may be done by using an analysis of time-activity curves. These curves are analyzed as indicator dilution curves.[12] A useful model in the analysis of indicator-dilution curves is that of a linear, time-invariant system (LTI). In particular, LTI models are useful in describing the transformation of a curve detected upstream into the curve detected further downstream.[2]

Consider the system illustrated in Figure 1. Fluid is flowing through the tube at a constant rate. Radioactivity is recorded by detectors A and B. Detectors A and B are identical and count over the same volume of fluid. It is useful to think of the pattern of fluid flow in the segment of tubing between the detectors as a system that transforms the time-activity curve recorded at detector A into the curve recorded at detector B. The curves, recorded at detectors A and B, are considered to be the input and output of the system. We shall term these curves I(t) and O(t), respectively.

Suppose one activity unit of a radiopharmaceutical is instantaneously injected from the syringe into the tubing at time 0. The time-activity curves obtained from this experiment are shown in Figure 2*A*. A curve of the form of I(t) is termed a "unit impulse." The area under this curve is equal to 1, and activity is present only at time 0. The curve O(t) demonstrates the dispersion of radiopharmaceutical in the segment of tubing between detectors A and B after a unit impulse injection. It is therefore termed the "unit impulse response" (UIR) of the system. We shall denote the UIR as U(t). If the detectors have a uniform counting efficiency, each will record a total number of counts proportional to the total amount of radiopharmaceutical passing beneath the detector. Since no radiopharmaceutical is lost, the total counts recorded by detectors A and B and hence the areas under the curves I(t) and O(t) are equal.

We shall assume that the segment of tubing between A and B can be modeled as an LTI with the curves I(t) and O(t) as the input and output, respectively. Given known input-output pairs, I(t) − O(t) and I′(t) − O′(t) the following facts are true for an LTI:

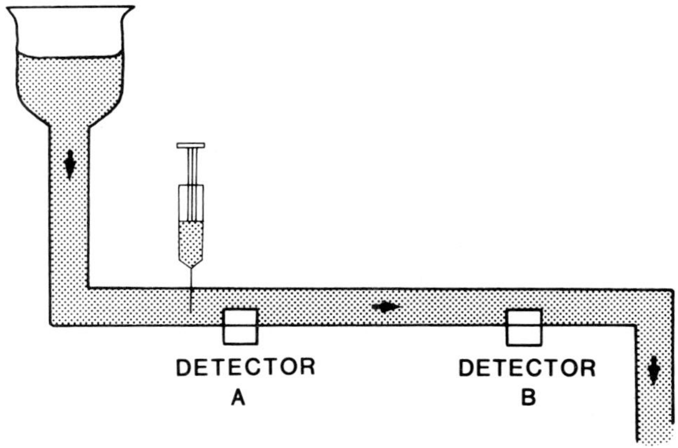

Figure 1. An example of a simple linear time-invariant system.

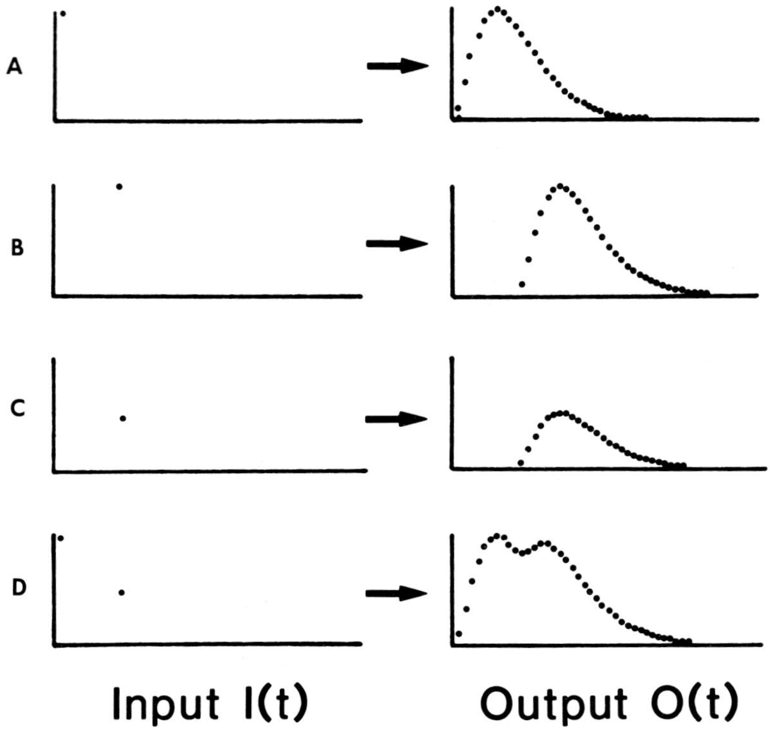

Figure 2. Examples of input-output pairs recorded from the system shown in Figure 1. The input, I(t), and output, O(t), curves are recorded from detectors A and B, respectively. U(t) is the output corresponding to a unit impulse input as shown in *A*.

1. An input equal to a time-shifted replica of I(t) would result in an output equal to an equivalently time-shifted replica of O(t) (Figs. 2*A* and 2*B*).
2. An input equal to a scaled replica of I(t) would result in an output equal to an equivalently scaled replica of O(t) (Figs. 2*B* and 2*C*).
3. An input equal to the sum of I(t) and I′(t) would result in an output equal to the sum of O(t) and O′(t). (Figs. 2*A*, 2*C*, and 2*D*).

It follows that the output due to an arbitrary input can be calculated from the input and a knowledge of the UIR. The output is equal to the sum of the scaled, time-shifted UIR replicas corresponding to each point of the input function. For example, Figure 3*B* shows an input-output pair with a more complex input function. Such an input function might be produced by an injection of radiopharmaceutical from a syringe further upstream than the syringe shown in Figure 1. The process of combining the input and UIR to obtain the output of an LTI is known as convolution. We say that O(t) is equal to the convolution of I(t) with U(t). Given I(t) and U(t), O(t) may be calculated explicitly from the formula:

$$O(t) = \sum_{j=0}^{t} I(t - j)\, U(j) \quad (t = 0, N)$$

where the sampling interval is, for convenience, taken as 1. More concisely, we have O(t) =

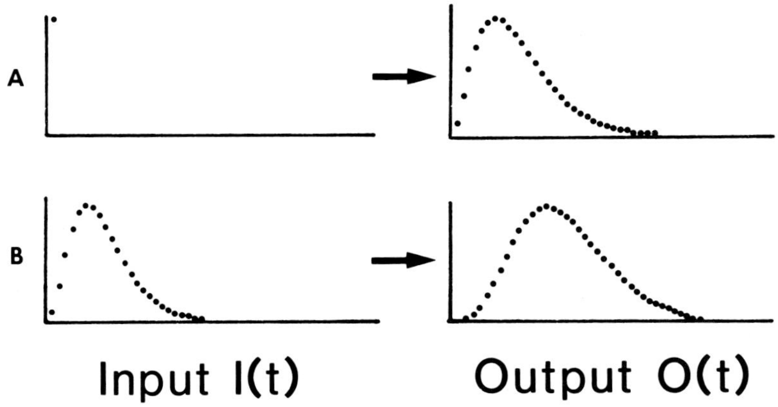

Figure 3. The output in *b* is calculated by convolving the input in *b* with the unit impulse response of the system, shown as the output in *A*.

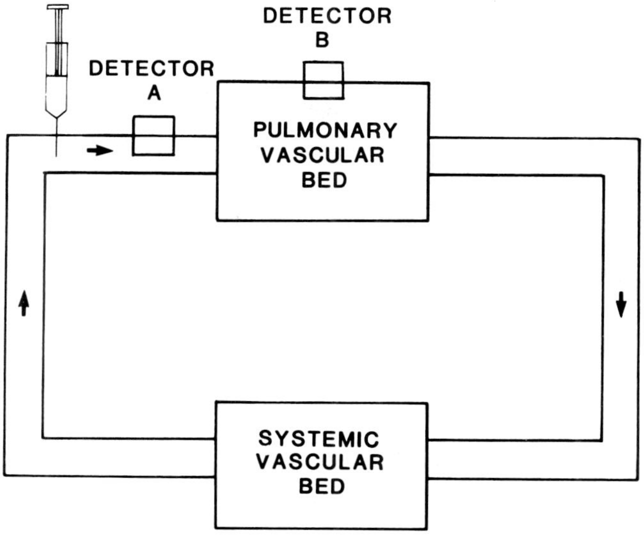

Figure 4. Conceptual model of the circulatory system in a normal subject.

I(t)*U(t) where * represents the operation of convolution. An important property of the operation of convolution is that the area under O(t) is equal to the product of the areas under I(t) and U(t). In other words, area is multiplicative under convolution.

An LTI Model of Left-to-Right Shunting. A model useful in the description of a radionuclide angiocardiogram obtained in a normal patient is shown in Figure 4. A radiopharmaceutical is injected from the syringe, passes through the pulmonary vascular bed, and is recorded by detector B. The radiopharmaceutical then passes through the remainder of the circulatory system and returns to the pulmonary vascular bed, where it is again recorded by detector B. This process continues indefinitely. The time-activity curve recorded at detector B is shown in Figure 5. This curve is composed of several sequentially appearing components. The first component, appearing at time t_p, is due to detection of the radiopharmaceutical passing through the pulmonary vascular bed before ever entering the systemic circulation. We shall term this component "P(t)." The second component, appearing at time t_{r1}, is due to detection of the radiopharmaceutical passing through the pulmonary vascular bed after one circuit of the systemic circulation. We shall term this component "R1(t)." R1(t) is equal to the convolution of P(t) with the UIR of the remainder of the circulatory system. In other words, R(t) describes the transformation of P(t) into R1(t). Conceptually, R(t) may be found by injecting a unit impulse of radiopharmaceutical at detector B and recording the curve obtained after a single passage of the systemic circulation. Since no radiopharmaceutical is lost, the area under R(t) is equal to one. Third and later components, appearing at times t_{r2}, t_{r3}, . . . are due to the detection of radiopharmaceutical passing through the pulmonary vascular bed after more than one circuit of the systemic circulation. We shall term these components "R2(t)," "R3(t)," . . . . The observed pulmonary curve O(t) may therefore be described by the formula:

$$O(t) = P(t) + R1(t) + R2(t) + \ldots$$

In the case of a patient with a left-to-right shunt, radiopharmaceutical leaving the pulmonary vascular bed may bypass the systemic circulation by travelling through a defect. We therefore need to add an additional pathway to our model as shown in Figure 6. After leaving the pulmonary vascular bed, a fraction K of the

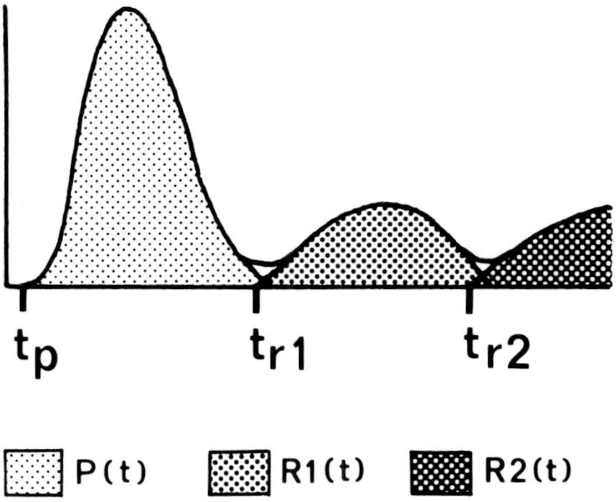

Figure 5. Components of the pulmonary curve obtained in a normal subject.

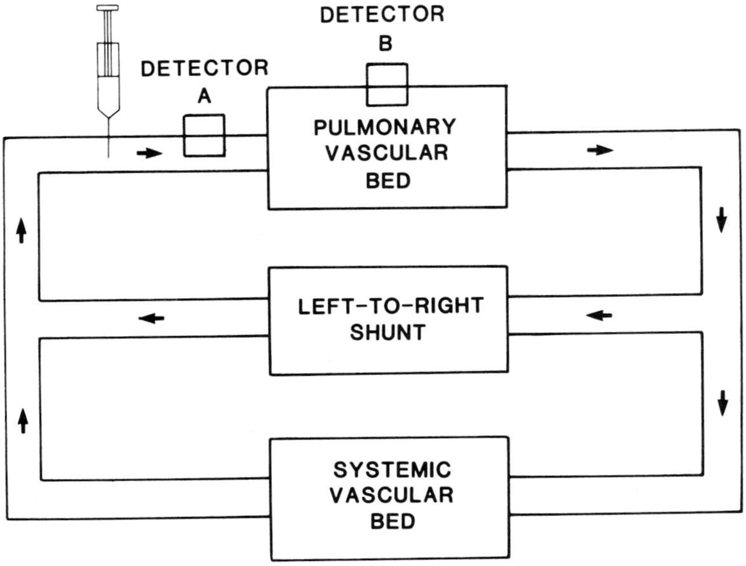

Figure 6. Conceptual model of the circulatory system in a patient with a left-to-right shunt.

radiopharmaceutical will pass through the shunt. The remaining fraction (1–K) of the radiopharmaceutical will pass through the systemic circulation. If the radiopharmaceutical is well mixed, these proportions are equivalent to the respective blood flows. The pulmonary-to-systemic flow ratio (Qp:Qs) is therefore equal to 1/(1–K).

The time-activity curve recorded at detector B is shown in Figure 7. The first component of the observed pulmonary curve is again P(t), which is due to detection of the radiopharmaceutical passing through the pulmonary vascular bed before ever passing through the shunt or systemic circulation. The minimal transit time of the circulatory pathway containing the shunt is generally less than that of the systemic circulation. Therefore, the second component of O(t), appearing at time t_{s1}, is due to detection of radiopharmaceutical passing through the pulmonary vascular bed after one circuit of the shunt. We shall term this component "S1(t)." S1(t) is equal to the convolution of P(t) with the UIR of the circulatory pathway containing the shunt, which we term "S(t)." S(t) may be characterized in a similar manner as was R(t). However, since only a fraction K of the radiopharmaceutical travels through the shunt pathway, the area under S(t) is equal to K. The area under S1(t) is equal to K times the area under P(t). Later components of O(t), appearing at times t_{s2}, t_{s3}, . . . are due to detection of radiopharmaceutical passing through the pulmonary vascular bed after more than one circuit of the shunt. We shall term these components "S2(t)," "S3(t)," . . . . The remaining components of O(t) are due to radiopharmaceutical passing through the pulmonary vascular bed after one or more circuits of the systemic circulation as well as combination circuits of the shunt and systemic circulation. The observed pulmonary curve is equal to:

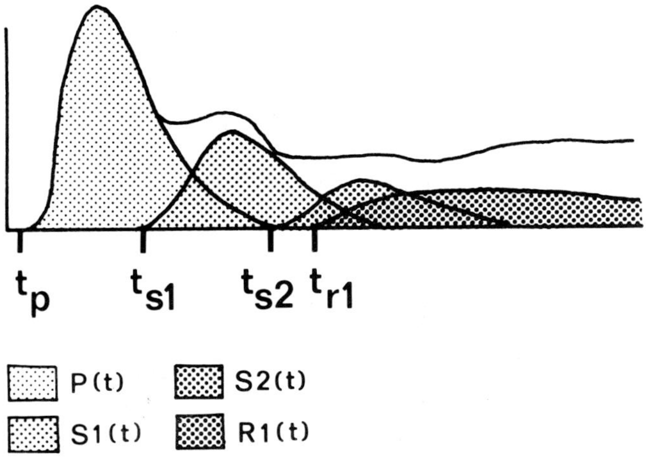

Figure 7. Components of the pulmonary curve obtained in a patient with a left-to-right shunt.

$$O(t) = P(t) - S1(t) + R1(t) + S2(t) + S1R1(t) + R2(t) + \ldots$$

where the notation SnRn is used to denote combination circuits through the shunt and systemic circulation.

Shunt quantitation is the problem of determining K or equivalently the area under S(t). K may be found by dividing the area under S1(t) by the area under P(t). Thus, by recovering P(t) and S1(t) from O(t), we can obtain an estimate of K.

Left-To-Right Shunt Quantitation Using the Gamma Variate Method. A commonly used method for recovering P(t) and S1(t) from the observed pulmonary curve O(t) is the gamma variate method. Consider the O(t) obtained from a normal person (Fig. 5). The portion of O(t) for $t_p \leq t \leq t_{r1}$ is due solely to the component P(t). At time t_{r1}, the component R1(t) appears. In most cases, almost the entire area of P(t) is to the left of t_{r1}. It is therefore possible to almost completely recover P(t).

It has been found experimentally that the P(t) obtained after a compact bolus injection of radiopharmaceutical can be closely approximated by a gamma variate function of the form:

$$P(t) = C(t-t_0)^{A}e^{-(t-t_0)/B}$$

where t_0 is the time at which activity first appears, and C, A, and B are variable parameters.[12] The gamma variate function can be fit to an observed data curve by a weighted least squares technique.[16] Thus, it is possible to estimate P(t) as a gamma variate function by fitting a gamma variate function to O(t) for $t_p \geq t \geq t_{r1}$ and extrapolating.

Now consider the O(t) obtained from a patient with a left-to-right shunt (Fig. 7). The initial portion of the curve is again solely due to the component P(t). At time t_{s1}, the component S1(t) begins to appear. In this case, t_{s1} is smaller than t_{r1}, and a substantial portion of P(t) occurs after t_{s1}. However, it is possible to recover P(t) approximately by fitting a gamma variate to O(t) for $_{tp} \leq t \leq t_{s1}$. One can then extrapolate from the gamma variate fit to recover P(t). We denote the area under P(t) as A1. In practice, it is necessary to infer the limits of the gamma variate fit from O(t). This can be done by visually interpreting the curve and manually choosing the points. Alternatively, the limits can be chosen automatically by using a rule such as fitting from 10 per cent of the maximum activity on the upslope of O(t) to 70 per cent of the maximum activity on the downslope.[12]

We now need to recover the component S1(t). Subtracting the gamma variate fit for P(t) from O(t), we obtain the recirculation curve:

$$RC(t) = S1(t) + R1(t) + S2(t) + S1R1(t) + R2(t) + \ldots$$

RC(t) is equal to S1(t) for $t_{s1} \leq t \leq \text{Min}(t_{s2}, t_{r1})$. We shall denote $\min(t_{s2}, t_{r1})$ as t_{rc}. A gamma variate function is fit to this portion of the recirculation curve. This gamma variate fit is extrapolated to recover S1(t). We denote the area under S1(t) as A2. Again, in practice it is necessary to infer manually or automatically the limits of the fit from RC(t). One automatic rule is to fit from 10 per cent of a specially defined maximum on the upslope to one point after this maximum. This maximum is defined as that point above which the rise of activity failed to remain monotonic, that is, the last point on the upslope whose value was greater than 105 per cent of the previous value.[12]

K is equal to the ratio A2/A1. Pulmonary-to-systemic flow ratio (Qp:Qs) is equal to 1/(1–K). Multiplying by the area under P(t), we obtain the formula:

$$Qp{:}Qs = A1/(A1-A2).$$

Several alternative methods to estimate Qp:Qs from pulmonary time-activity curves have been suggested. Some of these are reviewed by Parker and Treves.[14] Some promising results have been reported for a recently proposed method based on an LTI model of the circulation similar to that described here. This method uses a signal processing known as homomorphic deconvolution to recover P(t) and S1(1).[13]

It is often possible to determine the level of a left-to-right shunt by visually analyzing time-activity curves generated from the superior vena cava, right atrium, right ventricle, and the lungs, thus defining the site of recirculation. A left anterior oblique projection with a 30° caudal tilt is useful for this purpose. For example, in partial anomalous pulmonary venous return to the superior vena cava, there is early recirculation in the superior vena cava, right atrium, right ventricle, and lungs. In atrial septal defect, there is early recirculation in the right atrium, ventricle, and lungs. In ventricular septal defect, there is early recirculation in the right ventricle and the lungs. In patent ductus arteriosus, there is early recirculation only in the lungs. If more than one shunt is present, it is possible to localize only the most proximal.

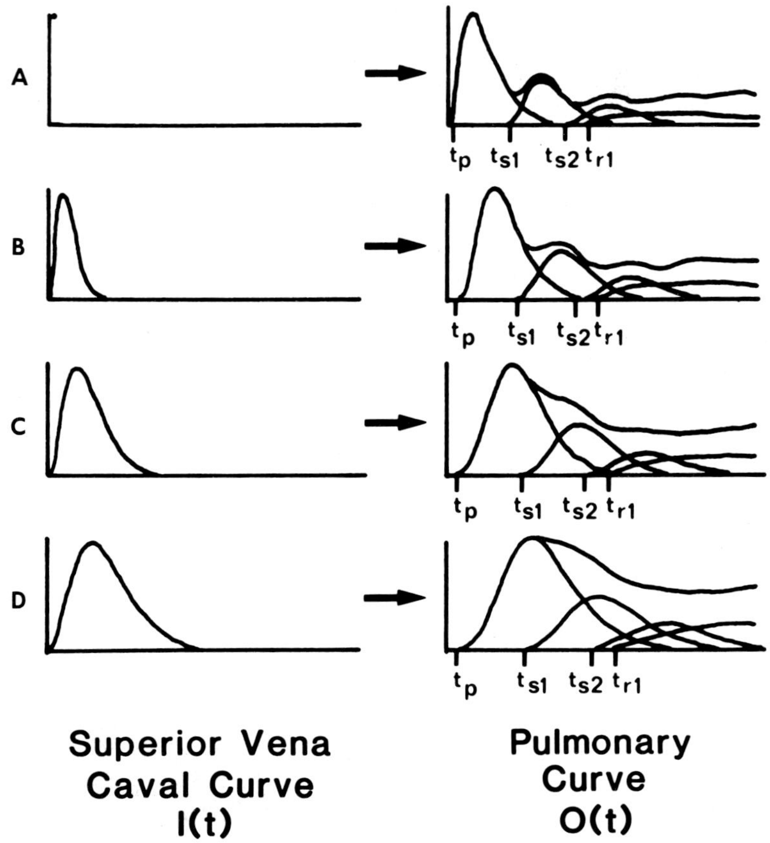

Figure 8. Effect of prolonged delivery of a radiopharmaceutical on the observed pulmonary curve.

Correction for Irregularities in the Delivery of Radiopharmaceutical to the Cardiopulmonary System. Shunt quantitation by the gamma variate method assumes that P(t) and S1(t) can be described by gamma variate functions. In addition, the method assumes that sufficiently large portions of P(t) and S1(t) occur before t_{s1} and t_{rc}, respectively, to allow accurate extrapolation. The validity of both of these assumptions depends upon the time course of delivery of the radiopharmaceutical to the cardiopulmonary system. This delivery can be monitored by using a region of interest over the superior vena cava. This is shown schematically as detector A in Figures 4 and 6. The time-activity curve obtained from over the superior vena cava is termed "I(t)." D(t) is the curve that would be produced from a unit impulse injection at the superior vena cava. An example of such a unit impulse-UIR pair is shown in Figure 8*A*. O(t) may be expressed at the convolution of I(t) with D(t).

Figure 8*B* shows time-activity curves recorded from detectors A and B in Figure 6. The I(t) shown in Figure 8*B* represents the delivery of radiopharmaceutical as a compact bolus. The components P(t) and S1(t) of the resulting pulmonary curve may be accurately described by gamma variate functions. In addition, sufficiently large portions of P(t) and S1(t) occur before t_{s1} and t_{rc}, respectively, to allow accurate extrapolation. Figures 8*C* and 8*D* represent studies where I(t) has become increasingly prolonged. In these studies, P(t) and S1(t) may still be accurately described by gamma variate functions. However, increasingly smaller portions of P(t) and S1(t) now occur before t_{s1} and t_{rc}. This reduces the accuracy of the extrapolation necessary in recovering P(t) and S1(t). Figures 9*C* and 9*D* represent studies where I(t) has become fragmented. In these studies, P(t) and S1(t) are no longer accurately described by gamma variate functions. In this case, shunt quantitation may become inaccurate or impossible.

Ideally, one would like to deliver radiopharmaceutical to the cardiopulmonary system as a unit impulse because this best facilitates shunt quantitation by the gamma variate method. This would result in an observed pulmonary curve equal to the unit impulse response of the system, D(t). In practice, it is impossible to deliver a unit impulse I(t) by intravenous injection. However, it is possible to estimate D(t) from I(t) and O(t) by undoing the operation of convolution. This is known as deconvolution.

Exact solution of the convolution equation for D(t) is an unstable process in the sense that small errors in the recorded data can result in large errors in the computed UIR.[5] This can be illustrated by considering the special case of I(t) equal to a unit step function.

$$I(t) = \begin{array}{ll} 0 & t < \emptyset \\ 1 & t \geq \emptyset \end{array}$$

Figure 10*A* shows a unit impulse-UIR pair; 10*B* shows the O(t) obtained by convolution of the unit step function with the UIR shown in 10*A*. In this case, the convolution I(t) and D(t) is equivalent to integration of D(t). It follows that in this case deconvolution is equivalent to point-by-point differentiation of O(t). Figure 10*C* shows the O(t) in 10*B* degraded with 1 per cent pseudorandom noise. Figure 10*D* shows the UIR estimate obtained from point-by-point differentiation of the O(t) in 10*C*. Note that O(t) in Figures 10*B* and *C* is almost identical, whereas the corresponding UIR in Figures 10*A* and *D* are markedly different. In this case, the instability of deconvolution manifests itself as the sensitivity of point-by-point differentiation to small data errors.

In practice, it is necessary to incorporate some characterization of what constitutes an acceptable estimate of D(t) into the deconvolution process, thereby obtaining a well-behaved, approximate solution to the deconvolution problem. As discussed previously, D(t) may be expressed as the sum of a set of component curves. Using such a characterization of an acceptable UIR, one can obtain accurate UIR estimates from noise-degraded data.[11] The D(t) obtained by deconvolution may be analyzed in the same manner as O(t). The analysis is facilitated as the assumptions of the gamma variate method become more accurate.

Studies on dogs and humans have shown that deconvolution may improve the accuracy of

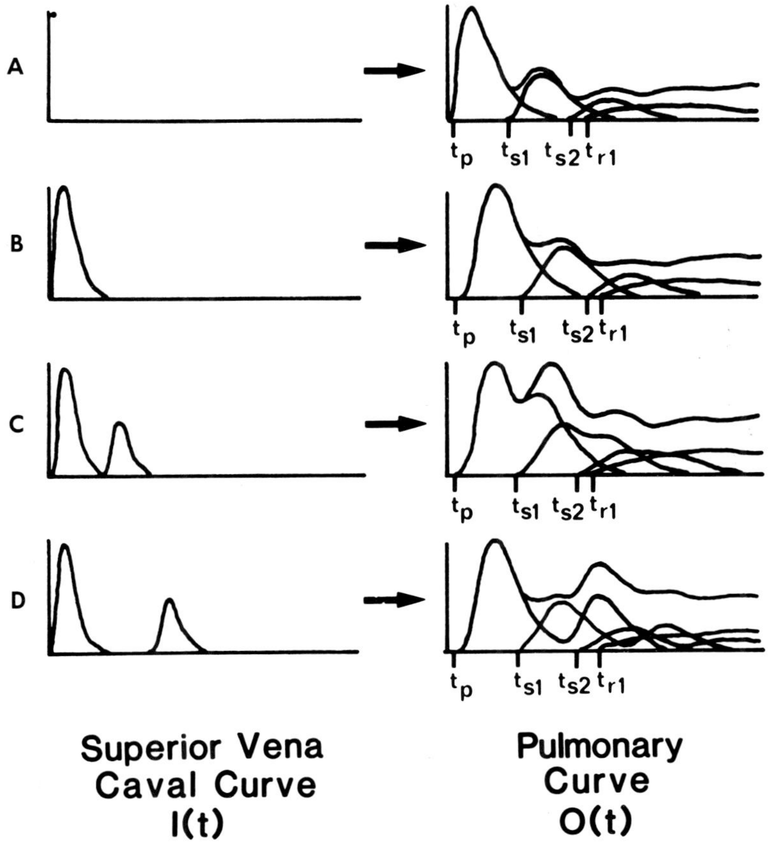

Figure 9. Effect of fragmented delivery of a radiopharmaceutical on the observed pulmonary curve.

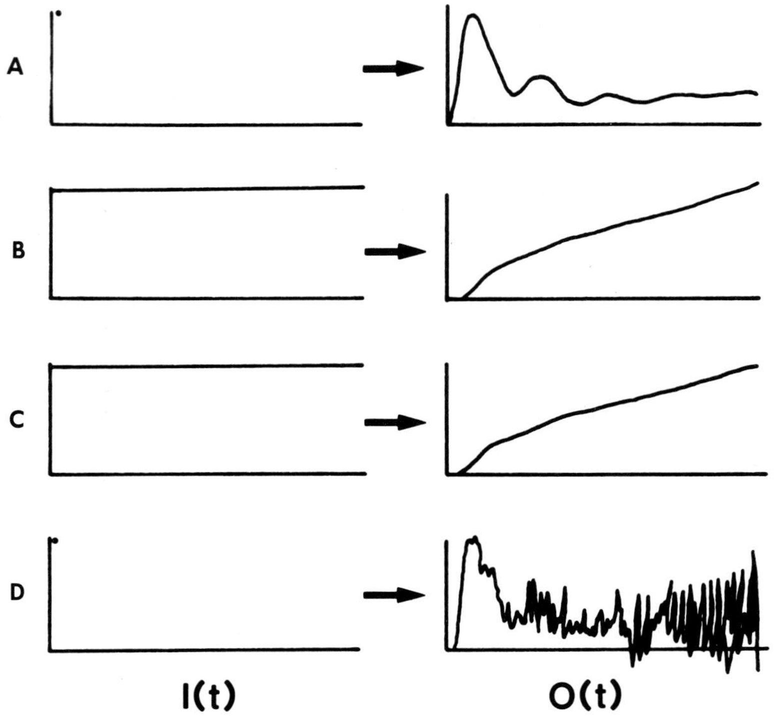

Figure 10. Effect of random data errors on exact deconvolution.

shunt quantitation by radionuclide angiocardiography.[1, 6, 10] Figure 11 shows the effect of deconvolution on radionuclide angiocardiography performed on a normal dog. Without deconvolution, the pulmonary curve obtained from a study performed with a fragmented injection shows a pattern suggestive of a left-to-right shunt. After deconvolution, the pulmonary curve is suggestive of a normal subject. Note the similarity of UIR estimates obtained from studies performed with single and fragmented injections on the same animal. Figure 12 shows that effect of deconvolution on radionuclide angiocardiography performed on a dog with a left-to-right shunt. The pulmonary curve obtained from a study performed with a fragmented injection is distorted relative to the pulmonary curve obtained from a study performed with a compact injection on the same animal. After deconvolution, both lung curves are nearly identical.

Right-To-Left Shunting. Right-to-left shunting may be quantified by using a method that in principle is almost identical to the method previously described for left-to-right shunting. In this case, a time-activity curve from the left ventricle is used rather than the pulmonary curve. In a patient with a right-to-left shunt, the left ventricular curve will be composed of several sequentially appearing components.

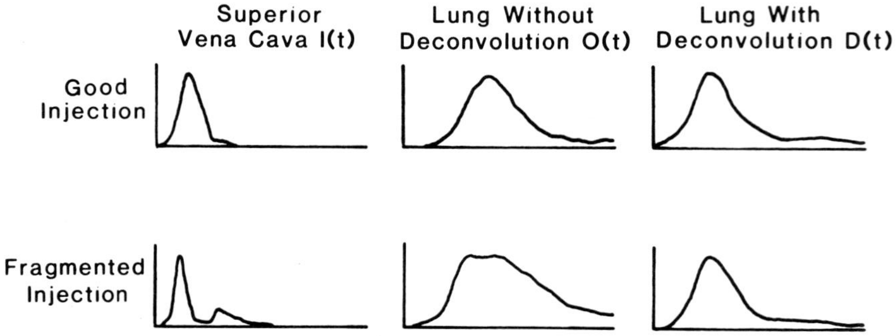

Figure 11. Effect of deconvolution on radiouclide angiocardiography performed on a normal dog.

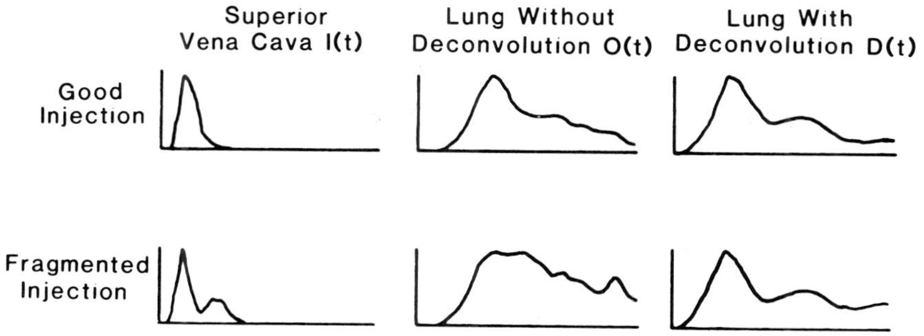

Figure 12. Effect of deconvolution on radionuclide angiocardiography performed on a dog with a left-to-right shunt.

The first component is due to detection of radiopharmaceutical passing through the defect. The second component is due to detection of radiopharmaceutical passing through the left ventricle that has travelled through the pulmonary vascular bed rather than through the defect. Several other components corresponding to the various recirculation pathways follow subsequently.

Shunt size may be calculated from the area under the first and second components of the left ventricular curve, A3 and A4, respectively. These components are recovered from the observed left ventricular curve by extrapolating their initial portions in a manner similar to that used in left-to-right shunt quantitation. Qp:Qs is calculated using the formula:

$$Qp:Qs = A4/(A3 + A4)$$

Several other theoretical approaches to the quantitation of right-to-left shunting involve the use of diffusable indicators and radiolabelled microspheres. Some of these are reviewed by Parker and Treves.[14]

RADIONUCLIDES

Radionuclide angiography is most commonly performed using Tc-99m-sodium pertechnetate, eluted with sterile saline from a molybdenum-99-technetium-99m generator. Technetium-99m, with a physical half-life of 6 hr, decays by way of a monoenergetic gamma ray of 140 kev, which can be imaged with the gamma scintillation camera. A collimator with high sensitivity should be used to maximize the recorded count rate. A dose of 200 μCi/kg body weight is used, with a minimum total dose of 2 mCi necessary for adequate counting statistics even in the smallest infants. To have the injected activity approximate a bolus, the volume administered must be between 0.1 and 0.5 ml; therefore, there must be 20 to 40 mCi of technetium-99m per milliliter of generator eluent. After intravenous injection, Tc-99m sodium pertechnetate is rapidly distributed within the extravascular and intravascular spaces with active uptake in the choroid plexus, thyroid gland, salivary glands, and stomach. A portion of the radiopharmaceutical is rapidly excreted in the urine, and a larger amount eliminated via the intestines 24 hr later. Before its administration, the patient is given a dose of 3 to 6 mg/kg of body weight of sodium perchlorate (intravenous) or potassium perchlorate (oral) in order to block the concentration of the radionuclide in the thyroid gland, the stomach, and other organs and to speed its removal from the body.

The use of technetium-99m in radionuclide angiography has several drawbacks: (1) The patient receives radiation for a longer time than is necessary. The isotope has a 6 hr half-life; the typical angiogram is completed in 20 to 30 sec. In a one-year-old patient given 3 mCi of Tc-99m-sodium pertechnetate, the whole body absorbed radiation dose is about 200 mrad, and the critical organ (intestine) dose is 1500 mrad. (2) With currently accepted dosimetry, Tc-99m yields relatively low photon flux. High photon flux is important because it allows one to obtain improved temporal resolution without sacrificing anatomic resolution. (3) There is a lack of capacity for performing serial studies within a short period of time because of the increasing radiation to the patient and background activity within the body. Multiple or serial radionuclide angiograms would be useful in localizing a shunt by the use of multiple projections, for investigating the effects of pharmacologic agents and/or exercise on cardiac function, in assessing abnormalities of myocardial wall motion, and for evaluating the anatomic relationships of the large vessels.

A radionuclide of very short half-life would

obviate some of the above limitations. In our laboratory, progress has been made in the development of an osmium-191 → iridium-191m generator for clinical use. Osmium-191, which is reactor produced, has a physical half-life of 16 days and decays by internal conversion to iridium-191m. The latter isotope has a half-life of 4.96 sec and decays to stable iridium-191 with the emission of 65 and 129 kev photons (60 per cent and 25 per cent abundance, respectively). These energies can be efficiently detected with the gamma scintillation cameras currently available. In the present generator, an anionic osmium(VI) complex is loaded on a strongly basic anion exchange resin and eluted with 0.9 per cent sodium chloride at pH 1. The eluate is then rapidly buffered to pH 4 before injection.

There are several advantages to the use of iridium-191m: (1) There is very low radiation exposure to the patient even with the administration of multimillicurie amounts. In the newborn, the whole body absorbed dose is about 0.056 mrad/mCi. This is approximately 2500 to 4000 times less of a radiation dose on a millicurie per millicurie basis than that from technetium-99m. With the current levels of osmium-191 breakthrough in the generator eluent, however, there is only 8 to 40 times less radiation to the patient. (2) The low radiation dose per millicurie permits safe use of larger amounts of activity for the study. The high photon flux produced permits the rapid recording of serial images of higher information density than is practical with technetium-99m, resulting in more accurate quantitation of cardiac function and improved spatial resolution in the scintigram image. (3) The very short half-life of iridium-191m permits repeated or serial studies without background activity, whereas with technetium-99m a wait of several hours to one day is necessary between studies. Because of the low radiation dose, multiple studies may be done with a cumulative patient dose less than that incurred from one technetium-99m injection.[3, 17]

A preliminary evaluation of the effectiveness of iridium-191m for the detection and quantitation of left-to-right shunts has been carried out in 135 patients, ranging in age from four days to 67 years. The clinical diagnoses were ventricular septal defect (63), atrial septal defect (33), evaluation of Mustard procedure (4), and patent ductus arteriosus (15). The studies were satisfactory in the majority of the cases, although in four patients, shunt quantitation was not possible. In 20 additional patients, Qp:Qs was determined by both oxymetry at catheterization and iridium-191m radionuclide angiography. Comparison of the estimates obtained using these two methods yielded a correlation coefficient of 0.87 (Qp:Qs range 1.2 to 2.7, slope = 0.78, standard error of the estimate ± 0.237). From 10 to 80 mCi of iridium-191m were administered for these studies. No adverse reactions or electrocardiographic changes were observed.

CLINICAL APPLICATIONS

Radionuclide angiography for the detection and quantitation of shunts is nontraumatic and can be done simply and repeatedly. If the patient is too ill to be moved from an intensive care unit, imaging can be accomplished with a mobile scintillation camera/computer system. In the presence of valvular insufficiency, severe congestive heart failure, multiple cardiac lesions, or large bronchial collaterals, quantitative analysis of left-to-right shunting may be impossible.

Premature and Newborn Infants

Pulmonary Versus Cardiac Disease. Cyanosis in the newborn may be caused by cardiac disease, pulmonary disease, or a combination of both. Radionuclide angiography can help differentiate the causes. Cardiac disease with right-to-left shunting, such as the transposition of the great arteries or tetralogy of Fallot, will be indicated by the appearance of the radionuclide in the aorta before the lungs. Cardiac disease with left-to-right shunting, such as patent ductus arteriosus, will be indicated by the prolonged presence of the radionuclide in the lungs. In pulmonary disorders, the angiocardiogram may appear normal, although in cases of increased vascular resistance, it may show evidence of right-to-left shunting through a patent foramen ovale, a patent ductus arteriosus, or both. After the ligation of a patent ductus arteriosus, continuing respiratory distress syndrome suggests lung disease or a complication of surgical technique. One can distinguish between these alternatives with radionuclide angiography. A normal study points to a pulmonary cause: the persistence of a left-to-right shunt (1) with equal visualization of both lungs to incomplete closure of the ductus arteriosus or to the presence of additional cardiac defects (for example, aortic pulmonary window or ventricular septal defect) or (2) without visualization of the left lung to inadvertent ligation of the left pulmonary artery at the time of the attempted closure of the ductus.[19]

Patent Ductus Arteriosus. At least 15 percent of all premature infants with a birth weight less than 1800 gm have a hemodynamically significant patent ductus arteriosus. The diagnosis is suggested by the following: systolic or continuous murmur, wide pulse pressure, tachycardia, and often congestive heart failure. Even without clinical evidence of congestive heart failure, the left-to-right shunt through a patent ductus arteriosus can lead to a complicated course of respiratory distress syndrome and in combination with congestive heart failure can require prolonged artificial ventilation. The shunt flow can be accurately assessed with radionuclide angiography to determine whether surgical intervention is indicated.[18]

Ventricular Septal Defect. In newborns with this defect, the radionuclide angiogram may initially appear normal because of a relatively high pulmonary vascular resistance leading to a small left-to-right shunt. After a few days when the vascular resistance decreases, left-to-right shunting will increase and will be revealed on the radionuclide angiogram. The administration of pure oxygen in the inspired air may help diagnose left-to-right shunting since it acts as a vasodilator, thus decreasing the pulmonary vascular resistance.[4]

Older Infants and Children

Atrial Septal Defects. Patients with a secundum atrial septal defect have characteristic findings on physical examination, chest x-ray films, and electrocardiography. In our institution, surgical closure of these defects is usually undertaken without further diagnostic procedures. If confirmation becomes necessary, a combination of subxiphoid two-dimensional echocardiography and radionuclide angiography can localize the defect and quantitate the shunt flow. These two techniques are also helpful in differentiating pulmonary stenosis from atrial septal defects.[8]

Ventricular Septal Defects. The size of a ventricular shunt can be approximated by auscultation, electrocardiography, and chest x-ray film. However, radionuclide angiography can accurately quantitate Qp:Qs if greater than 1.2. Serial quantitation of left-to-right shunt flow in patients with a small ventricular septal defect can show changes in Qp:Qs and can document spontaneous closure. When a large ventricular septal defect is suspected, cardiac catheterization is necessary to obtain precise anatomic definition and to measure pulmonary arterial pressure and pulmonary vascular resistance. If serial evaluation of a patient reveals a diminution in shunt flow, the question of pulmonary hypertension may be raised. First pass radionuclide angiography cannot differentiate increased pulmonary vascular resistance from spontaneous shunt closing. A thallium-201 scintigram at rest will show increased uptake of this radionuclide in the right ventricular myocardium because of right ventricular hypertrophy secondary to pulmonary hypertension.[15]

Evaluation of the Postoperative Patient. Radionuclide angiography using mobile detection equipment can be performed postoperatively in the intensive care unit when cardiac catheterization would be contraindicated. Persistent murmurs or the appearance of new murmurs postoperatively would suggest residual lesions, detachment of the patch, or valve abnormalities. In such cases, the technique permits rapid, safe, and accurate detection and quantitation of any residual shunt.

Total correction of transposition of the great arteries can be accomplished early in life with use of the Mustard operation. Radionuclide angiocardiography can assist in the early and late postoperative evaluation. A successful Mustard procedure provides a characteristic angiocardiographic pattern. Complications of the Mustard procedure recognized with radionuclide angiocardiography include residual shunting through the atrial baffle, which can occur early or late in the postoperative period. Obstruction of the atrial baffle in either pulmonary or systemic circuits is indicated rather dramatically with radionuclide angiocardiography.[7]

Patency or occlusion of palliative shunts (Blalock-Taussig, Potts, Waterston) can be demonstrated in visual evaluation of pulmonary dilution curves. The curve obtained over the lung on the side of the anastomosis reflects a larger early pulmonary recirculation than that of the contralateral lung when the anastomosis is patent.[9]

REFERENCES

1. Alderson PO, Douglass KH, Mendenhall KG, et al: Deconvolution analysis in radionuclide quantitation of left-to-right shunts. J Nucl Med, *20*:502–506, 1979.
2. Bassingthwaighte JB: Circulatory transport and the convolution integral. Mayo Clin Prac, *42*:137–154, 1967.
3. Cheng C, Treves S, Samuel A, et al: A new osmium-191 → iridium-191m generator. J Nucl Med, *21*:1169–1176, 1980.
4. Fujii AM, Rabinovitch M, Keane JF, et al: Radionuclide angiocardiographic assessment of pulmonary vascular reactivity in patients with left-to-right shunt and pulmonary hypertension. Am J Cardiol, *49*:356–361, 1982.
5. Gamel J, Rousseau WF, Katholi CR, et al: Pitfalls in

digital computation of the impulse response of vascular beds from indicator-dilution curves. Circ Res, *32*:512–523, 1973.
6. Ham HR, Dobbeleir A, Viart R, et al: Radionuclide quantitation of left-to-right cardiac shunts using deconvolution analysis. J Nucl Med, *22*:688–692, 1981.
7. Hurwitz RA, Papanicolaou N, Treves S, et al: Radionuclide angiocardiography in evaluation of patients after surgical repair of transposition of the great arteries. Am J Cardiol, *49*:761–765, 1982.
8. Hurwitz RA, Treves S, Keane JF, et al: Current value of radionuclide angiocardiography for shunt quantification and management in patients with secundum atrial septal defect. Am Heart J, *103*:421–425, 1982.
9. Keane JF, Williams R, Treves S, et al: Assessment of the postoperative patient by non-invasive techniques. Prog Cardiovasc Dis, *18*:57–75, 1975.
10. Kuruc A, Treves S, Parker JA, et al: Radionuclide angiocardiography. An improved deconvolution technique for improvement after suboptimal bolus injection. Experimental results in dogs with and without atrial septal defects. Radiology, *148*:233–238, 1983.
11. Kuruc A, Treves S, Parker JA: Accuracy of deconvolution algorithms assessed by simulation studies. J Nucl Med, *24*:258–263, 1983.
12. Maltz DL, Treves S: Quantitative radionuclide angiocardiography. Determination of Qp:Qs in children. Circulation, *47*:1049–1056, 1973.
13. Nakamura M, Suzuki Y, Nagasawa T, et al: Detection and quantitation of left-to-right shunts from radionuclide angiocardiography using the homomorphic deconvolution technique. IEEE Trans Biomed Eng, *29*:192–201, 1982.
14. Parker JA, Treves S: Radionuclide detection, localization and quantitation of intracardiac shunts and shunts between the great vessels. Prog Cardiovasc Dis, *20*:121–149, 1977.
15. Rabinovitch M, Fischer KC, Treves A: Quantitative thallium-201 myocardial imaging in assessment of right ventricular pressure in patients with congenital heart defects. Br Heart J, *45*:198–205, 1981.
16. Starmer CF, Clark DO: Computer computation of cardiac output using the gamma function. J Appl Physiol, *28*:219–220, 1970.
17. Treves S, Cheng C, Samuel A, et al: Iridium-191m angiocardiography for the detection and quantitation of left-to-right shunting. J Nucl Med, *21*:1151–1157, 1980.
18. Treves S, Collins-Nakai R, Ahnberg D, et al: Quantitative radionuclide angiocardiography (RAC) in premature infants with patent ductus arteriosus (PDA) and respiratory distress syndrome (RDS). J Nucl Med, *17*:554, 1976.
19. Treves S, Fyler D, Fujii A, et al: Low radiation iridium-191m radionuclide angiography: Detection and quantitation of left-to-right shunts in infants. J Pediatr, *101*:210–215, 1982.

6

RADIONUCLIDE STUDIES OF THE CIRCULATION

Special Technical Considerations for Children

WESLEY COVITZ, M.D., and CASIMIR EUBIG, Ph.D.

With the technical assistance of BONNIE G. HADDEN

Radionuclide imaging of the infant and child is not a new development. However, the introduction of high-resolution portable gamma cameras interfaced to powerful computers has transformed nuclear imaging of children into a complex and vital modality. In the adult, the recent thrust of radionuclide investigations has been to examine the patient with coronary artery disease.[8] Pediatric applications were limited to shunt quantitation[25] and qualitative angiography[19] until recently. Today the full range of diagnostic nuclear imaging has been applied to children with congenital and acquired heart disease.

Children are anything but small adults. Size may be a problem, but the obstacles encountered when trying to gain the cooperation of a young child during injection of an isotope cannot be overstated. The children selected for study may have multiple lesions involving shunts and valvular obstruction or regurgitation. They often have rapid heart rates, and concern over the potential long-term effects of radiation precludes use of the larger radioisotope doses administered to adults. The pediatric patient, however, does offer some advantages for nuclear imaging. The detector may be positioned closer to the heart in the small patient, with improved resolution and less attenuation of activity by intervening tissues. Although the heart beats rapidly, at higher rates cycle lengths are more regular.[16] It is the objective of this chapter to describe the special technical considerations that come into play when performing radionuclide examinations of the heart on children.

THE PEDIATRIC RADIONUCLIDE PROTOCOL

The following is a detailed description of the protocol for a comprehensive radionuclide examination of the heart as performed in the Pediatric Cardiology Nuclear Laboratory at the Medical College of Georgia. An extensive discussion of the protocol will follow, providing an opportunity to examine the rationale behind this approach.

Description of the Radionuclide Protocol. The study is performed with a high-resolution, small-field-of-view, single-crystal Anger camera interfaced to a dedicated computer system and an electrocardiographic gating device. A first-pass study is performed during injection of the radioactive bolus. An equilibrium study follows once the imaging agent has equilibrated throughout the blood pool.

The first-pass study is performed with the subject supine in the anterior projection. The

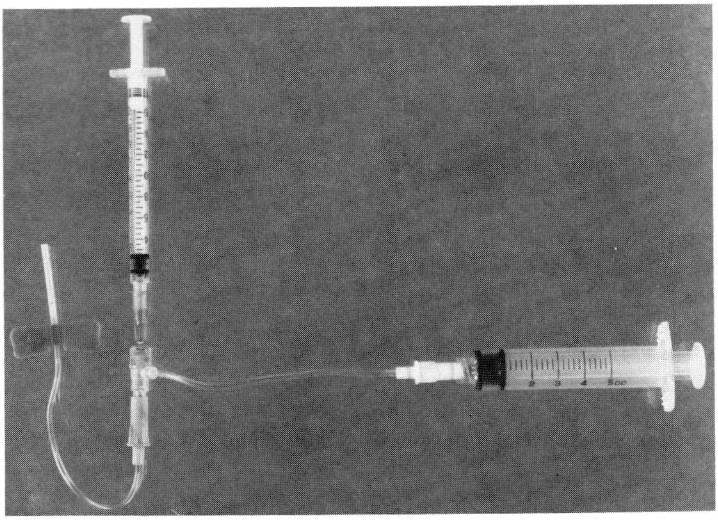

Figure 1. Intravenous injection set for bolus administration. The butterfly is inserted into a medial antecubital vein. The radionuclide is injected from the 1-ml syringe that enters the system via a needle that punctures the rubber bulb of the connector.

camera is positioned to image the heart and both lungs. The radiopharmaceutical is administered via a medial antecubital vein. A butterfly intravenous set (21 or 23 gauge), an injection tubing, and two syringes are used, as shown in Figure 1. The pediatric dose is made up into approximately 0.5 ml and injected rapidly; a syringe containing 5 ml of normal saline is used to flush the bolus into the circulation (this may be scaled down for the newborn and expanded for the adolescent). Care must be taken to prevent backflow into the dose syringe by holding the plunger firmly until all the flushed solution has been injected. The pharmaceutical used in our laboratory is technetium-99m albumin. A high-resolution or all-purpose parallel-hole collimator is used to record the passage of the radioactive bolus through the heart and lungs. Zoom or magnification mode is used for infants weighing less than 10 kg. Word mode frame images are taken at two to three per second for 30 sec. Without moving the patient, a 10-sec static image is obtained 3 min after injection of the radioisotope.

The patient is then repositioned in the left anterior oblique position so that the plane of the gamma camera is perpendicular to the interventricular septum. This plane varies from 30 to 60°; the angle tends to be greater in young children and is altered by ventricular dilatation. A parallel-hole, high-sensitivity collimator is used for gated equilibrium blood pool scanning. Magnification or zoom mode is utilized in patients weighing less than 15 kg. Care must be taken to center the camera over the heart. Images are obtained at the rate of 14 frames per cardiac cycle. The camera is triggered by the R wave of the patient's electrocardiogram. A 10-min acquisition is obtained.

The first-pass study is processed as follows: Frames acquired during the passage of the bolus from the superior vena cava to its ejection from the left ventricle are combined to produce a composite image. Two additional composites are made of the bolus passing through the right atrium and of the bolus passing through the left ventricle. These two composites are subtracted from each other, providing excellent delineation of those portions of the right side of the heart and left ventricle that do not overlap (Fig. 2). Areas of interest are selected over a portion of the superior vena cava, right atrium, right lung, and left ventricle. Time-activity curves are generated for each of those areas. The superior vena cava and right lung curves are used for shunt quantitation.[25] The curves over the right atrium and left ventricle are used for quantitation of cardiac output (Fig. 2*B*). The 10-sec static image obtained at 3 min after injection is used to determine counts per second at equilibrium over the identical right atrial and left ventricular areas of interest. Cardiac output over these two sites is derived from the following relationship:

> Cardiac output = equilibrium counts × blood volume/the area under the time-activity curve.[24]

Computer processing of the multiple gated acquisition or MUGA scan requires the combining of information obtained from hundreds of cardiac cycles (Fig. 3). A box is placed around the area that contains the left ventricle. The computer automatically selects the edge of the ventricle and an area in the inferior posterior quadrant of the left ventricle as background activity. The selection program permits automated edge detection during each frame of the composite cardiac cycle. The operator may intervene at any time during processing to make corrections. Ejection fraction, counts in the end-diastolic frame, time per frame, and cycles processed are measured. Relative stroke volume in counts ejected per beat and cardiac output in counts ejected per minute are derived. A continuous loop of the gated equilibrium scan is displayed in movie format to view wall motion.

Discussion of Radionuclide Protocol

The First-Pass Study. A medial antecubital vein is selected as the site of injection for a variety of reasons. First of all, unless the patient is critically ill or sedated, placing intravenous lines more centrally usually results in an uncooperative patient who is difficult to restrain. This makes delivery of an intact bolus somewhat unpredictable. A Valsalva maneuver is all that is necessary to propel a bolus that has already passed into the right atrium back into the superior vena cava, resulting in a double-peaked time-activity curve that may be mistaken for a left-to-right shunt (Fig. 4). The more lateral antecubital vessels are avoided because of the possibility of delaying the bolus at the shoulder. Ideally, the time between which a bolus appears and disappears in a right lung activity curve for shunt analysis should be less

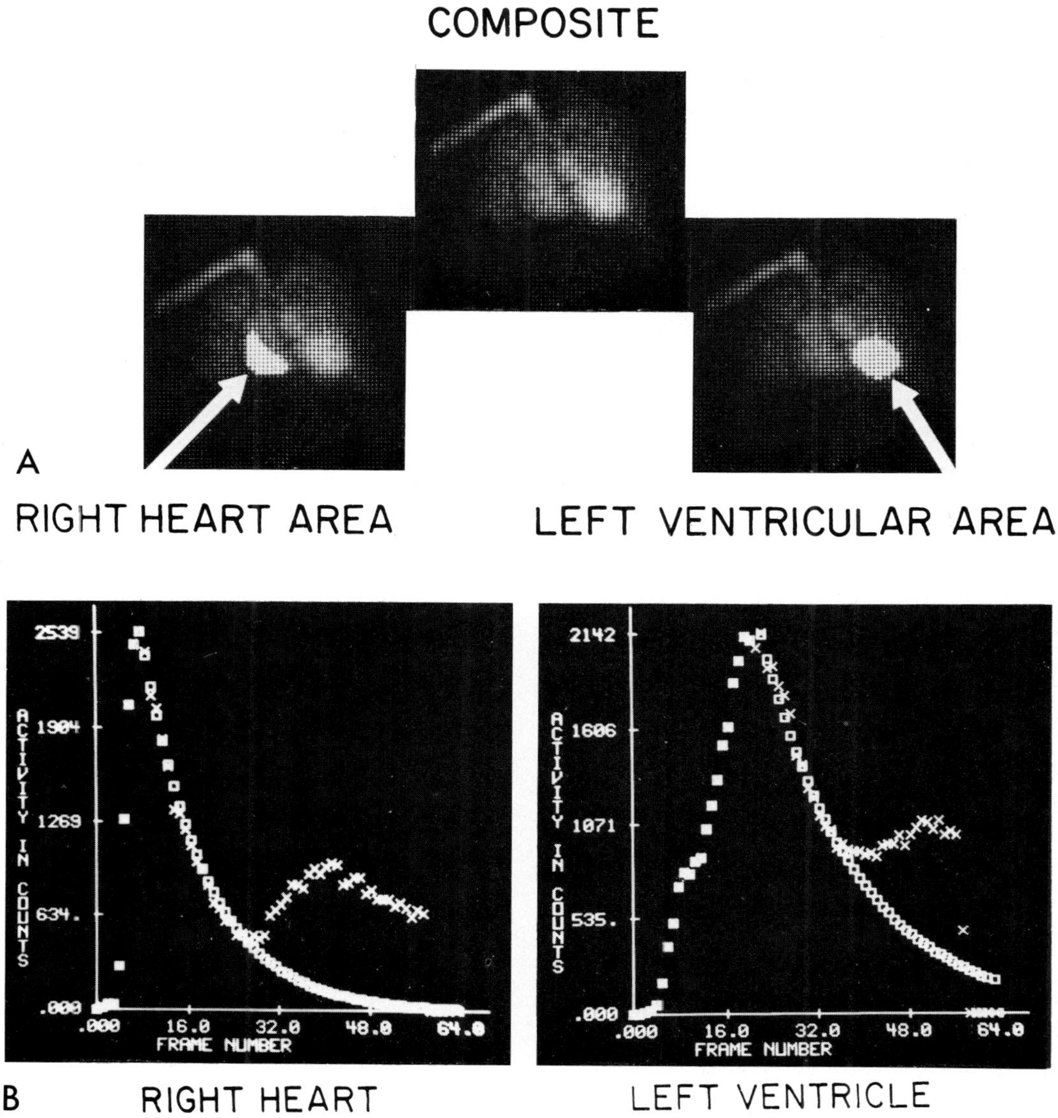

Figure 2. *A*, Area selection for cardiac output determination. The composite shows areas of right and left sides of the heart after subtraction of overlapping structures. *B*, Curves for cardiac output determination. Time-activity curves obtained from areas of the right and left sides of the heart are shown with exponential fitting of the washout portion of the curves.

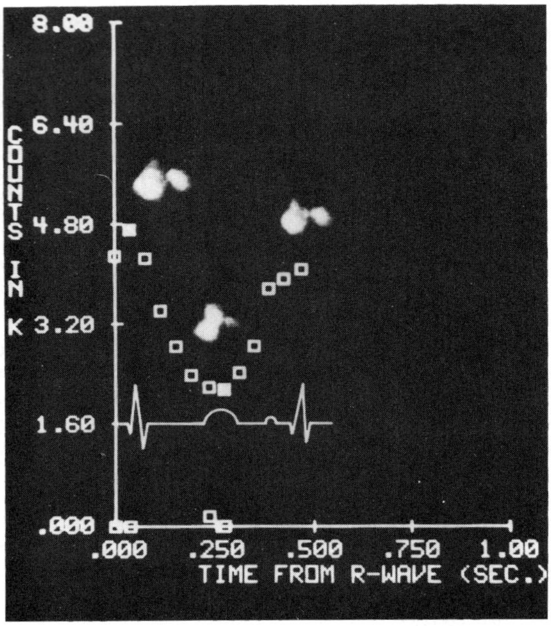

Figure 3. The MUGA scan. The left ventricle is separated from other cardiac structures by positioning. Hundreds of cardiac cycles are combined to form a representative cardiac cycle. The cycle is broken into 14 frames. Activity in the left ventricle after background subtraction is displayed.

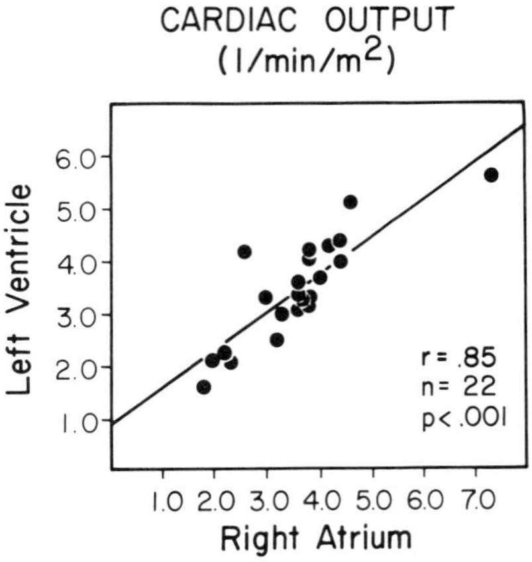

Figure 5. Comparison of cardiac output over right atrium and left ventricle. The excellent internal correlation of outputs derived from the area under time-activity curves would be impossible if adequate mixing of the bolus was not accomplished at the level of the right atrium. Six patients with ventricular septal defects or patent ductus arteriosus were included. Right atrial output was multiplied by Qp:Qs to correlate with left ventricular output. Excellent agreement was found.

than 2½ sec. Since only 80 per cent of boluses administered to children meet these criteria.[2] it is helpful to be able to quantify shunts with an alternate method. Studies in our laboratory suggest that mixing of the bolus is complete at the level of the right atrium with antecubital vein injection (Fig. 5). This may not hold true for more central injections. The opportunity to compare cardiac outputs over right atrium and left ventricle provides an alternate method for quantitating left-to-right shunts when boluses are imperfect, since the cardiac output curve-fitting method is less dependent on a narrow, single-peaked bolus for quantitation.

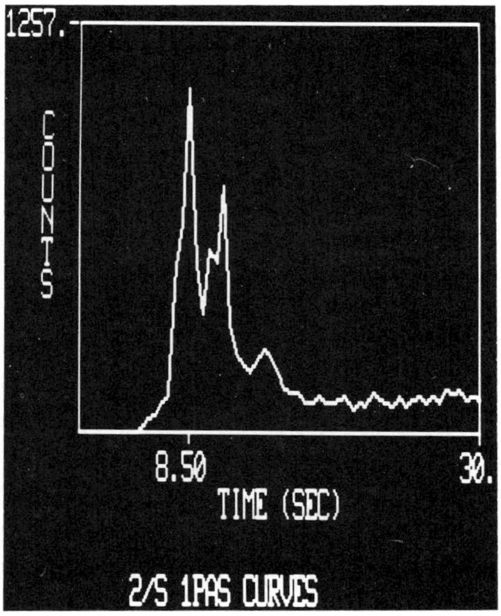

Figure 4. Time-activity curve generated over the right atrium in a child who made a Valsalva maneuver during bolus injection, resulting in a double peak.

The choice of pharmaceutical agent includes technetium in the pertechnetate form, technetium-labeled human serum albumin, and in vivo or in vitro labeled red blood cells. The pertechnetate may be used for angiography or first-pass shunt quantitation but is not suitable for cardiac output or gated blood pool scanning. Thyroid uptake is also greater when technetium is used in the salt form. In vitro red blood cell labeling is a time-consuming process. In vivo red blood cell labeling is the method of choice in adult cardiac studies because it is easy to perform and results in an improved target-to-background ratio of activity.[36] In pediatric studies, human serum albumin is preferred because it requires a single injection, whereas in vivo red blood cell labeling requires pretreatment with stannous pyrophosphate before the injection of technetium pertechnetate. The likelihood of obtaining cooperation from a child after two separate injections is small. The materials cannot be administered via the same intravenous line. If the stannous pyrophosphate extravasates and is thereby incompletely introduced into the circulation or if red blood cell uptake is reduced owing to severe anemia[12] or sickle hemoglobin,[31] labeling may be incomplete. Human serum albumin is commercially available in unit-dose or five-dose kits to which the technetium is added before injection.

Radionuclide pharmaceutical dosages are based on weight. The activity is distributed throughout the body. Sufficient activity must remain in the target organ so that after penetration through the tissues, adequate numbers of emissions will reach the detector. Relatively small doses may be used for cardiac studies of children because these subjects tend to be thin, permitting the detector to be placed very close to the heart and providing little subcutaneous tissue to attenuate the radioactive emissions. Potentially harmful effects of radiation are related to dosage per body weight, organ uptake, and radiosensitivity. Factors such as years of life expectancy in which to develop cancer, and the potential for genetic alterations in an individual who may subsequently bear children, increase the risk from radioactivity for the pediatric population. The recommended dosage for cardiac studies in pediatric patients is 0.2 to 0.3 mCi/kg.[5] There is, however, a limit to how small a dose will produce adequate activity for imaging. A minimum dose of 2 mCi for term infants and 1 mCi for premature infants is given. Table 1 provides a comparison of estimated radiation exposure from 0.2 mCi/kg of technetium-labeled human serum albumin and four plain x-rays of the abdomen. As one can see, the radionuclide studies compare quite favorably with x-ray examinations when the patient is more than ten years of age. The decision whether to perform such an examination must be based on the relative benefit to the child. The radionuclide study is justified if the information to be gained will result in a significant improvement in the patient's management.

Table 1. *Comparison of Radiation Effect in mRads of Technetium-99m HSA (200 μCi/kg) and Four X-Rays of the Abdomen*

Target	Radiation Source	Age (yr) 1	5	10	15	Adult
IMMEDIATE EFFECT						
Blood	Nuclear	605	650	630	660	672
Skin	X-ray	200	320	720	1000	1200
LONG TERM—CANCER EFFECT						
Whole Body	Nuclear	150	162	174	187	210
Bone Marrow	X-ray	—	—	—	—	88
LATENT—GENETIC EFFECT						
Ovary	Nuclear	549	548	650	715	756
Ovary	X-ray	—	—	—	—	204

Administering small doses of radionuclide in first-pass studies offers an advantage, since camera efficiency is dependent upon count rate. Failure to perceive all the scintillations that reach the gamma camera in the time allotted is called dead time loss. Time-activity curves obtained as the radioactive bolus enters the central circulation will be blunted initially when counts are lost owing to dead time. Subsequently, as the bolus is diluted, all of the activity will be counted. Dead time corrections are often necessary in patients who receive large doses. This type of correction is usually not necessary in pediatric studies.

Some degree of magnification is often necessary in first-pass studies of children. A high-resolution parallel-hole collimator is usually sufficient. A highly converging collimator is suggested for infants. Other techniques such as computer zooming may be inappropriate for first-pass studies in which a large field is to be examined. This type of study utilizes only the central field of the gamma camera for acquisition. If the bolus is to be checked before it enters the heart and the lungs are to be included for shunt determination, the central portion of the detector may be too small to view the necessary area.

Framing rates vary on computer systems; however, a rate of two frames per sec is adequate for patients with heart rates less than 100 beats per min; for faster rates, three frames per sec may be utilized. More rapid framing rates do not provide additional information and result in noisy images and increased processing time. The gamma camera is turned on just before injection of the radionuclide to be certain that the earliest entry of the bolus is recorded. The study must not be terminated before the bolus has cleared the left ventricle. Thirty sec is usually more than enough time to accomplish these goals.

First-pass studies are acquired in word mode to avoid overflow of pixels. If pixels are permitted to overflow owing to the concentrated activity of the bolus, information is lost. The static image obtained a few minutes after injection represents the distribution of the technetium-labeled albumin after equilibration. The image is needed for the cardiac output determination. Equilibration of albumin has been reported to be complete 10 min after injection.[38] In patients with low cardiac output, equilibration may take as long as 20 min.[15] In the majority of children studied in our laboratory, very little additional equilibration occurs after 3 min (Fig. 6). The

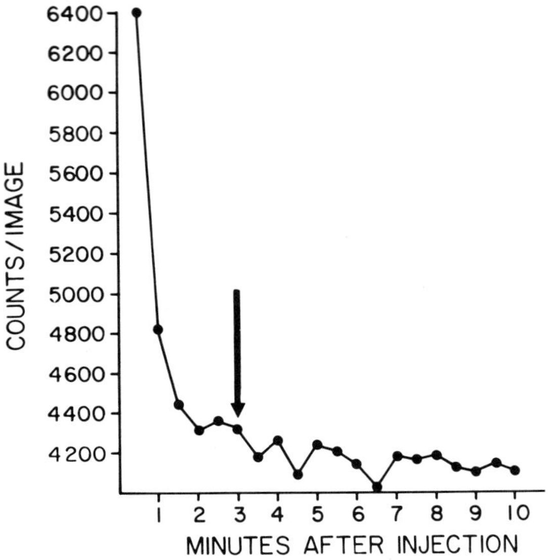

Figure 6. Equilibration of technetium-99m albumin. Activity from the left ventricular region of interest is plotted. Little additional equilibration occurs after 3 min.

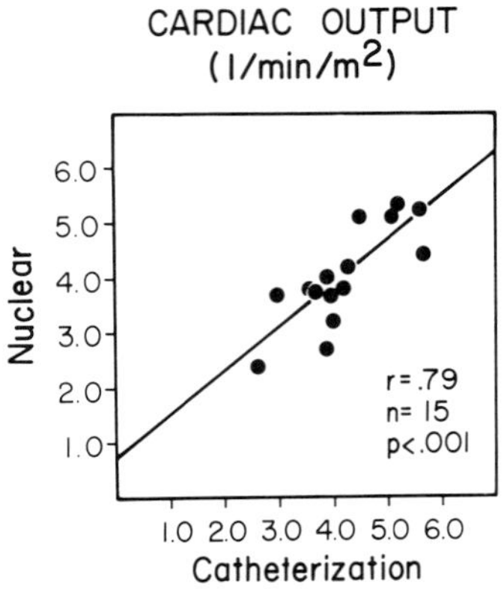

Figure 7. Comparison of cardiac output determined from first-pass time-activity curves and by the Fick method. A fair correlation was found.

likelihood of successfully immobilizing a child for more than 3 min is so small that we prefer to obtain our equilibrium image early rather than risk introducing error from movement of the patient.

Image processing is performed in a standard manner. The technique by which frames are added to produce a composite image and to identify the right atrium and left ventricle has been described. Time-activity curves over these two locations reflect cardiac output of the right and left sides of the heart. The washout phase of curves over the right atrium and left ventricle are fit exponentially by the computer and thus do not have to conform as rigorously as do curves for shunt analysis. Lesions that cause left ventricular volume overload, such as ventricular septal defect and patent ductus arteriosus, result in a proportional increase in left ventricular cardiac output, whereas atrial septal defects cause a relative increase in right atrial output. Although the absolute measurement of cardiac output by this technique has only a fair correlation with cardiac output determined by the Fick method (Fig. 7), the internal relationship between right atrial and left ventricular output is quite consistent (Fig. 5). Curves over the right lung are analyzed for left-to-right shunt by the gamma variant method of Maltz and Treves.[25] Comparison of right atrial, right lung, and left ventricular curves provides a useful method for detection of left-sided valvular regurgitation. The absence of detectable recirculation at right atrial and right lung levels and the presence of such a recirculation in the left ventricle suggest mitral or aortic regurgitation (Fig. 8).

The MUGA Scan. After equilibration of technetium-labeled albumin, changes in activity within the left ventricular chamber may be

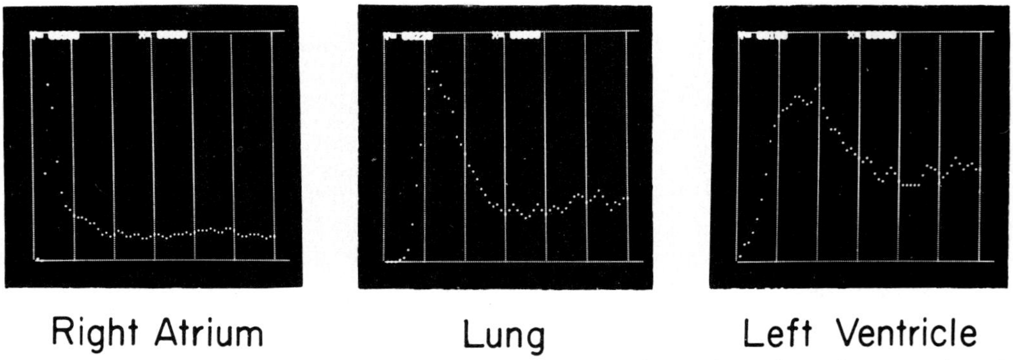

Figure 8. Time-activity curves from right atrium, lung, and left ventricle are shown for qualitative analysis. The left ventricular curve with delayed clearance of activity suggests recirculation of radionuclide. The absence of recirculation proximal to the left ventricle narrows the possible diagnoses to aortic or mitral insufficiency.

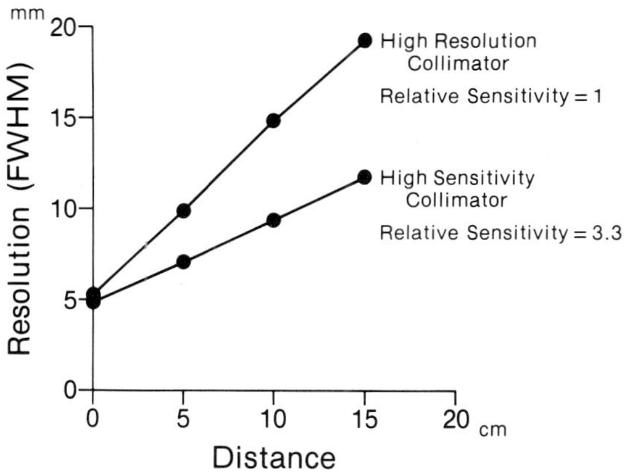

Figure 9. Comparison of the effect of collimator type on resolution (FWHM), as the detector is brought closer to a radioactive line source. When the structure to be imaged (left ventricle) is close to the detector (as in a child), a high-sensitivity collimator offers nearly the same resolution as a high-resolution collimator with three times the sensitivity. FWHM: full width at half maximum.

measured to reflect left ventricular function. Whereas first-pass studies rely upon temporal separation of cardiac structures, the gated equilibrium scans require physical separation of the left ventricle from overlying structures. The ventricles are separated in a left anterior oblique projection, which directs the plane of the collimator perpendicular to the interventricular septum. Optimum separation of the left atrium from the left ventricle requires a 10 to 15° caudal tilt. In infants, if the caudal tilt is too steep, the cardiac apex and liver may overlap. Because the left atrium is separated from the crystal by other structures, attenuation reduces its contribution to the calculated ejection fraction.

Gamma camera collimator design is usually such that the sensitivity of a parallel-hole collimator remains constant independent of distance but varies greatly from collimator to collimator. On the other hand, the resolution of these collimators changes with distance from the collimator, as shown in Figure 9. The high-sensitivity collimator can be used on children, whose bodies are much smaller than those of adults, thus gaining sensitivity but not losing much resolution as long as the organ to be imaged remains close to the collimator face. If, however, the left ventricular chamber is so small that it covers too few pixels to delineate the edges of the ventricle adequately, then magnification becomes essential. In children weighing less than 15 kg, automated edge detection may be inadequate to outline the left ventricle in end systole. In children of this size, acquisition must be performed in zoom mode. This is an electronic method that permits information received at the center of the crystal to be spread over a large number of computer pixels. The same number of events spread over a larger area increases the ease with which the computer can determine the borders of the left ventricle, especially if the data are filtered to eliminate noise. For the newborn—in particular, the premature infant—additional magnification is necessary. This may be accomplished through collimation. Figure 10 shows a gated equilibrium scan on a 1200-gm infant obtained with a 4-mm

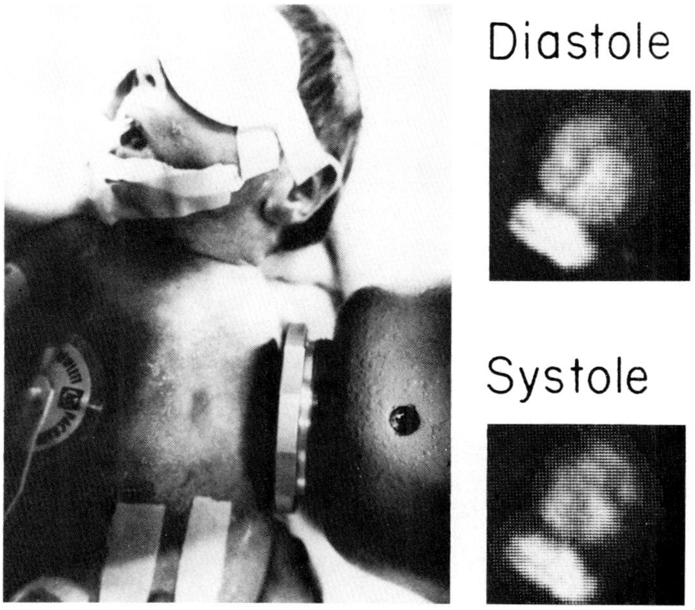

Figure 10. MUGA scan of a 1200-gm infant obtained with a pinhole collimator.

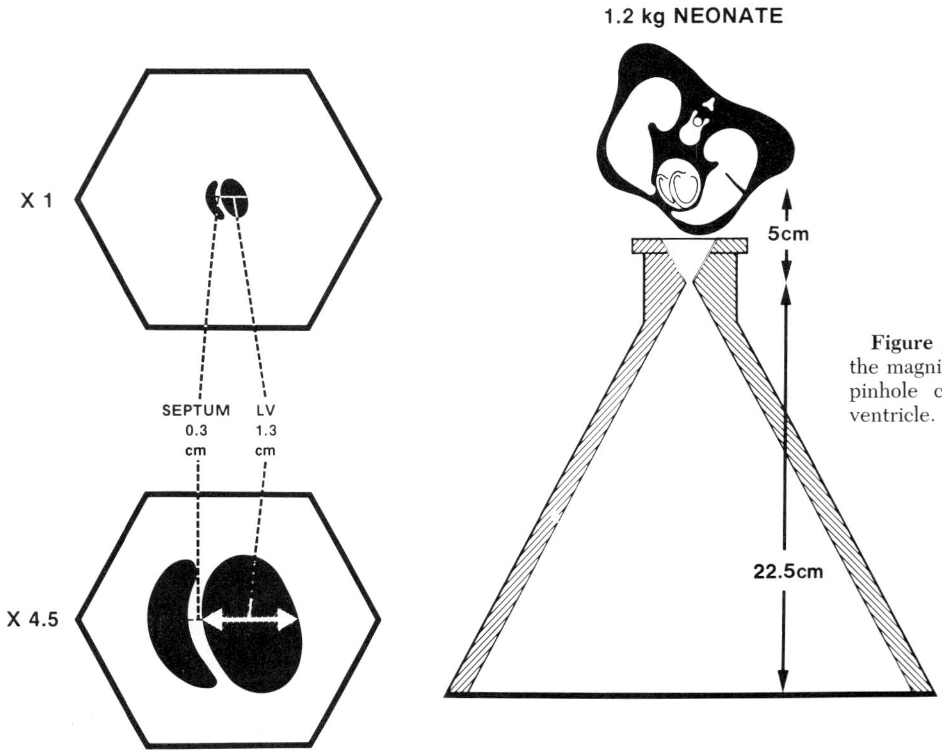

Figure 11. Demonstration of the magnification possible with pinhole collimation. LV: left ventricle.

pinhole collimator. The left ventricle is magnified 4.5 times on the surface of the crystal (Fig. 11). When applying this technique, if one is not careful to center the area of interest in the field of view of the pinhole collimator, peripheral structures may be distorted owing to a lack of field uniformity. In spite of an inherent limitation of resolution of the gamma camera (3 to 4 mm), size in itself does not prohibit imaging even the smallest heart.

In children the dose of radiopharmaceutical is adjusted for body weight and thus is relatively constant per milliliter of blood volume. However, cardiac volumes are smaller, so there is the problem of trying to image a smaller amount of activity, which leads to increased noise. A frame rate of 12 to 14 frames per cycle is used to increase counts per image and still gives adequate temporal resolution for ejection fraction calculation.[17] A 10-min acquisition results in 20 to 30,000 counts over the left ventricle in the end-diastolic frame. Attainment of counts per frame that result in statistically reliable studies requires a trade-off between acquisition time and radioactive dose. Since we are restricted by safety considerations in pediatric practice in the amount of radioactivity to be administered, an increased acquisition time may be necessary to provide high-quality images. In the critically ill or unconscious patient, this increase represents no problem. However, in the ambulatory child it may be difficult and sometimes impossible to immobilize the patient long enough to obtain a study of quality. For this reason, we perform a series of 1-min gated acquisitions. Afterward, we combine those 1-min acquisitions to obtain up to 10 min worth of data. If the patient moves or has a significant change in heart rate, the preceding acquisition is unaffected. This minimizes the necessity for having the child be still for 10 consecutive min.

A standardized approach to processing of scans and the use of automated edge detection programs result in highly reproducible measurements of left ventricular ejection fraction. Inter- and intraobservation errors are small.[28] Little error is introduced from short acquisition times or left atrial overlap.[28] The alternative to the gated equilibrium technique is the first-pass study with rapid framing rates. This technique, however, suffers from low count images and all the problems associated with bolus administration in children.

Ejection fraction and the change in ejection fraction with interventions such as exercise are valuable indicators of cardiac performance. Changes in counts ejected per beat or per minute also reflect alterations in cardiac performance. In the absence of a known relationship between counts and volume of blood, relative measurements of a stroke volume (counts ejected/beat) and cardiac output (counts ejected/min) may be obtained after correcting each image for the number of cardiac cycles processed and the time per frame.[34] A comparison of the output in counts per frame of the right and left ventricles provides additional valuable information. The stroke volumes of the ventricles should be equal in the absence of intracardiac shunting or valvular regurgitation. Comparison of right and left ventricular stroke counts provides a tool for shunt quantitation[9] or quantitation of valvular regurgitation.[30] With our technique, in which we routinely follow a bolus injection with a static image at 3 min and a MUGA scan, we thus have three opportunities to quantitate left-to-right shunt. We obtain the typical right lung curve for shunt analysis, we obtain a first-pass cardiac output over the right atrium and left ventricle, and we obtain left versus right ventricular stroke counts. This increases the likelihood of obtaining an accurate shunt determination in the child. The quantitation of valvular regurgitation may play a critical role in the evaluation of the pediatric patient. Such a situation is demonstrated in Figure 12, in which an infant who developed low cardiac output after total repair of an atrioventricular (AV) canal defect was identified as having severe mitral regurgitation due to a breakdown, in the repair of the anterior mitral leaflet. No left-to-right shunt was present on first-pass study.

Utilizing count information to make absolute measurements such as end-diastolic volume is not as reliable as comparing chambers within an image or changes from moment to moment on an equilibrium scan. In adults, attenuation of counts through the chest wall is of major concern. The pediatric patient is ideal in that the child is usually quite thin. The proximity of areas of concentrated activity represents a source of error in pediatric patients because of scatter. The wide range of body shape and size also contributes to the difficulty in relating left ventricular activity to volume. The area-length method is unsuitable in the smaller patient unless adequate magnification is obtained and counts are high enough for accurate edge detection. Two additional methods are in use. The first technique involves obtaining a blood sample and counting it.[33] The second method involves imaging the left ventricle at two different angles to derive a correction for attenuation.[23] An excellent correlation of radionuclide-derived ventricular volume with angiography has been found in children, but the standard error of the estimate is quite large.[27]

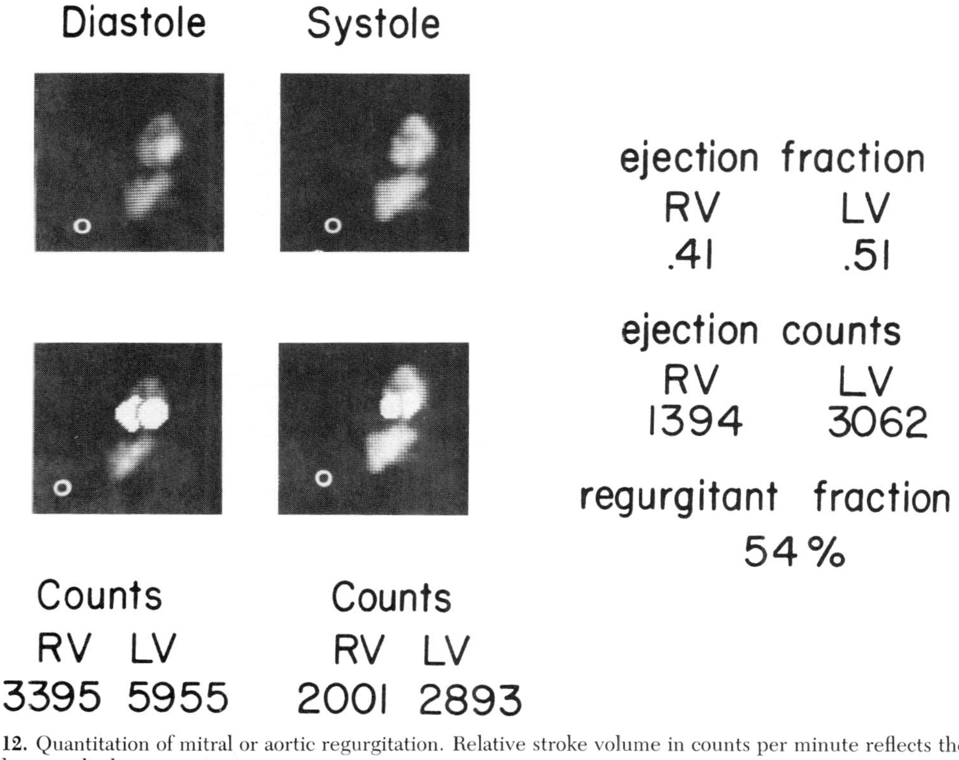

Figure 12. Quantitation of mitral or aortic regurgitation. Relative stroke volume in counts per minute reflects the volume overload due to valvular regurgitation.

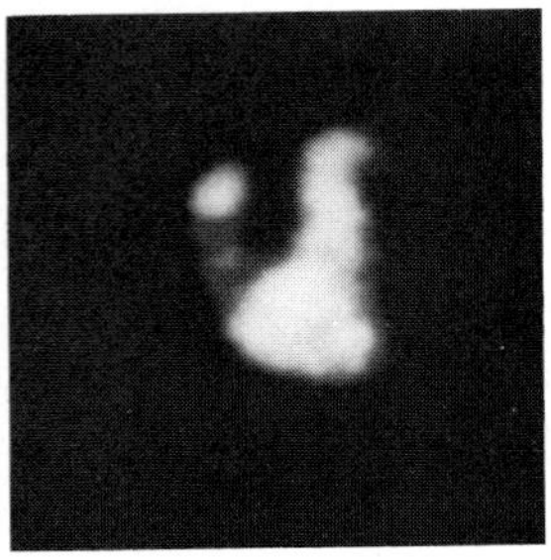

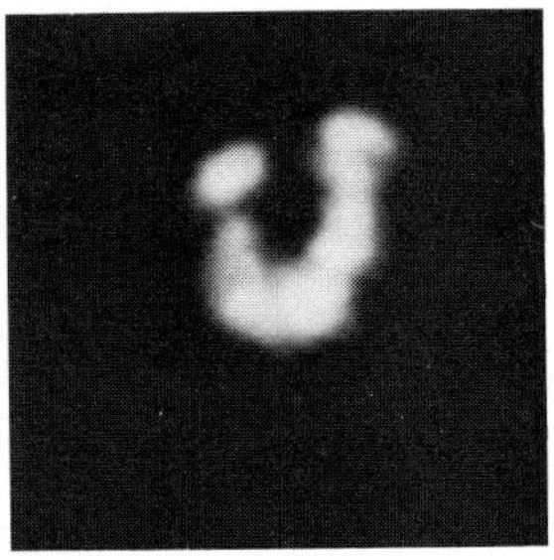

Figure 13. Composite end-diastolic and end-systolic images obtained from electrocardiographic gating of the passage of a bolus through the right ventricle. The images represent the average of three to five cardiac cycles.

Ejection fraction may be measured for the right ventricle as well as the left from a MUGA scan.[27] Reasonable results may be obtained if care is taken in positioning. The right atrial contribution to the right ventricular ejection fraction may be significant. If highly reliable, right ventricular ejection fractions are desired, it is preferable to perform a gated first-pass study (Fig. 13). The end-diastolic and end-systolic images represent a composite of three to five cardiac cycles. No background correction is necessary. Separation of right atrium and right ventricle is accomplished with ease.

The MUGA scan is of value in detecting wall motion abnormalities. This analysis is, however, infrequently used in the evaluation of the pediatric patient. Wall motion is assessed in the right anterior oblique projection as well as in the usual left anterior oblique view obtained for ejection fraction determination. Qualitative assessments are made from a movie of the cardiac cycle displayed in an endless loop. Abnormalities may be defined further by overlaying edge images from end-systolic and end-diastolic frames. A variety of quantitative methods for study of regional wall motion are available. These methods generally depend upon dividing the left ventricle into quadrants and measuring regional ejection fractions.[11]

Diastolic left ventricular function may be assessed from an equilibrium radionuclide scan.[6] Because the scan results from the combination of hundreds of cardiac cycles of varying length, events occurring in diastole may not be adequately examined from a routine study. List mode computer techniques allow one to examine diastolic filling by selecting data taken with a minimal variation in cycle length, by reformatting with reverse gating, and by acquiring data at a rapid rate.

PEDIATRIC EXERCISE TESTING

Information to Be Obtained During Exercise. Much progress has been made since the initial observation that the stress ejection fraction is of value in detecting patients with coronary artery disease.[8] The radionuclide ejection fraction, however, remains the most achievable and valuable measure of global left ventricular function. The radionuclide ejection fraction determination is free of geometric assumptions and requires no external calibration, since it represents a ratio. Count-related changes in left ventricular end-diastolic volume and cardiac output may be measured during exercise, greatly enhancing the interpretation of the radionuclide exercise test.[34] Regional left ventricular function is assessed using wall motion analyses[11] and diastolic function with filling rates.[6] Right ventricular ejection fraction may also be measured during exercise if the study is designed appropriately.[27]

Myocardial perfusion or thallium scanning during exercise is of limited value in pediatric practice. The isotope is normally injected 1 to 2 min before reaching maximum exercise. The exercise is completed, and then the patient, in the supine position, is imaged from several projections. Several hours later, redistribution images are obtained. A cold spot in the left ventricular myocardium, which resolves after redistribution, suggests coronary insufficiency. The resolution of the gamma camera is suitable for detecting transmural defects but inadequate for detecting subendocardial ischemia. Although coronary anomalies are rare in childhood, the test is of value as a screening test for coronary arteriography (Fig. 14) in the child with a provocative history (exercise-induced chest pain or syncope) and a negative stress electrocardiogram.

Technique. A continuous, graded, maximal exercise test has been developed that is well suited to making the radionuclide measurements and interpreting them. Physical working capacity varies widely in childhood and depends on age, height, weight, muscle mass, sex, strength, and endurance.[1] To make comparisons between patients with heart disease and heter-

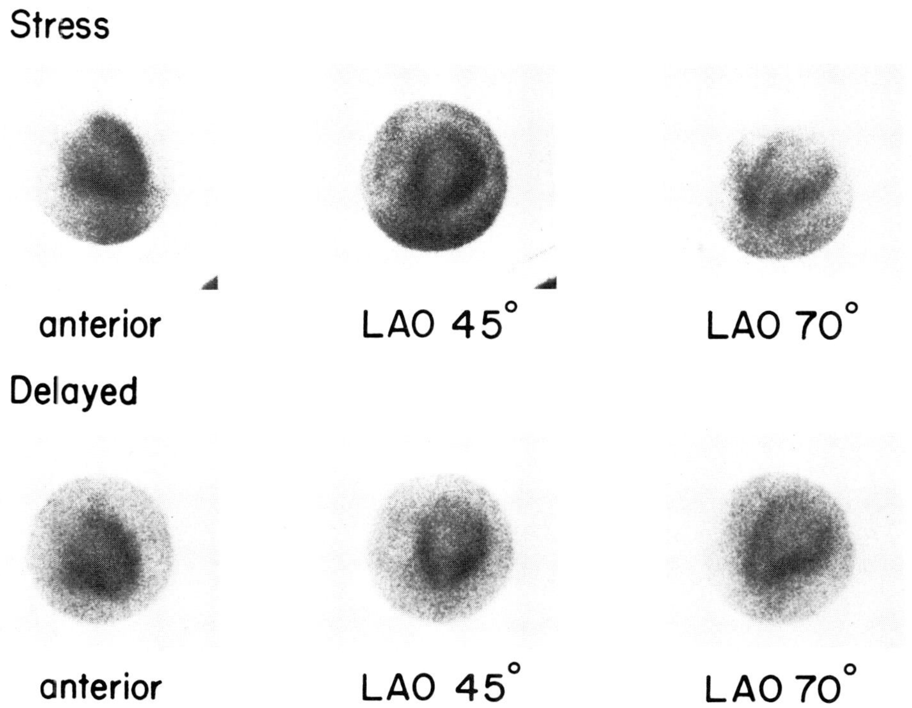

Figure 14. Thallium stress test. Above: Thallium was injected during the last minute of a maximal test. The immediate recovery images for three projections are shown. There is an apical cold spot that improves somewhat on the delayed images. Below Delayed images were obtained several hours later. The improvement suggests that the area involved was ischemic during exercise. This eight-year-old boy had an aberrant left coronary artery and apical akinesis on angiography. LAO: left anterior oblique.

ogeneous controls, a meaningful end point such as maximal voluntary effort is necessary. A continuous protocol was chosen because children are more likely to cooperate during a single large effort than during repeated efforts with breaks between.

First-pass or equilibrium radionuclide techniques may be used during exercise. First-pass studies require an injection of radioisotope as a bolus for each determination. The radiation dose is thereby increased, and the patient must exercise with an intravenous line in place. Equilibrium techniques are, therefore, better suited for pediatric patients. Serial measurements may be made for several hours after the injection of technetium-labeled human serum albumin into a peripheral vein. Owing to background activity, however, the ejection fraction obtained is of necessity an average of hundreds of cardiac cycles. Equilibrium measurements are thus sensitive to patient motion and changes in heart rate during the acquisition of a study. A graded test consists of several 3-min exercise stages. The subject exercises at a predetermined work load based on height or weight, which is increased with every stage. Heart rate equilibrates during the first minute of each exercise stage, and radionuclide measurements are made during the last 2 min.

A variety of exercise techniques are in use. Little work has been done using treadmill exercise, however, owing to the difficulty of imaging in this position. The procedure calls for the patients to lie down for imaging immediately after a maximum test. An intravenous bolus is administered, before the heart rate falls, to obtain a first-pass ejection fraction.

Supine exercise is popular because the patient's position under the detector is easily maintained. The patient lies on his or her back with a cycle ergometer mounted over the exercise table. Shoulder blocks eliminate motion. The camera is rotated to the proper obliquity.

A radionuclide exercise test is more difficult to accomplish in the sitting position, but the rewards are great. The ejection fraction response to exercise is more consistent and of a greater magnitude in the sitting position.[32, 35] Immobilization of the patient is generally accomplished by having the patient sit on a table with the table back upright so that the patient is supported. The subject's chest is wedged between the backboard and camera. This position is somewhat restrictive, however, since children usually bob when performing sitting cycle exercise. For this reason, the adjustable wedge mold and harness were developed to hold the patient's chest to the camera in the

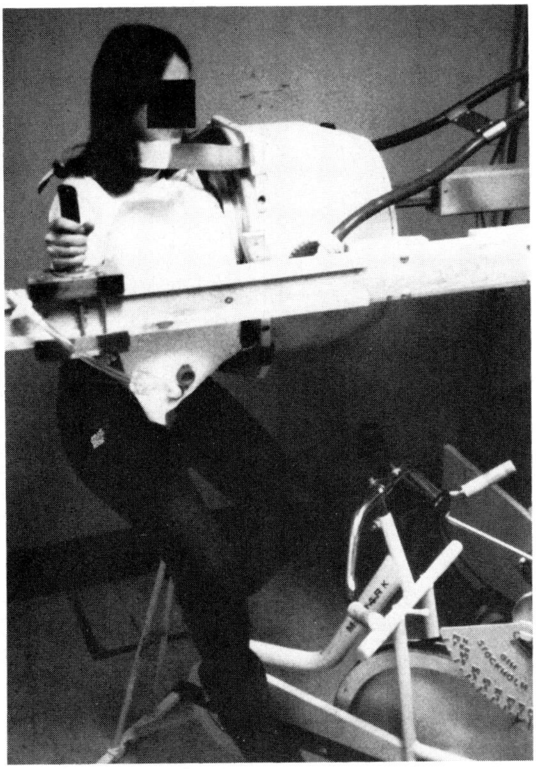

Figure 15. The adjustable wedge mold and harness are displayed. The subject is harnessed to the gamma camera and sits on the cycle ergometer. The wedge mold maintains the proper obliquity for equilibrium imaging and eliminates patient-detector motion.

proper obliquity for equilibrium blood pool imaging (Fig. 15). The camera-patient assembly moves together as the patient pedals on the cycle ergometer.

The effectiveness of the adjustable wedge mold was tested in a series of experiments. A radioactive point source was fastened to the chest of volunteers who exercised with the wedge mold or with other restraining devices. The full width at half maximum activity of the point source was obtained during exercise, with the gamma camera, to determine if motion was eliminated (Fig. 16). The results of this study are shown in Table 2. The adjustable wedge mold and harness successfully eliminated patient-detector motion in both horizontal and vertical directions. Without this device, motion was significant, especially in subjects with less strength and when fatigue developed.

A parallel-hole, high-sensitivity collimator is used to maximize count rates owing to the necessity of a short acquisition time. The wedge mold is kept flat over the left precordium so that the camera is no more than 2 cm from the chest wall. A Brattle physiologic electrocardiographic gate triggers the computer (Medical Data Systems*), which records what the gamma camera observes during the last 2 min of each 3-min exercise stage.

The Normal Response to Exercise. No data have been published as yet for radionuclide measurements during exercise for normal children. It is difficult to justify administering radionuclides to normal children, so standards for our laboratory are based on a group of children whose condition approximates a normal one. Twelve adolescents who underwent cardiac catheterization because of chest pain or mild valvular obstruction or insufficiency, or for postoperative assessment, made up our control group. Left ventricular function was normal on angiography, and a nonnuclear exercise test was normal. Resting ejection fraction was 0.67 ± 0.08 (mean ± SD). At maximum, upright exercise ejection fraction rose to 0.81 ± 0.07. End-diastolic volume was unchanged with exercise, becoming 1.0 ± 0.10 times resting diastolic volume at maximum exercise. Cardiac output was 2.78 ± 0.26 times resting output at maximum exercise.

The normal ejection fraction response was a stepwise increase with increasing work. Abnormal responses for our laboratory included an ejection fraction at maximum that was less than the resting value; a decline in ejection fraction greater than 0.05 during increasing exercise and heart rate; and no change in ejection fraction with exercise. The abnormal patterns were seen with poor cardiac output responses, decreased work capacity, and/or electrocardiographic signs of ischemia. One patient with a flat ejection fraction curve had a normal exercise test, but all the ejection fractions, including the resting value, were greater than 0.80.

Interpretation of the radionuclide exercise test depends upon the subject's reaching maximum voluntary effort. Since abnormal tests are often associated with a reduced heart rate response, it is important to differentiate an abnormal test from a submaximal effort. Observing the subject when exercise is terminated can be very helpful in determining whether a maximal effort has been made. Oxygen consumption measurements may be obtained to see if the patient has exceeded his or her anaerobic threshold.

The Effect of Position on Exercise Responses. The cardiac output achieved at maximum during supine exercise is slightly greater than that for sitting exercise. Stroke volume is greater at rest during supine exercise and

*Medical Data Systems, 2311 Green Rd., Ann Arbor, Michigan 48105.

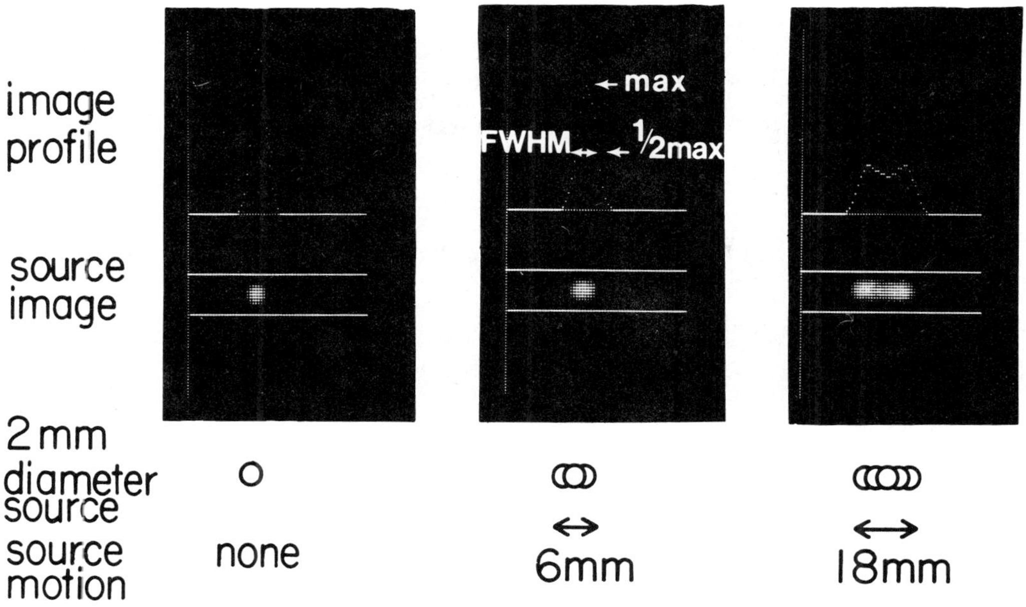

Figure 16. Technique for assessing patient-detector motion. A radioactive point source was placed on the chest of volunteers to detect motion or blurring of images. This illustration demonstrates the appearance of a point source that was mechanically oscillated and the significance of changes in the full width at half maximum (FWHM) of the distribution of counts when the source was imaged. The greater the blurring due to motion, the larger the FWHM will be.

changes little with exercise. Stroke volume increases significantly during sitting exercise.[35] The cardiac output response to maximum exercise is therefore achieved differently, depending upon the position in which the subject exercises. These differences must be taken into account in the evaluation of subjects with heart disease because the physiologic adaptation to the patient's abnormality may be different, depending upon the position. Furthermore, the adaptation may or may not be as successful for the same work load in a given position. Exercise studies on children with aortic stenosis provide an example of this phenomenon. We exercised four children with aortic stenosis in the upright position. Ejection fractions were high even at rest. During exercise, the ejection fractions were so high that fluctuations were meaningless. The obstructed left ventricles were virtually disappearing during systole. The patient with the most severe obstruction had a fall in ejection fraction at maximum exercise. Whereas changes in ejection fraction were not helpful in the assessment of the degree of aortic stenosis except in the most severely affected individual, physiologic adaptation was accomplished by dilating the left ventricle to increase stroke volume. In fact, the percentage increase in left ventricular end-diastolic volume was related to the degree of aortic stenosis (Fig. 17). An echocardiographic study of left ventricular performance during supine exercise in children with aortic stenosis revealed a significant increase in contractility in response to submaximal exercise.[10] A possible explanation for the discrepancy between findings on exercise performed in upright and supine positions in children with aortic stenosis is as follows: Patients with aortic stenosis, when lying supine, will experience a slight increase in left ventricular end-diastolic volume. A lower ejection fraction will be required at rest to maintain the resting cardiac

Table 2. *Comparison of Wedge Mold and Harness with Other Methods of Eliminating Patient-Detector Motion*

	FOAM WEDGE/TAPE			FOAM WEDGE/HARNESS			MOLD/HARNESS		
	Mean	*SD*	*Max*	*Mean*	*SD*	*Max*	*Mean*	*SD*	*Max*
Horizontal motion (mm)	4.4	4.6	13.0	4.3	5.3	18.8	0.5	0.6	1.6
Vertical motion (mm)	2.4	3.2	8.4	1.1	2.2	7.8	0.7	1.7	4.2

SD: standard deviation; Max: maximum.

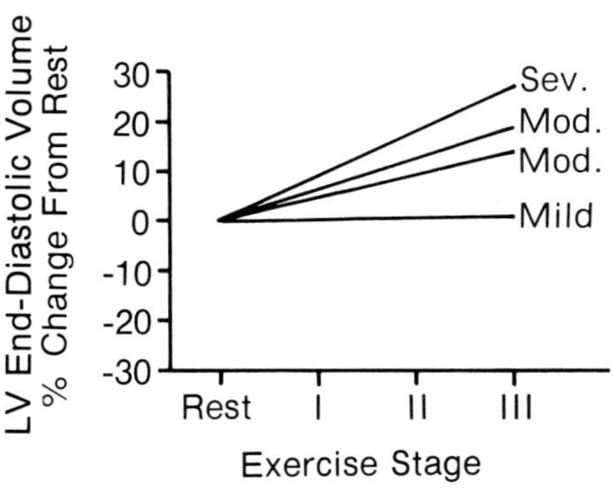

Figure 17. Change in left ventricular (LV) end-diastolic volume with exercise. The degree of aortic stenosis is displayed as mild, moderate (mod.), or severe (sev.) based on catheterization findings. A greater degree of left ventricular dilatation developed with exercise in patients with more severe aortic stenosis.

output. As the subject exercises, ejection fraction may increase from the lower resting level to result in an appropriate increase in cardiac output.

Reliability of Radionuclide Measurements. The radionuclide ejection fraction performed from an equilibrium blood pool study is the most reproducible of the radionuclide determinations. Accurate results may be obtained with as little as 1½ to 2 min of acquisition. Interobserver differences of 1 to 2 per cent have been encountered in interpretation of studies. Less than 2 per cent variation was encountered when a single observer processed the same study on different occasions.[28] Count-related changes in end-diastolic volume and cardiac output during exericse have been validated by Fick cardiac outputs with measured oxygen consumption.[34] Absolute measurements of left ventricular end-diastolic volume have an excellent correlation with volumes obtained from left ventricular angiograms in pediatric patients.[27] The standard error of the estimate, however, is quite large. The measurement of absolute cardiac output from first-pass technique has only a fair correlation with Fick cardiac outputs (Fig. 7). Cardiac outputs so derived are only reasonable approximations. Right ventricular ejection fraction is less reliable than left ventricular measurements using equilibrium technique owing to right atrial overlap. A computer technique called phase analysis may be helpful to demonstrate the degree of overlap of right atrium and right ventricle.[22] First-pass gated right ventricular ejection fractions are not plagued by this problem because the chambers may be separated temporally as well as spatially.

Applications. Radionuclide exercise testing has been applied to patients with aortic and mitral valvular insufficiency to describe the pathophysiology, to aid in the timing of surgery, and to evaluate the postoperative patient.[7] Several studies have been performed in children after repair of cyanotic congenital heart defects. Reduto et al.[29] performed first-pass right and left ventricular ejection fractions during upright exercise on 16 children after repair of tetralogy of Fallot. In spite of excellent hemodynamics and normal left ventricular ejection fraction responses, an exercise-induced drop in right ventricular ejection fraction was observed in 13 patients. Only one patient had an abnormal right ventricular ejection fraction at rest. Parrish et al.[26] reported a drop in right ventricular ejection fraction in two of three children who had Mustard's operation for repair of transposition of the great arteries. Harder et al.[18] studied 20 children with tricuspid atresia. Equilibrium left ventricular ejection fractions were performed during supine exercise. Of 13 children with normal resting ejection fractions, 2 had a fall in ejection fraction with exercise. Five of the 7 children with abnormal resting ejection fractions had a further decrease with exercise. The radionuclide stress test may also be useful in the assessment of cardiac rehabilitation programs for children who have surgery for congenital heart disease.

The radionuclide stress test is of value in the assessment of children with chest pain. Only those patients with a provocative history should be studied. An abnormal ejection fraction response has been described in patients with mitral valve prolapse.[4]

Left ventricular ejection fractions have been measured during submaximal supine exercise in children with cystic fibrosis.[13] An ischemic response was noted in two children with normal resting ejection fractions.

Radionuclide exercise tests have been performed to assess patients with thalassemia[21] and sickle cell anemia[14] and individuals undergoing chemotherapy with cardiotoxic drugs such as doxorubicin hydrochloride (Adriamycin).[3] The test provides information to evaluate the natural history of disease, the efficacy of treatments such as transfusion programs, and the ability of patients to engage in recreational sports activities.

Usage. Radionuclide studies may be performed in any hospital whose nuclear medicine department has a computer dedicated for nuclear imaging and an ECG gating device. The equipment, although expensive, is universally available at this time. A radionuclide exercise test is, of necessity, an expensive procedure because of the large capital outlay for equipment. The test is time-consuming, taking nearly an hour to perform. The studies are justified, however, owing to the high density of information to be obtained noninvasively.

In summary, a radionuclide exercise test may be performed in either the upright or the supine position. The continuous, graded, maximal test is recommended for pediatric patients. Equilibrium techniques offer the advantage of serial measurements from a single dose of radionuclide. The interpretation of an ejection fraction response is dependent upon the end point of the test. Relative changes in cardiac output and end-diastolic volume provide complementary information to aid in the cardiac assessment. Valuable information may be obtained if patients are selected appropriately and studies are performed with proper design and attention to detail.

REFERENCES

1. Adams FH, Linde LM, Meyake H: The physical working capacity of normal school children. Pediatrics, *28*:55–64, 1961.
2. Alderson PO, Jost RG, Straus AW, et al: Radionuclide angiocardiography. Improved diagnosis and quantitation of left to right shunts in children using area ratio techniques. Circulation, *51*:1136–1143, 1975.
3. Alexander J, Dainiak N, Berger J, et al: Serial assessment of doxorubicin cardiotoxicity with quantitative radionuclide angiocardiography. N Engl J Med, *300*:278–283, 1979.
4. Andrews EJ Jr, Fleming JW, Mello M: Pitfalls in the diagnosis of myocardial ischemia using radionuclide techniques. Clin Nucl Med (abstract), *6*:144, 1981.
5. Ashburn WL, Alazraki NP: Cardiovascular: Shunt quantitation. *In* Handmaker H, Lowenstein JM (eds): Nuclear Medicine in Clinical Pediatrics. New York, Society of Nuclear Medicine, 1975, pp. 81–88.
6. Bonow RO, Bacharach SL, Green MV, et al: Impaired left ventricular diastolic filling in patients with coronary artery disease: Assessment with radionuclide cineangiography. Circulation, *64*:315–323, 1981.
7. Borer JS, Bacharach SL, Green MV, et al: Exercise induced left ventricular dysfunction in symptomatic and asymptomatic patients with aortic regurgitation: Assessment with radionuclide cineangiography. Am J Cardiol, *42*:351–357, 1978.
8. Borer JS, Bacharach SL, Green MV, et al: Real-time radionuclide cineangiography in the noninvasive evaluation of global and regional left ventricular function at rest and during exercise in patients with coronary artery disease. N Engl J Med, *296*:839–844, 1977.
9. Bough EW, Gandsman EJ, Benham ID, et al: Detection and quantitation of atrial shunts in adults by gated radionuclide angiography. Am J Cardiol (abstract), *45*:409, 1980.
10. Breitweser JA, Boerth RC, Graham TP Jr, et al: Divergent left ventricular response to exercise in children with left ventricular pressure or volume overload. Am J Cardiol (abstract), *47*:446, 1981.
11. Brown EJ, Wynne J, Holman BL, et al: Regional ejection fraction during exercise: A quantitative measurement to localize coronary artery stenosis. J Nucl Med (abstract), *22*:79, 1981.
12. Callahan RJ, Froelich JW, McKusick KA, et al: Factors affecting the rate and extent of incorporation of Tc 99m into pre-tinned red blood cells. J Nucl Med (abstract), *23*:109, 1982.
13. Chipps BE, Alderson PO, Roland JA, et al: Noninvasive evaluation of ventricular function in cystic fibrosis. J Pediatr, *95*:379–384, 1979.
14. Covitz W, Eubig C, Balfour IC, et al: Exercise induced cardiac dysfunction in sickle cell anemia: A Radionuclide study. Am J Cardiol, *51*:570–575, 1983.
15. Figueras J, Weil MH: Blood volume prior to and following treatment of acute cardiogenic pulmonary edema. Circulation, *57*:349–355, 1978.
16. Green MV, Bacharach SL, Douglas MA, et al: Sources of virtual background in multi-image blood pool studies. *In* Sorenson JA (ed): Nuclear Cardiology: Selected Computer Aspects. New York, Society of Nuclear Medicine, 1978, pp. 97–106.
17. Hamilton GW, Williams DL, Caldwell JH: Frame-rate requirements for recording time-activity curves by radionuclide angiocardiography. *In* Sorenson JA (ed): Nuclear Cardiology: Selected Computer Aspects. New York, Society of Nuclear Medicine, 1978, pp. 75–83.
18. Harder JR, Gilday DL, deSouza M, et al: Radionuclide assessment of left ventricular function in patients with tricuspid atresia. Am J Cardiol (abstract), *47*:458, 1981.
19. Hurley PJ, Wesselhoeft H, James AE Jr: Use of nuclear imaging in the evaluation of pediatric cardiac disease. Semin Nucl Med, *2*:353–372, 1972.
20. Kereiakes JG, Feller PA, Ascoli FA, et al: Pediatric radiopharmaceutical dosimetry. *In* Cloutier RJ, Coffey JL, Snyder WS, et al (eds): Radiopharmaceutical Dosimetry Symposium. Washington, D.C., U.S. Department of Health, Education and Welfare, Publication (FDA) 76–8044, 1976.
21. Leon MB, Borer JS, Bacharach SL, et al: Detection of early cardiac dysfunction in patients with severe beta-thalassemia and chronic iron overload. N Engl J Med, *301*:1143–1148, 1979.
22. Links JM, Douglass KH, Wagner HN Jr: Patterns of ventricular emptying by Fourier analysis of gated blood-pool studies. J Nucl Med, *21*:978–982, 1980.
23. Links JM, Becker LC, Schindledecker JG, et al: Measurement of absolute left ventricular volume from gated blood pool studies. Circulation, *65*:82–91, 1982.
24. MacIntyre WJ: In vivo tracer studies by external gamma ray counting. *In* Hine GJ (ed): Instrumentation in Nuclear Medicine. New York, Academic Press, 1967, pp. 353–364.
25. Maltz DL, Treves S: Qualitative radionuclide angiocardiography. Determination of Qp:Qs in children. Circulation, *47*:1049–1056, 1973.
26. Parrish MD, Graham TP Jr, Born ML, et al: Radionuclide evaluation of RV and LV function in children—cineangiographic validation and observations in transposition of the great arteries. Am J Cardiol (abstract), *47*:458, 1981.
27. Parrish MD, Graham TP, Born ML, et al: Radionuclide ventriculography for assessment of absolute right and left ventricular volumes in children. Circulation, *66*:811–819, 1982.
28. Pfisterer ME, Ricci DR, Schuler G, et al: Validity of left ventricular ejection fractions measured at rest and peak exercise by equilibrium radionuclide an-

giography using short acquisition times. J Nucl Med, *20*:484–490, 1979.
29. Reduto LA, Berger HJ, Johnstone DE, et al: Radionuclide assessment of right and left ventricular exercise reserve after total correction of tetralogy of Fallot. Am J Cardiol, *45*:1013–1018, 1980.
30. Rigo P, Alderson PO, Robertson RM, et al: Measurement of aortic and mitral regurgitation by gated cardiac blood pool scans. Circulation, *60*:306–312, 1979.
31. Riordan F, Nelp WB: Binding capacity of normal and sickle cell hemoglobin for technetium atoms. J Nucl Med (abstract), *23*:91, 1982.
32. Slutsky R: Response of the left ventricle to stress: Effects of exercise, atrial pacing, afterload stress and drugs. Am J Cardiol, *47*:357–364, 1981.
33. Slutsky R, Karliner J, Ricci D, et al: Left ventricular volumes by gated equilibrium radionuclide angiography: A new method. Circulation, *60*:556–564, 1979.
34. Sorenson SG, Ritchie JL, Caldwell H, et al: Serial exercise radionuclide angiography: Validation of count-derived changes in cardiac output and quantitation of maximal exercise ventricular volume change after nitroglycerin and propranolol in normal men. Circulation, *61*:600–609, 1980.
35. Thadani V, Parker JO: Hemodynamics at rest and during supine and sitting bicycle exercise in normal subjects. Am J Cardiol, *41*:52–59, 1978.
36. Thrall JH, Fredos JE, Swanson D, et al: Clinical comparison of cardiac blood pool visualization with technetium 99m and blood cells labelled in vivo and with technetium 99m human serum albumin. J Nucl Med, *19*:796–803, 1978.
37. Webster EW, Alpert NM, Brownell GL: Radiation doses in pediatric nuclear medicine and diagnostic x-ray procedure. *In* James AE, Wagner HN, and Cook RE (ed): Pediatric Nuclear Medicine. Philadelphia, W. B. Saunders, 1974, pp. 34–58.
38. Yang SSL, Nickoloff EL, McIntyre PA, et al: Tc-99m human serum albumin: A suitable agent for plasma volume measurement in man. J Nucl Med, *19*:804–807, 1978.

7

RADIONUCLIDE EVALUATION OF CARDIOCIRCULATORY PERFORMANCE AT REST AND WITH EXERCISE

ROBERT A. SLUTSKY, M.D.

Evaluation of cardiac contraction by qualitative and quantitative techniques has been of particular interest to physicians involved in the care of children with heart disease. The development of radionuclide techniques for evaluating right and left heart hemodynamics has been extensively validated in adults and has recently been applied to the pediatric patient population with increasing frequency. The purpose of this article will be (1) to discuss the types of radionuclide studies performed; (2) to analyze methods of evaluating left and right ventricular ejection fraction and volumes; (3) to review methods for calculating regurgitant valvular lesions; (4) to examine the effects of exercise and disease states on cardiac dynamics; and (5) to relate cardiac and pulmonary dynamics during disease conditions and forms of stress.

TECHNICAL CONSIDERATIONS

Global ventricular function and ventricular volume can be derived from radionuclide angiograms by geometric or count-based techniques. Much of the original work in adults with radionuclide imaging involved application of traditional area-length formulae to left ventricular images to derive left ventricular volumes and ejection fraction.[1, 3, 25, 26, 34, 39, 48, 49] While apparently reproducible, area-length calculations are difficult and by definition depend upon geometric assumptions. Thus, count-based methods for evaluation of left ventricular size and function have been developed and are currently the most commonly used approaches. These techniques involve imaging of the cardiac blood pool with an external imaging device, such as a probe or gamma scintillation camera.[3]

In general, two methods of radionuclide data analysis have been used. One involves evaluating the transit of a bolus of a radionuclide material as it passes through the central circulation (first-pass technique). The other approach involves evaluating the cardiac chambers while various radioactive substances circulate in the blood pool in a steady state. This is the so-called "equilibrium" or gated blood pool technique and involves analysis of multiple R-R intervals, producing a summed composite cardiac cycle.[3]

A variety of technetium-99m-labeled radiopharmaceuticals may be used for either of these procedures. First-transit studies can be done with virtually any agent that does not settle in the lungs (such as technetium-99m bound to protein macroaggregates). Any radiopharmaceutical that can be injected in a tight bolus is suitable. If repeated studies need be performed, the agents may be varied so that one agent is excreted by the kidneys and one excreted by the liver. For equilibrium studies, any blood pool imaging agent is suitable. The possibilities include technetium-99m bound to human serum albumin, in vitro labeled red cells, or in vivo labeled red blood cells.[34]

In general, first-transit studies can be performed with standard single-crystal Anger cameras. The use of multicrystal cameras increases statistical accuracy of the procedure with some loss of resolution. Simple dedicated nuclear computer systems are available for these analyses. Gated or equilibrium studies are usually performed with single-crystal cameras and dedicated computer systems, which are usually part of most general purpose nuclear computer software packages. Regions-of-interest can be placed over both the right and left ventricle, and time-activity curves produced for both chambers (Figs. 1 and 2).

By and large, most children will allow radionuclide imaging without significant sedation. Usually, a small (21 gauge) butterfly needle is adequate for rapid and tight bolus injections. Discomfort is minimized when antecubital veins are used, though an external jugular vein can be injected when alternative sites are not available. When gated equilibrium imaging is planned, the site and speed of injection are less important. During these studies, because it is not necessary or even advisable to acquire data rapidly after the administration of the radioisotope, it is somewhat less important that the child is neither crying nor breathing irregularly, though obviously patient motion and alterations in cardiac loading conditions may invalidate data obtained during short acquisition periods. In fact, the advantage of blood pool imaging in children is that it allows the child to become calm between the injection of the radioisotope and the actual acquisition of radionuclide data.

While the acceptable amount of the radionuclide is somewhat variable, we recommend using more than 2 mCi of technetium even in the smallest of children. A general dosage rule of 150 to 200 μCi/kg is followed for first-transit studies. Potassium perchlorate should be administered before injection of technetium-99m pertechnetate to minimize thyroid uptake. A minimum of 3 to 5 mCi of technetium-99m may be used for gated blood pool studies if in vitro red blood cell labeling is performed. Better images with short acquisition times can be obtained when the dosage approximates 10 mCi in a larger child or adolescent. The radiation exposure (whole body) is not markedly different with the gated or first-transit technique, though target organ exposure obviously may vary somewhat. With the advent of short-lived radioisotopes, frequent first-transit studies with almost negligible radiation exposure may become available and preferable for pediatric cardiac nuclear imaging. In particular ^{195m}Au may completely change the nature of first-transit radionuclide angiography. Its widest use may be in the pediatric patient because of its extremely short half-life (approximately 30 sec).

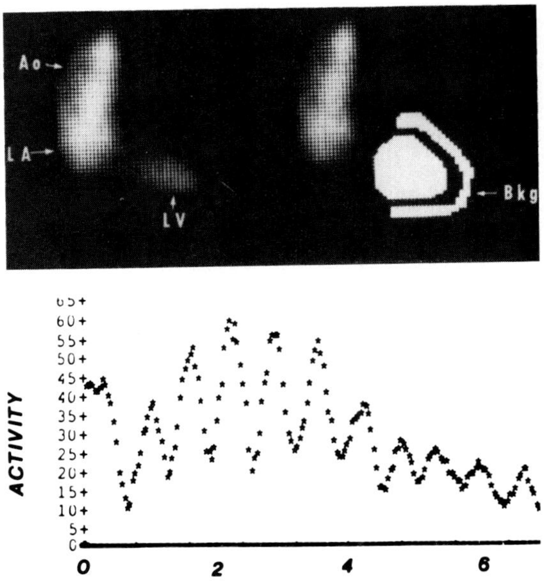

Figure 2. Left ventricular ejection fraction. Similar to Figure 1 in design. This illustration depicts a left ventricular region-of-interest assignment and the subsequent time-activity curve.

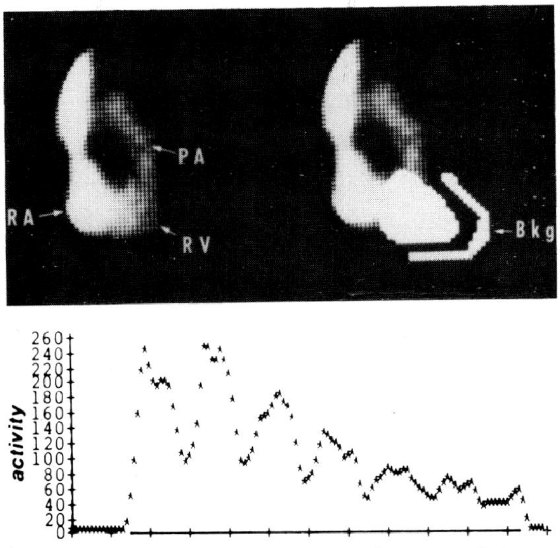

Figure 1. Right ventricular ejection fraction. A light pen algorithm is used to assign the right ventricle, and a background-corrected, time-activity curve produced. From the peaks (end-diastolic counts) and valleys (end-systolic counts), the ejection fraction can be calculated.

EVALUATION OF CARDIAC FUNCTION AND SIZE

First-Transit (First-Pass) Approach. This method requires the evaluation of the radioactive bolus as it passes in sequence through the right and left ventricle. A variety of camera projections can be used, the requirement being that the ventricles can be clearly seen and the valve planes located. Data are acquired in list or serial mode at a sampling frequency equal to or greater than 20 frames per second. Usually, the right and left ventricular time-activity curves are separated temporally. The computer operator then assigns either an end-diastolic left ventricular or right ventricular region-of-interest and the corresponding background region-of-interest. From these data, a background-corrected time-activity (volume) curve is generated. Ejection fraction can thus be calculated by evaluating multiple end-diastolic and end-systolic data points. In this situation, ejection fraction is a composite of [(end-diastolic counts − end-systolic counts) ÷ end-diastolic counts] for between 3 to 10 heart beats. This technique has been shown to correlate well with contrast ventriculography.[26]

The particular value of this approach is that it allows for both quantitative and qualitative analysis of the cardiac structures. The bolus can be followed as it travels sequentially through the various chambers and great vessels of the central circulation. This allows the examiner to characterize chamber and great vessel orientation along with localization of intracardiac shunts. For example, right-to-left shunts can be discerned by the early appearance of radioactivity in the left side of the circulation. Left-to-right shunts are made evident by prolonged recirculation in the right side of the heart (lungs), and regional obstruction such as in the superior vena cava or the pulmonary artery can be discerned if the bolus appears to "hang up" in certain portions of the circulation as it passes through the heart.

With the single-crystal camera, the first-pass angiogram can reliably estimate both right and left ventricular ejection fraction.[12, 31, 44] Analysis of absolute ventricular volume is even more difficult, although area-length methods have been successfully applied to first-pass angiograms derived from multicrystal cameras.[26] Intervention studies, however, require multiple injections and thus additional doses of radiotracers. Thus, these studies are limited by the number of data points that can be obtained.

Equilibrium Techniques. After the blood pool imaging radiotracer reaches a stable isotopic concentration, an electrocardiographic gate is used to time events in the cardiac cycle (Fig. 3). The electrocardiographic gate is used to accumulate multiple frames throughout the entire cycle, based on short acquisition intervals phased from the peak of the QRS complex. When multiple R-R intervals are summed and the resulting frames viewed in sequence, a cine format produces the illusion of ventricular contraction. The left ventricle can be assigned

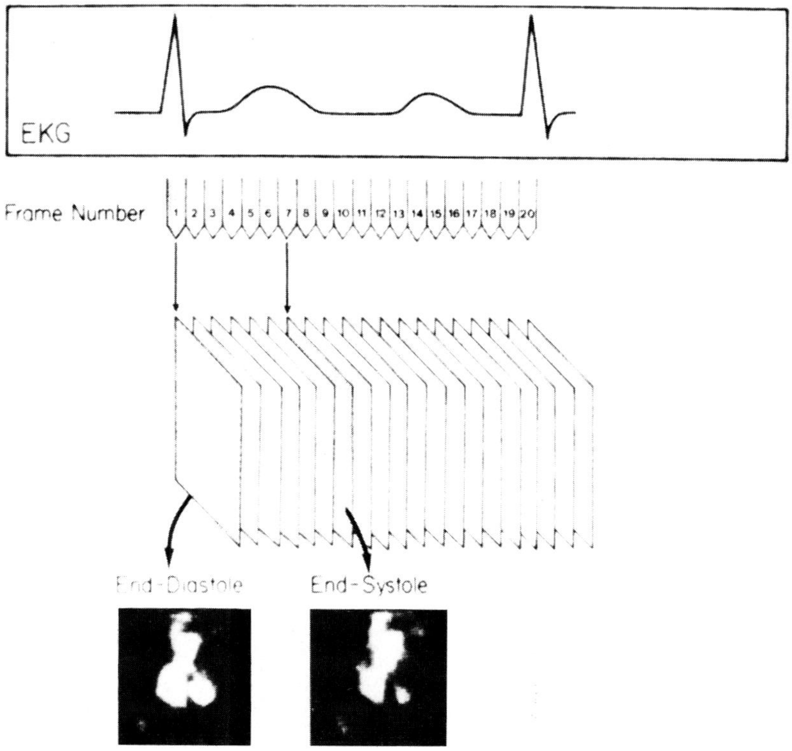

Figure 3. ECG-gated blood pool images are assembled on line to produce a composite cardiac cycle. Each R-R interval is divided into a fixed number of frames based on its temporal location from the peak of the R wave. Each temporally matched frame is then added to produce a summed image.

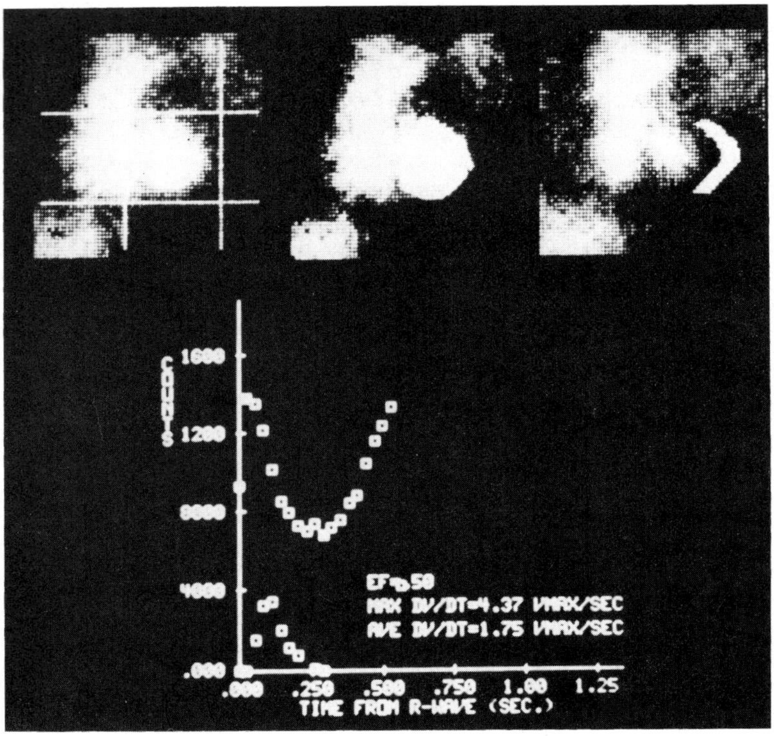

Figure 4. Edge detection algorithms require the computer operator to locate the left ventricle. An edge is located based on simple threshold (first derivative) and rate of change of counts (second derivative) on a pixel-by-pixel basis.

manually or with a variety of edge detection algorithms that are provided in most standard general nuclear medicine computers (Fig. 4). Ejection fraction and ventricular volume can be quantitated from the time-activity (volume) curves with a high degree of accuracy and reproducibility.[8, 10, 12, 31, 44, 45]

Gated radionuclide studies are performed in the left anterior oblique projection for evaluating global left ventricular function, where the right and left ventricle are more clearly separated. One dose of a radiotracer can produce multiple studies (and thus data points) for up to 4 hr after the initial injection.[44] In general, the right ventricle is best evaluated by the first-transit (pass) technique in the anterior or right anterior projection, where the tricuspid valve plane can be visualized, as well as the pulmonary valve and right ventricular outflow tract. Because the right ventricle is identified before the remainder of the central circulation, background is relatively unimportant. In a recent review of 30 first-pass angiograms, we could not demonstrate any improvement in our right ventricular ejection fraction values by background subtraction.

Additionally, when right ventricular performance needs to be serially followed, it is possible to use krypton^{81} or xenon^{133} as the radioisotope. Once these substances (dissolved inert gases) reach the pulmonary bed, they are expired. Thus, there is also potential for the evaluation not only of right heart function but also of regional pulmonary perfusion and the subsequent ventilatory washout of the radioisotope. The radiation exposure is very small because little of the radioisotope leaves the pulmonary bed.

Recent reports have suggested that equilibrium angiograms can produce accurate estimates of right ventricular ejection fraction and volume.[22, 31, 40, 42] Nonetheless, substantial variability occurs in adults using 45° left anterior oblique images of the right ventricle for analysis of right ventricular ejection fraction when compared with that of biplane right ventriculograms.[13] Parrish et al.[30, 31] have not found this true in children, although further validation of these count-based methods seems mandatory (Figs. 5 and 6).

Although chamber volumes may be obtained from standard geometric formulae during first-pass studies, volumes can be derived nongeometrically from equilibrium images.[7] The hypothesis that left ventricular volume can be calculated independent of geometry is based on the known characteristics of conventional radionuclide materials. Thus, radioactive materials used in equilibrium studies are distributed in such a manner that there is a stable concentra-

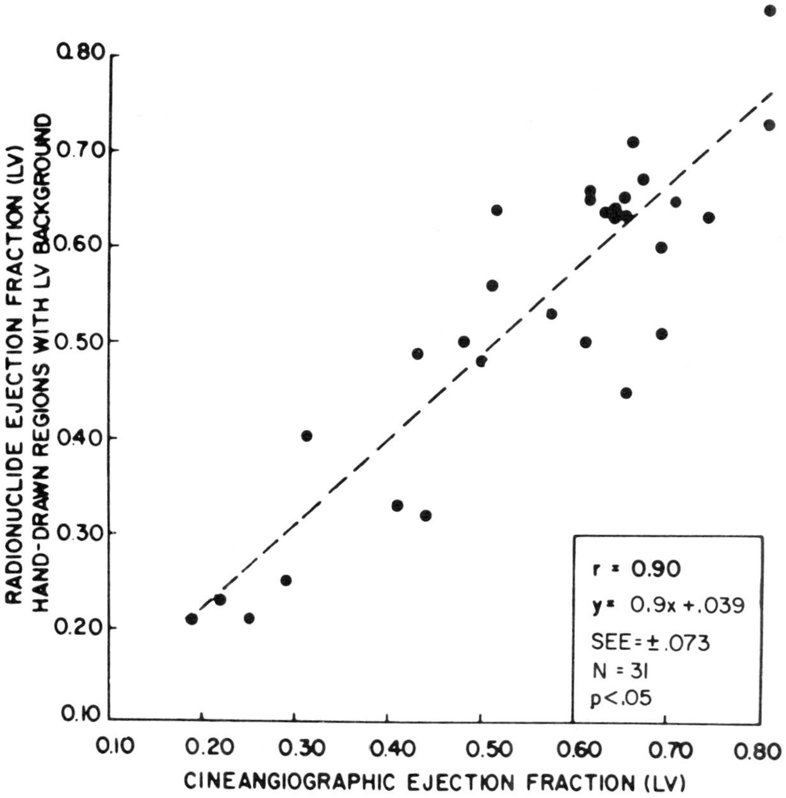

Figure 5. A comparison of equilibrium radionuclide and contrast ventriculographic estimates of left ventricular function are shown in 31 children prospectively studied. (*From* Parrish M, Graham T, Born M, et al: Radionuclide evaluation of right and left ventricular function in children: Validation of methodology. Am J Cardiol, *49*:1241–1247, 1982, with permission.)

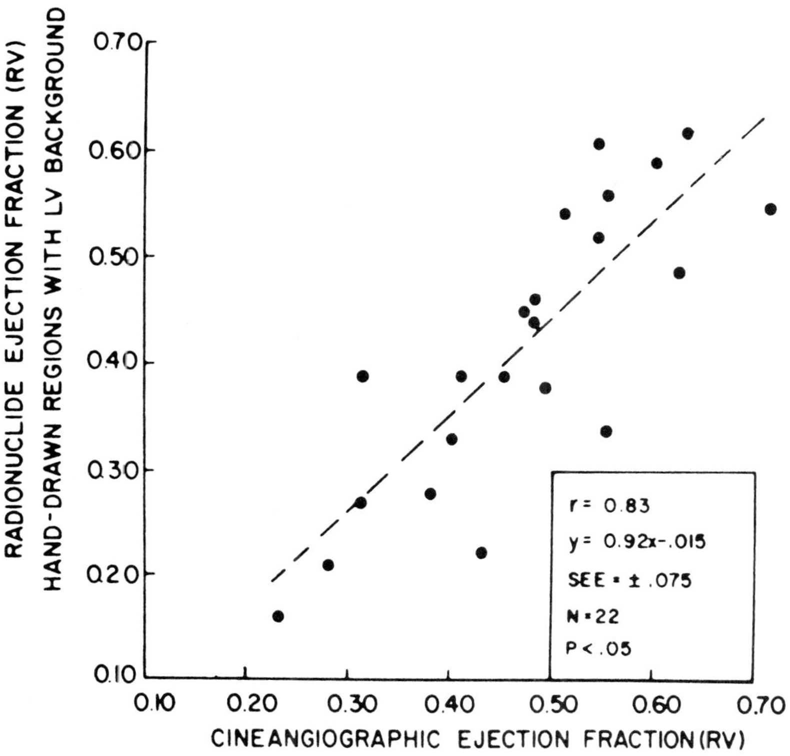

Figure 6. Similar to Figure 5, equilibrium radionuclide and contrast ventriculographic estimates of right ventricular function are shown. (*From* Parrish M, Graham T, Born M, et al.: Radionuclide evaluation of right and left ventricular function in children: Validation of methodology. Am J Cardiol, *49*:1241–1247, 1982, with permission.)

tion of isotopic activity for brief periods. If C = D/V (where C is concentration, D is administered dose, and V is volume of distribution), and C is a constant or can be determined, then V may be calculated. Similarly, the volume of a particular region-of-interest should be proportional to the amount of radiotracer in that region-of-interest. Variation in attenuation from patient to patient will detract from the constancy of this relationship between patients. Units of cardiac chamber volume can be derived from the following equation (and used for any chamber of interest with some degree of success):

$$\text{Volume (units)} = \frac{\dfrac{\text{EDC or ESC} \times \text{normalized frame time}}{\text{heart beats}}}{\text{reference venous counts}}$$

where EDC is the end-diastolic counts, and ESC is the end-systolic counts. All studies need to be normalized to a constant frame duration. We happen to have chosen 0.04 sec because it was the most convenient value for achieving up to 28 points in each composite time-activity (volume) curve when the heart rate was 54 to 71 beats per min (the standard framing rate for out-gated scintigraphic reconstruction software). For faster heart rates, shorter times for each frame were selected, thus producing respectively shorter sampling and acquisition times. Since a 0.04 sec per frame was the most commonly used in our rest population, it served as the "standard," and normalization to this convenient time was made when briefer time frames were found. Alternative frame corrections have been successfully used by others.

This technique has been successfully applied to the evaluation of children with simple and complex congenital heart lesions.[45] A multiplicity of approaches for attenuation correction have been attempted in large part to obviate the need for regression equation relationships between the radionuclide and contrast volumes, to facilitate comparison between children of varying sizes, and to minimize the variability of the technique. Most correction techniques assume that the space between the heart and the skin (composed of blood pool, heart muscle, lung constituents, air, and the respective chest wall components) can be approximated by the attenuation coefficient of water. The attenuation correction then equals:

$$e^{-u(d)}$$

where u is the attenuation coefficient of water and d is the distance of the heart from the skin. Most attenuation correction techniques then involve determining this distance. All appear to improve somewhat on the reliability of the equilibrium method. Which will provide the most accurate and reproducible method with the minimum amount of time and work is at present uncertain.

ANALYSIS OF VALVULAR REGURGITATION

While substantial literature has become available on the evaluation of left-to-right and right-to-left intracardiac shunt calculations using first-transit radionuclide angiography (see article by Treves), little information is available on the evaluation of valvular regurgitation.

In adults, regurgitation can be calculated using both the first-pass and equilibrium technique by use of the "constancy" concept. That is to say, the cardiac output on the right and left side of the heart is assumed to be constant and to approximate unity. Thus, the ratio of left- to right-sided stroke volume or cardiac output should increase with left-sided regurgitation and decrease with right-sided regurgitation.

At present, most studies have involved adult patients[4, 9, 14, 19, 35, 52] with left-sided disorders (mitral regurgitation and aortic insufficiency), though data in pediatric patients are forthcoming (Parrish, personal communication).

Nonetheless, little data are available on regurgitant indexes at rest or during interventions in pediatric patient populations.

RADIONUCLIDE EVALUATION OF ISOLATED DISEASE STATES

Hemodynamic evaluation of congenital heart disease generally occurs at direct cardiac catheterization. Recent advances in quantitative echocardiography have also led to the use of ultrasound imaging to sequentially evaluate right and left ventricular dynamics. To date, little objective data are available on using radionuclide techniques in children. While validation studies have been performed and experiences detailed,[14, 17, 26, 30, 50] little cumulative data are available for either prognostic or therapeutic purposes in specific diseases at rest or during interventions.

Reduto and co-workers[33] examined radionuclide measures of left and right ventricular function at rest and during exercise in 16 postoperative patients after total correction of the

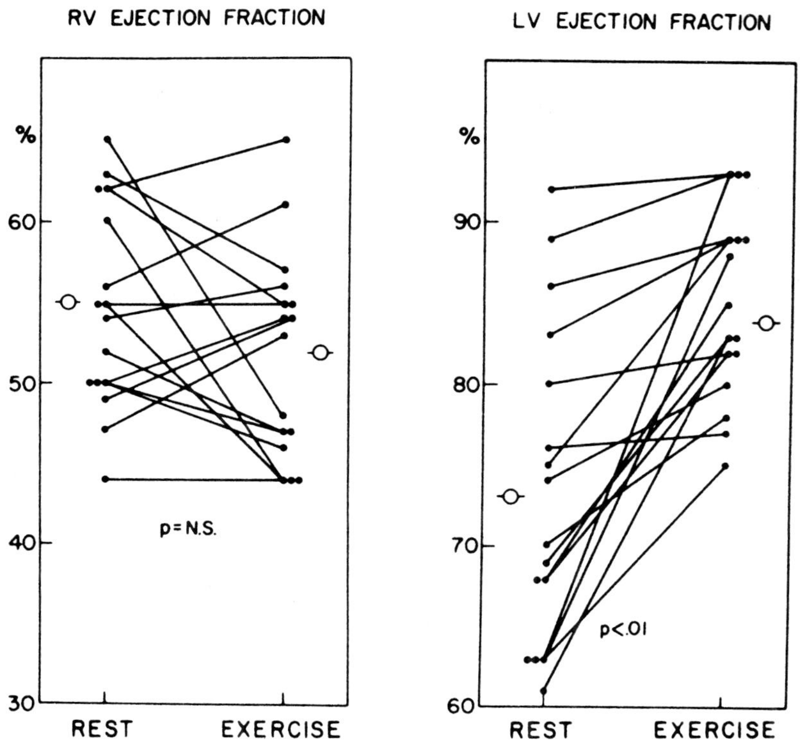

Figure 7. Rest and exercise cardiac function are shown from 16 asymptomatic patients after surgical correction of the tetralogy of Fallot. Though the patients were asymptomatic, note the frequent abnormal reduction in RV ejection fraction during exercise. (*From* Reduto L, Berger H, Johnstone D, et al: Radionuclide assessment of right and left ventricular exercise reserve after totoal correction of tetralogy of Fallot. Am J Cardiol, *45*:1013–1018, 1980, with permission.)

tetralogy of Fallot. All the patients were asymptomatic, most (15 of 16) had normal right ventricular function (ejection fraction) at rest, and all had normal left ventricular function (ejection fraction) at rest. During exercise, the right ventricular response was abnormal in 13 of the 16 subjects and was associated on additional radionuclide stress studies with scintigraphic evidence (increased thallium uptake) of residual right ventricular hypertrophy (Fig. 7). While the prognostic importance of this finding remains uncertain, particularly in patients with clinical evidence of an adequate surgical repair, the potential utility of observing the patient both pre- and postoperatively may be worthwhile in this as well as other diseases. Others have characterized the effects of operative repair of the tetralogy of Fallot on regional pulmonary blood flow[36] and the effects of d-transposition on a regional lung function.[32] The clinical importance of these findings, however, has never been demonstrated.

Recently, Benson et al. evaluated the right ventricular response to exercise by using equilibrium technique in patients who had undergone a Mustard procedure for d-transposition of the great arteries.[5] Prognosis in this circumstance depends on the ability of the right ventricle to behave as the systemic ventricle. They found that children clinically well after Mustard's procedure often have abnormal right ventricular volume and function responses. This raises questions about the long-term capacity of the chamber to maintain cardiac output (Fig. 8).

In a short report, Novetsky and co-workers[27] detailed their experience with ECG-gated blood pool imaging in a patient with Ebstein's anomaly. They observed that the subjective radionuclide findings were similar to those observed during contrast angiography, and objective evidence of tricuspid regurgitation was demonstrated by the scintigraphic studies. They recommended radionuclide evaluation before direct invasive studies in order to minimize the time and risk of the invasive procedures.

While congenital abnormalities are the most common cause of cardiac ailments in children, acquired illnesses occur and are also suitable for radionuclide evaluation. Children with myocarditis and with valvulitis (rheumatic, infectious, and so on) would be suitable for both rest and exercise hemodynamic monitoring for the purpose of prognosis and potential therapeutic interventions.

Patients with hemoglobinopathies often receive large amounts of blood transfusions. As their iron load increases, the risk of deposition of cardiac iron and dysfunction increases. Leon and colleagues[20] demonstrated a marked reduction in left ventricular contractile reserve in anemic patients who had received over 100 transfusions (Fig. 9). The implications for iron

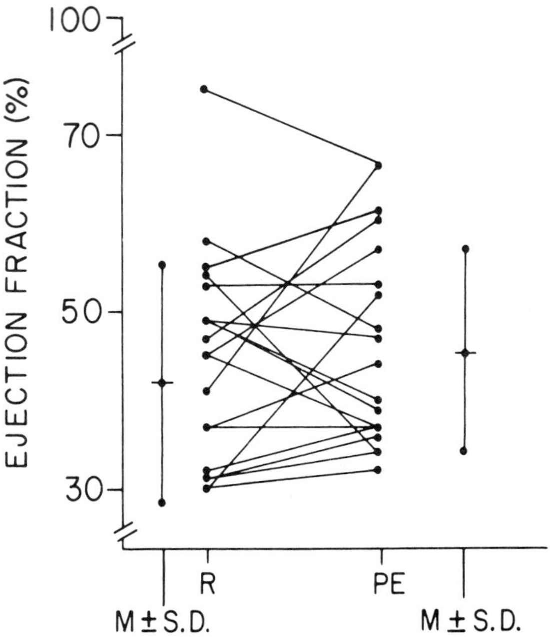

Figure 8. This figure shows the abnormal right ventricular (<5 ejection fraction unit increase in ejection fraction) response to exercise in asymptomatic children after Mustard's operation for d-transposition of the great vessels. (*From* Benson L, Bonet J, McLaughlin P, et al: Assessment of right ventricular function during supine bicycle exercise after Mustart's operation. Circulation, *65*:1052–1059, 1982, with permission.)

chelation therapy before the development of congestive cardiomyopathy were readily apparent, though results were not available.

Matthay et al.[24] examined the effects of chronic pulmonary parenchymal disease (cystic fibrosis) on right heart function in children. While many patients with cystic fibrosis predominantly experience recurring pulmonary infections, cardiac complications often contribute to both morbidity and mortality. Although left ventricular ejection fraction was normal in most patients, right ventricular function was often abnormal (9 of 22 patients). Five of these nine subjects with reduced right ventricular function at rest went on, within two years, to develop cor pulmonale. Radionuclide angiography has been also used to select therapeutic modalities for patients with cystic fibrosis.[11]

Finally, the response of cardiac function to increasing dosages of cardiotoxic chemotherapeutic agents has been studied (Fig. 10) in order to minimize cardiotoxicity and maximize the amount of drug able to be used.[2] This technique has already altered the clinical approach to both the adult and pediatric patients receiving Adriamycin and other anticancer drug regimens.

RADIONUCLIDE ANALYSIS OF THE HEART DURING EXERCISE

The hemodynamic response of the heart to various forms of stress, including exercise, has recently been reviewed.[38] In the normal adult, the left and right ventricular ejection fraction will rise 0.05 units or greater during bicycle exercise. End-diastolic volume increases minimally usually when exercise is performed with the patient in the erect position, and end-systolic volume declines. Right ventricular volumes behave similar to left ventricular volumes.[41] In patients with coronary disease, the left ventricular ejection fraction usually behaves abnormally during exercise, with some increase in end-diastolic volume. With elevation of pulmonary pressures or in patients with isolated right coronary artery disease, the right ventricle may fail, and right ventricle dilatation can oc-

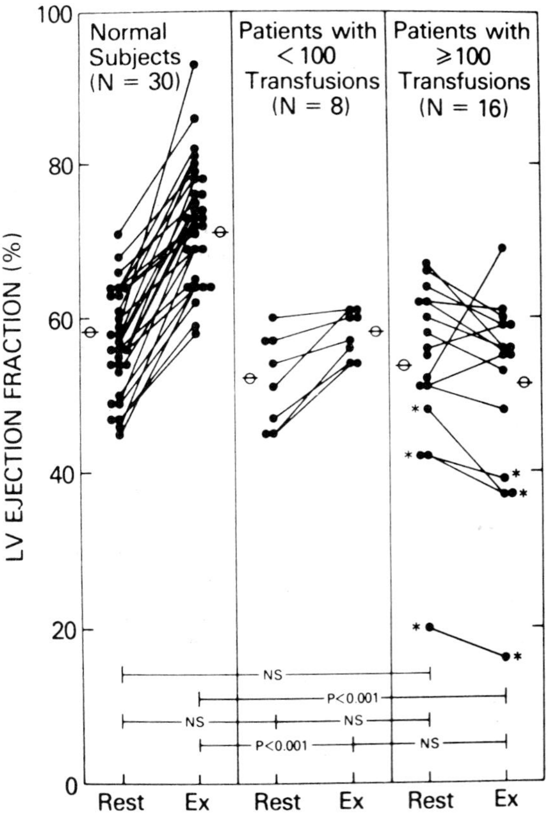

Figure 9. The left ventricular response to supine exercise is given in normal subjects and in patients who had received varying amounts of transfusions due to congenital anemias. Note the evidence of greater LV dysfunction with more transfusions. The asterisks indicate the presence of regional wall motion abnormalities. (*From* Leon M, Borer J, Bacharach S, et al: Detection of early cardiac dysfunction in patients with severe beta-thalassemia and chronic iron overload. N Engl J Med, *301*:1148–1149, 1979, with permission.)

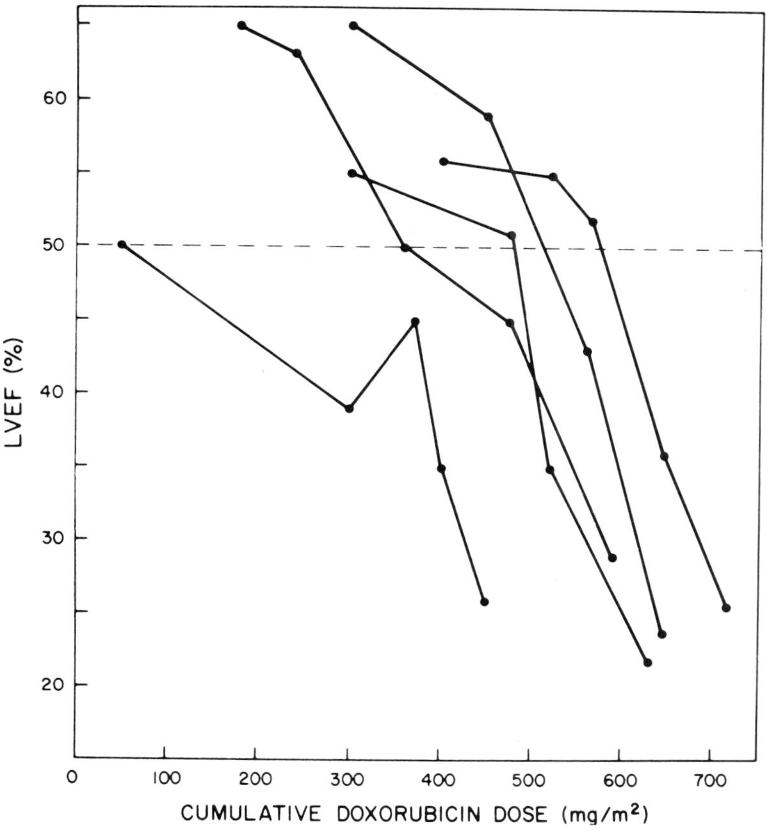

Figure 10. Serial LVEFs (left ventricular ejection fraction) were obtained in five subjects who had congestive heart failure after the administration of doxorubicin. Congestive heart failure occurred only after the LVEF was reduced below 0.30. (*From* Alexander J, Dainiak N, Berger H, et al: Serial assessment of doxorubicin cardiotoxicity with quantitative radionuclide angiocardiography. N Engl J Med, *300*:278–285, 1979, with permission).

cur.[6, 15, 23, 44] In patients with lung disease, right ventricular and pulmonary pressures rise during exercise, resulting in dilatation and dysfunction of the right side of the heart.

Only a few small series of radionuclide hemodynamic measures during exercise have been reported from pediatric patient populations.[30, 33] Right and left ventricular dysfunction during exercise has been shown in patients operated on for tetralogy of Fallot and in subjects with transposition of the great vessels, congenital mitral stenosis, and idiopathic congestive cardiomyopathy (Figs. 11 and 12). It might be anticipated that the degree of right ventricular dysfunction (and volume changes) during exercise might help predict the severity of pulmonic obstruction preoperatively in patients with tetralogy of Fallot and in patients with varying forms of pulmonic stenosis. These postulates will require further confirmation. Nonetheless, radionuclide stress scintigraphy in children has vast potential, which, at present, is virtually unexplored.

RELATION OF CARDIAC AND PULMONARY DYNAMICS

Reduced systolic pump performance often is associated with pulmonary vascular engorgement, particularly during acute changes in left atrial pressure. The heart has been found to adapt pharmacologically to induced increases in aortic pressure and afterload by increasing preload and maintaining stroke volume. The dysfunctional ventricle may respond with a less substantial cardiac output and stroke volume response, particularly when the degree of left ventricular filling pressures needed to develop appropriate degrees of ejection is considered. When phenylephrine is administered, pulmonary congestion can occur in patients with latent failure of the left side of the heart.

During the induction of acute heart failure during atrial pacing in patients with heart disease, elevations in filling pressure are associated with a prolongation of pulmonary transit time and an increase in pulmonary blood volume (and presumably lung water). During acute myocardial injury, pulmonary symptoms and radiographic signs are well represented by increases in cardiac filling pressures and reductions in arterial pressure and cardiac output. Finally, during exercise, pulmonary congestion may result at lower levels of exercise in noncompliant chambers or when evidence of valvular obstruction is present.

Pulmonary dynamics, aside from shunt calculations, can be analyzed with radionuclide function studies (first-transit or equilibrium).

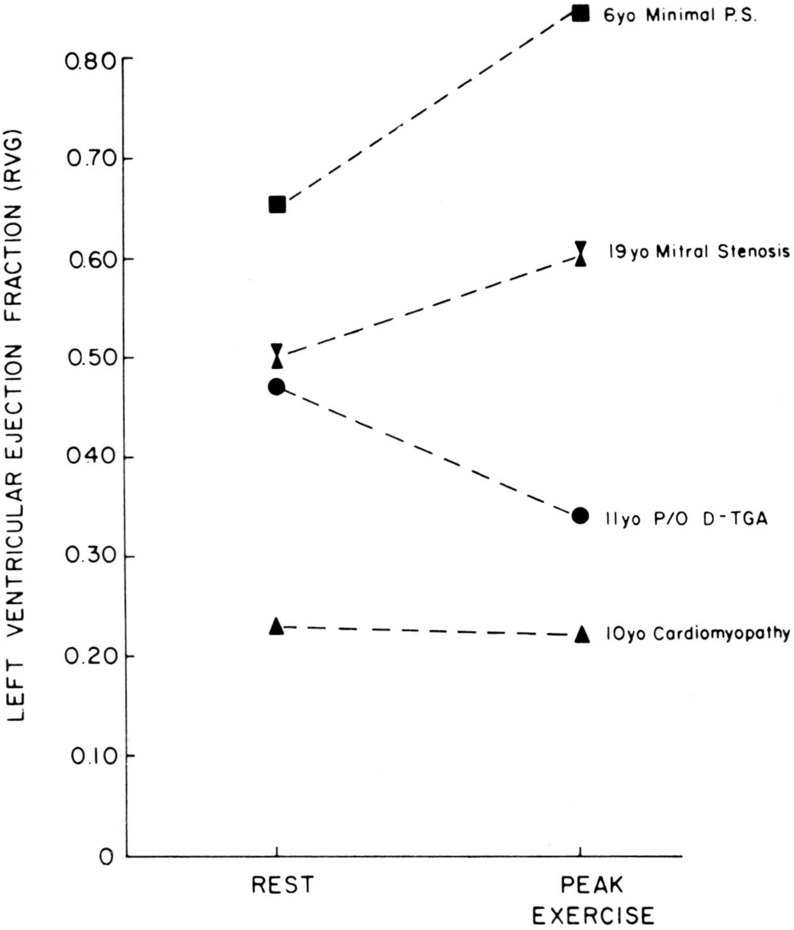

Figure 11. The left ventricular response to exercise in four patients with congenital disease (PS: pulmonic stenosis; D-TGA: dextrotransposition of the great vessels; P/O: Postoperative; RVG: equilibrium radionuclide). (*From* Parrish M, Graham T, Born M, et al: Radionuclide evaluation of right and left ventricular function in children: Validation of methodology. Am J Cardiol, *49*:1241–1247, 1982, with permission.)

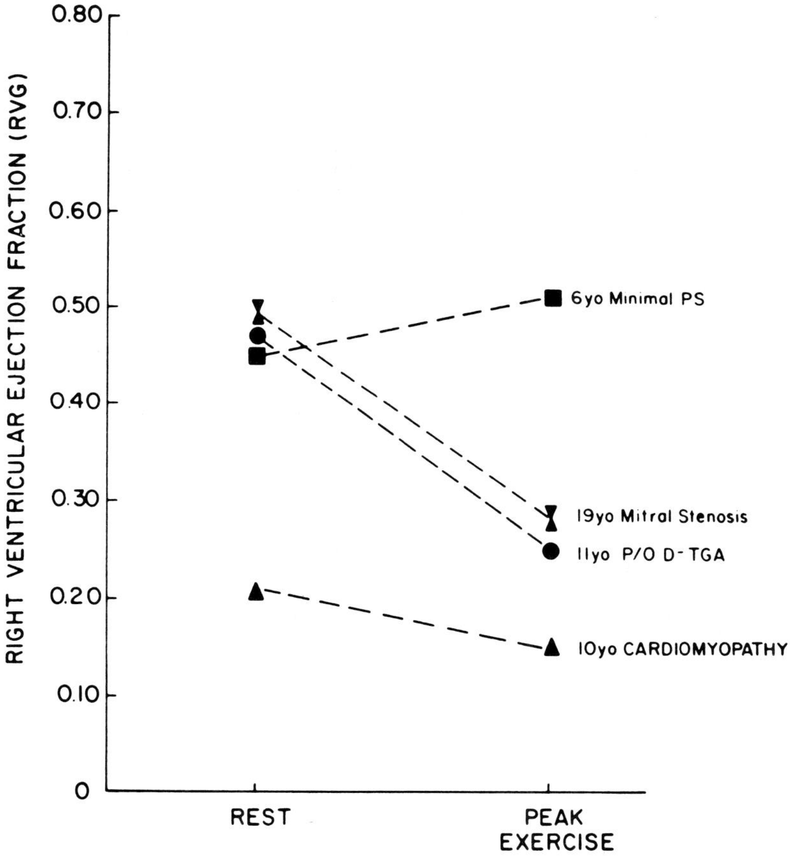

Figure 12. Right ventricular response in the patients described in Figure 11. (*From* Parrish M, Graham T, Born M, et al: Radionuclide evaluation of right and left ventricular function in children: Validation of methodology. Am J Cardiol, *49*:1241–1247, 1982, with permission.)

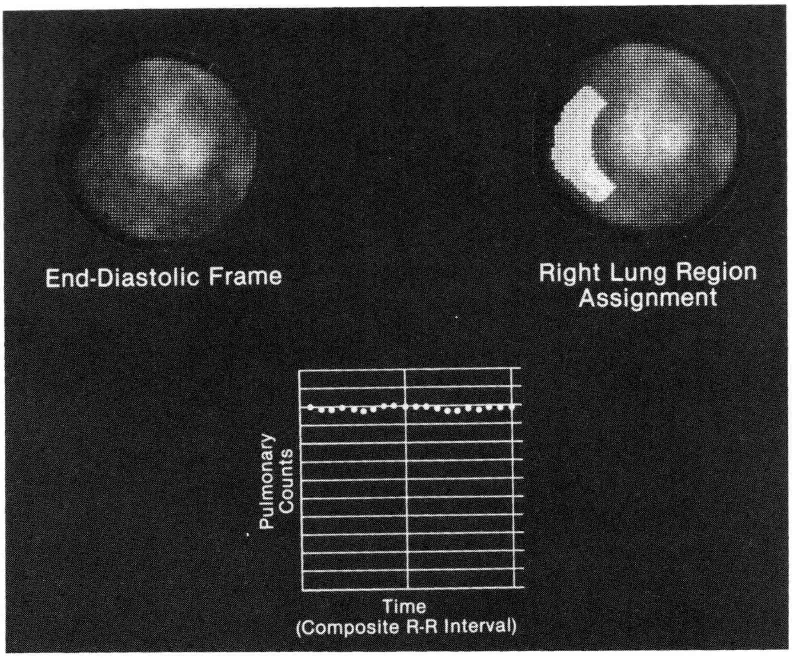

Figure 13. A standard pulmonary region-of-interest is shown in the end-diastolic equilibrium. A typical pulmonary time activity curve is shown in the lower panel.

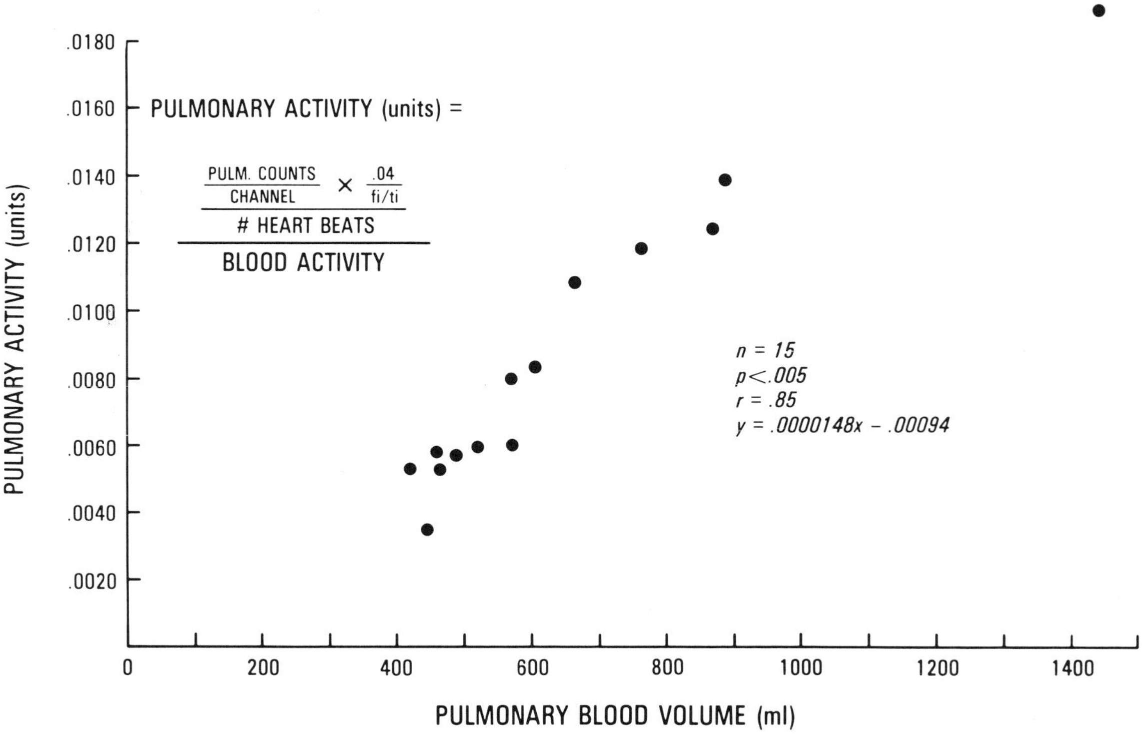

Figure 14. The relationship between the number of counts from the lungs and green dye estimates of pulmonary blood volume is shown in 15 patients undergoing transeptal cardiac catheterization.

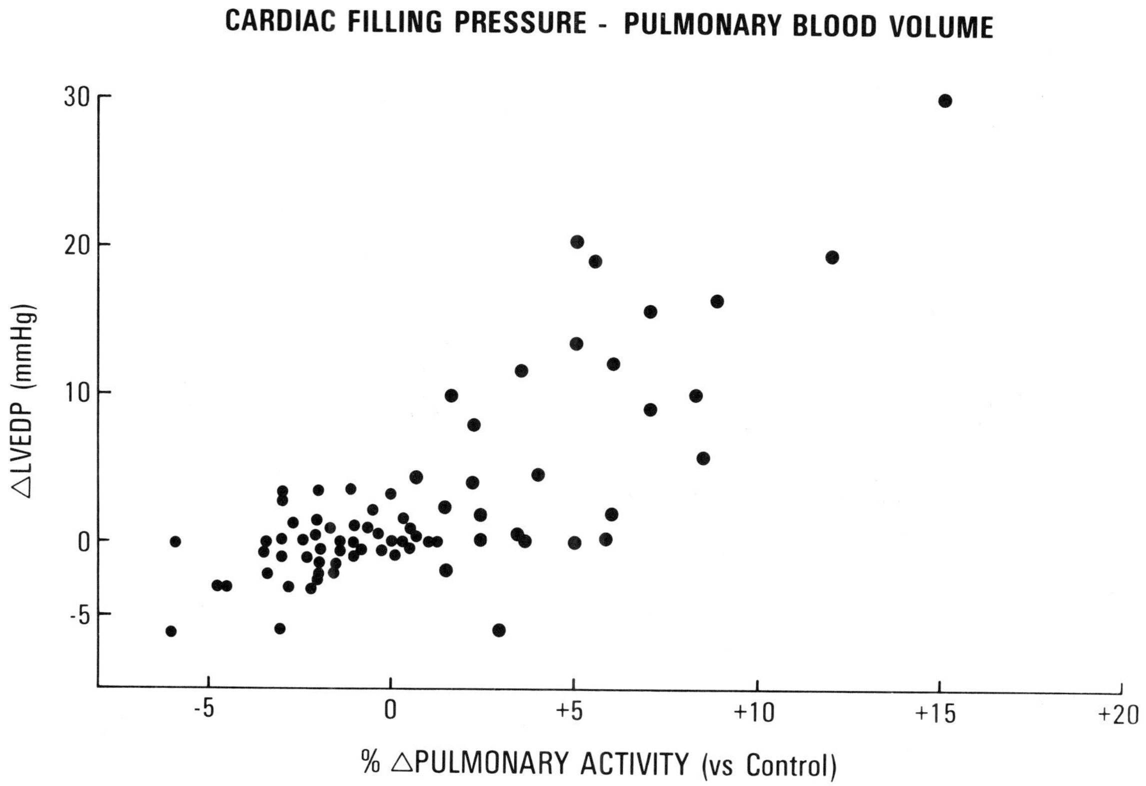

Figure 15. In 11 patients, the relationship between lung counts and left ventricular end-diastolic pressure is shown during atrial pacing.

Intravascular pulmonary blood volume can be assessed by standard indicator dilution methods by using the first-transit approach. Regions-of-interest over the left ventricle (atrium) and right ventricle allow indicator curves (time-activity) to be devised and mean transit time calculated. Cardiac output can also be derived from first-transit data. Pulmonary blood volume then equals transit time multiplied by the cardiac output.[6]

Okada and co-workers[28] used regions-of-interest placed over the lung in gated blood pool cardiac images to analyze regional pulmonary blood volume changes. We have found that these measures of pulmonary intravascular volume correlate well with standard indicator dilution techniques (Figs. 13 and 14).[29] During pacing, changes in radionuclide measures of pulmonary blood volume relate to changes in pressure of the left side of the heart (Fig. 15).[51] Others have had similar experiences relating cardiac pressure and pulmonary blood volume during exercise.[28] We have found this technique simple to use and clinically valuable for drug interventions,[46] phenylephrine stress studies,[37] and during exercise.[47] Lindsey and Guyton[21] have additionally demonstrated that occlusion of the pulmonary outflow tract produces a reduction of pulmonary blood volume determined by radionuclide techniques. This technique thus appears to be a noninvasive approach for sequentially evaluating cardiopulmonary dynamics and pressures. Its potential in children with pulmonic stenosis and tetralogy of Fallot remains unexplored. At present, little extension of these physiologic principles or radionuclide approaches has been extended to the pediatric population.

CONCLUSION

Relatively few studies using radionuclide techniques are available for evaluating cardiac performance at rest or during exercise. These techniques have been frequently and successfully used in large numbers of adult patients and in all likelihood can be expanded to aid in the management of pediatric patient populations. With the introduction of short-lived radiotracers, these studies will undoubtedly increase in number and improve our understanding of cardiac hemodynamics pre-

and postoperatively, as well as during many forms of stress and interventions in children with acquired congenital heart disease.

REFERENCES

1. Alderson, P, Bernier D, Ludbrook P, et al: Serial radionuclide determinations of the ejection fraction with ^{99m}Tc-labelled red blood cells. Radiology, *119*:729, 1976.
2. Alexander J, Dainiak N, Berger H, et al: Serial assessment of doxorubricin cardiotoxicity with quantitative radionuclide angiocardiography. N Eng J Med, *300*:278–285, 1979.
3. Ashburn W, Schelbert H, Verba J: Left ventricular ejection fraction—a review of several radionuclide angiographic approaches using the scintillation camera. Prog Cardiovasc Dis, *20*:267, 1978.
4. Baxter R, Becker L, Alderson P, et al: Quantification of aortic valvular regurgitation in dogs by nuclear imaging. Circulation, *61*:404–410, 1980.
5. Benson L, Bonet J, McLaughlin P, et al: Assessment of right ventricular function during supine bicycle exercise after Mustard's operation. Circulation, *65*:1052–1059, 1982.
6. Berger H, Matthay R, Pytlik L, et al: First-pass radionuclide assessment of right and left ventricular performance in patients with cardiac and pulmonary disease. Sem Nucl Med, *9*:275–292, 1979.
7. Berger H, Reduto L, Johnstone D, et al: Global and regional left ventricular response to bicycle exercise in coronary artery disease. Assessment by quantitative radionuclide angiography. Am J Med, *66*:13, 1979.
8. Borer J, Backarach S, Green M, et al: Real-time radionuclide cineangiography in the non-invasive evaluation of global and regional left ventricular function at rest and during exercise in patients with coronary artery disease. New Engl J Med, *296*:839, 1977.
9. Bough E, Gandsman E, North D, et al: Gated radionuclide angiographic evaluation of valve regurgitation. Am J Cardiol, *60*:581–589, 1979.
10. Burow R, Strauss HW, Singleton R, et al: Analysis of left ventricle function from multiple gated acquisition (MUGA) cardiac blood pool imaging: A comparison with contrast angiography. Circulation, *56*:1024, 1977.
11. Chipps B, Alderson P, Roland J, et al: Noninvasive evaluation of ventricular function in cystic fibrosis. J Pediatr, *95*:379–384, 1979.
12. Dehmer G, Lewis S, Hillis LD, et al: Nongeometric determination of left ventricular volumes from equilibrium blood pool scans. Am J Cardiol, *45*:293, 1980.
13. Hooper W, Horn M, Moser K, et al: Right ventricular size and function: The discrepancy between blood pool imaging techniques. Cathet Cardiovasc Diagn, *8*:597, 1982.
14. Janowitz W, Fester A: Quantitation of left ventricular regurgitant fraction by first pass radionuclide angiography. Am J Cardiol, *49*:85–92, 1982.
15. Johnson L, McCarthy D, Sciacca R, et al: Right ventricular ejection fraction during exercise in patients with coronary artery disease. Circulation, *60*:1284–1300, 1979.
16. Jones R, Sabiston D, Bates B, et al: Quantitative radionuclide angiography for determination of chamber to chamber transit times. Am J Cardiol, *30*:855–864, 1972.
17. Kurtz D, Ahnberg D, Freed M, et al: Quantitative radionuclide angiography—determination of left ventricular ejection fraction in children. Br Heart J, *38*:966–973, 1976.
18. Laks H, Mudd J, Standeven J, et al: Long-term effect of the superior vena cava-pulmonary artery anastomosis on pulmonary blood flow. J Thorac Cardiovasc Surg, *74*:253–260, 1977.
19. Lam W, Pavel D, Byrom E, et al: Radionuclide regurgitant index: Value and limitations. Am J Cardiol, *47*:292–298, 1981.
20. Leon M, Borer J, Bacharach S, et al: Detection of early cardiac dysfunction in patients with severe beta-thalassemia and chronic iron overload. N Engl J Med, *301*:1148–1149, 1979.
21. Lindsey A, Guyton A: Continuous recording of pulmonary blood volume: Pulmonary pressure and volume changes. Am J Physiol, *197*:959–963, 1959.
22. Maddahi J, Berman D, Matsomoko D, et al: A new technique for assessing right ventricular ejection fraction using multiple-gated equilibrium cardiac blood pool scintigraphy. Description, validation, and findings in coronary artery disease. Circulation, *60*:581, 1979.
23. Maddahi J, Berman D, Matsuoka D, et al: Right ventricular ejection fraction during exercise in normal subjects and in coronary artery disease patients: Assessment by multiple-gated equilibrium scintigraphy. Circulation, *62*:133–140, 1980.
24. Matthay R, Berger H, Loke J, et al: Right and left ventricular performance in ambulatory young adults with cystic fibrosis. Br Heart J, *43*:474–480, 1980.
25. Mullins C, Mason D, Ashburn W, et al: Determination of ventricular volume from radioisotope angiography. Am J Cardiol, *24*:72, 1968.
26. Newman G, Benson D, Anderson P, et al: Comparison of catheterization and radionuclide cardiac volume in children. In press.
27. Novetsky G, Turner O, Codini M, et al: Ebstein's anomaly: Demonstration by ECG-synchronized radionuclide cineangiography. Clin Nucl Med, *6*:341–343, 1981.
28. Okada R, Osbakken M, Boucher C, et al: Pulmonary blood volume response to exercise: A non-invasive determination of exercise-induced changes in pulmonary capillary wedge pressure. Circulation, *65*:126–133, 1982.
29. Okada R, Pohost G, Kirshenbaum H, et al: Radionuclide determined changes in pulmonary blood volume with exercise. N Engl J Med, *301*:569–576, 1979.
30. Parrish M, Graham T, Born M, et al: Radionuclide evaluation of right and left ventricular function in children: Validation of methodology. Am J Cardiol, *49*:1241–1247, 1982.
31. Parrish M, Graham T, Born M, et al: Radionuclide ventriculography for the assessment of absolute right and left ventricular volumes in children. Circulation, *66*:811, 1982.
32. Rabinovitch M, Rosenthal A, Sade R, et al: Regional lung function studies and radionuclide angiography in D-transposition of the great arteries. Pediatr Res, *11*:1117–1121, 1977.
33. Reduto L, Berger H, Johnstone D, et al: Radionuclide assessment of right and left ventricular exercise reserve after total correction of tetralogy of Fallot. Am J Cardiol, *45*:1013–1018, 1980.
34. Rhodes B: Radiopharmaceuticals. *In* Strauss HW, Pitt B (eds): Cardiovascular Nuclear Medicine. St. Louis, C. V. Mosby Company, 1979, pp. 57–76.

35. Rigo P, Alderson P, Robertson R, et al: Measurement of aortic and mitral regurgitation by gated cardiac blood pool scans. Circulation, *60*:306–311, 1979.
36. Sade R, Sloss L, Treves S, et al: Repair of tetralogy of Fallot after aortopulmonary anastomosis. Ann Thorac Surg, *23*:32–38, 1977.
37. Slutsky R: Pulmonary blood volume: The response to afterload in normal subjects and patients with previous myocardial infarction. Invest Radiol, *17*:241, 1982.
38. Slutsky R: The response of the left ventricle to stress: A discussion of the effects of atrial pacing, afterload, exercise and drugs. Am J Cardiol, *47*:357–364, 1981.
39. Slutsky R, Ackerman W, Karliner J, et al: Right and left ventricular dysfunction in patients with chronic obstructive lung diseases. Am J Med, *68*:205, 1980.
40. Slutsky R, Ashburn W, Karliner J: A method for the analysis of right ventricular volume by equilibrium radionuclide angiography. Chest, *80*:471, 1981.
41. Slutsky R, Hooper W, Ackerman W, et al: Right ventricular size, function and pressure: The response to supine bicycle exercise in normal subjects and patients with severe obstructive lung disease. Eur J Nucl Med, *7*:553, 1982.
42. Slutsky R, Hooper W, Gerber K, et al: Assessment of right ventricular function at rest and during exercise in patients with coronary artery disease: A new approach using equilibrium radionuclide angiography. Am J Cardiol, *45*:63, 1980.
43. Slutsky R, Hooper W, Gerber K, et al: Assessment of right ventricular function at rest and during exercise in patients with coronary artery heart disease: A new approach using equilibrium radionuclide angiography. Am J Cardiol, *45*:63–71, 1980.
44. Slutsky R, Karliner J, Battler A, et al: The reproducibility of ejection fraction and ventricular volume by gated radionuclide angiography after acute myocardial infarction. Radiology, *132*:153, 1979.
45. Slutsky R, Karliner J, Ricci D, et al: Left ventricular volumes by gated equilibrium radionuclide angiography: A new method. Circulation, *60*:556, 1979.
46. Slutsky R, Mancini GBJ, Costello D, et al: Pulmonary blood volume: Response to spontaneous angina pectoris and sublingual nitroglycerin in patients with coronary heart disease. Am Heart J, *105*:243, 1983.
47. Slutsky R, Shabetai R, Mancini GBJ, et al: Pulmonary blood volume: Analysis during exercise in patients with left ventricular dysfunction. Eur J Nucl Med, *8*:523, 1983.
48. Straus HW, Zaret B, Hurley P, et al: A scintiphotographic method for measuring left ventricular ejection fraction in man without cardiac catheterization. Am J Cardiol, *28*:575, 1971.
49. Tobrinick E, Schelbert H, Henning H, et al: Right ventricular ejection fraction in patients with acute anterior and inferior myocardial infarction. Circulation, *57*:1078, 1978.
50. Treves S, Fogle R, Lang P: Radionuclide angiography in congenital heart disease. Am J Cardiol, *46*:1247–1255, 1980.
51. Tubau J, Slutsky R, Gerber K, et al: Pulmonary blood volume: Relationship to changes in left ventricular end-diastolic pressure during atrial pacing. Am Heart J, *105*:940, 1983.
52. Urguhart J, Patterson R, Packer M, et al: Quantification of valve regurgitation by radionuclide angiography before and after valve replacement surgery. Am J Cardiol, *47*:287–291, 1981.

8

COMPUTED TOMOGRAPHY

The Technique and Its Use for the Evaluation of Cardiocirculatory Anatomy and Function

MARTIN J. LIPTON, M.D., and CHARLES B. HIGGINS, M.D.

Heart disease is one of the most difficult technical challenges for diagnostic imaging. It also represents the major medical problem of our time in terms of death and acute and chronic disability.[5] The total direct cost of heart disease in America exceeds 12 billion dollars each year, and the indirect costs have been estimated at 50 billion annually.[12] These statistics tend to indicate the relative inadequacy of presently available diagnostic methods in detecting heart disease early and in adequately evaluating it.

The traditional diagnostic gold standard is cardiac catheterization, a process that combines hemodynamic recording with angiocardiography. The major disadvantages of this approach are the invasiveness of the procedure, hospitalization, and cost. Such invasive procedures are far from ideal because they also frequently fail to provide critical information, such as myocardial blood flow, and suffer from a fundamental limitation of projection imaging, namely, the superimposition of structures. Significant improvements in x-ray imaging techniques during the past two decades have contributed greatly to the demonstration of cardiovascular anatomy and function. Historically, the major requirements for imaging cardiac structures have been equipment that provides high-speed (temporal resolution) and high-detail (spatial resolution) imaging. The quality of cardiac angiography has therefore undergone dramatic advances over a quarter of a century. This background should be remembered when examining the newer noninvasive modalities.

Rapid and impressive developments have been made in the evaluation of the heart using nuclear medicine techniques. Projection imaging of the distribution of an intravenously injected radioactive tracer has been the standard technique. More recently, single photon-emission tomography[7] and positron-emission tomography[30] have been introduced to provide cross-sectional cardiac imaging. These are discussed elsewhere in this issue. It should be noted, however, that the clinical utility of all these studies is limited by relatively poor spatial resolution (approximately 1 cm), which is characteristic of all nuclear imaging methods.

Echocardiography yields considerably higher spatial resolution than isotope methods and has become an established technique for clinical cardiac diagnosis. This modality, however, also has important limitations because only portions of the heart can be imaged owing to air in surrounding lung, because images depend greatly upon the skill and experience of the echocardiographic technician, and because adequate studies cannot be obtained in some persons because of body habitus or pulmonary hyperinflation. Furthermore, the method has fundamental limitations in defining tissue abnormalities and perfusion.

Computed tomographic (CT) scanning is a relatively new method for cardiac imaging. It can provide images that have the necessary spatial resolution for displaying anatomic structures in three dimensions—thus overcoming the problems associated with superimposition—

and in addition, can provide unique physiologic data. This article will describe some of the diagnostic capabilities unique to CT scanning that have already been demonstrated. So far, experience with CT scanning for cardiac diagnosis has been limited to only a few centers around the world. Although cardiac gating is critical for dimensional measurements of cardiac structures, diagnostic images of the heart can be obtained with relatively fast scanners (greater than 5 sec exposure time) without gating.

CT SCANNERS

CT scanners produce images of thin cross-sections of the body by using a computer technique known as image reconstruction from projections. The projection data are acquired by measuring the attenuation of a typical fan beam of radiation directed through a selected slice of the body from many angles. The scanner precisely measures density changes along each x-ray path and presents this digitized data as a two-dimensional image on a precise geometric matrix. The theory underlying this concept was developed and applied by Hounsfield and Cormack, who were awarded the 1979 Nobel Prize for their research. These studies resulted in the first available commercial CT head scanner in England in 1972.[8, 13]

CT technology has advanced rapidly during its first decade. The need for neuroangiography has declined over 40 per cent since the availability of CT scanning. On the other hand, the temporal requirements of cardiac imaging dictate that CT scanning must attain a scanning speed equivalent to cineangiography before its full potential is reached. It is then anticipated that computed tomography will perhaps have an even greater impact on the diagnosis and management of heart disease.

CURRENT CARDIAC CT TECHNIQUES

Present limitations of CT imaging of the heart are primarily technical; the major problem is the relatively long exposure time of whole body scanners compared with that of the cardiac cycle. The influence of cardiac motion and to a lesser extent respiratory motion is therefore significant, and more so in infants and children. The exposure time of the earliest EMI scanner in 1973 was 5 min. This time has rapidly been reduced, and several manufacturers now offer CT machines with scan times in the 1 to 5 sec range, which has made cardiovascular CT imaging feasible.[13]

CT SCAN REGISTRATION

The operator selects the anatomic level to be scanned as well as the thickness of each slice of tissue. Selection of thickness is accomplished by varying the width of the x-ray beam. Usually, 1 cm scans are the most useful for cardiac imaging, but half centimeter and even thinner slices are possible.

The correct determination of anatomic level is important for scan slice registration and is made possible by a digital chest radiograph obtained with the CT scanner at the onset of the scanning procedure. The patient is transported on the CT table while the x-ray tube is kept stationary and the x-ray tube is pulsed. This technique provides a slit digital radiograph as shown in Figure 1.

This computed radiograph, which resembles a conventional chest x-ray (see Fig. 1*B*), allows the CT computer to register each level in memory. The radiograph also displays a linear scale alongside the image (see Fig. 1*A*). This enables any given anatomic level to be located and rescanned; it is also useful for obtaining precise contiguous scans at multiple levels through the heart or, when necessary, the whole chest. This option is usually employed in conjunction with intravenous drip infusion of contrast medium, thereby permitting the acquisition of a cubic matrix of CT data stored in the CT computer. This cubic matrix allows any arbitrary sagittal, coronal, or oblique reconstruction to be selected from the transverse scans and generated. These projection images resemble those normally obtained with conventional angiocardiography.

ADMINISTRATION OF CONTRAST MEDIUM

Requirements of cardiac CT scanning include the administration of contrast medium because the CT densities of blood and myocardium are similar. Therefore, contrast enhancement is required to identify the lumina of all vascular structures and the cardiac chambers of the heart.

Considerably less contrast enhancement is required with CT methods than with either conventional angiography or digital subtraction systems for several reasons. First, the cross-

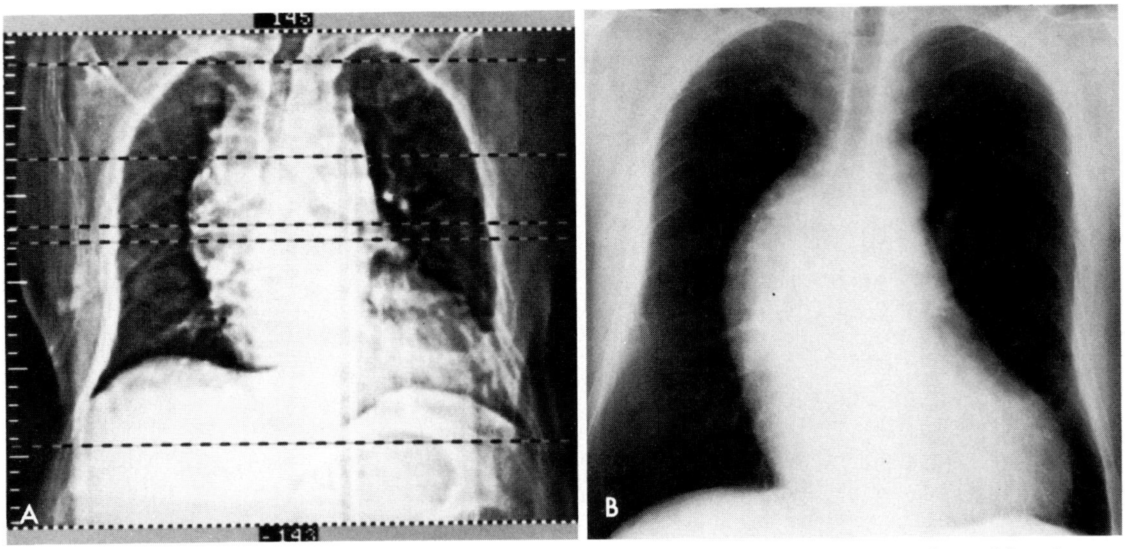

Figure 1. *A*, Computed chest radiograph of a patient with a wide mediastinum. This image was obtained by advancing the table through the pulsed x-ray fan beam while the x-ray tube was kept stationary. Each pulse generates one line of the image. The digital processor constructs the image by the juxtaposition of lines. The technique ensures accurate CT slice registration for selecting appropriate anatomic levels desired. Note adjacent linear scale. The horizontal dotted lines are selected and can be varied by the operator; they correspond to the scan levels to be exposed. This computed radiograph has a wide dynamic range. Bones and soft tissues can be seen by changing the CT window and level at the console. *B*, This regular chest radiograph is of the same patient as seen in *A* for comparison. The chest x-ray film has greater spatial resolution but does not have the flexibility of varying the contrast, since it is a fixed, exposed film.

sectional imaging format of a CT scanner avoids the problem previously discussed of superimposed structures. Second, a CT scanner has a remarkably high density resolution, which is an order of magnitude greater than that reached with conventional radiographic film-screen systems. This difference permits highly sensitive identification and localization of calcification that may not otherwise be possible. However, the major advantage of this contrast sensitivity is that relatively little intravenous contrast medium is required (usually 0.15 to 0.25 gm/kg yields diagnostic bloodpool CT images). Such small amounts would be generally inadequate for obtaining useful angiograms by the intravenous route.

Contrast agents used in cardiovascular CT studies are those with high iodine content (approximately 40 per cent iodine). Two methods are frequently used for administrating contrast medium. One, by bolus injection, is most useful for evaluating the dynamic aspects of the circulation. The other, by drip infusion, is used when a longer period of opacification is desired so that predominantly anatomic structures can be displayed.

In dynamic scanning, a bolus of contrast medium is injected at a flow rate of approximately 5 ml/sec while a series of sequential scans are rapidly exposed all at the same anatomic level. Dynamic CT scanning of this type results in the acquisition of an initial precontrast image, which is followed by contrast enhancement of the vascular structures in progressive sequence. First, the cardiac chambers on the right side are seen, then the pulmonary arteries, followed by the left atrium, and finally the left ventricle, and the aorta (Fig. 2).

The other method of contrast enhancement is performed by continuous gravity drip infusion of between 0.15 to 0.35 gm/kg of a conventional contrast agent containing a high concentration of iodine. Contiguous CT scans are commenced when approximately half the total volume of contrast agent has been administered so that a relatively steady bloodpool level is present. All scans are obtained during held inspiration. However, when this is not possible because of factors related to a person's health or disposition, the patient is allowed a breath between scan sequences and is then instructed to hold his or her breath again in deep inspiration. The resulting CT images, even in problem patients, are frequently diagnostic.

GATED CT SCANNING

A further development of CT scanning is the application of electrocardiographic gating,

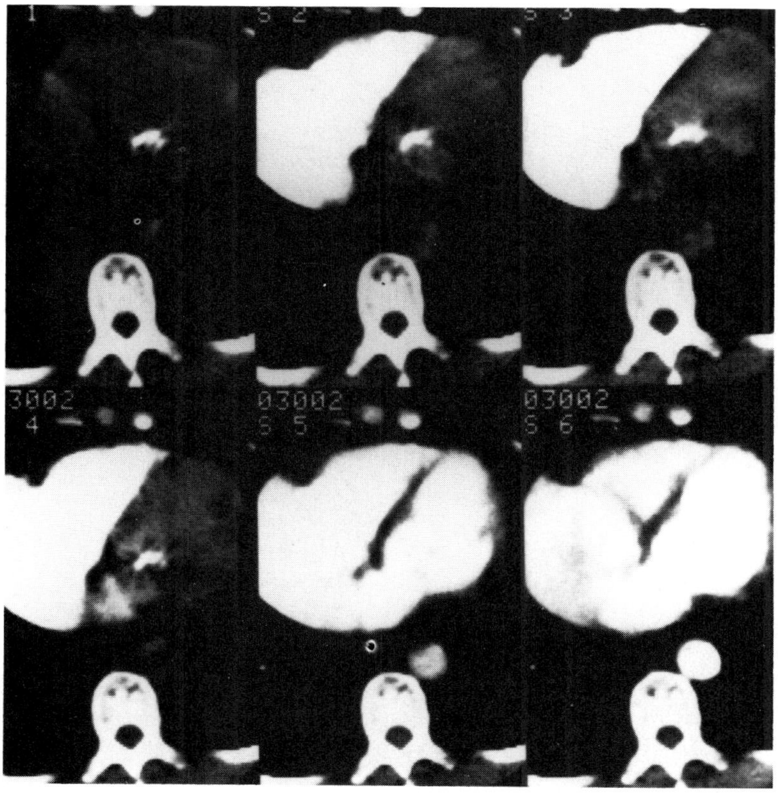

Figure 2. A dynamic sequence of nongated CT scans 1 cm thick during the passage of an intravenous bolus of contrast medium. Note how the right-sided structures are enhanced first and then progressively washout as the left side is enhanced. The white density in scan 1 is calcium in the mitral valve. The right atrium is large due to congestive heart failure. (*From* Lipton MJ, Brundage BH, Doherty PW, et al: Contrast medium-enhanced computed tomography for evaluating ischemic heart disease. Cardiovasc Med, *4*:1219–1229, 1979, with permission.)

which, although not routinely available with all CT scanners, is currently being explored in a number of centers.[9, 14, 21, 25, 26] This technique is one method to overcome the problem of cardiac motion and is critical to obtain quantitative dimensional data, ejection fraction, or extent of wall thickening during the cardiac cycle.

Gated CT scanning differs significantly from standard CT scanning. To obtain a reconstructed image of a stationary object by standard computed tomography, one must obtain a full complement of angular x-ray data over the full scanning circle from 0 to 360° without significant gaps in the angular data set. To image the heart, a rapidly moving structure, over one cardiac cycle (in ten serial images), multiple scans are required. Each scan covers multiple cardiac cycles; the standard scans (referenced to the ECG signal) must then be broken into multiple angular segments, each containing the angular data acquired for each 10 per cent of the cardiac cycle (Fig. 3). The angular segments that fall within the same portion of the cardiac cycle are then pooled together to reconstitute a new gap-free angular data set.

Currently, two gating techniques are used: retrospective[2] and prospective gating.[26, 29] With retrospective gating, the CT scan data and the ECG are merely simultaneously recorded, but the ECG signal does not guide the acquisition of x-ray data in any manner. Subsequently, the image is reconstructed from data obtained within a selected time window (biologic window), bracketing the desired portion of the ECG signal, such as a QRS complex for end-diastole.

The prospective gating system allows preselection of a fraction of the electrocardiographic R-R interval width to be monitored.[26] The biologic window width sets the fraction of the cardiac cycle to be represented by each image. Prospective gating assures the even distribution of the R-waves throughout the scanning circle in the minimum number of scans. This is accomplished by activating the x-ray tube at the appropriate time, relative to the R-wave on the ECG input, such that one of the following R waves falls in the largest gap in the already acquired angular x-ray data (see Fig. 3*A*). In our studies, the width of the biologic window has generally been set at 10 per cent of the R-R interval. Since the heart rate was maintained between 100 to 120 beats per minute, each frame represents 0.05 to 0.06 sec. With the

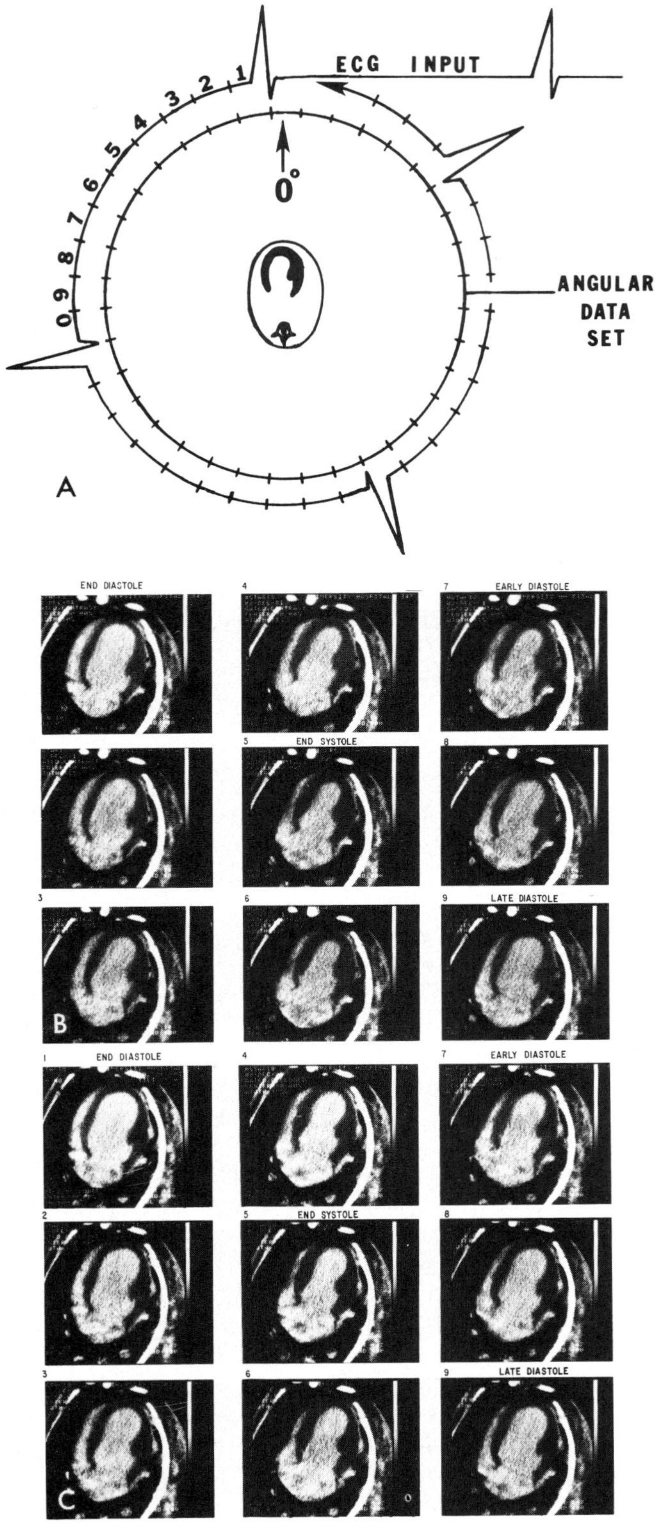

Figure 3. *A*, Schematic diagram demonstrating the operation of prospective ECG-gating system with the biologic window set at 10 per cent of the R-R interval. Also depicted is the concept that when the R wave is uniformly distributed over the scanning circle, one R wave per angular segment, sufficient data are obtained to reconstruct ten images in which each image corresponds to 10 per cent of the cardiac cycle. *B*, Series of gated CTT scans (approximately 60 msec images) through the mid left ventricle depicting one composite cardiac cycle obtained at rest. Images progress through the cardiac cycle vertically starting at the top left and ending on the bottom right. The tenth image in the series is not shown. *C*, Series of gated CTT scans (approximately 60 msec images) obtained after occlusion of the left anterior descending artery in the same dog shown in Figure *B* at the same left ventricular level. The sequence is similar to that of *B*. (*From* Mattrey RF, Slutsky RA, Long SA, et al: In vivo assessment of left ventricular wall and chamber dynamics during transient myocardial ischemia using prospectively ECG-gated computerized transmission tomography. Circulation, *67*:1245–1251, 1983, with permission.)

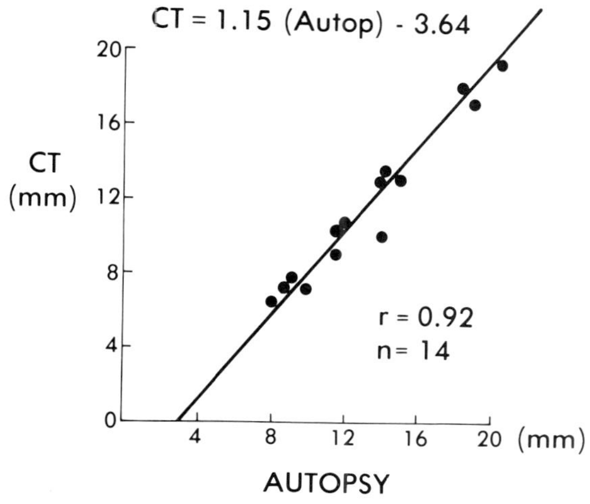

Figure 4. Linear regression for septal wall thickness; along the abscissa are measurements (mm) obtained at autopsy, and corresponding computed transmission tomographic estimates lie on the ordinate. (*From* Skioldebrand CG, Ovenfors C-O, Mavroudis C, et al: Assessment of ventricular wall thickness in vivo by computed transmission tomography. Circulation, *61*:960–965, 1980, with permission.)

biologic window set at 10 per cent of the R-R interval, approximately eight scans were required to obtain a full complement of gated angular data requiring approximately 45 sec of breath holding.

CT scanning has the advantage of being able to identify not only the inner endocardial walls but also the epicardial surface. Thus, wall thickness, as well as total myocardial mass, can be estimated even without ECG gating,[27, 28] but gating should enhance precision of dimensional quantitation by computed tomography. Initial results have shown a close correlation between CT measurements and postmortem anatomic measurements (Figs. 4 and 5). An even more exciting prospect for CT scanning is the quantitation of myocardial wall dynamics in terms of wall thickening and thinning during each heart cycle.[23] ECG-gated CT scanning is required with conventional body CT scanners for this purpose. Gated CT scans in an animal model of regional ischemia have identified the region of ischemia (see Fig. 3*B* and *C*) by demonstrating loss of wall thickening during the cardiac cycle.[29] This has also been observed in patients.[24]

CLINICAL APPLICATION IN HEART DISEASE

Various congenital and acquired cardiovascular disorders have been effectively examined by computed tomography.[6, 18, 22, 23] These are considered in the following sections.

Congenital Abnormalities Involving the Great Vessels and Venous Structures. The clinical findings and conventional chest radiographs may raise the question in a given patient of nonvascular or vascular mediastinal mass. CT scanning provides a most effective and almost

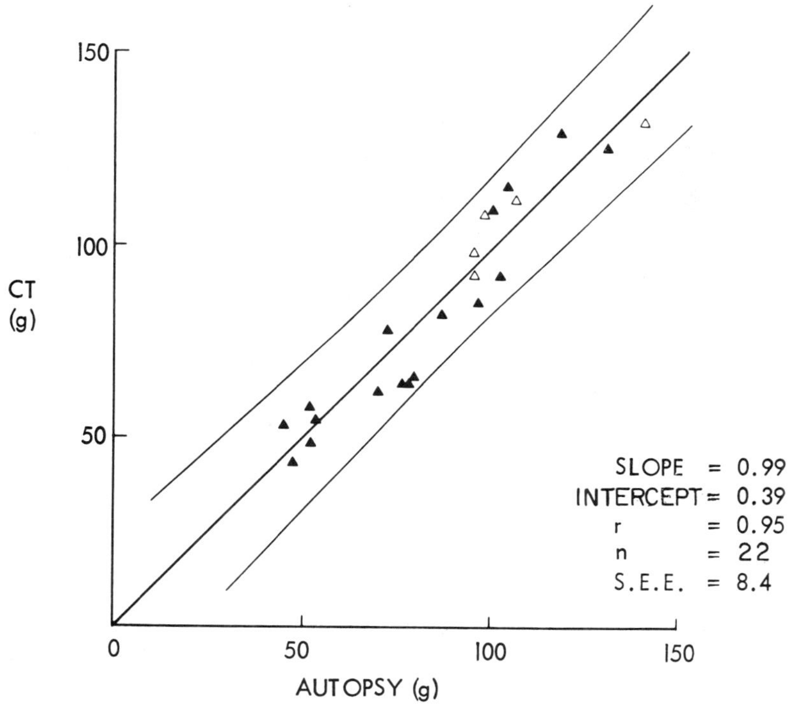

Figure 5. Relation between autopsy values and computed tomographic (CT) estimates of left ventricular (LV) mass. Filled triangles: normotensive dogs; open triangles: beagles with left ventricular hypertrophy. The lines on either side of the regression line indicate the 95 per cent confidence limits. (*From* Skioldebrand CG, Lipton MJ, Mavroudis C, et al: Determination of left ventricular mass by computed tomography. Am J Cardiol, *49*:63–70, 1982, with permission.)

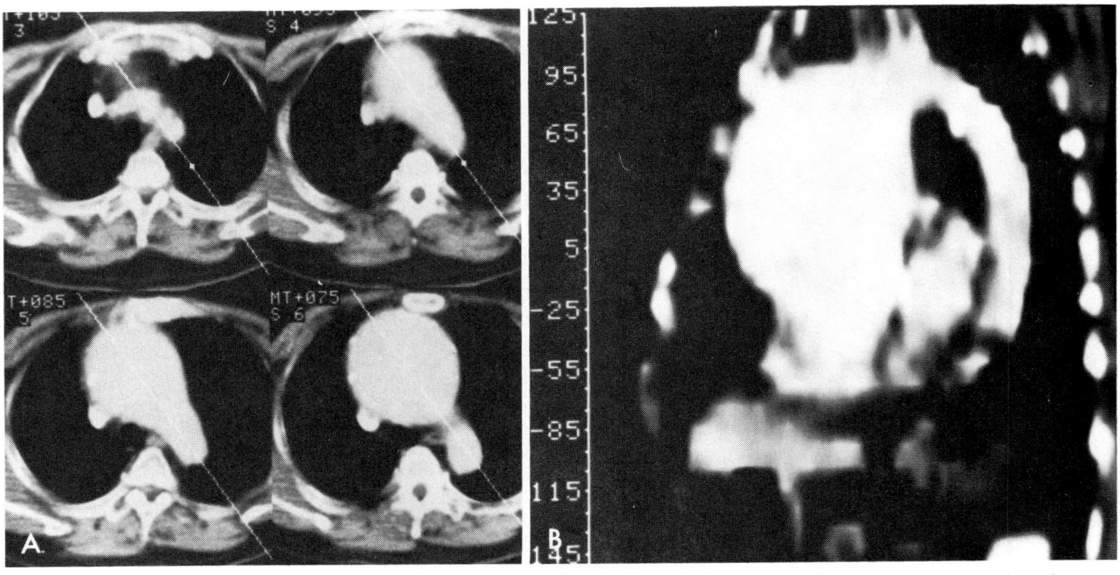

Figure 6. *A*, Four CT scans obtained at different anatomic levels through the aorta in the same patient as that shown in Figure 1. Note the peripherally situated, patchy calcifications around the markedly dilated lumen of the ascending aorta. Note also that the whole aorta is opacified as one homogeneous structure. The oblique line indicates the plane selected for oblique reconstruction. *B*, This is the oblique CT reconstruction through the plane indicated in *A*. This image illustrates the excellent demonstration possible of anatomic structures by CT. Note that the grossly dilated ascending aorta resumes a normal diameter at the origin of the great vessels and appears to maintain its normal caliber beyond them. This patient had a true aneurysm of the aorta.

noninvasive screening procedure in this setting. Such a case is illustrated in Figure 6. The transverse scans display a markedly dilated ascending aorta and depict areas of calcification along its outer margin. This can be seen before infusion of contrast medium, which confirms (by its uniform enhancement) that the mass is indeed vascular. An oblique reconstruction can then be generated from such multiple contiguous transverse scans as shown in Figure 6*B*. This image closely resembles a typical left anterior oblique projection obtained during a conventional angiogram.

True aortic aneurysms can be distinguished from classic aortic dissections.[20] Details of the findings in these conditions have been described in detail previously.[11] Dissecting aneurysms can also be diagnosed by CT scanning (Fig. 7). False and true lumina may opacify differentially. Calcifications, when present, may

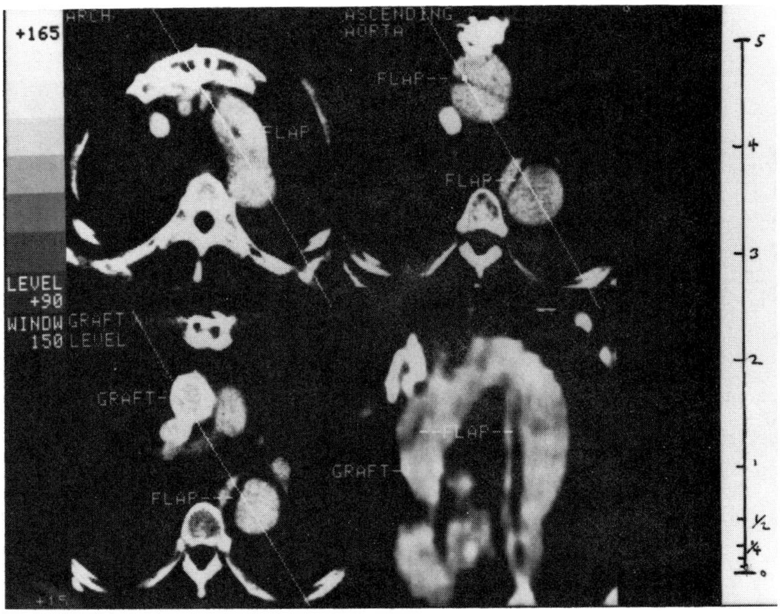

Figure 7. Shows a CT scan of a patient with an aortic dissection. The upper two panels (contrast-enhanced CT scans) show an intimal flap through the aortic arch and both the ascending and descending aortas. The left lower image is a CT scan through a previously placed teflon graft in the ascending aorta. The oblique CT reconstruction was created from multilevel cross-sectional images in the plane indicated by the white cursor line selected by the physician. The longitudinal intimal flap is labeled.

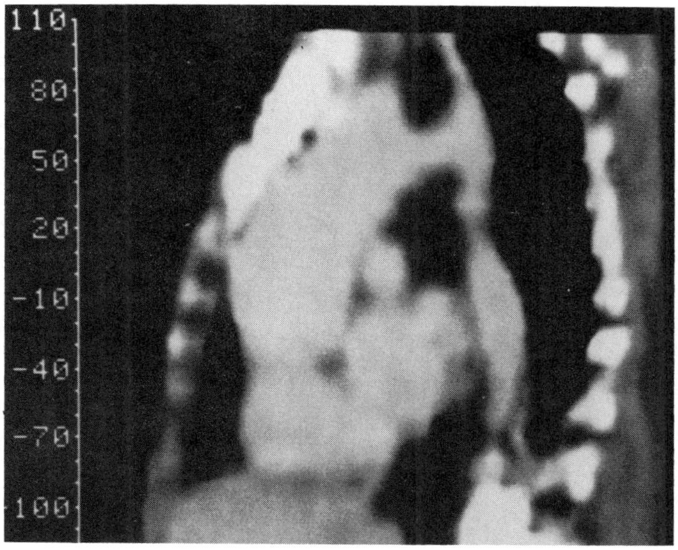

Figure 8. A contrast-enhanced oblique CT reconstruction of a coarctation of the aorta. Note the dilated ascending aorta and the small stenotic descending component. The position of origin of the left subclavian artery or any other vessel can be easily explored and displayed.

appear to lie centrally within the torn lumen, in contradistinction to true aneurysms. Coarctation of the aorta is also readily demonstrated by CT scans;[10] an example is shown in Figure 8. CT scans can provide—unlike angiography—any desired projection image of the aorta. Furthermore, questions about vessel origins (for example, the subclavian artery) can be studied in any projection long after the procedure is completed. The potential of a CT scan to estimate blood flow by means of time/density analysis is also exciting. It is still in its infancy, but there are compelling reasons to believe that this modality will become an important technique, particularly when fast cardiac CT scanners become available.[3, 19]

Malpositions, such as transposition of the great vessels, can also be demonstrated by CT scanning as shown in Figure 9. Venous anomalies in isolation or in association with congenital heart disease (Fig. 10) are also frequently noted during routine contrast-enhanced CT studies.[34]

Intracardiac Shunts. Computed tomography provides a flexible approach for displaying intra- and extracardiac anatomy. An example of an intact intraventricular septum is shown in Figure 11. The oblique plane of the reconstruction selected can then be generated and in this case yields an image equivalent to a left anterior oblique projection. Compare this image with the image shown in Figure 12 in which a ventricular septal defect was demonstrated. The ability to obtain dynamic CT scanning at one level with a bolus injection enables a CT computer program to generate time/density curves as illustrated in Figure 13. In this case, the region-of-interest was placed over the right ventricle. Note the biphasic nature of the curve, indicating the presence of left-to-right shunting. Contrast medium enhancement can be used with dynamic CT scanning for obtaining physiologic estimates of shunting. However, such applications are just emerging, and two requirements remain to be met before the full potential of computed tomography can be attained. These two needs are continuous subsecond exposures and simultaneous multilevel scanning. Such instruments are being constructed, and prototypes are being tested.[3, 19]

Cardiac Tumors. The presence and particularly the extent of intracardiac and paracardiac tumors can be determined by conventional noninvasive imaging techniques. By virtue of its excellent spatial and density resolution, CT scanning can identify intracardiac, myocardial, and pericardial masses, as well as the extracardiac component of such masses. An example of an intraatrial malignant thymoma is shown in Figure 14. Similarly, other mass lesions have been successfully demonstrated by CT scanning, including intraatrial and intraventricular thrombus. Comparison of these findings with two-dimensional echocardiography suggests that CT scanning may have an equal or greater diagnostic accuracy.[1, 15, 32, 33]

Pericardial Abnormalities. Established noninvasive techniques (notably echocardiography) have proved valuable in detecting such lesions as pericardial effusion and thickening. However, CT scanning is emerging as perhaps a

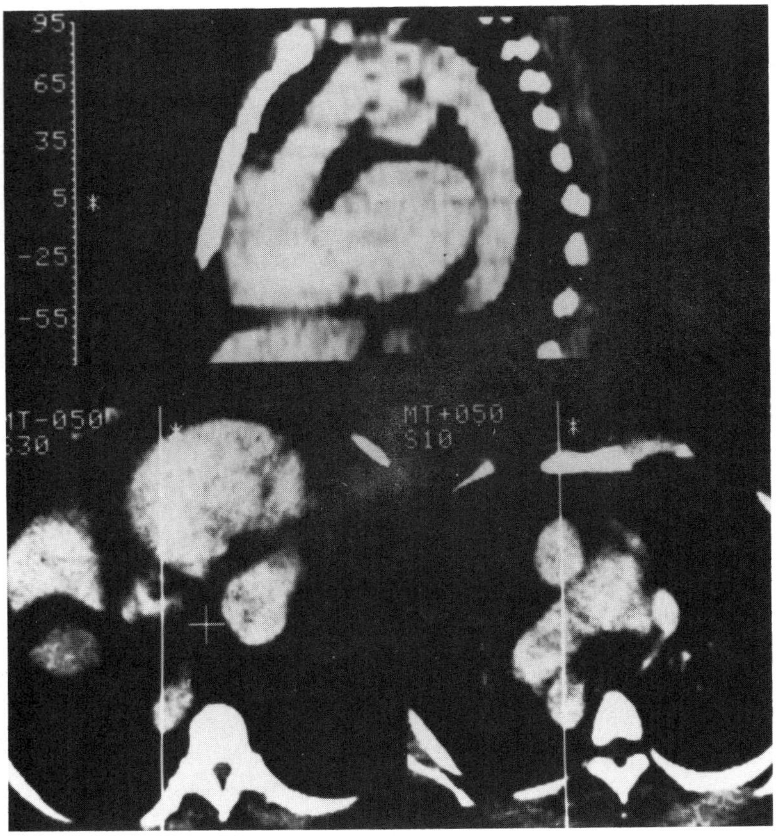

Figure 9. Lateral CT image reconstruction of a patient with transposition of the great vessels shows the aorta arising from the anterior ventricle. The combination of transverse images and any other selected arbitrary plane of reconstruction makes CT a powerful imaging modality.

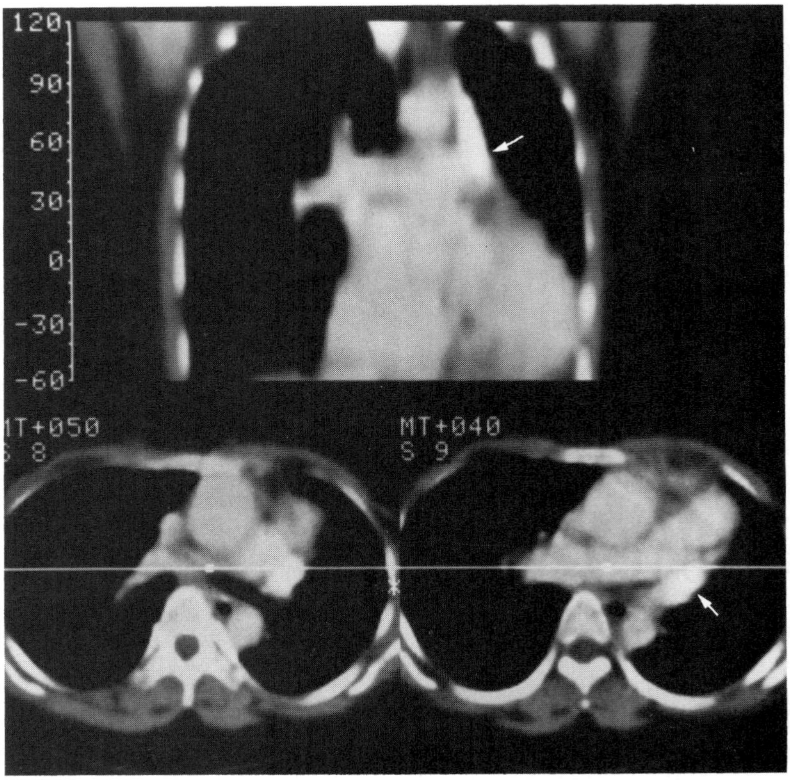

Figure 10. The lower panel illustrates CT scans at different levels with marked contrast enhancement of a left-sided mediastinal structure (arrow). The coronal reconstruction seen above confirms the presence of a left-sided superior vena cava (arrow). Other images showed that it drained directly into the coronary sinus.

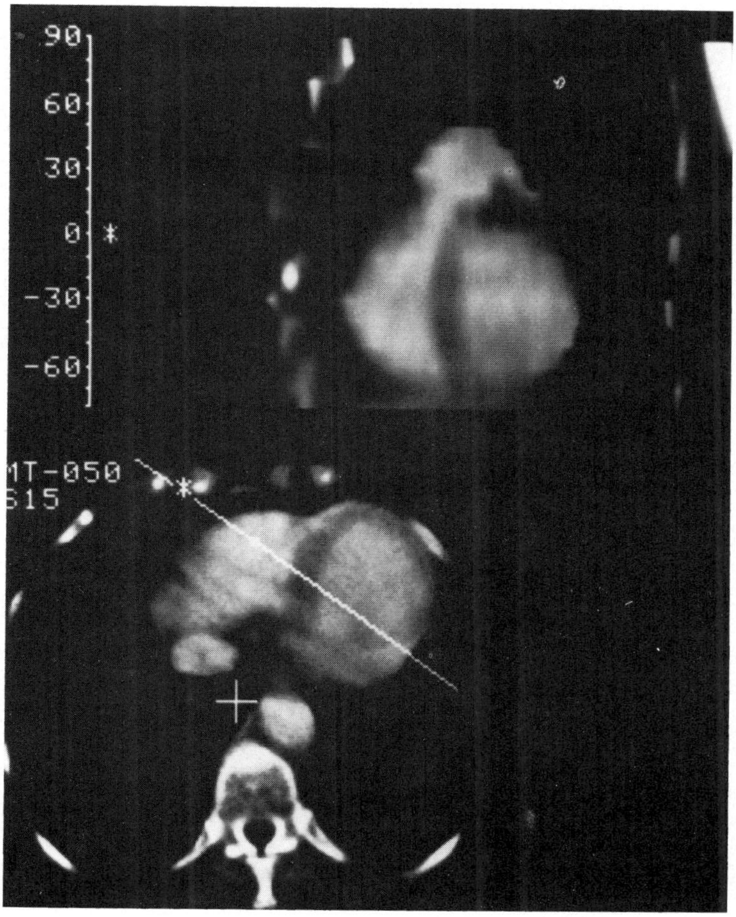

Figure 11. The lower panels illustrate a contrast-enhanced CT scan at the ventricular level. The cursor line is the oblique plane selected for reconstruction. The generated CT image (upper panel) is equivalent to the left anterior oblique projection and profiles a normal, well-defined interventricular septum; the left and right ventricular cavities are also elegantly seen and have relatively sharp boundaries. (*From* Lipton MJ, Brundage BH: Evaluation of ischemic heart disease in man by CTT. *In* Higgins CB, Carlsson E, Lipton MJ (eds): CT of the Heart and Great Vessels. Mt. Kisco, NY, Futura Publishing Co., 1983, pp. 255–261, with permission.)

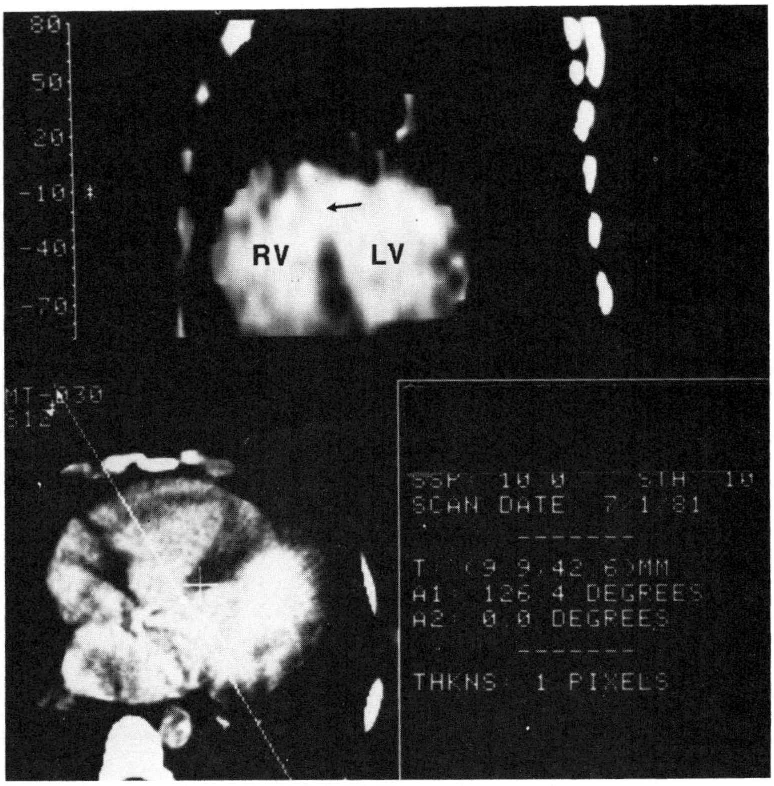

Figure 12. A large ventricular septal defect (arrow) is well demonstrated in this oblique reformat. rv: right ventricle; lv: left ventricle. (*From* Brundage BH, Lipton MJ: What is the role of CT scanning of the heart: *In* Rahimtoola SH (ed): Controversies in Coronary Artery Disease. New York, F.A. Davis and Co., 1982, pp. 91–112, with permission.)

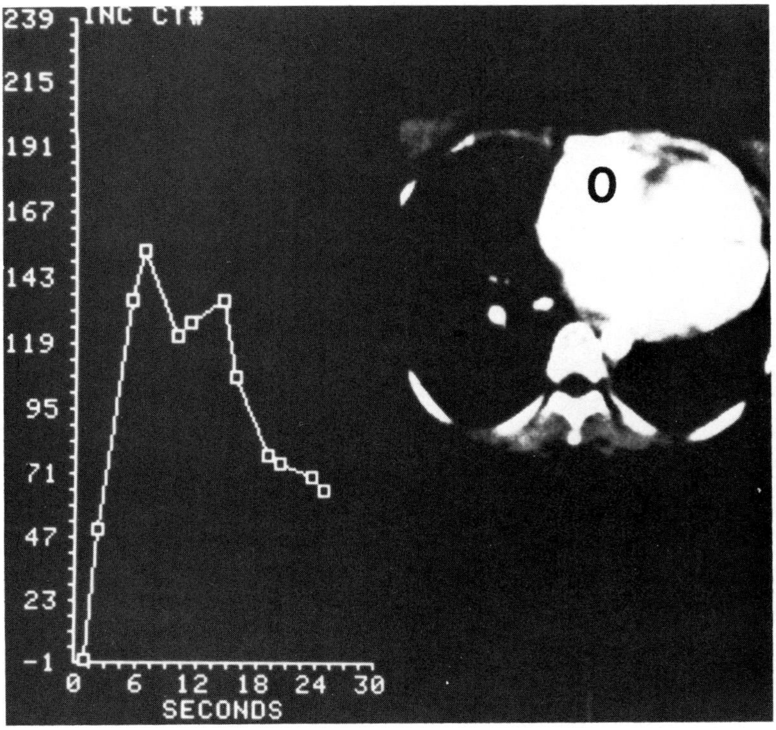

Figure 13. One CT scan from a dynamic sequence of scans during a bolus injection of contrast medium is shown. A region of interest (ROI) has been selected over the right ventricle, and a time/density curve has been generated using the average density change within the ROI on each scan and plotting this against time. The biphasic graph shown was obtained. This appearance is abnormal and indicates a left-to-right shunt lesion. This patient had a ventricular septal defect.

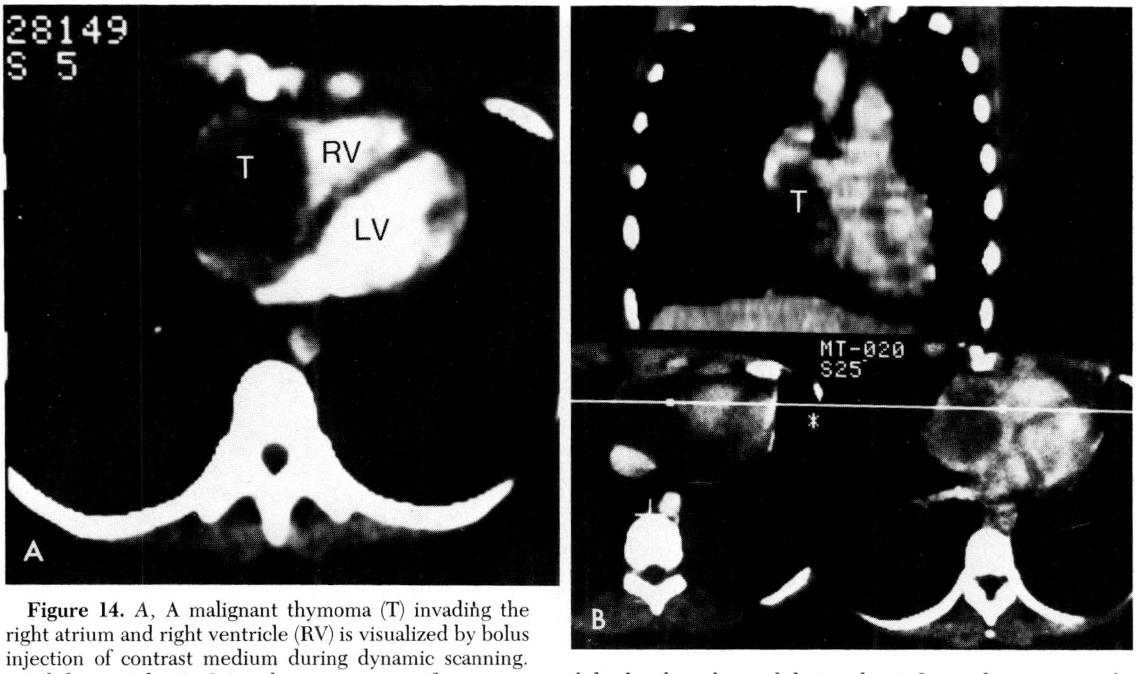

Figure 14. *A*, A malignant thymoma (T) invading the right atrium and right ventricle (RV) is visualized by bolus injection of contrast medium during dynamic scanning. LV: left ventricle. *B*, Coronal reconstruction of transverse axial display data obtained during drip infusion demonstrates the longitudinal extent of the tumor (T). (*From* Brundage BH, Lipton MJ: What is the role of CT scanning of the heart: *In* Rahimtoola SH (ed): Controversies in Coronary Artery Disease. New York, F.A. Davis and Co., 1982, pp. 91–112, with permission.)

more sensitive method for identifying constrictive pericarditis, congenital pericardial defects, and mediastinal mass lesions adjacent to the pericardium.[16] Figure 15*A* shows an abnormal cardiac silhouette in an asymptomatic patient. The bulge seen high along the left cardiac border was not adequately defined by two-dimensional echocardiography. A dynamic CT scan sequence through the left atrium is shown in Figure 15*B*. This revealed a greatly enlarged left atrial appendage. Additional multilevel CT scans were obtained, and a coronal CT image was then generated by using a reconstruction algorithm programmed into the CT computer. The images shown in Figure 15*C* indicate that the mass is due to an enlarged left atrial appendage that has herniated through a partial congenital defect in the left pericardium. Localized or generalized pericardial fluid can also be identified and quantitated by CT scanning.[17, 31] Pericardial cysts can be imaged in their entirety, and since the whole chest is readily scanned by computed tomography, associated abnormalities elsewhere can be detected routinely.

FUTURE DIRECTIONS

Once millisecond CT scanning is possible, the exceptional potential of CT scans for exploring cardiac anatomy and physiology should be realized. Present CT scanners not only are too slow but also can image only a single slice at a time. Two advanced scanners using different principles are currently under development. The Dynamic Spatial Reconstructor (DSR) at the Mayo Clinic is a research instrument employing numerous x-ray tubes placed in a circle around the patient. These tubes discharge in rapid millisecond sequences to provide the numerous projections needed. This device pioneered many of the ideas embodied in high-speed, three-dimensional imaging.[19]

An alternative and more practical approach to high-power x-ray generation is that incorporated in the cardiovascular CT (CVCT) scanner recently developed and constructed by Boyd and colleagues at the University of California, San Francisco, Medical Center.[3] This scanner employs a focused electron beam and sweeps a number of large hemicircles of tungsten, which effectively produce a number of x-ray fan beams. This approach does not suffer from heat loading limitations as do present body scanners; hence, continuous millisecond and simultaneous multislice scans are possible. The prototype unit is illustrated in Figure 16 and is now operational. The introduction of advanced CT scanners such as this should profoundly affect cardiovascular radiology. These units will ultimately compete directly with current noninva-

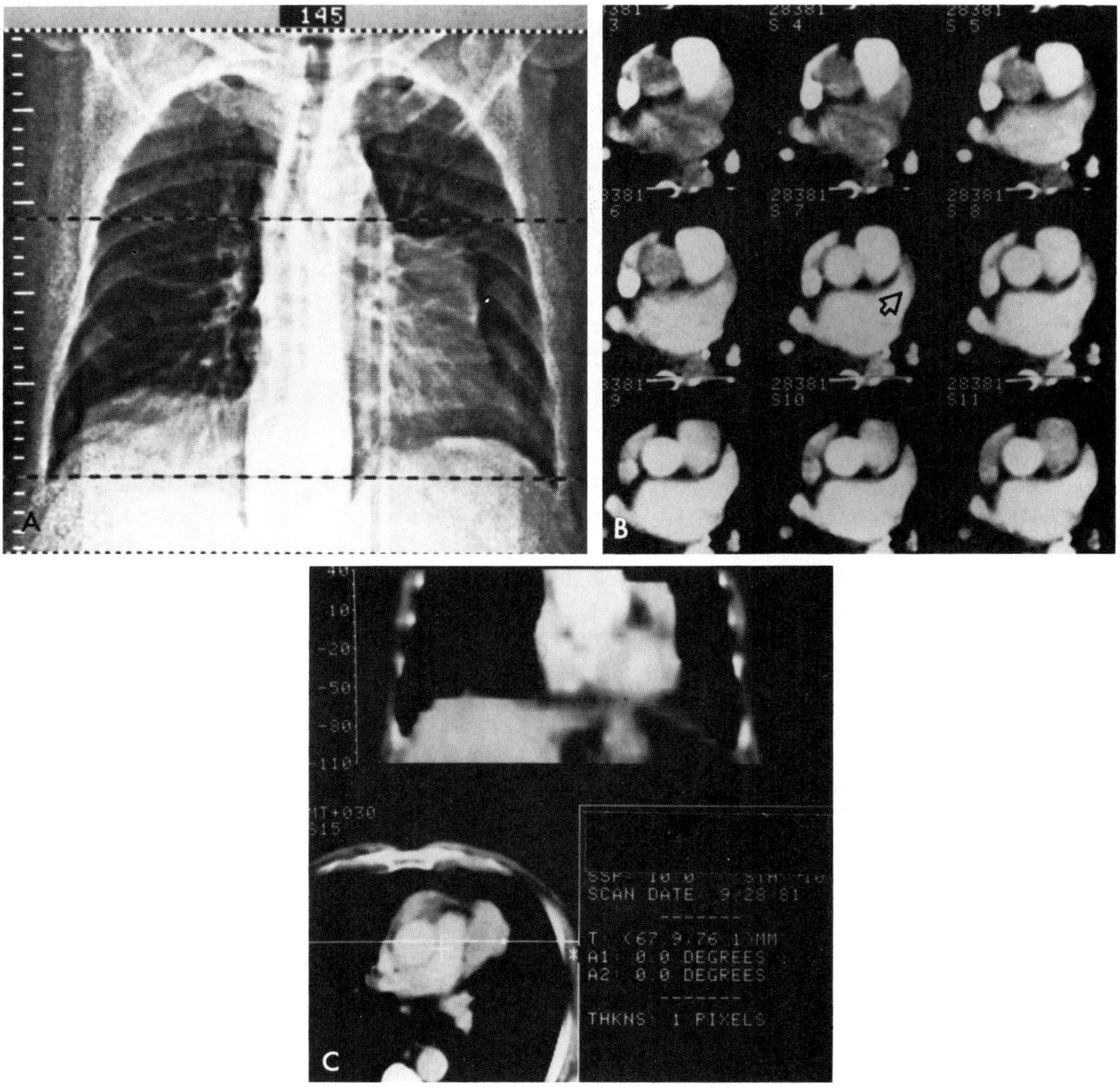

Figure 15. *A*, This computed radiograph of a young woman shows an abnormal bulge along the left cardiac border. The nature of this lesion could not be elucidated by echocardiography. A CT study is illustrated in *B* and *C*. *B*, A dynamic bolus study is shown through the level of the left atrium. Note the greatly enlarged left atrial appendage (arrows). *C*, Illustrates in the lower panel a CT scan from one level of a multilevel sequence of scans after infusion of contrast material. A coronal plane depicted (lower panel) was selected by the operator. The CT computer then generates the reconstructed image shown in the upper panel. This corresponds to a frontal projection. The abnormality is now seen to be an enlarged and herniated left atrial appendage through a partial congenital defect in the left pericardium.

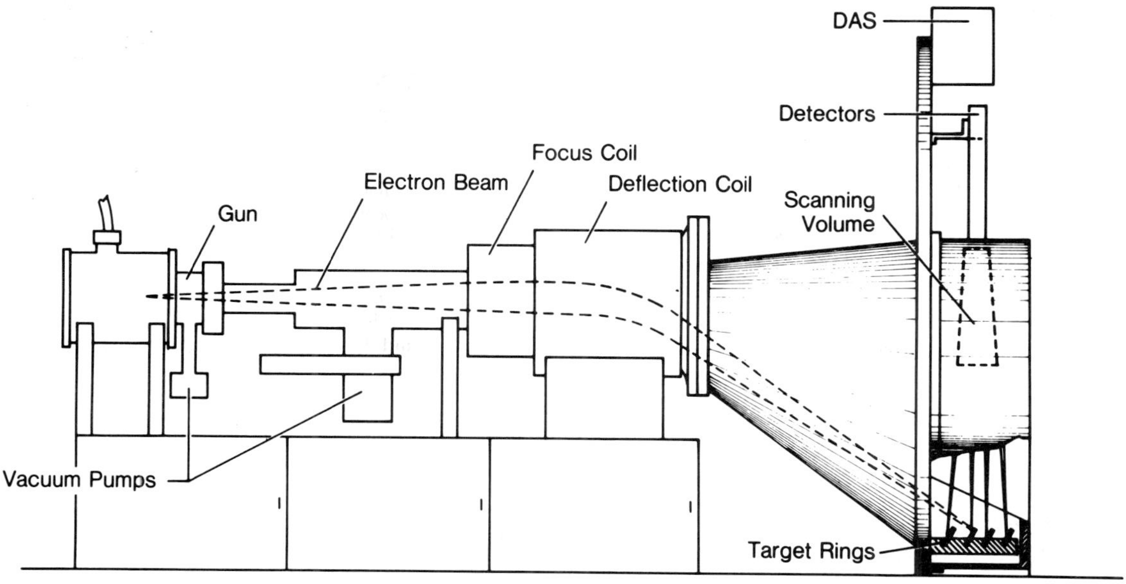

Figure 16. Cross-sectional view of the cine CT scanner (CVCT) currently under construction at the University of California, San Francisco. Electronic deflection of an intense beam of electrons replaces the mechanical gantry motion required in conventional CT scanners. X-rays are produced at a series of 180 cm diameter tungsten target rings that cover a half-circle below the patient. This design provides for high-scanning speed, multiplanar images, and continuous scanning capability with reduced heat-load limitations. (*From* Boyd DP, Lipton MJ: Cardiac computed tomography. Proc IEEE, *71*:298–307, 1983, with permission.)

sive as well as invasive angiographic techniques in the diagnosis and management of patients with all forms of heart disease.

SUMMARY

Computed tomography, a promising new imaging technique, has not yet been widely applied to cardiac disease. There is, furthermore, very little experience with CT scanning for patients with congenital cardiovascular malformations. Nevertheless, early studies with this remarkable modality indicate great promise for future application at low levels of radiation—approximately 10 to 15 per cent that of a conventional angiogram.[4]

The feasibility studies so far performed should be considered in that context. Nevertheless, relatively slow, whole body CT scanners can contribute useful clinical diagnostic information in patients with heart disease. Cardiac CT scanning is presently limited, as were all other conventional x-ray techniques at first, by relatively long exposure times. CT scan technology has made dramatic strides during its short existence of one decade, and there is strong evidence that this trend will continue in conjunction with rapid advances in high technology.

ACKNOWLEDGMENTS

We thank our colleagues Robert J. Herfkens, Bruce H. Brundage, Eric Carlsson, and Douglas P. Boyd at the University of California, San Francisco, and Robert F. Mattrey at the University of California, San Diego. We also thank Lauranne Cox for technical support during CT scanning procedures and Liz Braun for editing and typing the manuscript.

REFERENCES

1. Berninger WH, Redington RW, Doherty P, et al: Gated cardiac scanning in normal and experimentally infarcted canines. J Comput Assist Tomogr, *32*:155, 1979.
2. Berninger WH, Redington RW, Leue W, et al: Technical aspects and clinical applications of CT/X, a dynamic CT scanner. J Comput Assist Tomogr, *5*:206, 1981.
3. Boyd DP, Gould RG, Quinn JR, et al: A proposed dynamic cardiac 3-D densitometer for early detection and evaluation of heart disease. IEEE Trans Nucl Sci, NS-*26*:2724, 1979.
4. Brasch RC, Boyd DP, Gooding CA: Computed tomography scanning in children: Comparison of radiation dose and resolving power of commercial CT scanners. Am J Roentgenol, *131*:95, 1978.
5. Braunwald E (ed): Protection of the ischemic myocardium. Circulation (Suppl) *53*:1, 1976.
6. Brundage BH, Lipton MJ, Herfkens RJ, et al: Detection of patent coronary bypass grafts by computed tomography: A preliminary report. Circulation, *61*:826, 1980.

7. Budinger TF: Physical attributes of single-photon tomography. J Nucl Med, *21*:579, 1980.
8. Cormack AM: Nobel Prize Acceptance Speech. Med Phys, 7:277, 1980.
9. Godwin J, Herfkens R, Skioldebrand C, et al: Detection of intraventricular thrombi by computed tomography. Radiology, *138*:717, 1981.
10. Godwin JD, Herfkens RJ, Brundage BH, et al: Evaluation of coarctation of the aorta by computed tomography. J Comput Assist Tomogr, 5:153, 1981.
11. Godwin JD, Herfkens RJ, Skioldebrand CG, et al: Evaluation of dissections and aneurysms of the thoracic aorta by conventional and dynamic CT scanning. Radiology, *136*:125, 1980.
12. Heart Facts: 1981. Dallas, American Heart Association, 1981.
13. Hounsfield GN: Nobel Prize Acceptance Speech. Med Phys, 7:283, 1981.
14. Lackner K, Thurn P: Computed tomography of the heart: ECG-gated and continuous scans. Radiology, *140*:413, 1981.
15. Mavroudis C, Way LW, Lipton MJ, et al: Diagnosis and operative treatment of intracavitary liposarcoma of the right ventricle. J Thorac Cardiovasc Surg, *81*:137, 1981.
16. Moncada R, Baker M, Salinas M, et al: Diagnostic role of computed tomography in pericardial heart disease: Congenital defect, thickening, neoplasms and effusions. Am Heart J, *103*:263, 1982.
17. Refsum H, Skioldebrand CG, Lipton MJ, et al: Ventricular diastolic pressure-volume relations and the pericardium: Effects of changes in blood volume and pericardial effusion in dogs. Circulation, *64*:997, 1981.
18. Ringertz HG, Skioldebrand CG, Refsum H, et al: A comparison between the information in ECG gated and nongated cardiac CT images. J Comput Assist Tomogr, *6*:933, 1982.
19. Ritman EL, Robb RA, Johnson SA, et al: Quantitative imaging of the structure and function of the heart, lungs and circulation. Mayo Clin Proc, *53*:3, 1978.
20. Skioldebrand CG, Brasch RC, Lipton MJ: Utility of computed tomography in the diagnosis of thoracic aneurysm in childhood. Cardiovasc Radiol, *4*:30, 1981.
21. Lackner VK, Thurn P: EKG-gesteuerte kardiocomputertomographie. Fortsch Rontgenstr, *132*:164, 1980.
22. Lipton MJ, Brundage BH, Doherty PW, et al: Contrast medium enhanced computed tomography for evaluating ischemic heart disease. Cardiovasc Med, *4*:1219, 1979.
23. Lipton MJ, Higgins CB: Evaluation of ischemic heart disease by computerized transmission tomography. Radiol Clin North Am, *18*:557, 1980.
24. Lipton MJ, Napel S, Brundage B, et al: Electrocardiographic gated CT for regional myocardial motion analysis. Circulation, *64*:220, 1981.
25. Masuda Y, Yoshida H, Morooka N, et al: ECG-synchronized computed tomography in clinical evaluation of total and regional cardiac motion: Comparison of postmyocardial infarction to normal hearts by rapid sequential imaging. Am Heart J, *103*:230, 1982.
26. Mattrey RF, Higgins CB: Detection of regional myocardial dysfunction during ischemia with computerized tomography: Documentation and physiologic basis. Invest Radiol, *17*:329, 1982.
27. Skioldebrand CG, Lipton MJ, Mavroudis C, et al: Determination of left ventricular mass by computed tomography. Am J Cardiol, *49*:63, 1982.
28. Skioldebrand CG, Ovenfors CO, Mavroudis C, et al: Assessment of ventricular wall thickness in vivo by computed transmission tomography. Circulation, *61*:960, 1980.
29. Slutsky RA, Mattrey RF, Long SA, et al: In vivo estimation of myocardial infarct size and left ventricular function by prospectively ECG gated computerized transmission tomography. Circulation, in press.
30. TerPogossian MM, Phelps ME, Hoffman EJ, et al: A positron emission transaxial tomograph for nuclear imaging (PETT). Radiology, *144*:89, 1975.
31. Tomoda H, Hoshiai M, Furuya H: Evaluation of pericardial effusion with computed tomography. Am Heart J, 99:701, 1980.
32. Tomoda H, Hoshiai M, Tagawa R, et al: Evaluation of left atrial thrombus with computed tomography. Am Heart J, *100*:306, 1980.
33. Tomoda H, Mitsumoto H, Furuya H, et al: Evaluation of left ventricular thrombus with computed tomography. Am J Cardiol, *48*:573, 1981.
34. Webb WR, Gamsu G, Speckman JM, et al: CT demonstration of mediastinal venous anomalies. AJR, *159*:157, 1982.

9

COMPUTED TOMOGRAPHIC (CT) EVALUATION OF THE GREAT ARTERIES AND AORTIC ARCH MALFORMATIONS

RICHARD L. BARON, M.D., FERNANDO R. GUTIERREZ, M.D.,
and ROBERT C. McKNIGHT, M.D.

Recent technologic advances have resulted in many new noninvasive ways to evaluate congenital anomalies of the mediastinal great vessels. The use of two-dimensional cardiac ultrasound, computed body tomography (CT), and, more recently, digital intravenous angiography has resulted in a decrease in the number of invasive cardiac and great vessel angiograms as screening procedures.

Over the last few years it has become apparent that the cross-sectional anatomy at the base of the heart and the associated great vessels can be defined precisely by CT.[1, 2, 12, 14] The ability of CT scans to distinguish specific tissue densities and to display the mediastinum in a transverse plane, avoiding the overlapping mediastinal shadows seen on conventional chest radiographs, makes it an excellent tool for screening of structural abnormalities in the mediastinum. Because of the nature of the anatomic characteristics of these abnormalities, CT can play an important diagnostic role, not only as a complement to angiography but also in some cases as an effective screening examination, precluding further, more invasive evaluation. In addition, radiologists and referring physicians performing CT of the mediastinum in patients for other reasons must be aware of the CT appearance of congenital anomalies of the mediastinal great vessels in order not to mistake these normal structures for other abnormalities such as enlarged lymph nodes.

We currently use CT as the initial screening procedure in patients (over age five years) with a suspected mediastinal abnormality detected on standard chest radiographs. CT can determine whether the mediastinal abnormality is due to a vascular anomaly or to some other cause such as lipomatosis, lymphadenopathy or neoplasm, and congenital cysts, among others.

CT TECHNIQUE

Adequate imaging of mediastinal vascular structures requires "state-of-the-art" CT scanners with scan times of 4 sec or less to overcome the effects of respiration and motion artifacts. Although rapid advances with decreasing scan times have made CT more useful in very young patients, the visualization of the mediastinum in young children up to age five or six years is difficult owing to a paucity of mediastinal fat to outline smaller structures and to a lack of patient cooperation. Although sedation is being used in young children undergoing CT for evaluation of trauma and neoplasms, it has been our experience that if a patient is young enough to require sedation he or she will not be an optimal candidate for CT of the mediastinum to evaluate for congenital vascular anomalies. Other screening methods should be used in such young children.

Scans are obtained with the patient supine with maximal inspiration to separate the chest wall from the mediastinum. Sections 10 mm

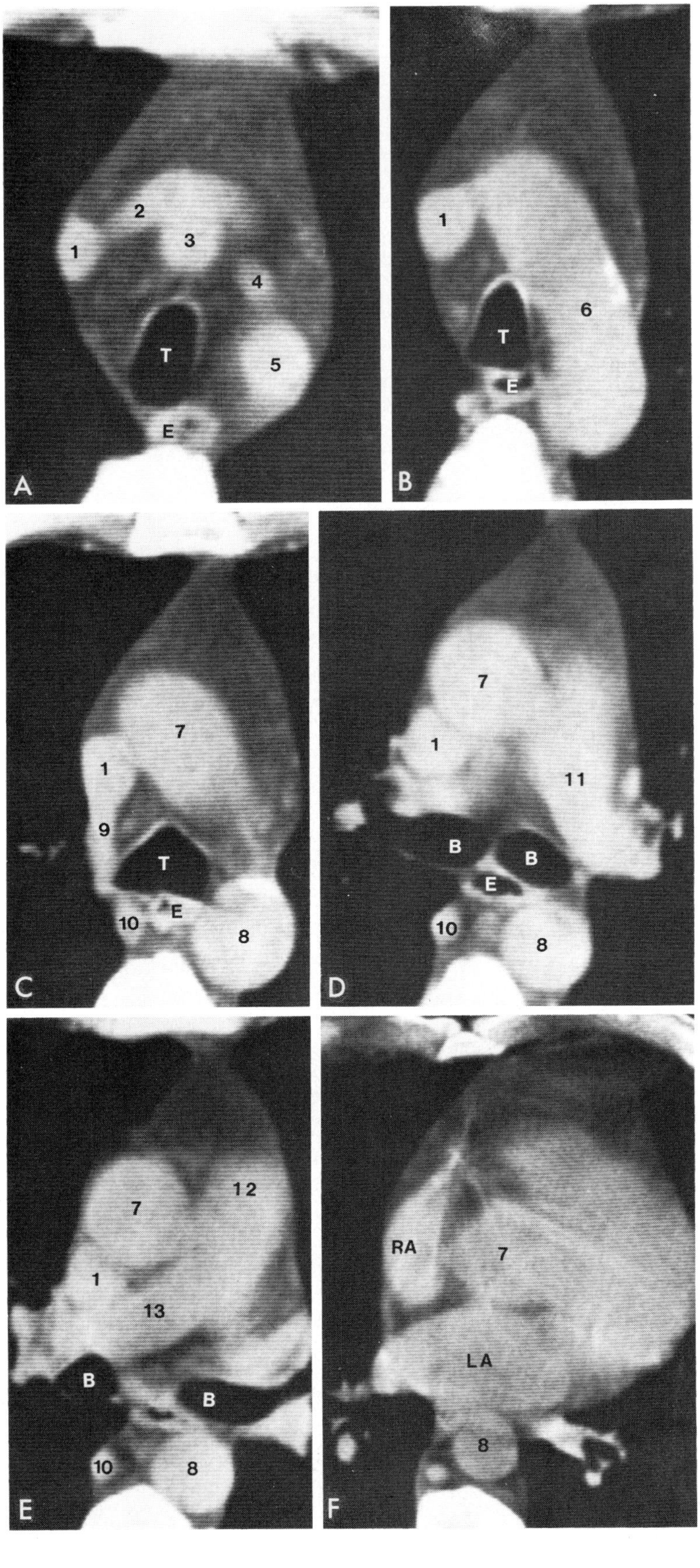

Figure 1. A series of normal CT scans in a 58-year-old man with exertional chest pain due to coronary artery disease. The lack of respiratory and other motion in this cooperative patient, as well as a large amount of mediastinal fat, provides easy recognition of the vascular structures without the use of intravenous contrast. *A*, Scan just above the aortic arch. *B*, Scan 2 cm lower at level of aortic arch. *C*, Scan 1 cm lower at level of agzygos arch. *D*, Scan 2 cm lower at level of left pulmonary artery. *E*, Scan 1 cm lower at level of right pulmonary artery. *F*, Scan 4 cm lower at level of aortic root. 1: superior vena cava; 2: left innominate vein; 3: innominate artery; 4: left common carotid artery; 5: left subclavian artery root; 6: aortic arch; 7: ascending aorta; 8: descending aorta; 9: azygos arch; 10: azygos vein; 11: left pulmonary artery; 12: main pulmonary artery; 13: right pulmonary artery; T: trachea; E: esophagus; B: bronchus; LA: left atrium; RA: right atrium.

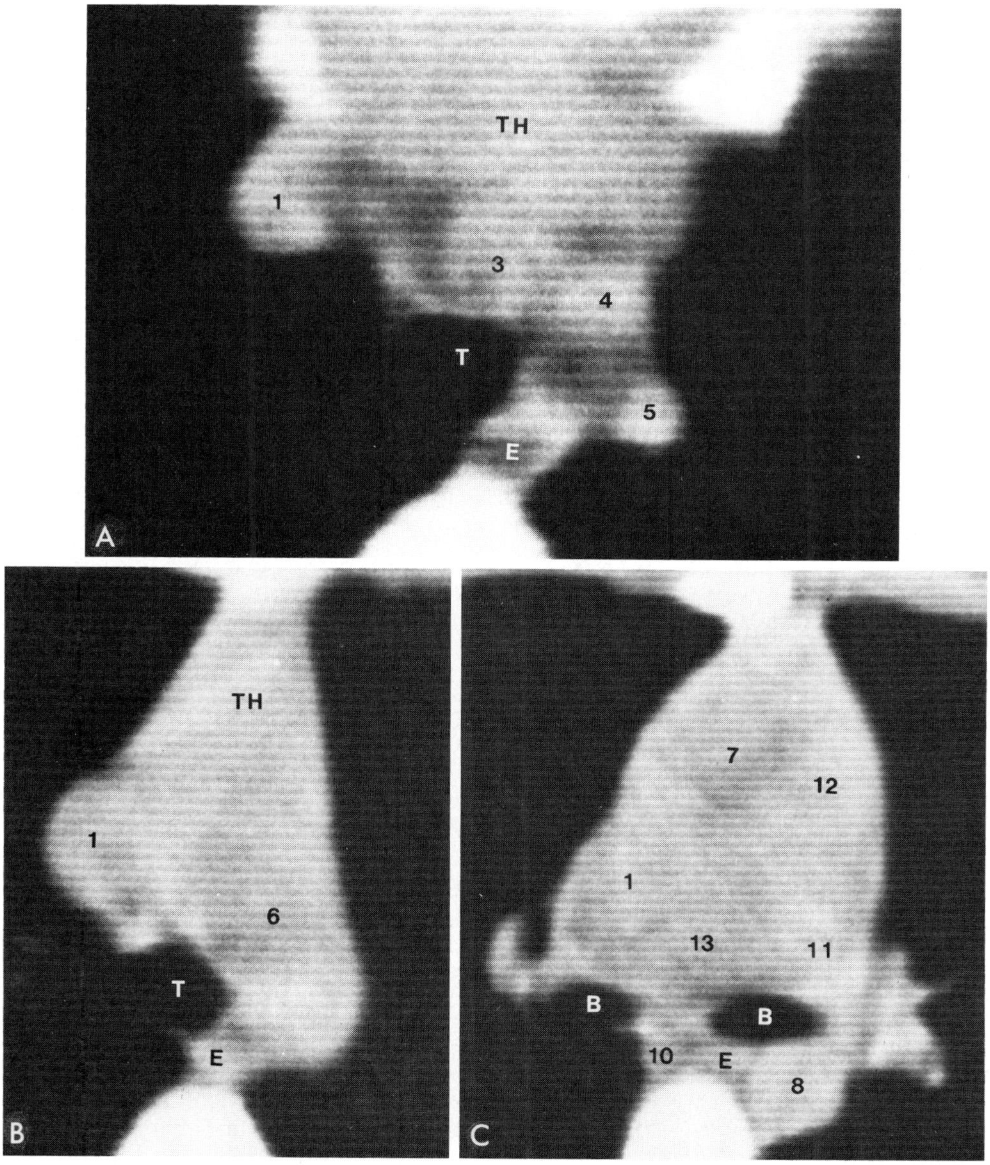

Figure 2. Normal mediastinum in a 7-year-old girl undergoing chemotherapy for osteogenic sarcoma. Note the lack of fatty separation of the mediastinal vessels in comparison with older patients. *A*, Scan just above the aortic arch. *B*, Scan at the level of the aortic arch. *C*, Scan at the level of the right pulmonary artery (compare with Figures 1*A*, *B*, and *E*). Abbreviations as in Figure 1; TH: thymus.

thick (collimation) at contiguous 10-mm intervals are used. Scanning with delayed processing of the scans to minimize motion of the patient between scans is optimal for subsequent reconstructions of the images in sagittal or coronal planes. If such reconstructions are considered necessary before scanning, some CT scanners produce more optimal sagittal and coronal reconstructions after CT scans are obtained at 5-mm intervals. A small field of view scan ("target scan") centered over the mediastinum may increase resolution in young patients.

Iodinated contrast enhancement is generally necessary to identify vessels and confirm the location of certain vascular structures. This can be done as a rapid intravenous drip infusion during the course of the CT study (in which case processing of the CT images should be deferred until the examination is completed to minimize the total volume of contrast media required for optimal vascular opacification). We use a drip infusion of Conray 60 to a maximum dose of 3 ml/kg or 150 ml total volume. Approximately one-half of the dose is administered before scanning and the remainder during the time the scan is performed. Alternatively, after non–contrast-enhanced imaging, certain CT levels may be selected for bolus injections of contrast, resulting in higher concentration of iodine achieved in the vascular structures and hence better opacification of selected CT levels of maximal interest.

CT OF THE NORMAL MEDIASTINUM

The unique cross-sectional imaging ability of CT allows for visualization of all the major mediastinal structures. Major vascular structures (aorta, superior vena cava, pulmonary arteries, and brachiocephalic vessels) are usually easily identified (Fig. 1), as are the other normal mediastinal structures. Direct visualization of the trachea, esophagus, and any other complicating soft tissue masses such as lymph nodes and duplication cysts complements the ability of CT to image the vascular structures.

In young patients with a paucity of mediastinal fat, the separation of vascular structures may be less than adequate despite cooperation of the patient (Fig. 2). Intravenous contrast media may be needed to delineate the individual vascular structures well (see Figs. 11 and 13). In most older children and adults, the vessels are separated by fat, and their size and configuration are readily recognizable.

CT EVALUATION OF MALFORMATIONS OF THE AORTIC ARCH AND GREAT VESSELS

Congenital Vascular Rings and Related Anomalies

Congenital anomalies of the aortic arch and its major branches may be asymptomatic, or, by the formation of vascular rings, they may produce symptoms due to esophageal or tracheal compression. The initial radiographic evaluation is usually accomplished by conventional chest radiographs supplemented occasionally by fluoroscopy combined with barium swallow examination. Precise anatomic evaluation of these anomalies with determination of the patency and size of each component of avascular ring has usually required contrast angiography.[5, 19, 20]

Recently it has become apparent that the cross-sectional anatomy depicted by CT may provide a noninvasive method for evaluating suspected aortic arch anomalies.[1, 2, 7, 11, 15, 24] These investigations have resulted from efforts to define mediastinal abnormalities initially detected on chest radiographs or barium swallow studies. Occasionally, although the initial radiograph suggests a vascular ring, the subsequent CT scan demonstrates a nonvascular mediastinal lesion accounting for the abnormality (Fig. 3). Thus, further vascular studies can be obviated by the CT findings.

Some of the more commonly encountered anomalies of the great arteries and their branches are shown in Table 1.[5, 19] The most common type of symptomatic vascular ring is the persistence of both right and left fourth embryonic arches forming a double aortic arch. Most often hypoplasia or atresia of the left arch is noted with this anomaly, although the two arches may be of similar caliber. CT images can accurately display the anatomy in such patients. The scans show the ascending aorta dividing into both left and right aortic arches, which then join again to form the descending aorta, entrapping the trachea and esophagus by a vascular ring (Fig. 4). The carotid and subclavian arteries each arise separately from the respective aortic arches without the formation of an innominate artery, as would be predicted by the preservation of the primitive double arch.[5, 19, 20]

A right aortic arch with aberrant left subclavian artery and left ductus ligament is the most common type of right aortic arch, occurring in 0.1 per cent of the population.[5, 20] The ring

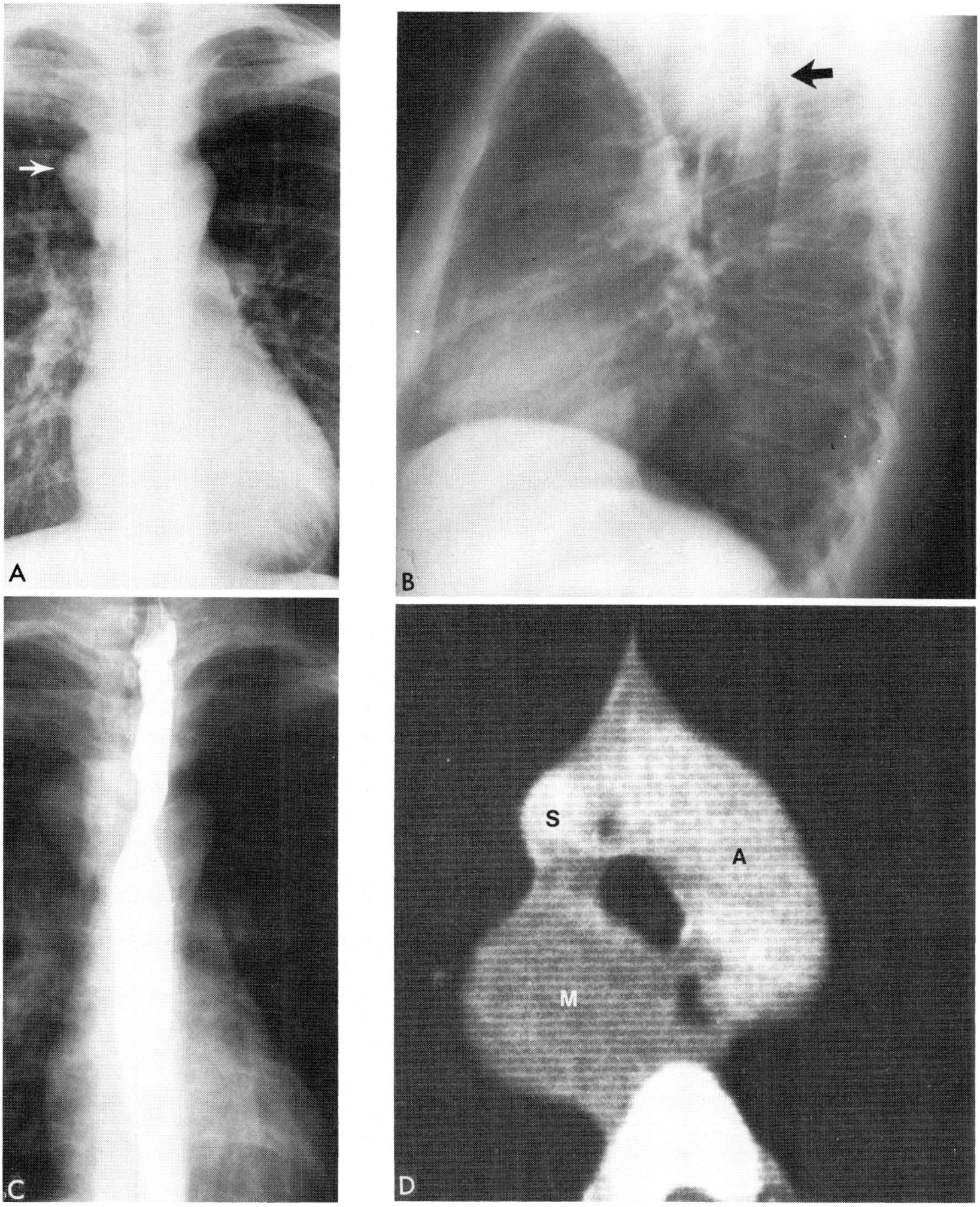

Figure 3. A 38-year-old woman with multiple vascular complications of juvenile onset diabetes mellitus. *A,B,* Chest radiographs show abnormal mediastium (arrow) with retrotracheal mass. *C,* Frontal barium swallow shows lateral compression of the esophagus. A lateral view failed to show retroesophageal compression. *D,* CT scan at the level of the aortic arch after intravenous contrast shows the mass to be nonvascular with a density of 10 EMI units and most likely a cyst. M: mass; A: aortic arch; S: superior vena cava.

Table 1. *Congenital Vascular Rings and Related Anomalies*

TRACHEAL AND/OR ESOPHAGEAL COMPRESSION FREQUENT:
1. Double arch
2. Right arch, aberrant LSA, left DA
3. Left arch, right descending aorta, right DA
4. Pulmonary artery sling
5. Left arch, anomalous distal innominate origin
TRACHEAL AND/OR ESOPHAGEAL COMPRESSION UNUSUAL:
1. Left arch, aberrant RSA, left DA
2. Right arch, mirror-image branching
3. Right arch, isolation LSA
4. Cervical arch

Abbreviations: LSA: left subclavian artery; RSA: right subclavian artery; DA: ductus arteriosus.

formed is loose, and most patients are not symptomatic, although rarely in young children a tight ring produces symptoms of tracheal and esophageal compression. Approximately 5 per cent of these children have associated congenital heart disease, and 2 per cent of patients with tetralogy of Fallot have this arch anomaly.[5] This anomaly is easily detected on CT imaging.[1, 2, 15, 24] Figure 5 illustrates the typical CT appearance of this arch anomaly in an otherwise asymptomatic older patient with an abnormal chest radiograph. In such cases, CT depicts the ascending portion and arch of the aorta in the right anterior mediastinum (Fig. 5*C*; compare with Fig. 1*B*), with the proximal descending aorta lying to the right of the spine. The aberrant left subclavian artery frequently has a dilated origin (diverticulum of Kommerell), which can cause increased density to the left and posterior to the trachea on standard radiographs. The cross-sectional CT images clearly illustrate the correct anatomic relationships and explain all abnormal mediastinal densities detected on standard chest radiographs. Occasionally a right aortic arch or very large diverticulum of Kommerell can cause confusion in evaluating a patient with another established disease process (Fig. 6). CT scans usually demonstrate the nature of the abnormal mediastinum and show no evidence for mediastinal tumor.

An anomalous left pulmonary artery originating from the right pulmonary artery (pulmonary artery sling) is a developmental defect in which the aberrant left pulmonary artery passes between the trachea and the esophagus to enter the left hilum. It frequently occurs in highly symptomatic young infants with stridor and wheezing because of compression of the right main stem bronchus, trachea, left main stem bronchus, or a combination of these structures, producing air trapping or collapse in the lung.[3, 5] Less frequently it has been reported as an incidental chest radiographic finding in asymptomatic children or adults.[3, 21] Stone et al.[21] have reported the CT findings in two cases of pulmonary sling. Figure 7 shows an asymptomatic patient with a retrotracheal mediastinal mass seen on chest radiography, tomography, and esophagography. CT scans show conclusively that the retrotracheal mass is an anomalous pulmonary artery and that no other nonvascular masses are present. Only mild airway compression is seen in this case.

Of the malformations that are usually not associated with symptomatic tracheal and/or esophageal compression, a left aortic arch with aberrant right subclavian artery and left ductus ligament is the most common malformation of the aortic arch and occurs in approximately 1 person in 200.[5, 19] Dysphagia, termed dysphagia lusoria, has been rarely attributed to this anomaly, although treatment is seldom, if ever, indicated. This anomaly is encountered at esophagography and occasionally during chest radiography when abnormalities of the mediastinum are seen (Fig. 8) that may be confused with aneurysm or other nonvascular masses. CT studies (Fig. 8*B*) may be helpful to demonstrate the aortic arch as well as the dilated infundibulum that gives rise to the aberrant subclavian artery. The CT image may not demonstrate the origin of the aberrant right subclavian artery from the aorta, but instead shows a contrast-enhancing structure located posterior to the esophagus and coursing cephalad in the right posterior aspect of the superior mediastinum on serial CT scans (Fig. 8*C*).

A right aortic arch with mirror-image branching of the great vessels, although not involved with vascular rings, is associated with cyanotic congenital heart disease in approximately 95 per cent of cases.[5] Commonly associated lesions include pulmonary atresia with ventricular septal defect, tetralogy of Fallot, truncus arteriosus, double outlet right ventricle, and single ventricle. The arch of the aorta can be seen on CT images passing to the right, with the descending aorta to the right of the spine and no retrotracheal vessel seen (see Fig. 13). The role of CT in this anomaly is limited to confirming the position of the aortic arch and its branch vessels within the chest and to evaluating the availability of proper sites for constructing shunts to the pulmonary arteries.

Cervical aortic arch is a rare and usually asymptomatic developmental anomaly thought to result from persistence of the second or third embryonic arches with regression of the normal

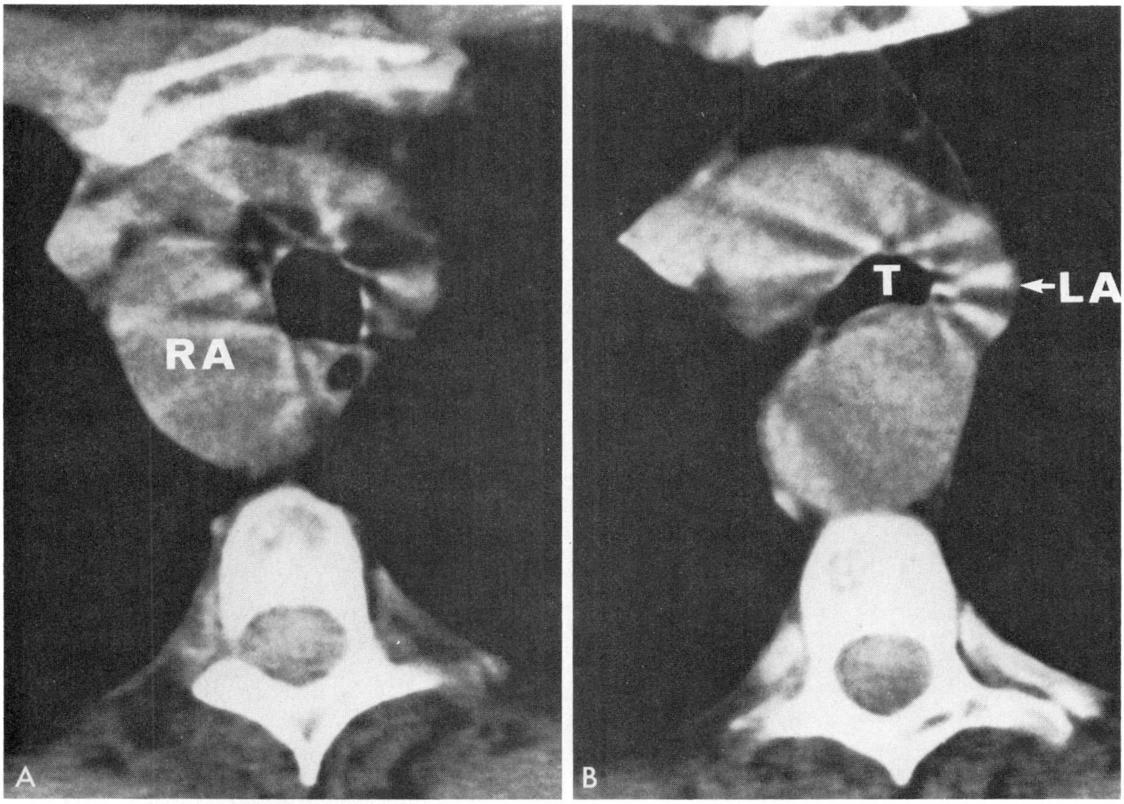

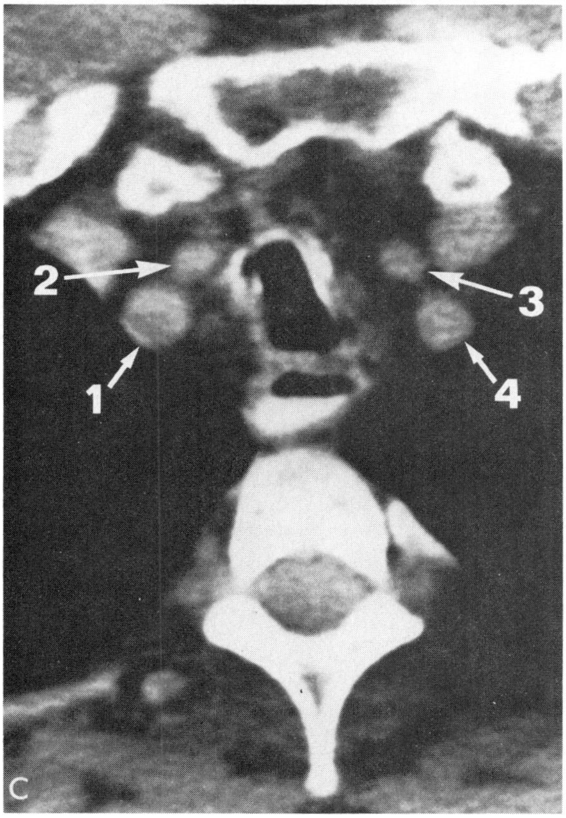

Figure 4. Double aortic arch in a 53-year-old man with respiratory symptoms and pulsatile narrowing of the trachea at bronchoscopy. A double aortic arch was confirmed by aortography. *A*, CT scan demonstrates a large right aortic arch (RA). *B*, Scan slightly inferior to A shows anteroposterior compression of the trachea (T) and a smaller left aortic arch (LA). *C*, Scan more cephalad than *A* shows a cross-section of the four major arteries grouped around the trachea ("four artery sign"). 1: right subclavian artery; 2: right common carotid artery; 3: left common carotid artery; 4: left subclavian artery. (Reproduced with permission from McLoughlin MJ, Weisbrod G, Wise DJ, et al: Computed tomography in congenital anomalies of the aortic arch and great vessels. Radiology, *138*:339, 1981.)

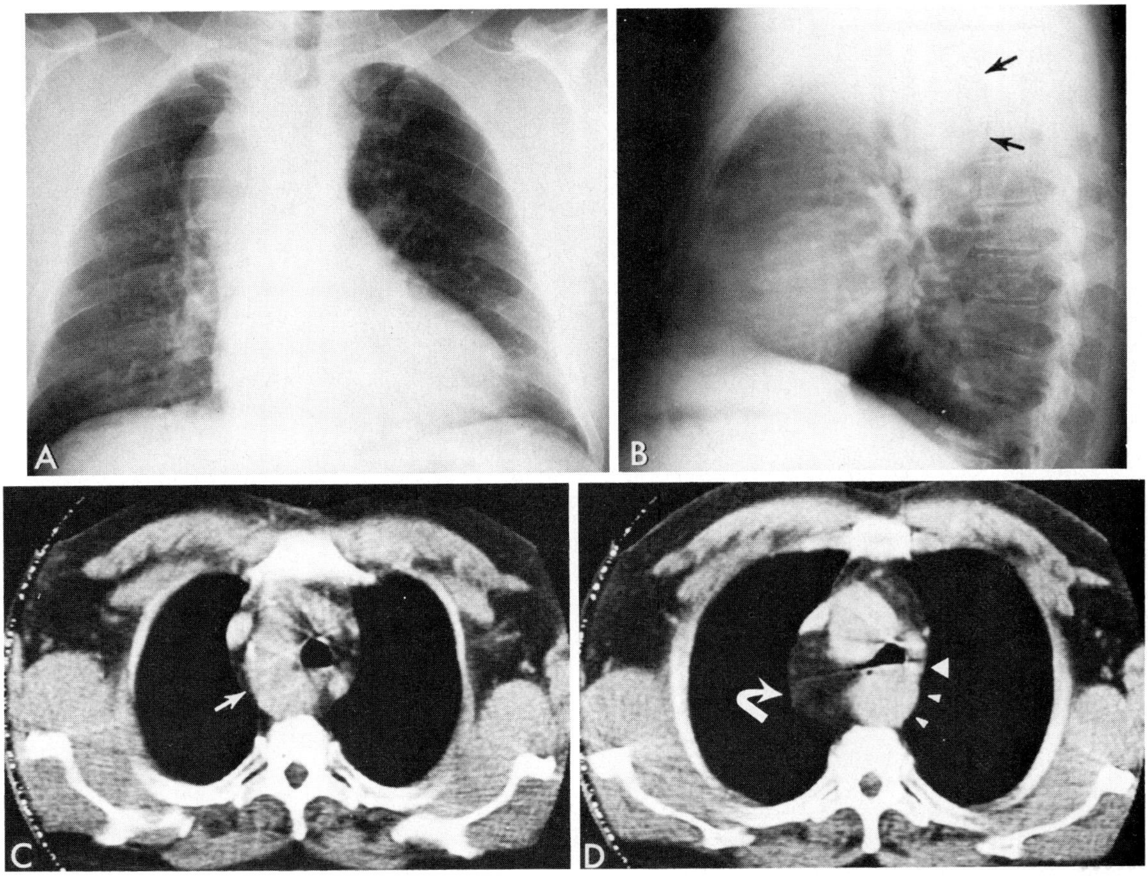

Figure 5. *A* and *B*, Posteroanterior and lateral chest radiographs of a 63-year-old man admitted for facial burns showing superior mediastinal widening and a retrotracheal density (arrows). *C*, Postcontrast CT scan demonstrates a right-sided aortic arch (straight arrow) accounting for a portion of the mediastinal widening. *D*, CT scan at 3 cm inferior to *C* demonstrates a focal mediastinal collection of benign fat (curved arrow) accounting for much of the widening. The descending portion of the right aortic arch (small arrowheads) is responsible for the retrotracheal density, as the left subclavian artery (large arrowhead) is small. The lower thoracic aortic descends on the left. (Reproduced with permission from Baron RL, Levitt RG, Sagel SS, et al: Computed tomography in evaluation of mediastinal widening. Radiology, *138*:107, 1981.)

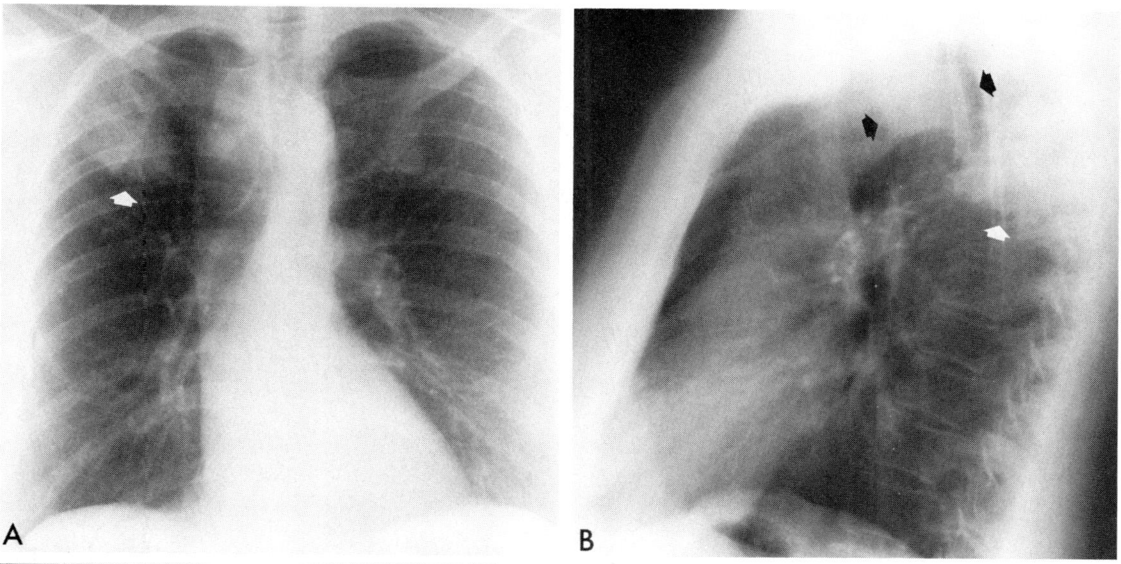

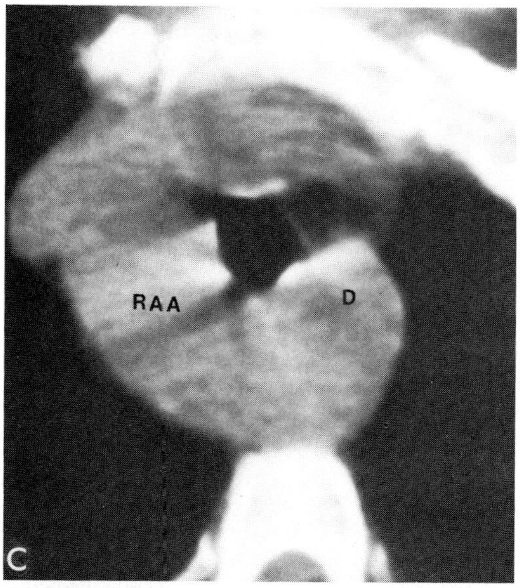

Figure 6. *A* and *B*, PA and lateral chest radiographs in a 47-year-old woman with chest pain and a right upper lobe mass diagnosed as adenocarcinoma (white arrows). There is abnormal widening of the mediastinum and a retrotracheal mass (black arrow). *C*, CT scan at the level of the aortic arch shows a right aortic arch (RAA) and a large diverticulum of Kommerell *(D)*, which give rise to the left subclavian artery. *D*, A scan 1 cm lower shows the descending aorta (DA) on the left and posterior to the trachea. *E*, A scan 5 cm lower at the level or the pulmonary artery (RPA) shows that the descending aorta has crossed back to the right side where it continues in the chest. AA: ascending aorta.

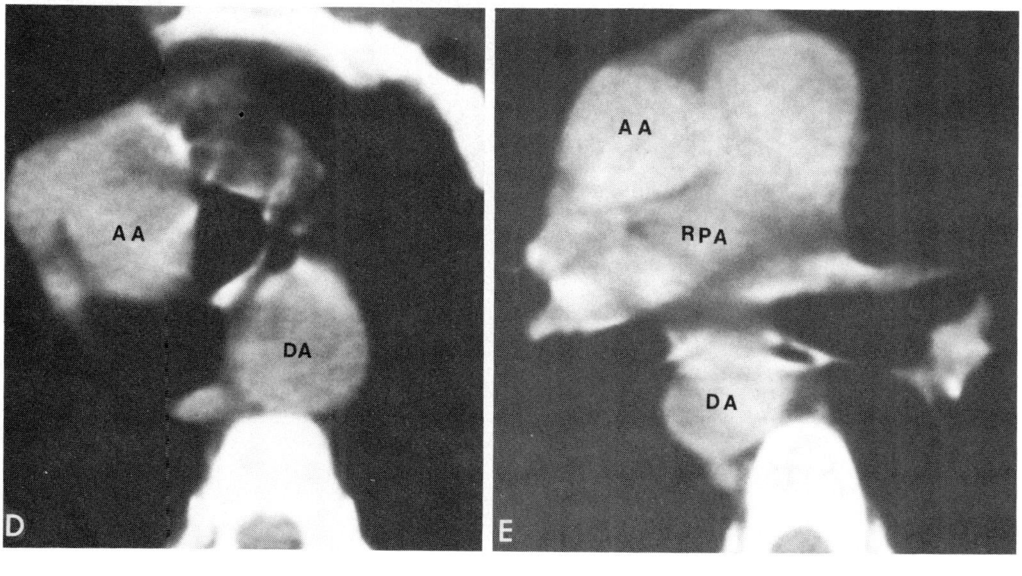

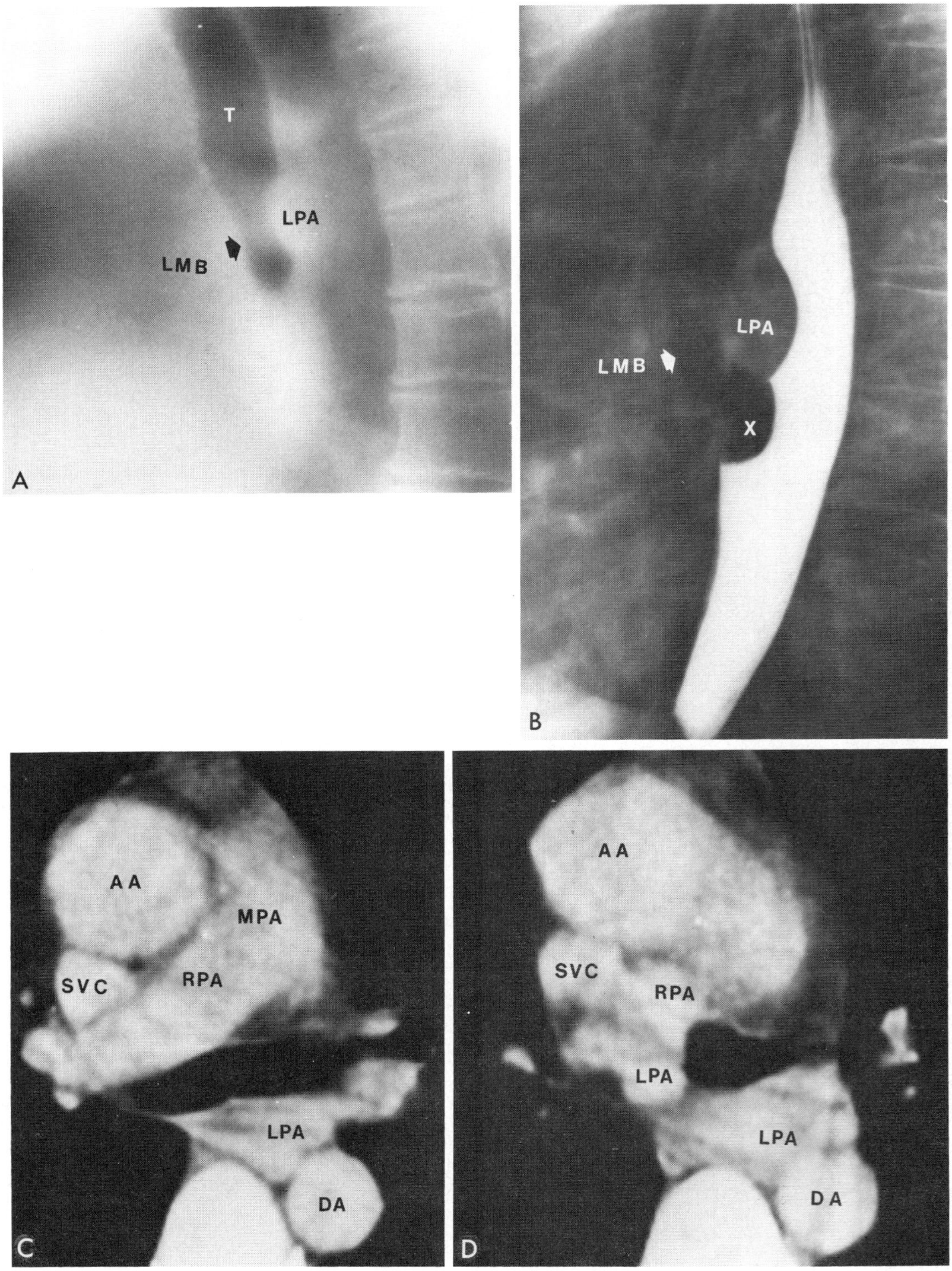

Figure 7. A 46-year-old asymptomatic man with abnormal chest radiographs *(A)* showing compression of the posterior aspect of his distal trachea by soft tissue mass. A barium swallow *(B)* showed indentation of the esophagus at the same level. CT scans at the level of the right pulmonary artery *(C)* and a more cephalad slice *(D)* show a normal right pulmonary artery and origin of the left pulmonary artery from the right pulmonary artery, which then passes up over the right bronchus as well as behind the trachea and anterior to the esophagus. AA: ascending aorta; DA: descending aorta; SVC: superior vena cava; RPA: right pulmonary artery; MPA: main pulmonary artery; LPA: left pulmonary artery; LMB: left main bronchus; X: air bubble. (Reproduced with permission from Stone DN, Bein ME, Garris JB: Anomalous left pulmonary artery: Two new adult cases. AJR, *135*:1259, 1980. Copyright ©, 1980, The Williams and Wilkins Company.)

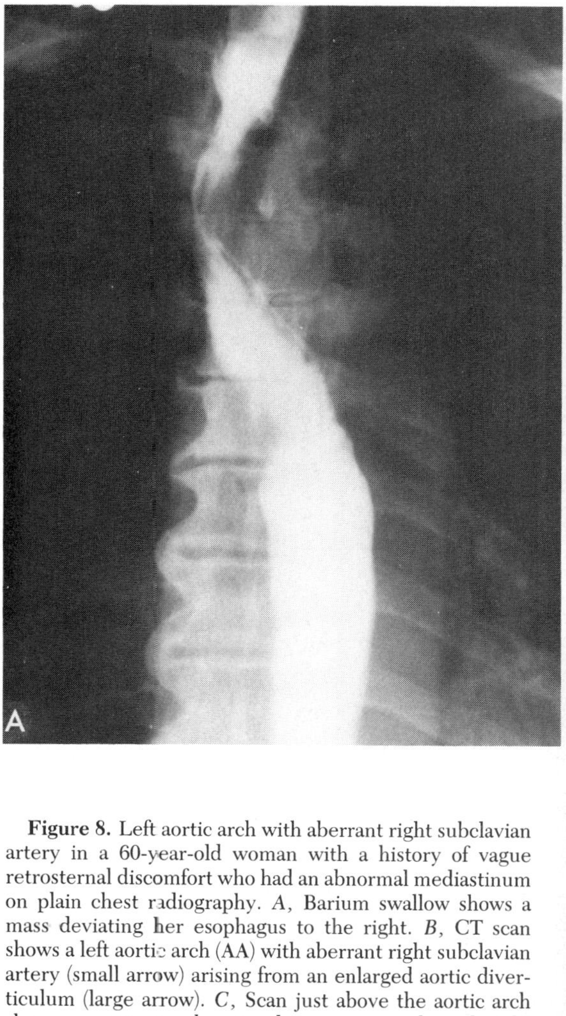

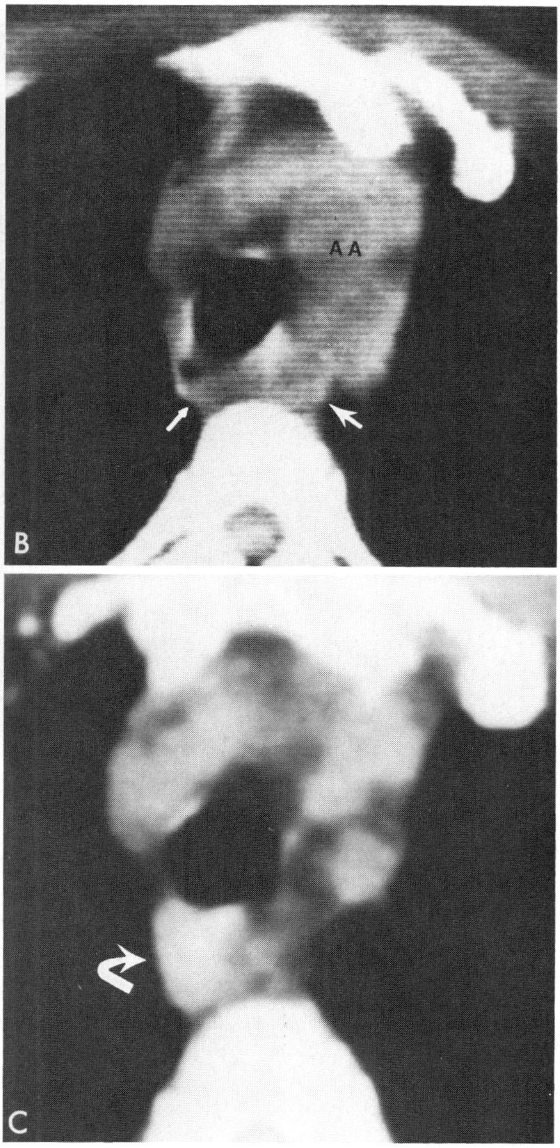

Figure 8. Left aortic arch with aberrant right subclavian artery in a 60-year-old woman with a history of vague retrosternal discomfort who had an abnormal mediastinum on plain chest radiography. *A*, Barium swallow shows a mass deviating her esophagus to the right. *B*, CT scan shows a left aortic arch (AA) with aberrant right subclavian artery (small arrow) arising from an enlarged aortic diverticulum (large arrow). *C*, Scan just above the aortic arch shows a contrast-enhancing large retroesophageal right subclavian artery (curved arrow).

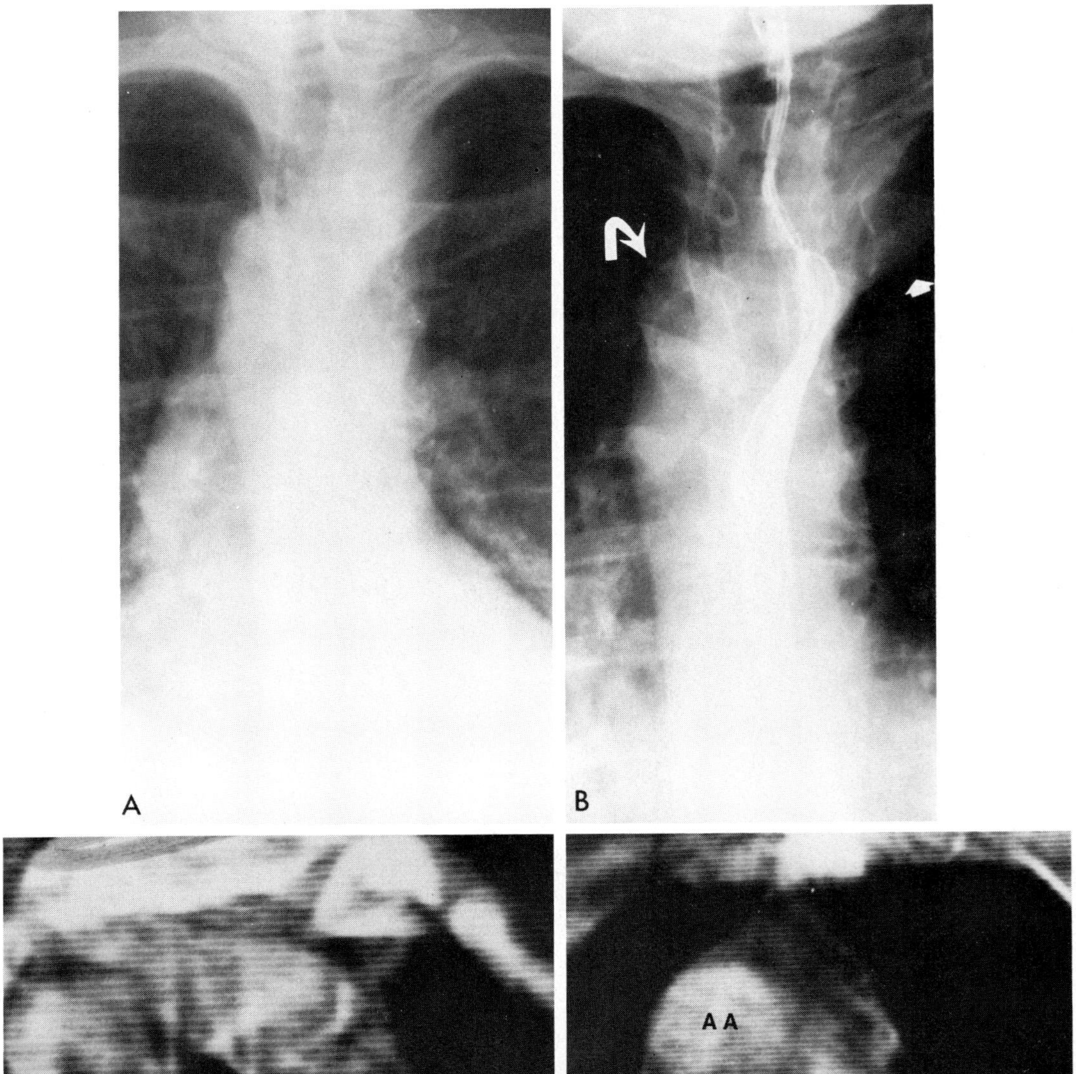

Figure 9. Left cervical arch in a 51-year-old woman studied because of abnormal chest radiograph *(A)*. *B*, Frontal esophagram shows compression of the esophagus and trachea by a high mediastinal mass on the left (arrow) and by an apparent aortic arch on the right (curved arrow). A contrast-enhanced CT scan *(C)* at level of lung apices shows the left cervical arch (CA). A more caudal scan *(D)* at the level of the left pulmonary artery (LPA) shows the right-sided ascending aorta (AA) and descending aorta (DA).

fourth arch. This anomaly is usually not associated with cardiac defects. Two-thirds of the arches are on the right side, and they may occasionally be linked with origins of the anomalous subclavian artery.[4] Abnormal pulsations in the neck as well as mediastinal abnormalities on chest radiography can be demonstrated to be due to a cervical aortic arch on the CT scan (Fig. 9).

Anomalies in Position of the Great Arteries

In great artery transposition complexes, the anatomy of conotruncal abnormalities and their relations to corresponding ventricles and inlet valves are usually determined by angiography.[8] Although these angiographic studies certainly demonstrate cardiovascular anatomy, they may occasionally be confusing when planning a surgical repair, in which the precise relation of vascular structures is important. CT has the advantage of demonstrating all the venous and arterial structures on the same film, allowing visualization of the side-to-side and front-to-back relationships of the great vessels and their position within the chest, information often difficult to ascertain from angiographic examination. Our surgical colleagues often find this additional information particularly helpful in

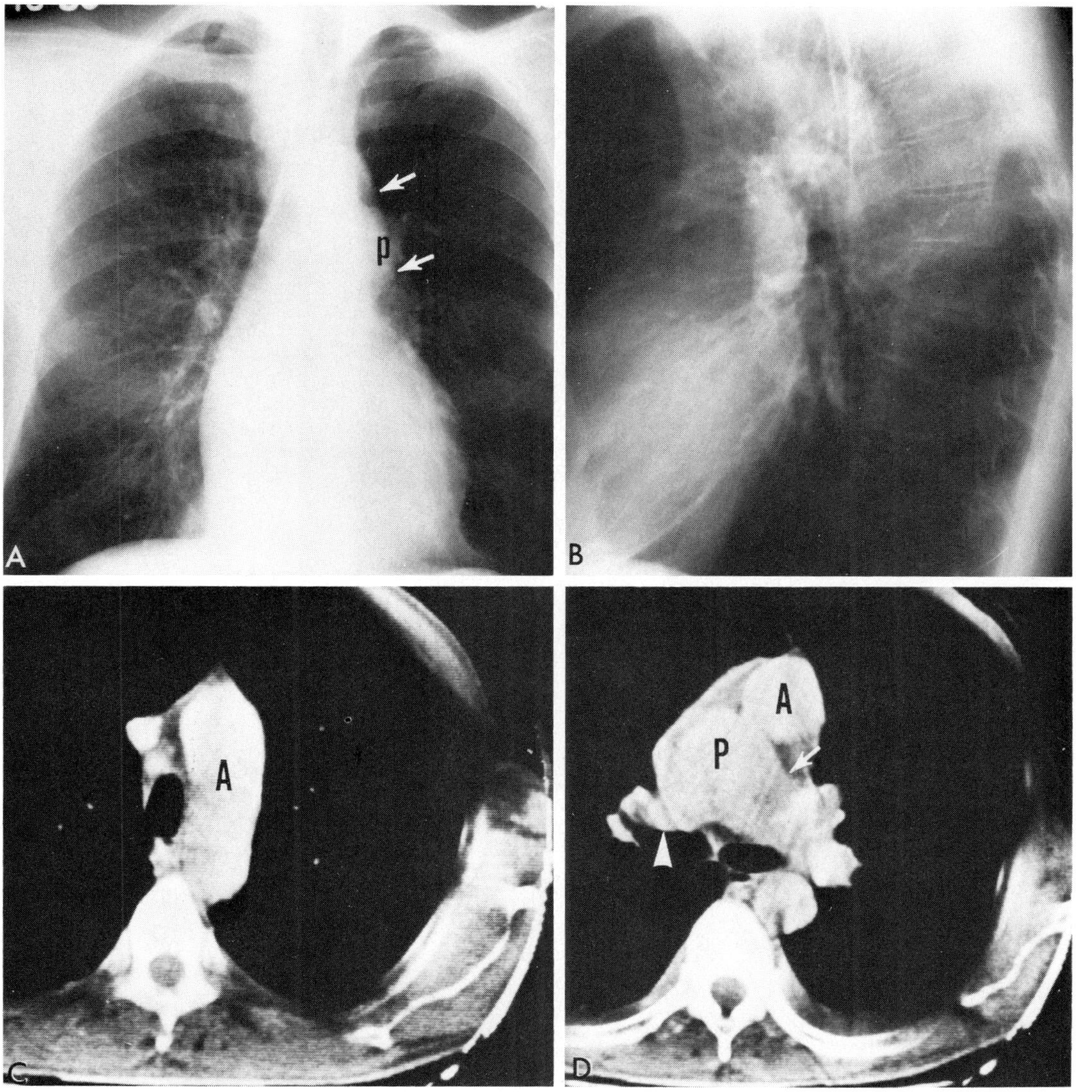

Figure 10. Corrected transposition of the great vessels in a 59-year-old with severe angina pectoris and systolic heart murmur thought to be of no clinical significance. Chest radiographs (*A* and *B*) show abnormal convexity in left mediastinum (arrows) and enlarged main pulmonary artery (p). *C*, Postcontrast CT scan. Abnormal axis of aortic arch *(A)* with leftward l-positioning of anterior part. *D*, Scan 4 cm inferiorly. Ascending aorta (A) anterior and left of main pulmonary artery (P), diagnostic of l (corrected)-transposition. Main and left pulmonary arteries (arrow) are dilated, whereas right pulmonary artery (arrowhead) is normal, indicating pulmonic valvular stenosis with poststenotic dilatation. This explains the murmur heard clinically. (Reproduced with permission from Baron RL, Gutierrez FR, Sagel SS, et al: CT of anomalies of the mediastinal vessels. AJR, *137*: 571, 1981. Copyright ©, 1981, The Williams and Wilkins Company.)

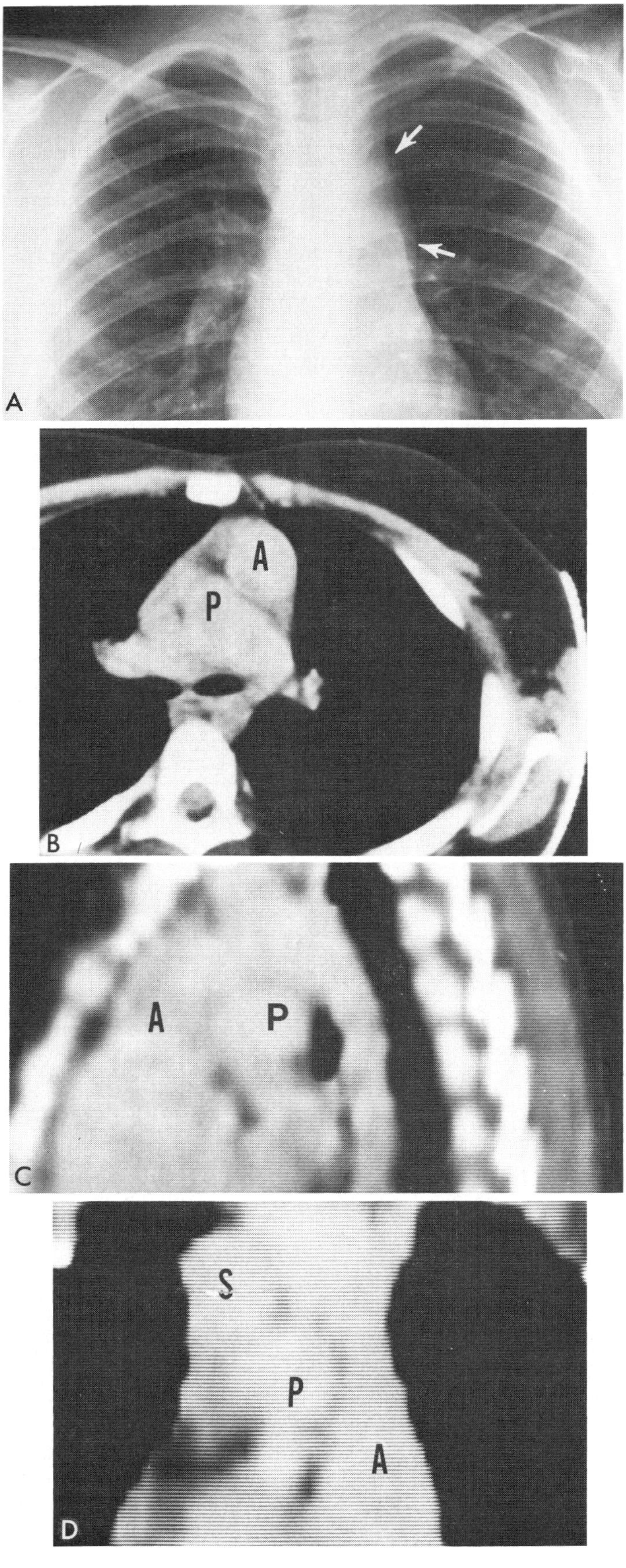

Figure 11. An 11-year-old boy with systolic heart murmur. Chest radiograph *(A)* shows a left paramediastinal density (arrows). Increased density in the retrosternal space noted on lateral projection. *B*, Characteristic changes of l-transposition, with ascending aorta (A) positioned to the left of the main pulmonary artery (P). Dilatation of the main and left pulmonary arteries. *C*, Sagittal multiplanar reconstructed CT. The aorta (A) arises from the anterior ventricle, and the pulmonary artery (P) arises from the posterior ventricle. *D*, Coronal multiplanar reconstruction CT. The aorta (A) arises on the left, and the pulmonary artery (P) arises on right. S: superior vena cava.

Illustration continues on opposite page.

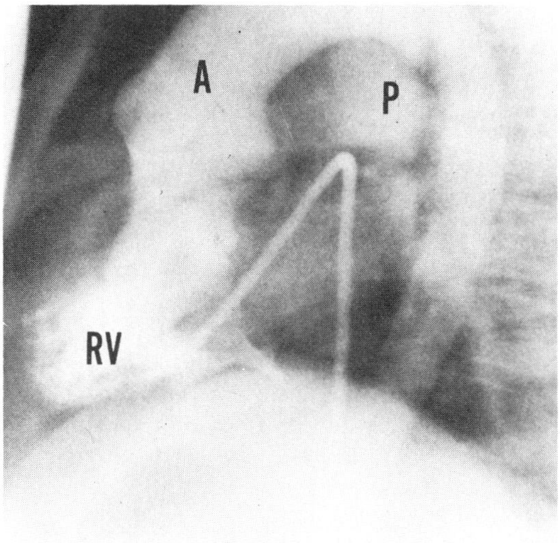

E

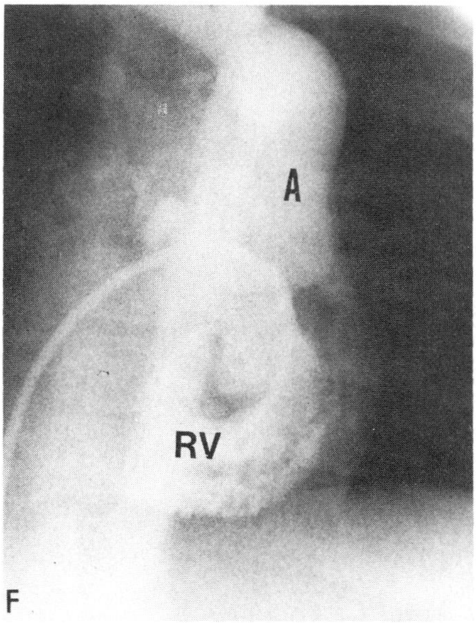

F

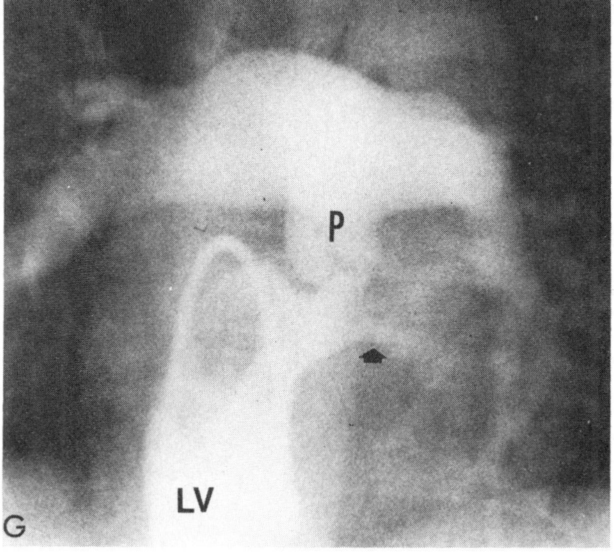

G

Figure 11 (*Continued*). Lateral *(E)* and frontal. *(F)* right ventricular angiograms. The aorta (A) arises on the left from the anterior (right) ventricle (RV). The pulmonary artery (P) opacifies from a small ventricular septal defect. *G*, Angiocardiogram after injection into posterior (left) ventricle (LV). Continuity with main pulmonary artery (P). Doming of pulmonic valve with poststenotic dilatation and small ventricular septal defect (arrow). (Reproduced with permission from Baron RL, Gutierrez FR, Sagel SS et al: CT of anomalies of the mediastinal vessels. AJR, *137*: 571, 1981. Copyright ©, 1981, The Williams and Wilkins Company.)

double outlet right ventricle, double outlet left ventricle, and single ventricle. Computed tomography is a noninvasive technique that can provide such information because of its cross-sectional image format.

A d-transposition accounts for approximately 5 per cent of congenital heart disease, whereas an l-transposition with atrioventricular inversion ("corrected transposition") comprises considerably less than 1 per cent of all cases.[4] The CT findings in an adult patient with l-transposition of the great arteries are shown in Figure 10. The leftward and anterior position of the aorta with respect to the pulmonary artery is easily seen (Fig. 10*C* and *D*). Associated pulmonic stenosis is suggested by dilation of the main and left pulmonary arteries, and this finding was substantiated at catheterization. Similar findings in an 11-year-old child admitted for catheterization before definitive surgery are shown in Figure 11.

Occasionally, reconstruction of the CT images in the sagittal and coronal planes is helpful in understanding the complex relationships of the great vessels in these anomalies. Because of some unfamiliarity with cross-sectional images, the findings may be more easily comprehended on the reformatted sagittal images (Fig. 11*C* and *D*).

The findings in d-transposition of the great vessels are shown in Figure 12. In contrast to the previous cases of l-transposition, the position of the aorta anterior and to the right of the pulmonary artery is easily seen. In addition, hypoplasia of the main pulmonary artery secondary to subpulmonary stenosis can also be observed. The size of the proximal portions of the great vessels may imply valvular stenosis, subvalvular or infundibular hypoplasia, and a variety of other lesions, including pulmonary hypertension.[17]

Truncus arteriosus accounts for approximately 1 per cent of congenital heart disease.[4] The diagnosis of truncus arteriosus or of pulmonary atresia with ventricular septal defect (pseudotruncus) can be strongly suggested by the CT findings of a single enlarged arterial vessel. A more definite diagnosis of truncus

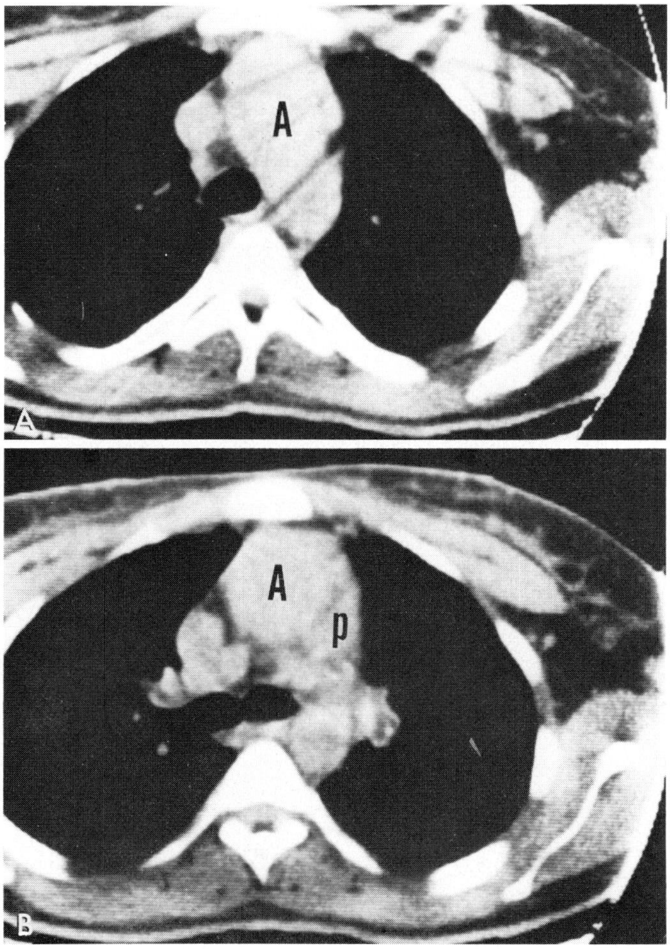

Figure 12. A 21-year-old woman with d-transposition. *A*, Axis of aortic arch (A) is normal (in contradistinction to the axis in l-transposition seen in Figure 10). Note streak artifact from brassiere clip. *B*, Scan 2 cm inferiorly. The ascending aorta (A) is positioned to the right of the pulmonary artery (p). Additional scans showed that the aorta arose from the anterior ventricle. Note the small size of the central pulmonary artery secondary to long-standing subpulmonary stenosis. (Reproduced with permission from Baron RL, Gutierrez FR, Sagel SS, et al: CT of anomalies of the mediastinal vessels. AJR, *137*:571, 1981. Copyright ©, 1981, The Williams and Wilkins Company.)

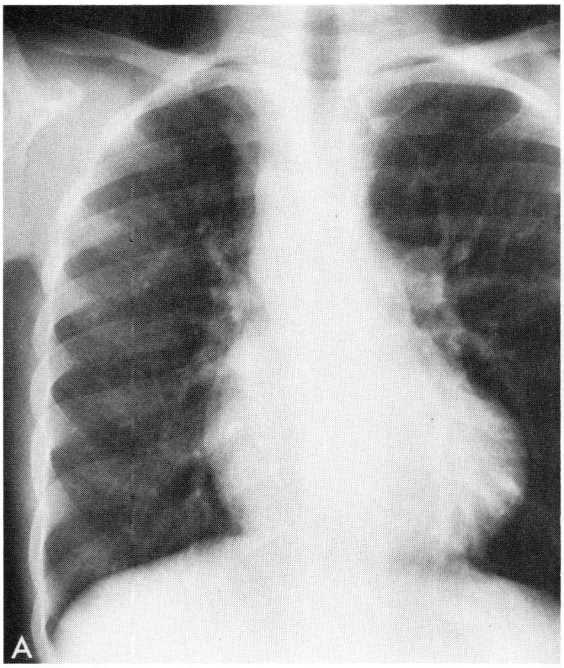

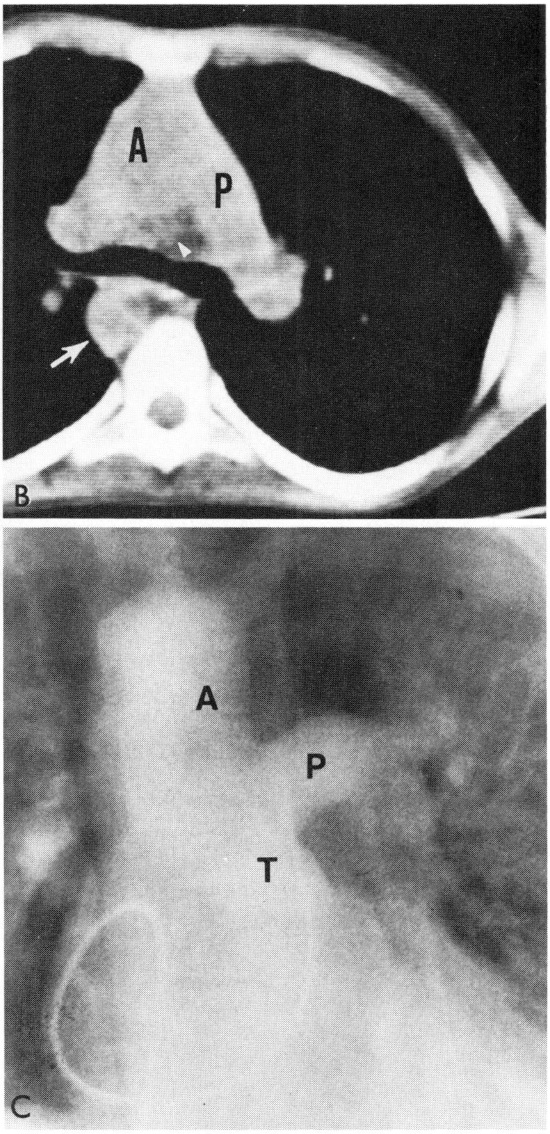

Figure 13. A 12-year-old girl with dizziness and exertional cyanosis. *A*, Right aortic arch, enlargement of left pulmonary artery and left peripheral pulmonary arteries, and uplifting of cardiac apex compatible with right ventricular hypertrophy. Truncus arteriosus was favored. *B*, Level of root of truncal vessel. It bifurcates into the left pulmonary artery (P) and the right ascending aorta (A). In the expected location of the right pulmonary artery (arrowhead), only some vague soft tissue densities intermixed with mediastinal fat are demonstrated. This explains discrepant pulmonary vascularity seen on plain chest radiograph. Right-sided descending aorta (arrow). *C*, Angiogram. Large truncal vessel (T) giving rise to aorta (A) and enlarged left pulmonary artery (P). No right pulmonary artery is seen. (Reproduced with permission from Baron RL, Gutierrez FR, Sagel SS, et al: CT of anomalies of the mediastinal vessels. AJR, *137*:571, 1981. Copyright ©, 1981, The Williams and Wilkins Company.)

arteriosus can be made if one or more pulmonary arteries are seen to arise directly from the aorta. A confirmed case of truncus arteriosus in a 12-year-old patient is shown in Figure 13. The size and origin of the pulmonary arteries, the continuity of right and left pulmonary arteries, and the occasional absence of a pulmonary artery originating from the common trunk (hemitruncus) (Fig. 13*B* and *C*) can be outlined in cross-section. All of these factors are of extreme importance in planning a definitive surgical repair of truncus arteriosus.

Coarctation of the Aorta

Coarctation of the aorta is a localized deformity of the aortic media, with infolding of the posterior wall producing an eccentric narrowing of the aortic lumen. It usually occurs just distal to the left subclavian artery but occasionally may be found elsewhere in the thoracic or abdominal aorta. Coarctation accounts for 2 to 8 per cent of congenital cardiovascular disease in infants and children.[5] The diagnosis is usually made clinically and is substantiated by chest radiography, and the precise anatomy is confirmed by aortography before surgery.[8]

Several reports have shown that CT may demonstrate coarctations of the aorta[11] or pseudocoarctation (incomplete or mild stenosis).[7, 9] Godwin et al.[11] stressed that reformatted CT images of the aorta in sagittal, coronal, or oblique paraxial planes may be helpful in demonstrating the lesion (Fig. 14). Such reconstructed images in the plane of the aortic arch

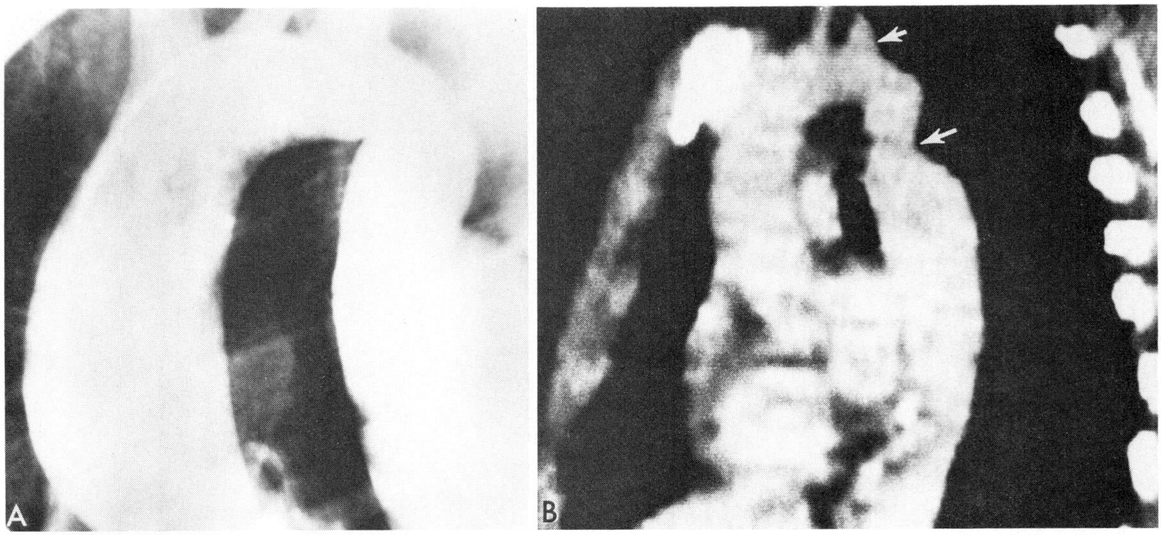

Figure 14. Coarctation of the aorta in a 27-year-old hypertensive man. The posteroanterior chest radiograph showed double contour of the aortic arch. No rib notching was apparent. Aortogram (A) in the right posterior oblique projection shows juxtaductal coarctation with poststenotic dilation and enlargement of the brachiocephalic arteries. Dilation of the ascending aorta is also present; other views showed a bicuspid aortic valve. *B*, Contrast-enhanced reformatted CT image in the plane of the aortic arch corresponding to the aortographic projection. Note coarctation (long arrow) with poststenotic dilation as well as large ascending aorta and large origin of the left subclavian artery (short arrow). (Reproduced with permission from Godwin JD, Herfkens RJ, Brandage BH, et al: Evaluation of coarctation of the aorta by computed tomography. J Comput Assist Tomogr, 5:153, 1981. Courtesy of Raven Press.)

resemble the right posterior oblique view obtained during aortography that surgeons are used to viewing. The low spatial resolution of CT and the lack of physiologic information provided by the CT study currently preclude the use of this technique except as a screening procedure or perhaps as a follow-up to definitive catheterization and aortography. CT may be particularly useful when preliminary clinical and radiographic findings are equivocal; this technique can thus serve as a noninvasive means for further screening patients. CT is not adequate for evaluating associated lesions such as bicuspid aortic valve or for assessing the pressure gradients across the stenosis. CT may be helpful postoperatively to assess for recurrent stenosis.[11] Pseudocoarctation may give a similar CT appearance and must be distinguished by catheterization.

Anomalies of the Great Veins

Many of the mediastinal venous anomalies appear initially as abnormal structures detected by standard chest radiographic procedures. Since most of these defects are unassociated with significant intracardiac anomalies, their recognition by noninvasive means such as CT may obviate the need for more invasive procedures, such as angiography, mediastinoscopy, or even thoracotomy. The great mediastinal veins can be portrayed in a three-dimensional manner by cross-sectional imaging in much the same way as the great arteries. Direct-contrast infusion in the appropriate extremity can opacify sequentially the left and right innominate veins and the superior vena cava. Reconstructed images in the coronal, sagittal, or oblique planes can also outline the full length of the structures to advantage.

Persistence of the left superior vena cava, the most common variant of mediastinal venous structures, occurs in approximately 0.3 per cent of the normal population.[6] Although most often the right superior vena cava arising from the embryologic cardinal vein persists in these patients as well, occasionally only the left superior vena cava persists. CT has been shown to be able to identify both types of persisting left superior vena cava.[1, 13, 23]

Most often, the left superior vena cava is smaller than the right superior vena cava. CT scans show the abnormal contrast-enhanced left superior vena cava situated lateral to the left common carotid artery; as it descends, it passes lateral to the aortic arch and left pulmonary artery to enter the coronary sinus or the right atrium via the hemizygous vein. On non–contrast-enhanced scans, such densities may be mistaken for adenopathy, but contrast enhancement equal to that of the other venous structures, coupled with a tubular structure on sequential CT scans, indicates the proper diagnosis (Fig. 15).

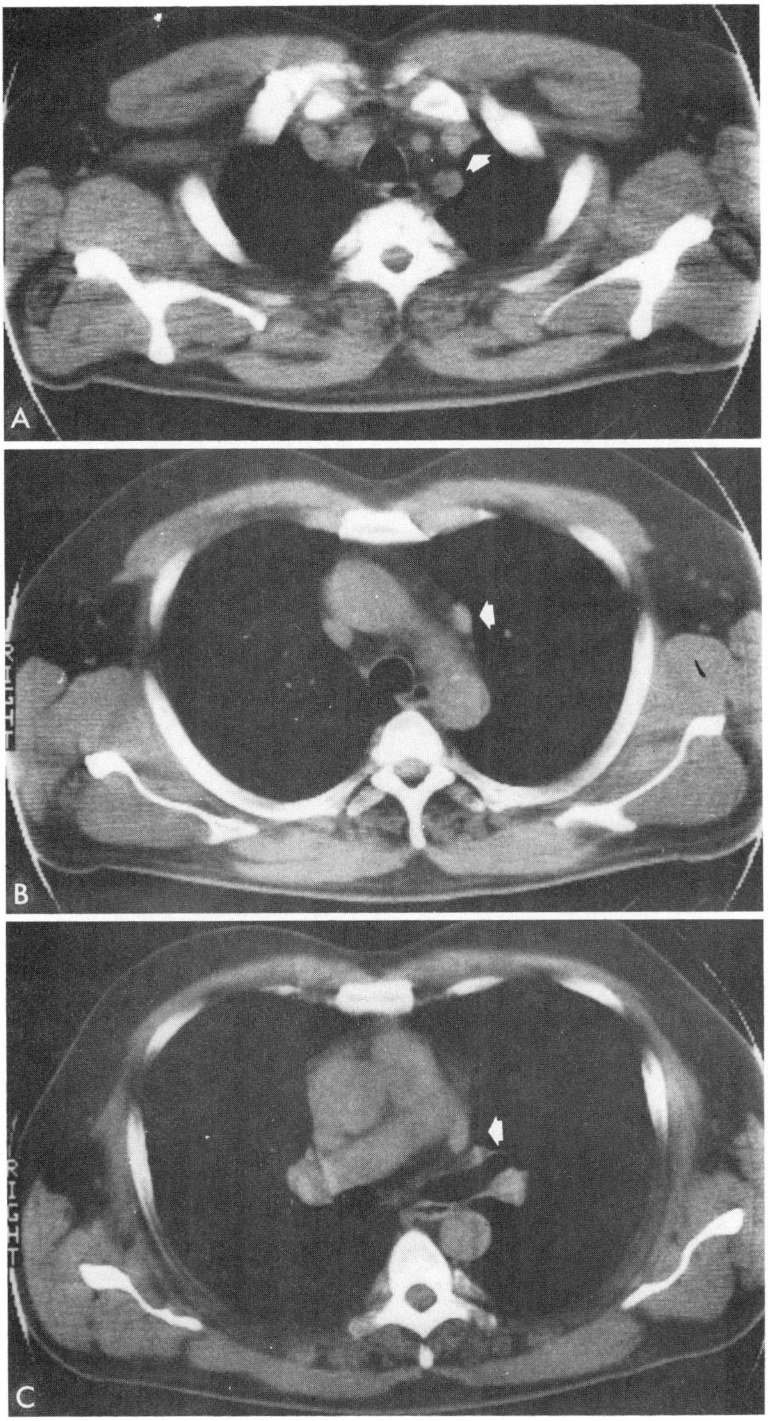

Figure 15. Persistent left superior vena cava. *A–C*, Sequential CT scans show the persistent left superior vena cava (arrows) as well as the right superior vena cava in the expected location to the right of the aorta. Bilateral upper extremity venogram confirmed the CT findings. (Reproduced with permission from Huggins TJ, Lesar ML, Friedman AC, et al: CT appearance of persistent left superior vena cava. J Comput Assist Tomogr, 6:294, 1982. Courtesy of Raven Press.)

When the right superior vena cava is absent, the CT images (Fig. 16) demonstrate a large vascular structure arising from the junction of the right and left innominate veins and continuing inferiorly to the left of the aortic arch without visualization of a normally positioned right-sided superior vena cava.

Diagnosing a persistent left superior vena cava is significant for several reasons. Most often, it explains an abnormal density detected on standard chest films, obviating the need for more invasive procedures. In addition, a correct diagnosis of persistent left superior vena cava is crucial because bilateral superior venae cavae have been a complicating factor during cannulation for open heart surgery. Finally, although

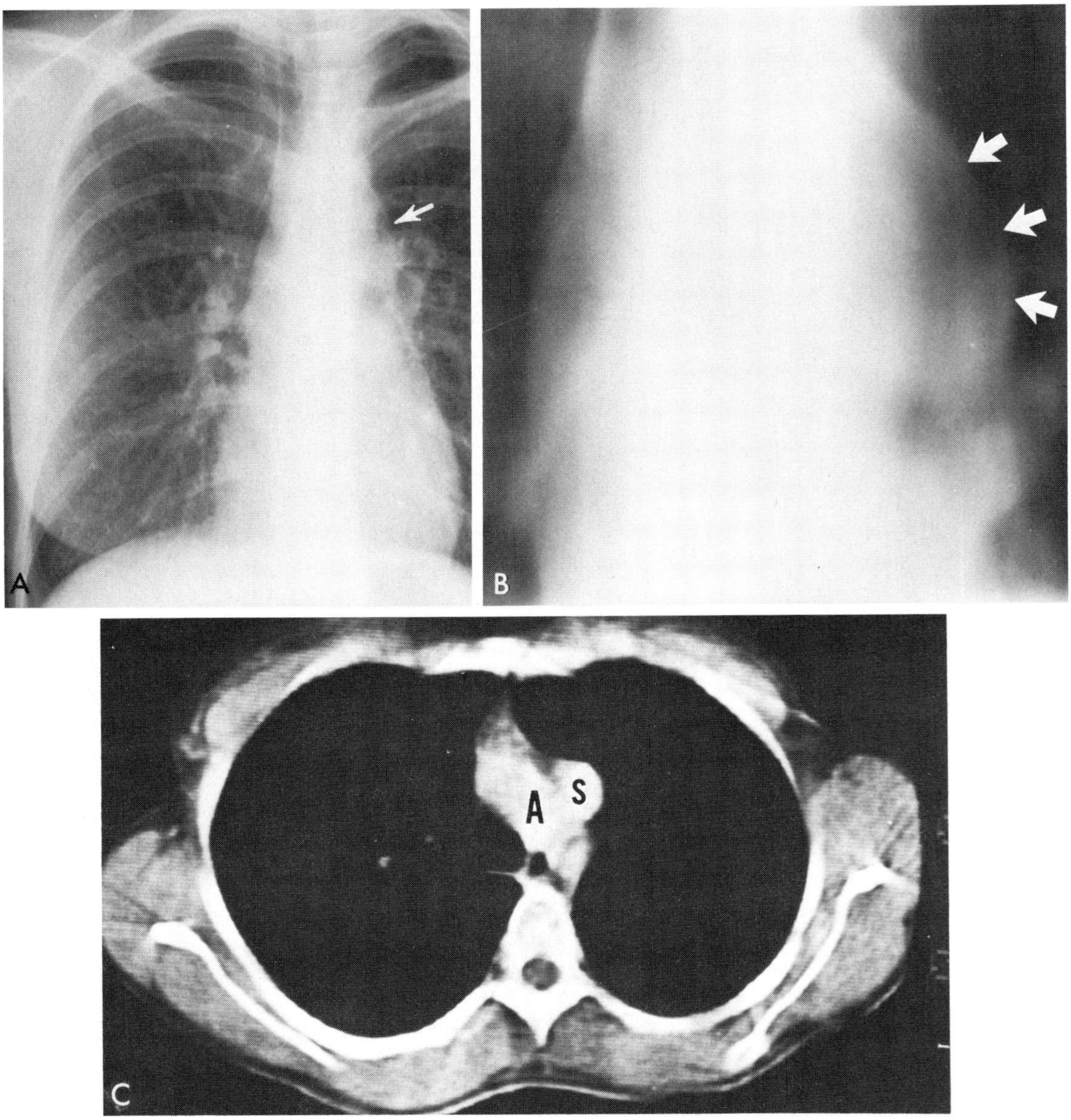

Figure 16. Persistent left superior vena cava. *A*, Chest radiograph shows a convex density (arrow) between the aortic knob and the pulmonary outflow tract. *B*, Anteroposterior tomogram confirms a convexity (arrows) in ductus area. A major diagnostic consideration was lymph node enlargement secondary to either granulomatous disease or neoplasm. *C*, Postcontrast CT scan is the level of the aortic arch (A). Enhancing structure is consistent with the persistent left superior vena cava (S). No caval structure is seen to the right of the aorta. (Reproduced with permission from Baron RL, Gutierrez FR, Sagel SS, et al: CT of anomalies of the mediastinal vessels. AJR, *137*: 571, 1981. Copyright ©, 1981, The Williams and Wilkins Company.)

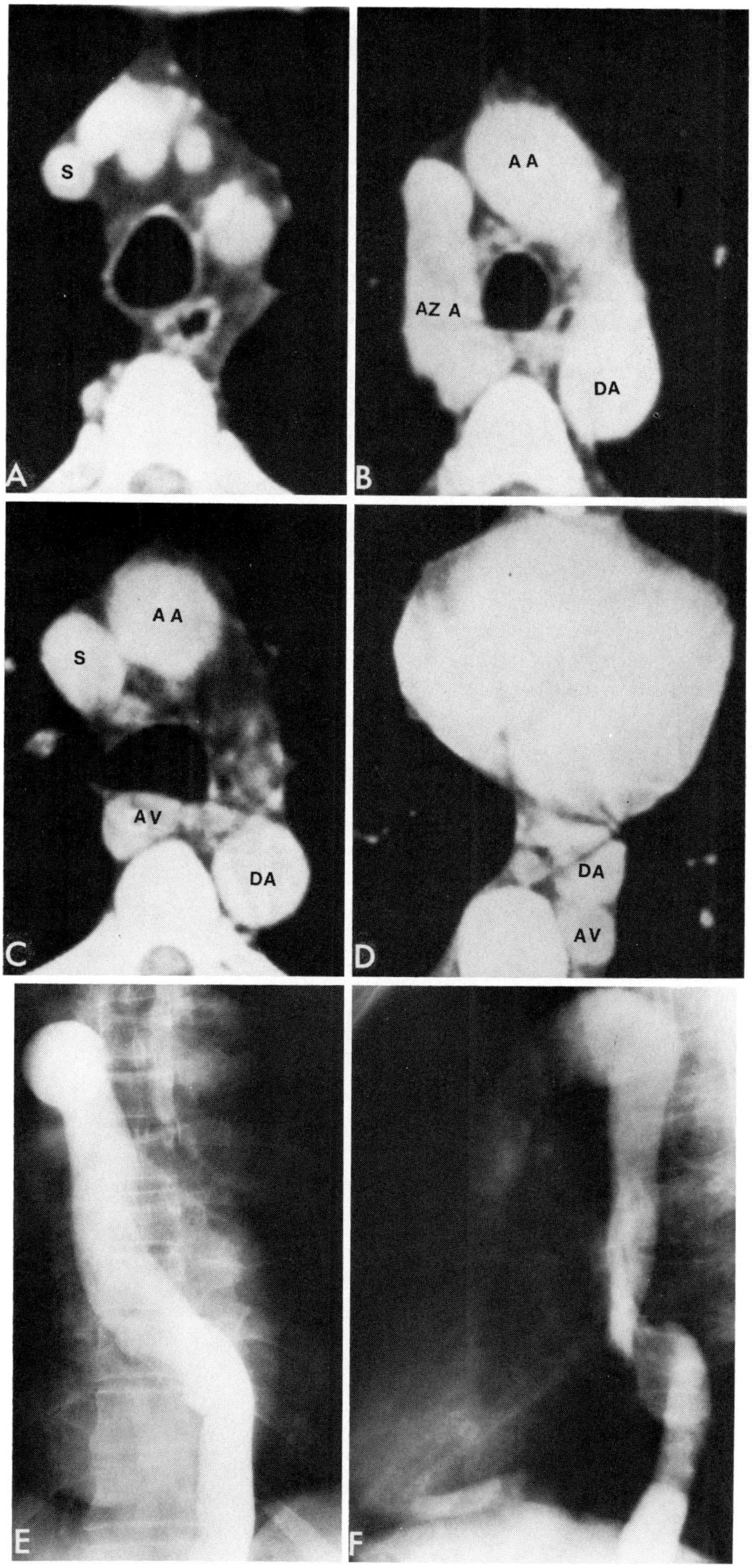

Figure 17. Azygos continuation of the inferior vena cava in a 51-year-old man. *A*, CT scan above the aortic arch shows a normal superior vena cava (S). *B*, Scan at level of azygos arch (AZ A) shows marked dilation of the azygos vein and arch. *C*, Scan at level below *B* shows azygos vein (AV) flattened and coursing to the left behind the trachea. *D*, Scan below *C* at the level of the heart shows the azygos vein lying behind the aorta on the left. Note the absence of normal right inferior vena cava. *E* and *F*, Frontal and lateral venograms confirm azygos continuation of a left inferior vena cava. AA: ascending aorta; DA: descending aorta.

most patients with persistent left superior vena cava do not have associated intracardiac anomalies, there is an increased incidence of such anomalies[6] when these patients are compared with the normal population.

Similarly, azygos and hemizygos venous drainage with interruption of the inferior vena cava may be demonstrated by CT scanning.[18] In such cases, the azygos or hemiazygos vein and the superior vena cava will dilate to accommodate the increased blood flow and should be readily detected on CT images (Fig. 17). CT evaluation may be used to advantage in certain cases of polysplenia and asplenia, in which knowledge of venous anatomy may be helpful in planning surgical procedures.

CONCLUSION

CT can play an important role both as a screening procedure and, in some cases, as an adjunct to angiography in defining the precise anatomy involved in congenital anomalies of the mediastinal vascular structures. Newer CT units with faster scan times and increased resolution will undoubtedly make this technique available for even younger patients.

REFERENCES

1. Baron RL, Gutierrez FR, Sagel SS, et al: CT of anomalies of the mediastinal vessels. AJR, *137*:571, 1981.
2. Baron RL, Levitt RG, Sagel SS, et al: Computed tomography in evaluation of mediastinal widening. Radiology, *138*:107, 1981.
3. Berdon WE, Baker DH: Vascular anomalies and the infant lung: Rings, slings, and other things. Semin Roentgenol, 7:39, 1972.
4. Brinsfield DE, Plauth WH: Clinical recognition and medical management of congenital heart disease. *In* Hurst JW, Logue RB, Schlent RC, et al (eds); The Heart, 4th ed. New York, McGraw-Hill, 1978, pp. 831–901.
5. Brinsfield DE, Shuford WH, Plauth WH, et al: Congenital anomalies of the aorta. *In* Lindsay J and Hurst JW (ed.): The aorta. New York, Grune and Stratton, 1979, p. 271.
6. Cha EM, Khoury GH: Persistent left superior vena cava, radiologic and clinical significance. Radiology, *103*:375, 1972.
7. Cholankeril JV, Ketyer S, Cholankeril MV: CT detection of coarctation of the aorta. J Comput Assist Tomogr, 5:355, 1981.
8. Elliott LP, Schiebler GL: The X-Ray Diagnosis of Congenital Heart Disease in Infants, Children and Adults. Springfield, IL, Charles C Thomas, 1979.
9. Gaupp RJ, Fagan CJ, Davis M, et al: Pseudocoarctation of the aorta. J Comput Assist Tomogr, 5:571, 1981.
10. Glanz S, Gordon DH: Right aortic arch with left descent. J Comput Assist Tomogr, 5:256, 1981.
11. Godwin JD, Herfkens RJ, Brundage BH, et al: Evaluation of coarctation of the aorta by computed tomography. J Comput Assist Tomogr, 5:153, 1981.
12. Guthaner DF, Wexler L, Harell G: CT demonstration of cardiac structures. AJR, *133*:75, 1979.
13. Huggins TJ, Lesar ML, Friedman AC, et al: CT appearance of persistent left superior vena cava. J Comput Assist Tomogr, 6:294, 1982.
14. Lackner K, Thurn P: Computed tomography of the heart: ECG-gated and continous scans. Radiology, *140*:413, 1981.
15. McLoughlin MJ, Weisbrod G, Wise DJ, et al: Computed tomography in congenital anomalies of the aortic arch and great vessels. Radiology, *138*:339, 1981.
16. Nada AS: Pediatric Cardiology, 2nd ed. Philadelphia, W.B. Saunders, 1963.
17. O'Callaghan JP, Heitzman ER, Somogyi JW, et al: CT evaluation of pulmonary artery size. J Comput Assist Tomogr, 6:101, 1982.
18. Rockoff SD, Druy EM: Tortuous azygos arch simulating a pulmonary lesion. AJR, *138*:577, 1982.
19. Shuford WH, Sybers RG: The Aortic Arch and Its Malformations. Springfield, IL, Charles C Thomas, 1974.
20. Stewart JR, Kincaid OW, Edwards JE: An Atlas of Vascular Rings and Related Malformations of the Aortic Arch System. Springfield, IL, Charles C Thomas, 1964.
21. Stone DN, Bein ME, Garris JB: Anomalous left pulmonary artery: Two new adult cases. AJR, *135*:1259, 1980.
22. Taber P, Chang LWM, Campion GM: Diagnosis of retroesophageal right aortic arch by computed tomography. J Comput Assist Tomogr, 3:684, 1979.
23. Webb WR, Gamsu G, Speckman JM, et al: Computed tomographic demonstration of mediastinal venous anomalies. AJR, *139*:157, 1982.
24. Webb WR, Gamsu G, Speckman JM, et al: CT demonstration of mediastinal aortic arch anomalies. J Comput Assist Tomogr, 6:445, 1982.

10

THE DEFINITION OF CARDIAC MALPOSITIONS WITH ECHOCARDIOGRAPHY AND COMPUTED TOMOGRAPHY

INA L. D. TONKIN, M.D.

Cardiac malformations associated with cardiac malpositions can present a diagnostic challenge. This chapter will outline a systematic approach to cardiac malpositions based upon the clinical, roentgenographic, ultrasonographic, echocardiographic, computed tomographic, and catheterization findings of 30 patients with some form of visceroatrial situs abnormality. Knowledge of the position of asymmetric abdominal and thoracic viscera gives a clue to the probable atrial positions[2, 8, 18, 30] (Figs. 1 and 2). Because of the progress in definitive repair of complex congenital heart disease in early infancy, it is now necessary to diagnose in full detail even the most complex lesions in the newborn period. This necessity has stimulated interest in diagnostic techniques and in the classification of congenital heart disease. The diagnosis of the types of visceroatrial situs and their implications will be reviewed in this chapter. The excellent classifications of atrioventricular and ventriculoarterial connections previously reported[2, 26, 28, 34] will not be reviewed.

Abdominal ultrasonography was performed on all 30 patients. In the author's experience, an accurate diagnosis of most visceroatrial situs abnormalities can be made on the basis of the chest radiograph with abdominal ultrasonography and/or echocardiography and computed tomography (CT) before cardiac catheterization, surgical correction, or necropsy results. In some instances, ultrasonography or CT or both may be the initial diagnostic procedure. Heterotaxic patterns—that is, anomalous placement of organs and major blood vessels within the abdomen—seen on ultrasonographic or CT examination should be recognized as indicating an abnormal situs and should not be confused with other pathologic conditions.

DEFINITIONS

Cardiac Positions. Normally, the major portion of the heart lies to the left of the midline. For the purpose of this review, any heart other than a left-sided heart in a situs solitus individual represents a cardiac malposition. This definition refers not only to the cardiac positions but also to the appropriateness of the cardiac position in relation to the total body situs. A right-sided heart with the cardiac apex to the right is clearly unusual, even though it may be appropriate or normal in an individual with situs inversus (Table 1). A left-sided heart, or levocardia, however, is inappropriate in a person with situs inversus and is also an example of cardiac malposition with an extremely high incidence of congenital heart disease (Table 1). In addition, in this review, all patients having situs ambiguus with either right isomerism (asplenia syndrome) or left isomerism (polysplenia syndrome) are regarded as having cardiac malpositions.

Levocardia, dextrocardia, and *mesocardia* are general terms indicating cardiac apex only. They do not give any indication of cardiac structure or body situs. Levocardia denotes a

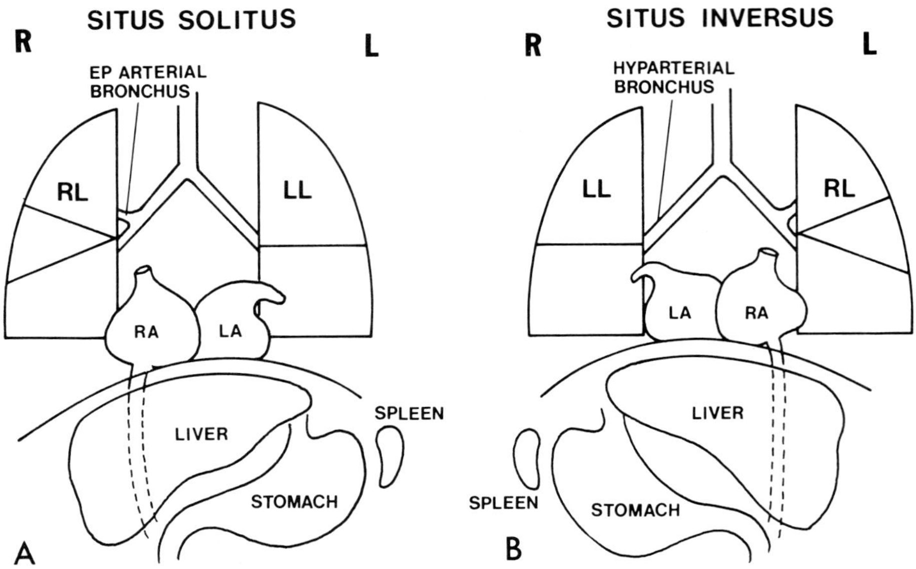

Figure 1. *A*, A schematic representation of situs solitus showing the eparterial bronchus on the right with the trilobed right lung (RL). On the left, there is a hyparterial bronchus because the pulmonary artery crosses over the bronchus. The left lung (LL) has two lobes. The left bronchus is longer than the right by about a 1.7 to 2:1 ratio. The right atrium (RA) is on the patient's right side, and the left atrium (LA) is on the left side. The abdominal viscera are normal, with the liver on the right and the spleen and stomach on the left. The inferior vena cava is to the right of the spine, and the aorta descends to the left of the spine in the normal or situs solitus situation. *B*, In the schematic representation of situs inversus, there is a mirror image, with the trilobed lung and eparterial bronchus on the left, a bilobed lung and hyparterial bronchus on the right, dextrocardia, and reversal of the abdominal organs and vessels.

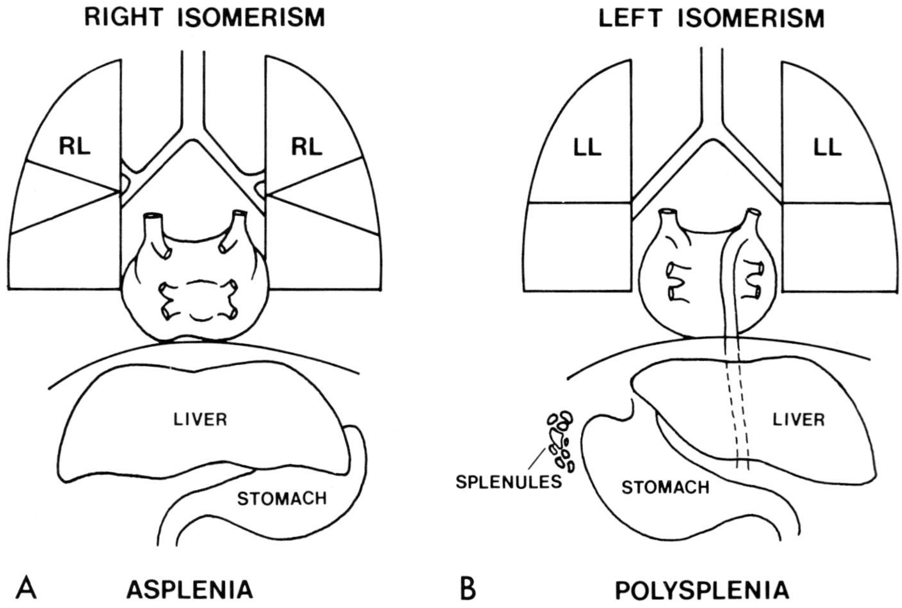

Figure 2. *A*, With situs ambiguus, there may be bilateral right isomerism with bilateral trilobed lungs and eparterial bronchi of the same short length. In the instance of right atrial isomerism, the atrial appendages are usually symmetric and resemble a broad-based right atrial appendage. The liver is frequently in the midline, as may be the stomach with absence of the spleen. The abdominal aorta and inferior vena cava cross to the same side of the spine in the abdomen with inferior vena cava–right atrial continuity. *B*, In left isomerism or polysplenia syndrome, there are bilateral hyparterial bronchi, bilobed lungs, and bilateral left atria or a common atrium. By definition, at least two spleens are along the greater curvature of the stomach. Left isomerism frequently involves interruption of the inferior vena cava with azygos or hemiazygos continuation to a superior vena cava. Heart disease is less severe in this syndrome, with a 5 to 10 per cent incidence of no congenital heart disease (Table 1).

Table 1. *Cardiac Malpositions*

VISCEROATRIAL SITUS	ASSOCIATION WITH CHD*
Situs solitus with levocardia	Normal, less than 1%
Situs solitus with dextrocardia	95%
Situs inversus with dextrocardia	3–5%
Situs inversus with levocardia	Very rare, 100%
Situs ambiguus—left isomerism (polysplenia syndrome)	90%
Situs ambiguus—right isomerism (asplenia syndrome)	99–100%

*CHD: congenital heart disease.

left-sided heart; dextrocardia denotes a right-sided heart with a right cardiac apex; and mesocardia denotes a midline heart.[12, 23, 26, 28, 34, 35]

Cardiac displacement is the shifting of the heart within the thorax by extracardiac factors, such as a hypoplastic lung or paralyzed hemidiaphragm. This has been referred to in the literature as dextroposition, mesoposition, or levoposition, depending on the direction of the shift.

Situs solitus indicates the normal position of the atria and viscera. The lungs, liver, spleen, stomach, and atria are usually asymmetric organs, and the term situs is used to define the position of the atria and viscera relative to the midline or sagittal plane. Situs solitus with levocardia is the normal situation, with less than 1 per cent incidence of congenital heart disease (Fig. 1*A*; Table 1).

Situs inversus is the mirror-image location of the atria and abdominal viscera. Situs inversus with dextrocardia is the usual situation, and persons with this condition have only a 3 to 5 per cent incidence of congenital heart disease. Situs inversus with levocardia is extremely rare but is almost always associated with congenital heart disease (Fig. 1*B*).

Heterotaxia is the abnormal arrangement of organs and major blood vessels different from the orderly arrangement of either situs solitus or situs inversus, i.e., malrotation of the bowel.[8, 21, 28, 30]

In *situs ambiguus*, the third abnormal type of situs, the relationship of the atria and viscera is inconsistent or heterotaxia is present. In this type of situs abnormality, structures that are usually asymmetric can be symmetric (i.e., both sides of the viscera, lung, and atria are nearly identical to one another[2, 8, 16, 18, 19, 21, 22, 26–28 30, 32–35] (Figs. 2*A* and *B*).

Isomerism is a term used to describe symmetric morphology.[27, 30, 32, 33] *Right isomerism* (asplenia syndrome) is characterized by situs ambiguus with bilateral right-sidedness[2, 26, 27, 33] (Fig. 2*A*). *Left isomerism* (polysplenia syndrome) is a second type of situs ambiguus characterized by bilateral left-sidedness[2, 26, 27, 33] (Fig. 2*B*).

CLINICAL MATERIAL

During the three-year period from August 1979 through August 1982, 30 patients with visceroatrial situs abnormalities were studied by ultrasonography, echocardiography, and CT in conjunction with chest and abdominal radiographs. One additional patient with visceroatrial situs solitus was used for comparative evaluation of the normal anatomy demonstrated by ultrasonography and computed tomography (Fig. 2*A–C*). In 22 of the 30 patients, the findings at diagnostic cardiac catheterization[6] were also correlated with the preoperative diagnosis of visceroatrial situs (Table 2). Ten of the 30 patients are deceased, with postmortem correlation in 5 patients (Table 2).

All patients were examined by echocardiography or ultrasonography or both using a Picker 80L B-mode Scanner with real-time capabilities, a Varian V3400 Sector Scanner, or a Technicare 8100 Auto Sector Scanner with 3.5 or 5 MHz transducers. Several patients were examined by CT using a GE 8800 CT/T Scanner. The patients were 1 day to 26 years old. Sedation with sodium thiopental administered rectally (Pentothal, rectal suspension, 25 mg/kg) was used occasionally for CT and ultrasonography of children under the age of three years.[3, 30] In six patients, radionuclide liver-spleen scans were obtained.

SITUS SOLITUS

An example of situs solitus in a normal patient without congenital heart disease is used for orientation and reference (Fig. 3*A* to *C*). With situs solitus and levocardia, the right atrium is normally located on the right and the left atrium on the left, with the inferior vena cava entering the right atrium in a usual fashion (Fig. 1*A*). On the transverse abdominal ultrasonogram, one sees the liver echo texture to the patient's right with a sonolucent inferior vena cava traveling through the liver to the right of the spine. In addition, normally there is a left-sided aorta, which descends in the chest to the left side of the spine within the abdomen (Fig. 3*B*). In a patient with situs solitus and a right aortic arch,

Table 2. *Clinical and Anatomic Features of Visceroatrial Situs Abnormalities*

ABNORMALITY/CASE NO.	CARDIOVASCULAR ANOMALIES	ABDOMINAL VESSELS	VISCERAL HETEROTAXIA	CLINICAL COURSE
Situs Solitus with Dextrocardia:				
1. 14m,F	Dextrocardia, none	IVC on R; aorta on L	Liver on R; stomach on L; spleen on L; G-B R	A&W
Situs Inversus with Dextrocardia or Mesocardia:				
2. 6y,M	Univentricular heart; two AV valves	IVC on L; aorta on R	Liver on L; stomach on R; spleen on R	A&W; R B-T shunt
3. 5y,F	AV disc; VA disc with pul atresia; VSD (ventricular inversion)	IVC on L; aorta on R	Liver on L; stomach on R	A&W; R Waterson shunt
4. 4y,F	AV disc; VA disc with pul atresia; VSD (ventricular inversion)	IVC on L; aorta on R	Liver on L; stomach on R; spleen on R	A&W; L B-T shunt
5. 6y,M	Univentricular heart; pul atresia; two AV valves, accessory chamber	IVC on L; aorta on R	Liver on L; stomach on R; spleen on R	A&W; R B-T shunt
6. 5y,M	AV disc; VA disc with pul atresia; VSD	IVC on L; aorta on R	Liver on L; stomach on R; spleen on R	A&W; R Waterson shunt; L B-T shunt
7. 20m,F	None	IVC on L; aorta on R	Liver on L; stomach on R	A&W
8. 2y,M	None	IVC on L; aorta on R	Liver on L; stomach on R	A&W
Left Isomerism (Polysplenia Syndrome):				
9. 3y,M	Levocardia; post repair partial AV canal	Azygos cont of IVC to R SVC; aorta on L	Liver on L; stomach on R; gallbladder midline	A&W; post–total repair
10. 6w,M	Levocardia; complete AV canal	Hemiazygos cont of IVC to L SVC; aorta on L	Liver on L; stomach on R	Deceased; postmortem at 2 y
11. 1w,M	Dextrocardia; univentricular heart; common atrium and common AV valve; interruption of aortic arch, type B	Hemiazygos cont of IVC to L SVC	Liver on R; stomach on L	Deceased
12. 6d,F	Levocardia; univentricular heart; common atrium and common AV valve; interruption of aortic arch, type B	Azygos cont of IVC to R SVC	Liver on L; stomach on R	Deceased
13. 26y,F	Levocardia	Azygos cont of IVC to R SVC; aorta on L	Liver on L; stomach on R	A&W
14. 6y,M	Levocardia; VSD	Azygos cont of IVC to R SVC; aorta on L	Liver on L; stomach on R; gallbladder on L	A&W
15. 2y,F	Levocardia; VSD?	Azygos cont of IVC to R SVC; aorta on L	Liver on R; stomach on L; gallbladder on R	A&W
16. 7d,F	Levocardia; common AV valve; DORV; PS	IVC on R; aorta on L	Liver on R; stomach on L	Deceased; postmortem
17. 11m,F	Levocardia; partial AV canal	Azygos cont of IVC to R SVC; aorta on L	Liver on R; stomach on L	A&W; post–total repair

Table continued on opposite page

Table 2. *Clinical and Anatomic Features of Visceroatrial Situs Abnormalities* (Continued)

ABNORMALITY/CASE NO.	CARDIOVASCULAR ANOMALIES	ABDOMINAL VESSELS	VISCERAL HETEROTAXIA	CLINICAL COURSE
18. 4y, F	Levocardia; moderate AS?	Azygos cont of IVC to R SVC; aorta on L	Liver on R; stomach on L	A&W
19. 10y, F	Levocardia; spontaneous closure of VSD at 10 y	Azygos cont of IVC to R SVC, aorta on L	Liver on R; stomach on L	A&W
20. 14y, F	Levocardia	Azygos cont of IVC to R SVC; aorta on L	Liver on L; stomach on R	A&W
Right Isomerism (Asplenia Syndrome):				
21. 4y, F	Levocardia; DORV with PS; TAPVC to R atrium; common AV valve	IVC on L; R arch crosses to L	R arch, type I; liver on L; stomach on R	Deceased; 5 y; L B-T shunt
22. 3d, M	Dextrocardia; DORV with large VSD and PS; common atrium; and common AV valve	IVC on R; R aortic arch	R arch; liver at midline; stomach at midline	Deceased; postmortem at 9 m; R B-T shunt
23. 4y, M	Dextrocardia; univentricular heart with PS; common atrium; and common AV valve	IVC crosses to R; R aortic arch	R arch, type I; liver on L; stomach on L	Deceased; postmortem; L B-T shunt
24. 14m, M	Levocardia; univentricular heart; common atrium; and common AV valve	IVC on L; aorta on L	L arch; liver on L stomach on L	A&W; CHF
25. 2d, F	Dextrocardia; TGA (AV conc, VA disc); pul atresia; multiple VSDs; common atrium	IVC on L; aorta on L	L arch; liver on L; stomach on R	Deceased; 10 m
26. 4y, M	Levocardia; univentricular heart; pul atresia	IVC on L; aorta on L	L arch; liver on L; stomach on R	A&W; R B-T shunt
27. 3y, M	Levocardia; univentricular heart; pul atresia; PAPVR; two AV valves	IVC on R; aorta on R	R arch, type I; liver on R; stomach on L	A&W; L B-T shunt
28. 1d, F	Levocardia; univentricular heart; pul atresia; common AV valve, bil PDAs	IVC crosses to L; aorta on L	L arch; liver midline; stomach on R	Deceased; 3 d
29. 1d, M	Levocardia; common AV valve; TAPVC; pul atresia; TGA	IVC on L; aorta on L	L arch; liver midline; stomach midline	Deceased; postmortem at 2 m; R B-T shunt
30. 2w, F	Levocardia univentricular heart; TGA; PS; common AV valve	IVC on L; aorta on L	L arch; liver midline; stomach on R	A&W

Note: F: female; M: male; m: months; y: years; w: weeks; d: days; AV: atrioventricular; VSD: ventricular septal defect; cont: continuation; IVC: inferior vena cava; SVC: superior vena cava; R: right; L: left; bil: bilateral; A&W: alive and well; G-B: gallbladder; DORV: double outlet right ventricle; TAPVC: total anomalous pulmonary venous connection; PS: pulmonic stenosis; AS: aortic stenosis; CHF: congestive heart failure; TGA (AV conc): atrioventricular concordance; VA disc: ventriculoarterial discordance (complete transposition of the great arteries); pul: pulmonary; B-T shunt: Blalock-Taussig shunt; R arch, type I: right aortic arch—type I with mirror image branching; PAPVR: partial anomalous pulmonary venous return; AV disc: atrioventricular discordance; VA disc: ventriculoarterial discordance (corrected transposition of the great arteries).

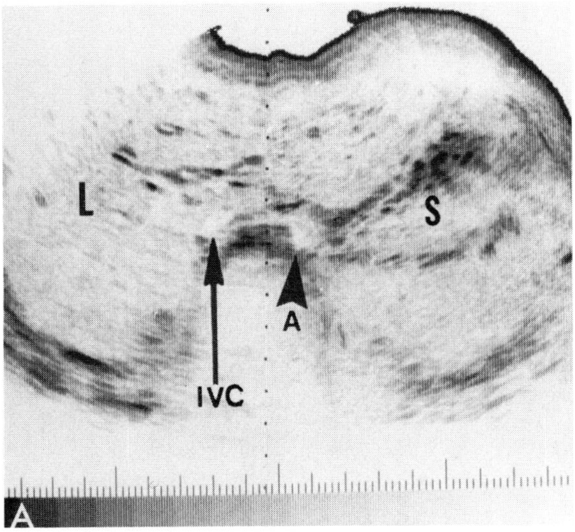

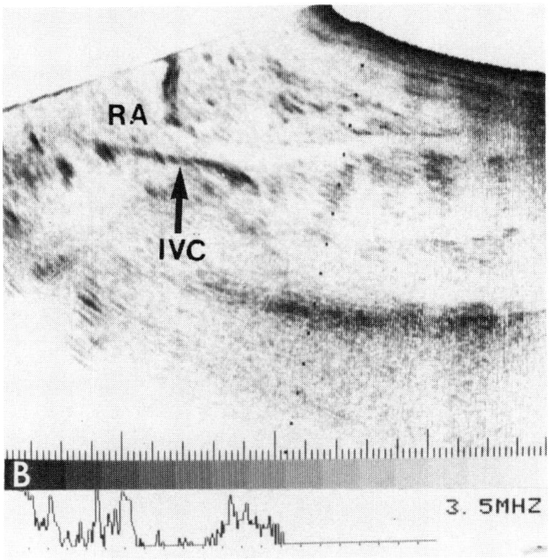

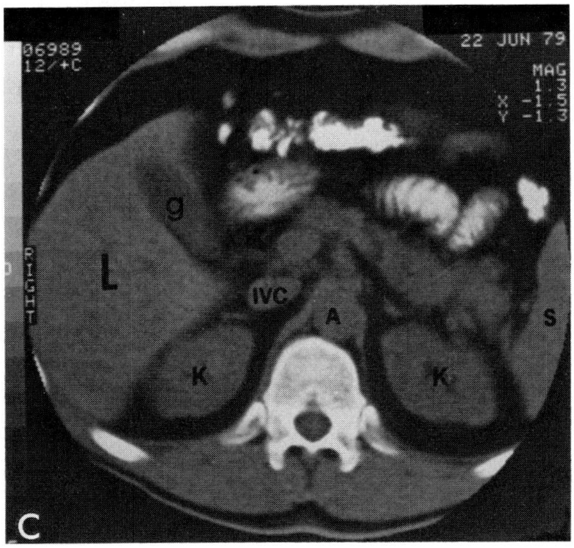

Figure 3. *A*, Visceroatrial situs solitus. The transverse upper abdominal ultrasonogram shows a right-sided liver (L) and right-sided inferior vena cava (IVC, arrow). The aorta (A, arrowhead) is to the left of the spine. The echogenic structure represents a fluid-filled stomach (S), which is on the patient's left side. *B* The longitudinal ultrasound examination in situs solitus shows the sonolucent inferior vena cava (IVC, arrow) entering the right atrium (RA) just to the right of midline in a normal location. There is mild pulsation of the inferior vena cava with respiration on real-time examination, compared with that of the aorta. *C*, The transverse CT examination of an additional patient with situs solitus; contrast material on the small bowel shows the inferior vena cava (IVC) to the right of the spine with a retrocrural aorta (A). The liver (L) and gallbladder (g) are to the patient's right. A small portion of the spleen (S) can be seen to the patient's left, with both kidneys (K) identified.

the aorta will usually cross to the left of the spine in the abdomen.

On longitudinal two-dimensional sector scanning or B-mode scanning, the inferior vena cava should enter the right atrium to the right of the spine (Fig. 3*B*). The normal vascular pattern and presence of the liver and spleen can also be seen in patients who are undergoing CT examinations (Fig. 3*C*). Ultrasonography or sector scanning is extremely helpful in patients with situs solitus and dextrocardia when visualization of the bronchial anatomy is too poor to determine bronchial or atrial situs on the posteroanterior (PA) and lateral chest radiographs.[2, 16, 18, 19, 27]

Normally, there is a 95 per cent incidence of congenital heart disease in patients with situs solitus and dextrocardia (Table 1). However, in evaluating the cardiac anatomy of a patient who is clinically normal but who has this condition, it is important to define the location and position of the inferior vena cava as it enters the right atrium as a sign of atrial isomerism.[2, 26] Occasionally, the patient may be one of those 5 per cent of patients having dextrocardia with situs solitus and no evidence of congenital heart disease (Case 1) (Fig. 4*A–D*).

SITUS INVERSUS

Seven patients with total situs inversus demonstrated mirror imaging on chest and abdominal radiographs (Fig. 5*A*). The ultrasonographic examination in each case showed mirror-image positioning of the abdominal viscera and vessels. In each case, the liver was located on the patient's left, with the inferior vena cava to the

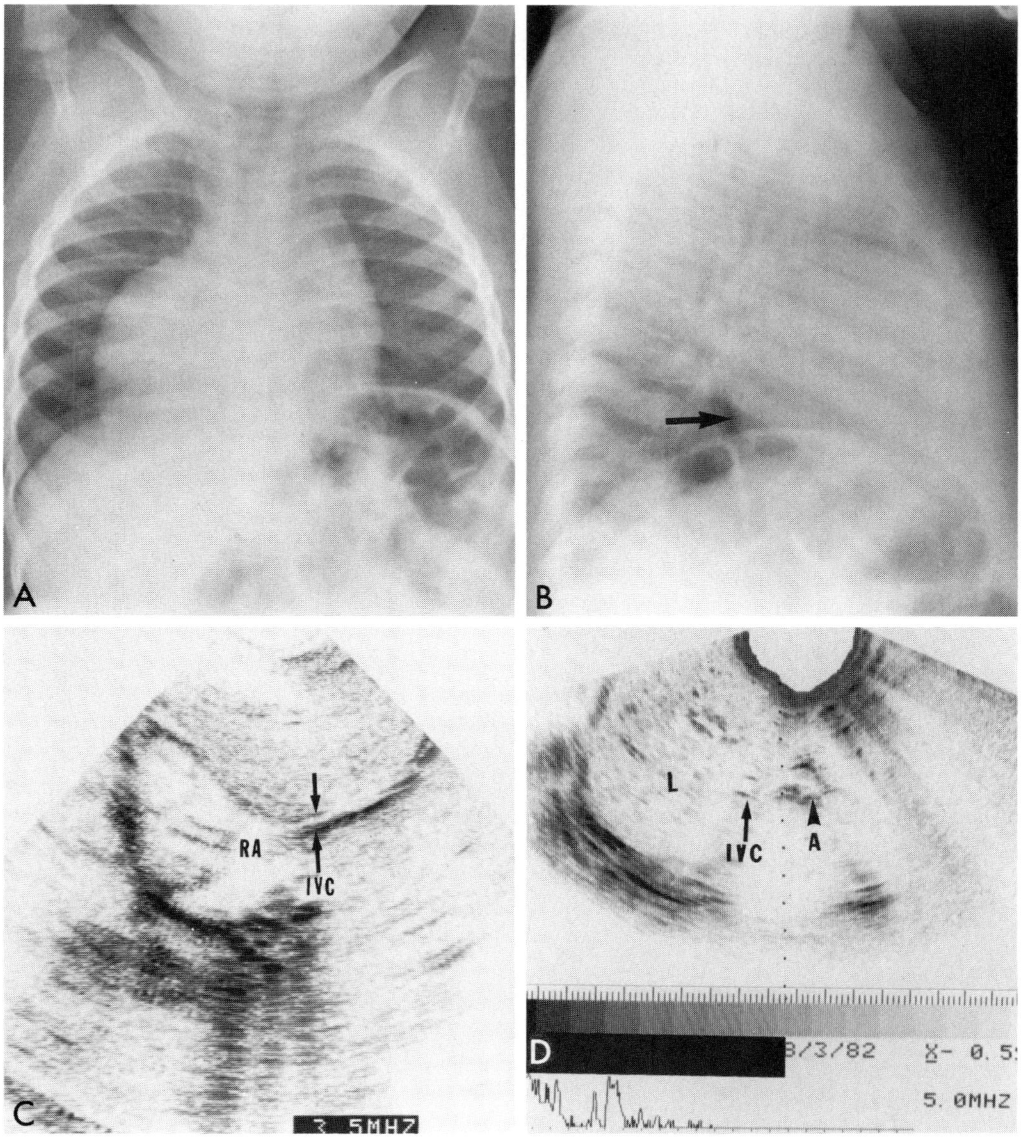

Figure 4. *A*, A 14-month-old girl (patient no. 1) had no clinical evidence of congenital heart disease. The posteroanterior (PA) chest radiograph shows bronchial anatomy, which probably indicates an eparterial bronchus on the right and total situs solitus with dextrocardia. The liver appears to be mostly to the right side with a left-sided stomach. There is a probable left aortic arch. The findings are compatible with situs solitus and dextrocardia, which is associated with a 95 per cent incidence of congenital heart disease. *B*, The lateral projection shows a probable inferior vena cava shadow (arrow) with poor definition of the pulmonary artery and bronchial anatomy. *C*, A real-time ultrasound examination was performed to evaluate the cardiac anatomy and to determine if the patient truly had situs solitus of the atria and viscera rather than situs ambiguus. The two-dimensional sector scan showed evidence of the inferior vena cava (IVC, arrows) as a sonolucent structure entering the right atrium (RA). Two-dimensional and M-mode examinations of the heart showed no abnormality. *D*, A transverse B-mode ultrasound examination demonstrated the liver (L) to the patient's right with faint visualization of the sonolucent IVC (arrow, IVC) to the right. The sonolucent and pulsating aorta (A, arrowhead) is to the left of the spine, indicating visceroatrial situs solitus and dextrocardia without evidence of congenital heart disease, which is unusual (see Table 1).

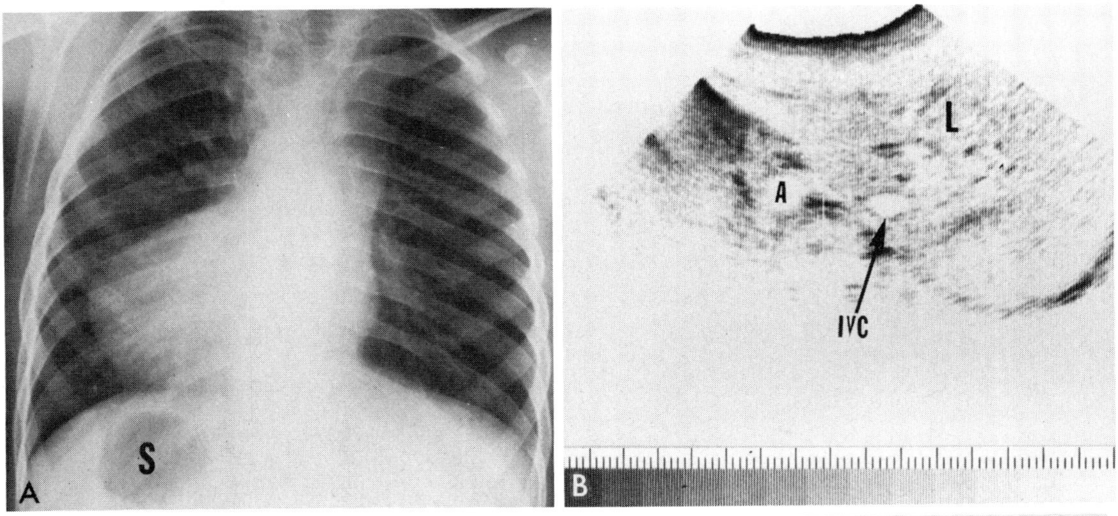

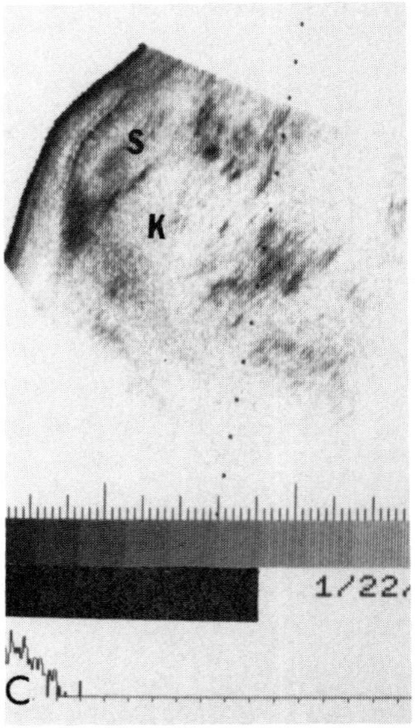

Figure 5. *A*, The PA chest radiograph of patient no. 5. A six-year-old boy had total visceroatrial situs inversus or situs ambiguus with dextrocardia, a right-sided aortic arch, right-sided stomach (S), and left-sided liver. With true situs inversus with dextrocardia, there is a 3 to 5 per cent incidence of congenital heart disease. However, there is severe congenital heart disease with corrected transposition of the great arteries, pulmonary atresia, and ventricular septal defect. The patient has undergone a right thoracotomy for a right Blalock-Taussig shunt. *B*, Transverse ultrasonogram of total situs inversus in patient no. 5, a six-year-old boy. The liver (L) is to the left with a left-sided inferior vena cava (IVC, arrow). The sonolucent pulsating aorta (A) is to the right of the spine. *C*, A coronal oblique ultrasound examination of this patient's right side demonstrated a homogeneous and normal-appearing spleen (S) and right-sided kidney (K). This indicates the patient had total visceroatrial situs inversus (see Tables 1 and 2).

(*B*, reproduced with permission from Tonkin IL, Tonkin AK: Visceroatrial situs abnormalities. Sonographic and computed tomographic appearance. AJR, *138*:509, 1982. Copyright ©, 1982, The Williams and Wilkins Company.)

left of the spine and the aorta descending to the right of the spine (Fig. 5*B*). In each case, the stomach was located on the patient's right, and in four cases, ultrasonography demonstrated the presence of a spleen in the patient's right upper quadrant. (Cases 2, 4, 5, and 6) (Fig. 5*C*). Five of the seven patients have severe cardiac anomalies, which are generally seen in only 3 to 5 per cent of patients with total situs inversus (Tables 1 and 2). This high incidence is, no doubt, due to the evaluation of patients at our institution with cardiovascular conditions. Two patients (Cases 7 and 8) were evaluated with ultrasonography after the incidental radiographic presentation of probable total situs inversus. Both of these patients had no evidence of congenital heart disease and presented with wheezing. In all seven cases, the ultrasonographic examination of the abdomen differentiated total situs inversus from situs ambiguus.

The rare condition of situs inversus has intrigued physicians since it was first described by Aristotle. Seventy-six of the 1,551,047 (0.00005 per cent) patients who registered at the Mayo Clinic from 1910 through 1947 were found to have complete situs inversus.[29] A diagnosis of abdominal situs inversus can be clearly made by abdominal arteriography, which can alleviate a complex and potentially dangerous surgical dilemma in emergency cases of gastrointestinal hemorrhage or blunt abdominal trauma.[29]

LEFT ISOMERISM (POLYSPLENIA SYNDROME)

During the three-year period of study, 12 patients with left isomerism or polysplenia syndrome were evaluated with chest radiography and ultrasonography or echocardiography. The plain chest radiographs in older patients were suggestive of left isomerism with abdominal heterotaxia, hyparterial bronchi, and no inferior vena cava shadow with probable azygos continuation (Fig. 6*A* and *B*). In most of the cases, absence of the inferior vena cava at the level of the liver was noted at ultrasonography (Fig. 6*C*). The longitudinal ultrasonographic examination also demonstrated no inferior vena cava

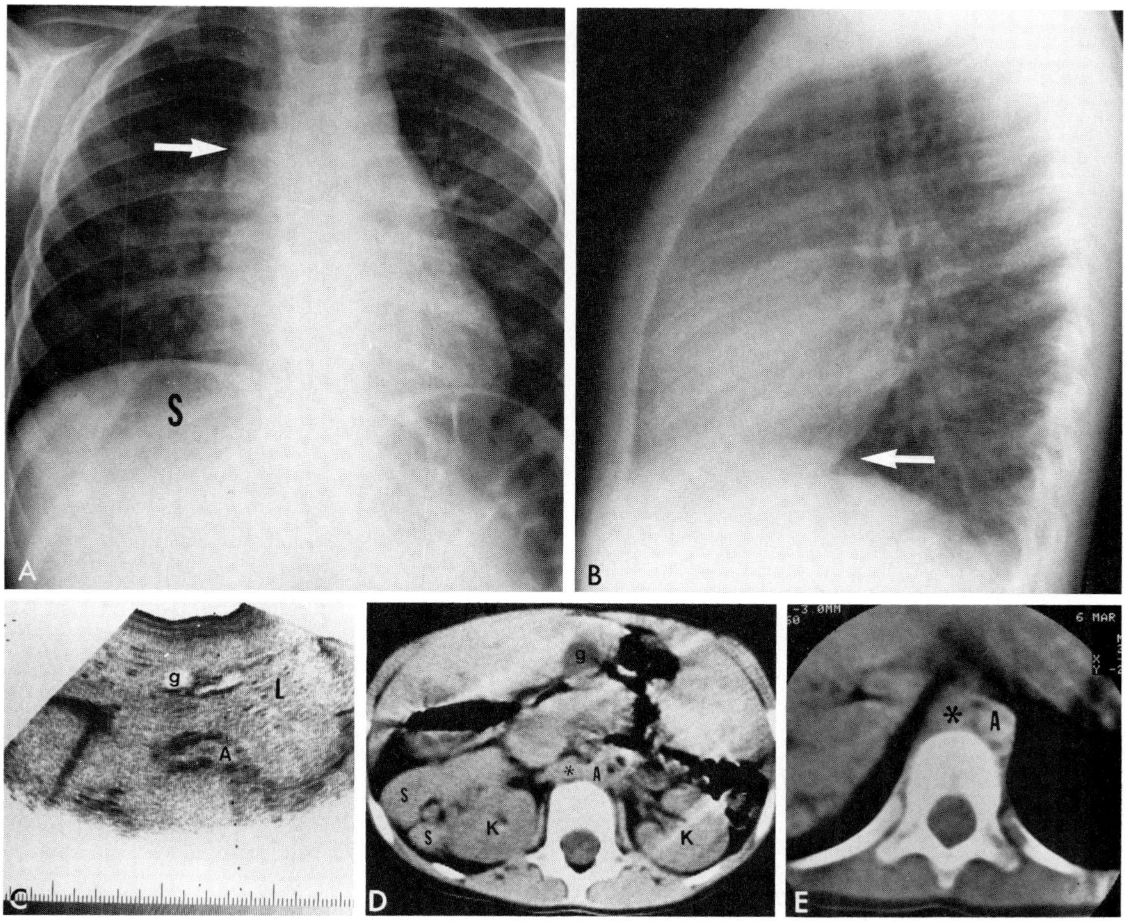

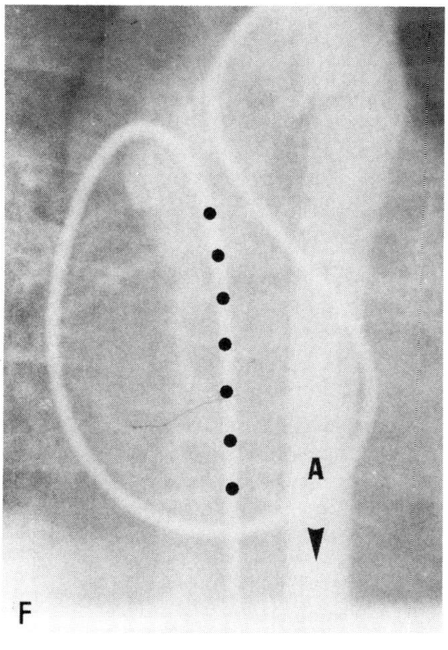

Figure 6. *A*, The PA chest radiograph of patient no. 9 shows evidence of probable situs ambiguus with left isomerism and bilateral hyparterial bronchi. In addition, to the right of the trachea, there is a density that may represent an azygos vein (arrow). The patient had a left-sided aortic arch with levocardia and a right-sided stomach (S). *B*, The lateral chest radiograph shows absence of the inferior vena cava shadow (arrow). *C*, Left isomerism (polysplenia syndrome) in patient no. 9, a three-year-old boy. The transverse ultrasonogram shows the liver (L) to the left and the aorta (A) to the left of the spine. The inferior vena cava is not seen with independent drainage of the hepatic veins into the atrium. There is a midline gallbladder (g). *D*, The CT scan without contrast enhancement shows a transverse liver with a midline gallbladder (g). The structures are thought to represent splenules (S). The aorta (A) with retrocrural azygos vein (asterisk) is seen. The kidneys are also identified (K). *E*, A magnified CT image of the vascular anatomy shows the aorta (A) to the left with a retrocrural venous structure (asterisk). *F*, Correlation with the vascular anatomy at the initial cardiac catheterization shows a femoral venous catheter (dots) that passes through the azygos vein with contrast material injected into the normal descending left-sided aorta (A, arrowhead). One year after total repair of a partial atrioventricular canal, this patient has a satisfactory result.

(*C–E* reproduced with permission from Tonkin, IL, Tonkin AK: Visceroatrial situs abnormalities: Sonographic and computed tomographic appearance. AJR, *138*:509, 1982. Copyright ©, 1982, The Williams and Wilkins Company.)

entering the right atrium with independent drainage of the common vein or hepatic veins into the right atrium.[12, 31] In this series, 7 of the 12 patients with left isomerism or polysplenia syndrome underwent cardiac catheterization, and the vascular anatomy was correlated with ultrasonographic and CT findings (Fig. 6*A–F*).

CT was performed on three patients (Cases 9, 10, and 13), with the position of the great abdominal vessels and multiple splenules demonstrated[5, 13, 20] (Figs. 6*D* and *E* and 7*A–G*). Results from ultrasonography and CT (Fig. 7*D* and *E*) were comparable.

Left isomerism or polysplenia syndrome may be seen in adulthood (Case 13), and some patients (Cases 13, 19, and 20) have no evidence of significant congenital heart disease (Table 2). Therefore, if ultrasonography or CT is the first imaging modality used (Fig. 7*D* and *E*), these abnormal vascular heterotaxic patterns should be recognized as such and should not be confused with additional pathologic conditions.[5, 13, 24, 30, 38]

In the newborn period it is essential to evaluate the infant with complex congenital heart disease using erect PA and lateral chest radiography and echocardiography (Fig. 8*A* and *B*). Ultrasonography even in the newborn period demonstrates complex vascular anatomy and allows the precatheterization diagnosis of left isomerism or polysplenia syndrome (Figs. 8*A–D* and 9*A–F*). Real-time or two-dimensional sector scanning can show the anomalous systemic veins and the exact vascular anatomy before catheterization so that a basilic vein cut-down can be planned, if necessary, to allow easy access into the cardiac chamber (Fig. 9*E* and *F*). In questionable or in mixed situs anomalies, a CT scan, even without contrast material will demonstrate polysplenia syndrome, with multiple splenules visualized[5, 20, 38] (Fig. 9*G* and *H*).

With left isomerism, interruption of the inferior vena cava between the renal veins and hepatic veins with azygos-hemiazygos continuation is usually seen.[2, 33] This sign may be suggested from evaluation of a plain chest radiograph that shows absence of an inferior vena cava shadow on the lateral projection and a widening of the paravertebral pleural reflection in the right or left paratracheal area, which may indicate a dilated azygos or hemiazygos vein[2, 23, 27] (Figs. 6*A*, 7*A*, and 12*A* and *C*). This venous anomaly may appear as a mediastinal mass in older patients. When this anomaly is

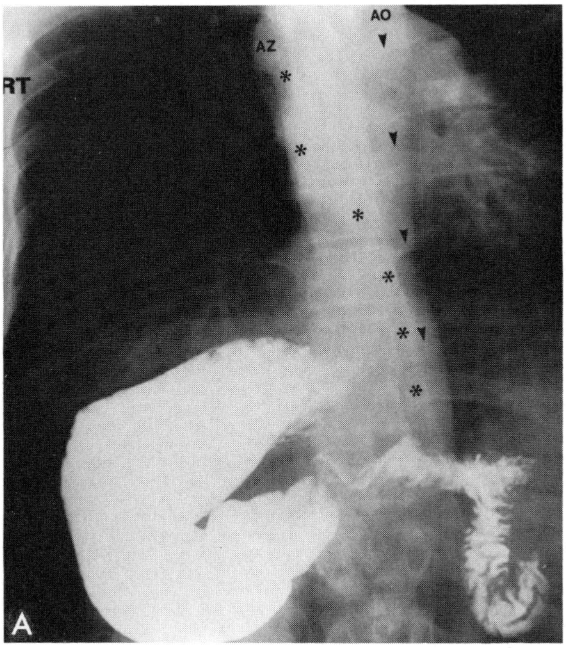

Figure 7. *A*, The anteroposterior (AP) supine overpenetrated radiograph of the lower chest and abdomen of a 26-year-old woman with right upper quadrant pain (patient no. 13). The study demonstrated barium in a right-sided stomach, which on the initial ultrasound examination was mistaken for a right upper quadrant mass. In addition, one can see an azygos vein (AZ, asterisks) that enters the superior vena cava and crosses in the abdomen to the left side. In addition, there is a left-sided aorta (AO, arrowheads) that descends to the left of the spine. The bronchial anatomy is not well seen, because a chest radiograph was not available. *B*, Left isomerism (polysplenia syndrome) in patient no. 13, a 26-year-old woman with right upper quadrant pain. The CT scan with oral contrast material showed a right-sided stomach (S) with three structures thought to represent multiple splenules (Sp, arrow) in the right upper quadrant. The liver is predominantly in the left upper quadrant. The aorta (A) is on the left, but there is no inferior vena cava in the usual position adjacent to the caudate lobe of the liver and anterior to the crus of the diaphragm. Instead, there is the retrocrural left-sided vessel (asterisk); also, the left kidney (K) is visualized. *C*, An additional CT slice of the same patient shows an additional and separate splenule (arrow, Sp) with no change in the vascular anatomy (A, asterisk). *D*, A higher CT slice again shows the aorta (A) and retrocrural azygos vein (asterisk) with the right-sided liver (L). *E*, A comparable transverse ultrasound examination demonstrates the vascular anatomy. The aorta (A, arrowhead) and hemiazygos veins (asterisk, arrow) are demonstrated to the left of the spine with the liver (L). *F*, A higher CT slice within the abdomen shows the course of the hemiazygos vein (asterisk) as it crosses behind the aorta (A) from left to right (arrow) to form the azygos vein, which ascends to enter the right superior vena cava. *G*, A higher CT slice at the dome of the diaphragm shows the now right-sided course of the hemiazygos vein (asterisk) as it ascends to enter the superior vena cava. The aorta (A) is unchanged in its course. (*B*, *E*, and *F* reproduced with permission from Tonkin IL, Tonkin AK: Visceroatrial situs abnormalities: Sonographic and computed tomographic appearance. AJR, *138*:509, 1982. Copyright ©, 1982, The Williams and Wilkins Company.)

Illustration continues on opposite page.

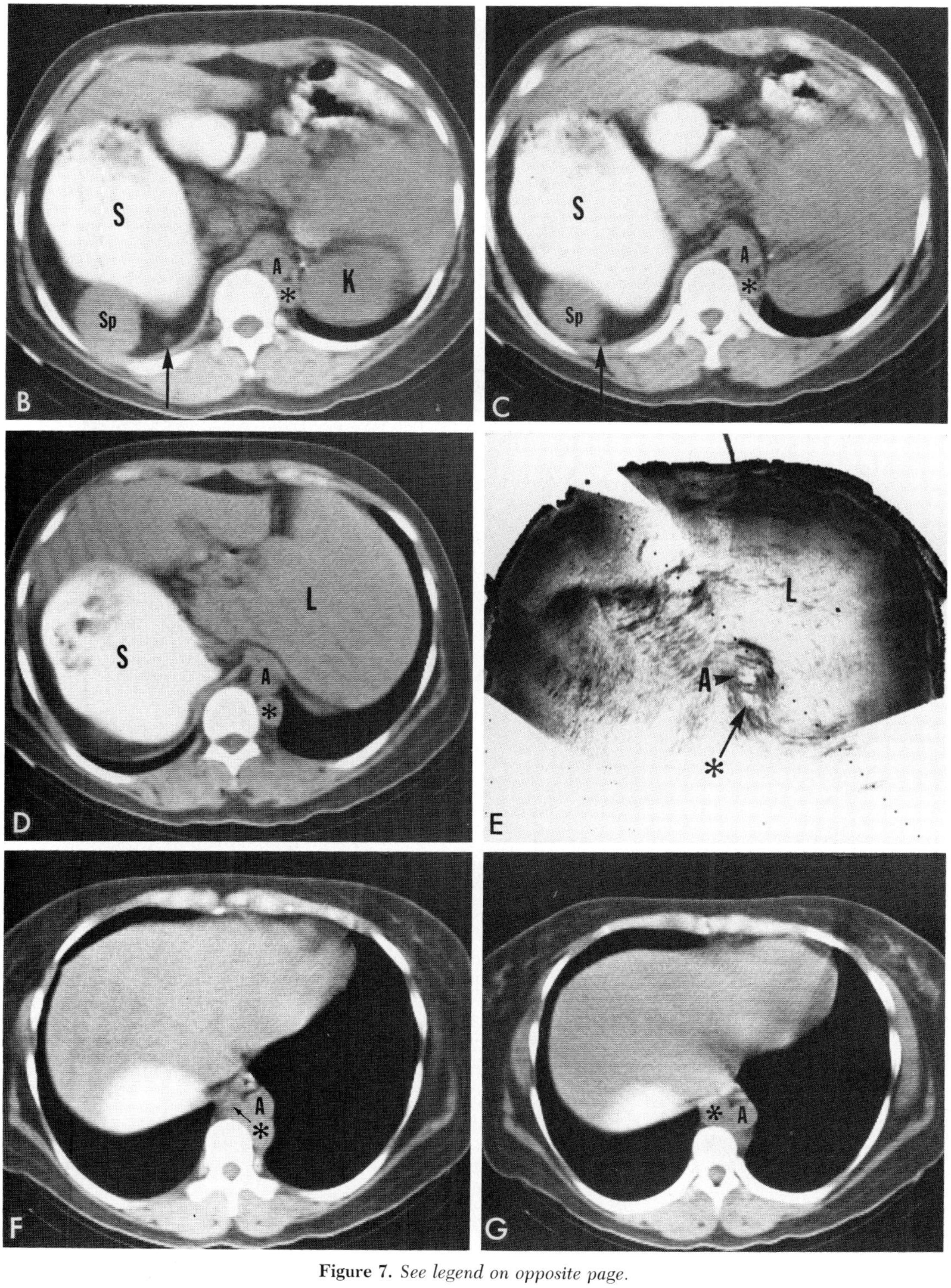

Figure 7. *See legend on opposite page.*

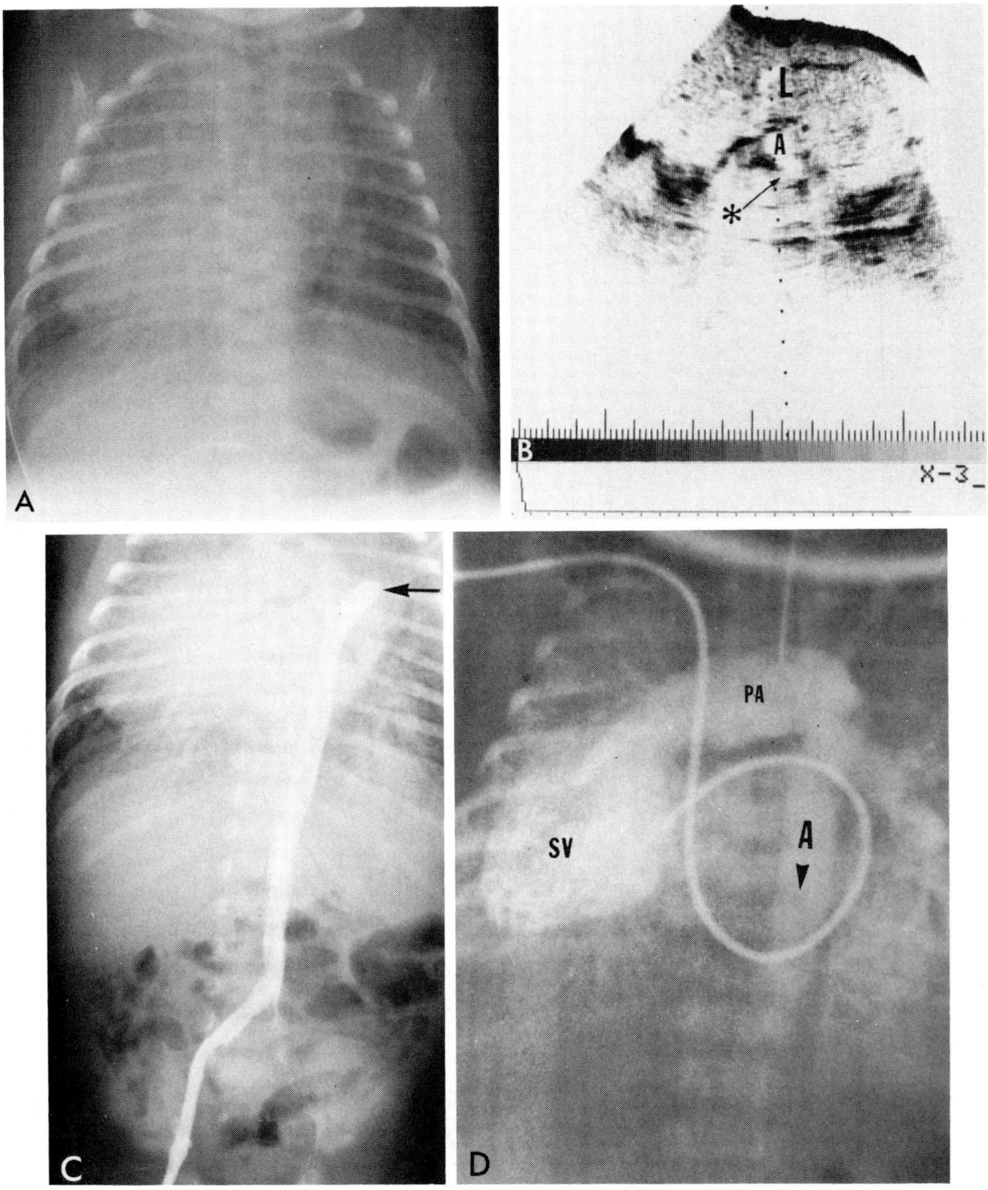

Figure 8. *A*, The PA chest radiograph of this one-week-old boy, patient no. 11, shows situs ambiguus with probable bilateral hyparterial bronchi, dextrocardia, and a right-sided stomach. An ultrasound examination was performed to determine if there was access to the heart from the femoral vein or if a venous cut-down in the arm would be necessary because of azygos continuation of the inferior vena cava in this infant at the time of catheterization. *B*, Left isomerism (polysplenia syndrome), patient no. 11. This one-week-old boy with congestive heart failure and situs ambiguus had a transverse ultrasonogram performed before cardiac catheterization. There was a large transverse liver (L). The aorta (A) is to the left of a venous structure (asterisk, arrow), presumed to be the left-sided inferior vena cava or hemiazygos vein to the left below the aorta. A normal inferior vena cava was not visualized entering the atrium. *C*, A foot vein injection was performed before cardiac catherization, because this was early in the evaluation of the abdominal visceroatrial situs. The study confirmed the ultrasonographic findings with a left-sided inferior vena cava and hemiazygos continuation to the left superior vena cava (arrow). Polysplenia syndrome with hemiazygos continuation of the inferior vena cava was diagnosed from the chest radiograph and abdominal ultrasonogram. *D*, At catheterization, a catheter was placed in the right basilic vein into the right-sided superior vena cava into an atrial structure and into the single ventricle (SV), where an injection was made in the straight PA projection. This study demonstrated a single ventricle or univentricular heart with a common AV valve and interruption of the aortic arch, type B. One can see the pulmonary artery filled (PA) with opacification of the descending aorta (A, arrowhead), which descends to the left of the spine.

(*B* and *C* reproduced with permission from Tonkin IL, Tonkin AK: Visceroatrial situs abnormalities: Sonographic and computed tomographic appearance. AJR, *138*:509, 1982. Copyright ©, 1982, The Williams and Wilkins Company.)

suspected on plain chest film, it is important to confirm the absence or presence of inferior vena cava–atrial communication with ultrasonography (or CT) of the abdomen before cardiac catheterization. Abdominal ultrasonography will show the exact location of the abdominal aorta as well as the absence of the inferior vena cava at the level of the liver with independent drainage of the confluence of hepatic veins into the right atrium.[12, 31] With real-time imaging capabilities, this anomaly can be demonstrated even in very small infants (Figs. 8 and 9).

One patient in this series posed a diagnostic dilemma (Fig. 10*A*) (Case 16). In this 7-day-old female, the AP supine chest radiograph showed cardiac enlargement and some decrease in pulmonary vascularity; the AP and lateral chest radiographs showed probable normal situs (Fig. 10*A* and *B*). The transverse ultrasonographic examination at one week of age showed an inferior vena cava to the right of the spine traveling its usual course and the abdominal aorta slightly to the left of the spine, indicating probable situs solitus (Fig. 10*C*). The longitudinal abdominal ultrasonogram also showed evidence of inferior vena cava–right atrial communication (Fig. 10*D*). At catheterization this patient was thought to have situs solitus with complex congenital heart disease consisting of some form of double outlet right ventricle with a common AV valve and pulmonic valvar stenosis. However, this patient died at seven days of age with multiple congenital anomalies, including duodenal stenosis, which was not recognized owing to placement of a nasogastric tube with suction, and necrotizing enterocolitis. At postmortem examination, the patient was also found to have severe complex congenital heart disease with a common atrioventricular canal, a double outlet right ventricle, and a hypoplastic left ventricle or outlet chamber. In addition, there was severe pulmonic stenosis, a small patent ductus arteriosus, and a persistent left superior vena cava. The right lung, consisting of three lobes, had an incomplete fissure between the upper and middle lobes. The left lung was unremarkable. There was malrotation of the intestines and an annular pancreas. The inferior vena cava and abdominal aorta were normal, as demonstrated on ultrasonographic examination. However, this patient was found to have 14 splenules at postmortem examination: 1 large, 1 medium-sized, and 12 small ones. This patient may be categorized as having the form of polysplenia syndrome entitled F-anisosplenia of Landing.[16] However, this patient may also represent some form of mixed situs syndrome (Fig. 10*A–E*).

In many cases, since patients with polysplenia syndrome frequently have abdominal heterotaxia, both ultrasonography and CT are useful in the diagnosis of visceral heterotaxia (Fig. 11*A–C*). In all patients who underwent cardiac catheterization, there was excellent catheter position and angiographic correlation (Fig. 11*D*). By definition, the person with polysplenia syndrome has two or more spleens.[22, 33, 34, 35] CT examination of the abdomen will demonstrate azygos or hemiazygos continuation of the inferior vena cava, with the vein localized behind the crus of the diaphragm, as well as show multiple splenules that are usually located along the greater curvature of the stomach[5, 13, 24, 38] (Figs. 6*D*, 7*B* and *C* and 9*G* and *H*). Partial or complete failure of rotation of the intestinal tract is common, and the mesentery may be located in the midline. The liver and an occasional midline gallbladder can be visualized[33] (Fig. 6*C* and *D* and Table 2).

Further help in establishing atrial situs may be obtained by noting the pattern of air bronchogram, particularly in films taken with high kilovoltage or tomography.[16, 18, 19, 27, 32, 33] (Fig. 12*C*). If the air bronchograms suggest bilaterally symmetric bronchi of the eparterial type (the normal right bronchus is an eparterial bronchus passing over the pulmonary artery; both bronchi are relatively short, approximately 1 cm, when measured from the carina; this is highly indicative of right isomerism, or asplenia syndrome, and hence of situs ambiguus. If the air bronchogram has a pattern resembling bilateral left-sided bronchi (hyparterial) (with the pulmonary artery crossing over the bronchus, which has a longer segment, measuring 1.7 to 2 cm from the carina), this is suggestive of left isomerism or polysplenia syndrome (Fig. 12*A–C*). The CT scout view of the chest can also easily demonstrate the bronchial anatomy. The ultrasonographic examination will confirm the CT diagnosis of the hyparterial bronchus by demonstrating azygos continuation of the inferior vena cava (Fig. 12*D*).

From the electrocardiogram (ECG) it is possible to deduce the atrial location by noting the abnormal P-wave sector.[23] This method is noninvasive and indirect. However, more precise location can be made by establishing that the inferior vena cava returns to the right atrium.[2, 17, 23]

It has been noted that complete atrial ventricular block can occur in patients with polysplenia syndrome, and a pacemaker may be required.[11]

The occurrence of Kartagener's syndrome (chronic sinusitis, bronchiectasis, and situs in-

Text continued on page 175

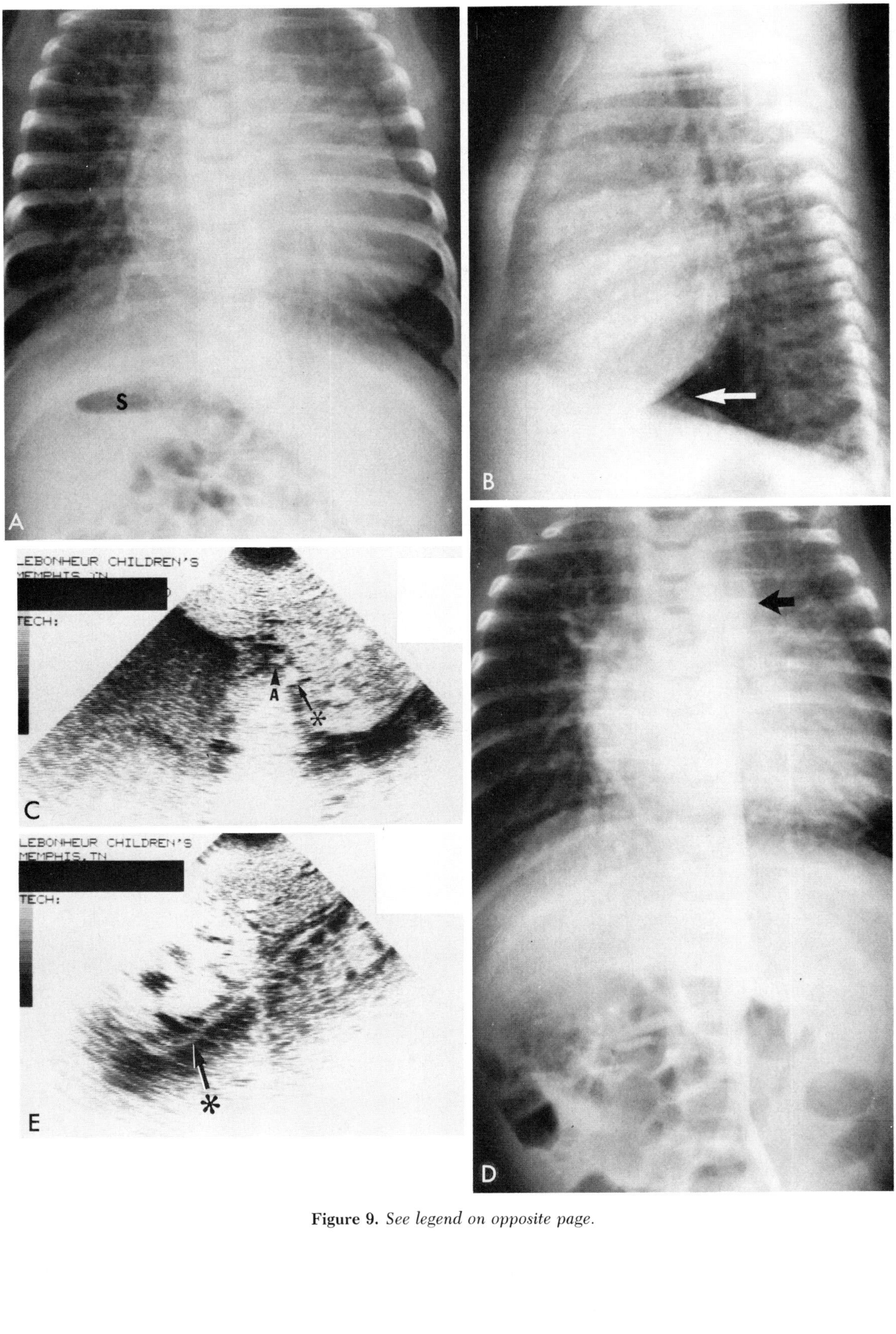

Figure 9. *See legend on opposite page.*

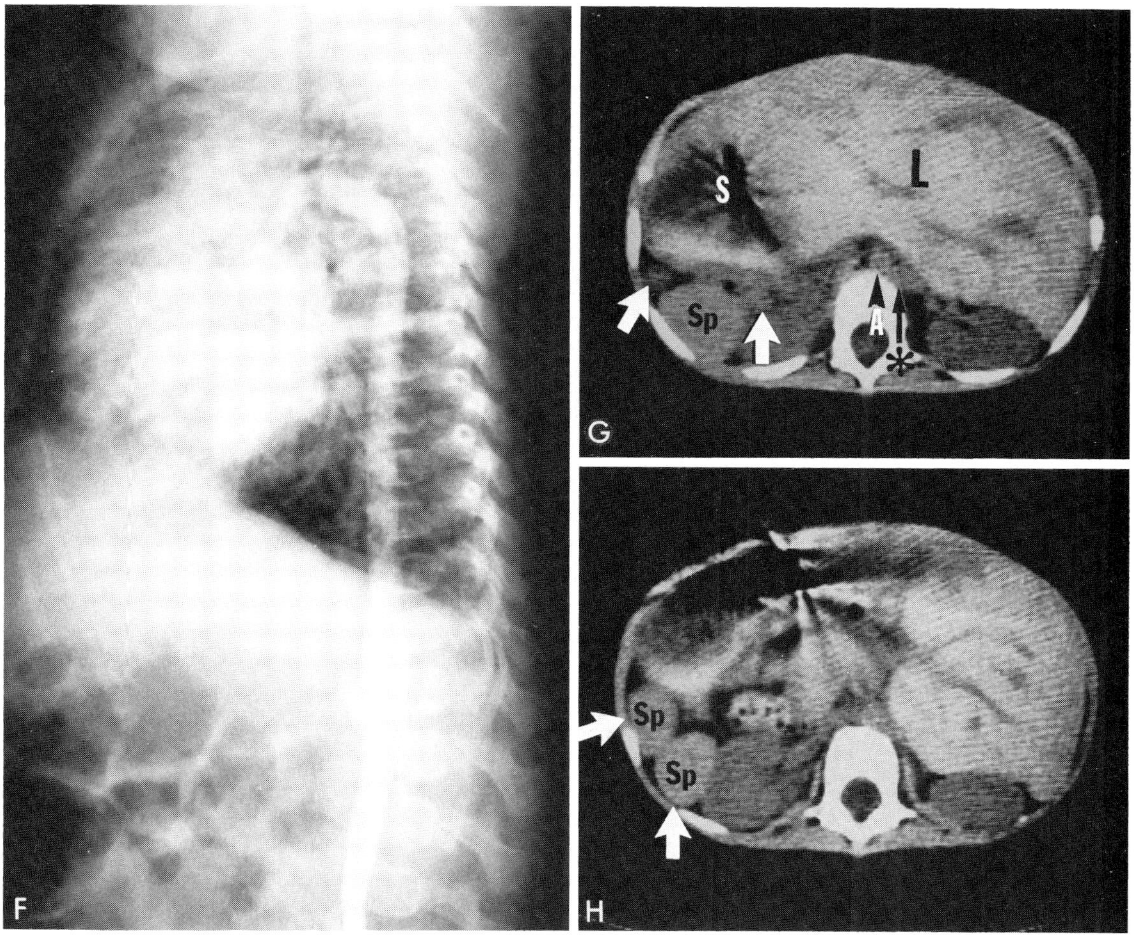

Figure 9. *A*, The PA chest radiograph of this six-week-old boy, patient no. 10, shows probable situs ambiguus with levocardia, left-sided aortic arch, a right-sided stomach (S), and the bulk of the liver to the patient's left side. The pulmonary vascularity is increased with cardiac enlargement and congestive heart failure. *B*, The lateral projection shows no evidence of an inferior vena cava shadow (arrow). *C*, A real-time, two-dimensional sector scan of the abdomen demonstrated two vascular structures to the left of the spine. The pulsating aorta (A, arrowhead) is visualized to the left of the spine, as is a retrocrural vascular structure with less pulsation, which probably represented a left-sided inferior vena cava with azygos continuation (arrow, asterisk). Polysplenia syndrome with interruption of the inferior vena cava was diagnosed from the chest radiographs and real-time ultrasonography. *D*, Injection into a vein of the foot was performed before cardiac catheterization to confirm the ultrasonographic findings. The study demonstrated a left-sided inferior vena cava with hemiazygos continuation to the left superior vena cava (arrow). *E*, The longitudinal sector scan nicely demonstrates the venous anatomy, showing the hemiazygos vein to the left of the spine as it enters the left-sided superior vena cava (arrow, asterisk). This patient has a complete AV canal defect. *F*, The lateral projection of the foot vein injection demonstrates the classic "candy cane" appearance of the left-sided hemiazygos vein as it enters the left superior vena cava. *G*, Transverse computed tomography without contrast material was performed for confirmation of the polysplenia syndrome. The study demonstrated multiple structures thought to represent splenules (Sp, arrows). In addition, one can see the right-sided stomach (S) with a large congested liver (L) to the left. One can also see the comparable vascular structures with the aorta (A, arrowhead) to the left of the spine and a hemiazygos vein (arrow, asterisk). *H*, A lower CT slice of the abdomen of the same patient again demonstrates multiple splenules (Sp, arrows).

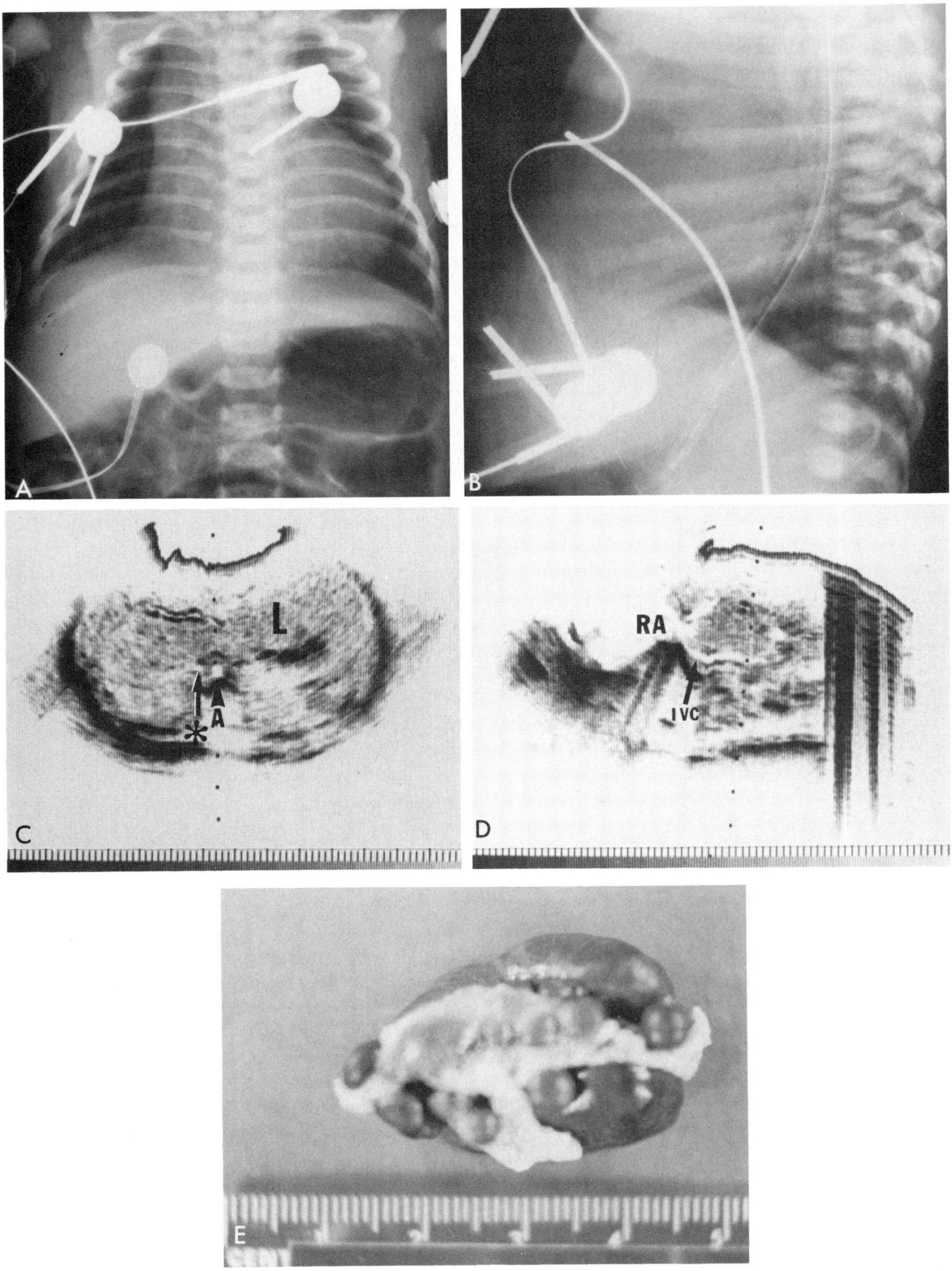

Figure 10. *A*, The AP chest radiograph of a three-day-old girl, patient no. 16, shows cardiac enlargement with levocardia and congestive heart failure. *B*, On the lateral projection, the inferior vena cava shadow is not seen. *C*, The transverse ultrasound examination shows evidence of possible situs solitus with the inferior vena cava (arrow, asterisk) and liver (L) to the right and the aorta (A, arrowhead) to the patient's left. *D*, The longitudinal ultrasound examination showed evidence of the inferior vena cava (IVC, arrow) entering into an atrial structure (RA). Therefore, cardiac catheterization could be performed from below. The plain film and ultrasound examination presented a confusing picture, but situs solitus of the atria and viscera with complex congenital heart disease was probable. *E*, However, at postmortem examination, the patient was found to have a questionable form of polysplenia syndrome or F-anisoplenia of Landing[16] with 14 splenules demonstrated. At postmortem examination, this patient was found to exemplify a variation of a typical polysplenia syndrome.

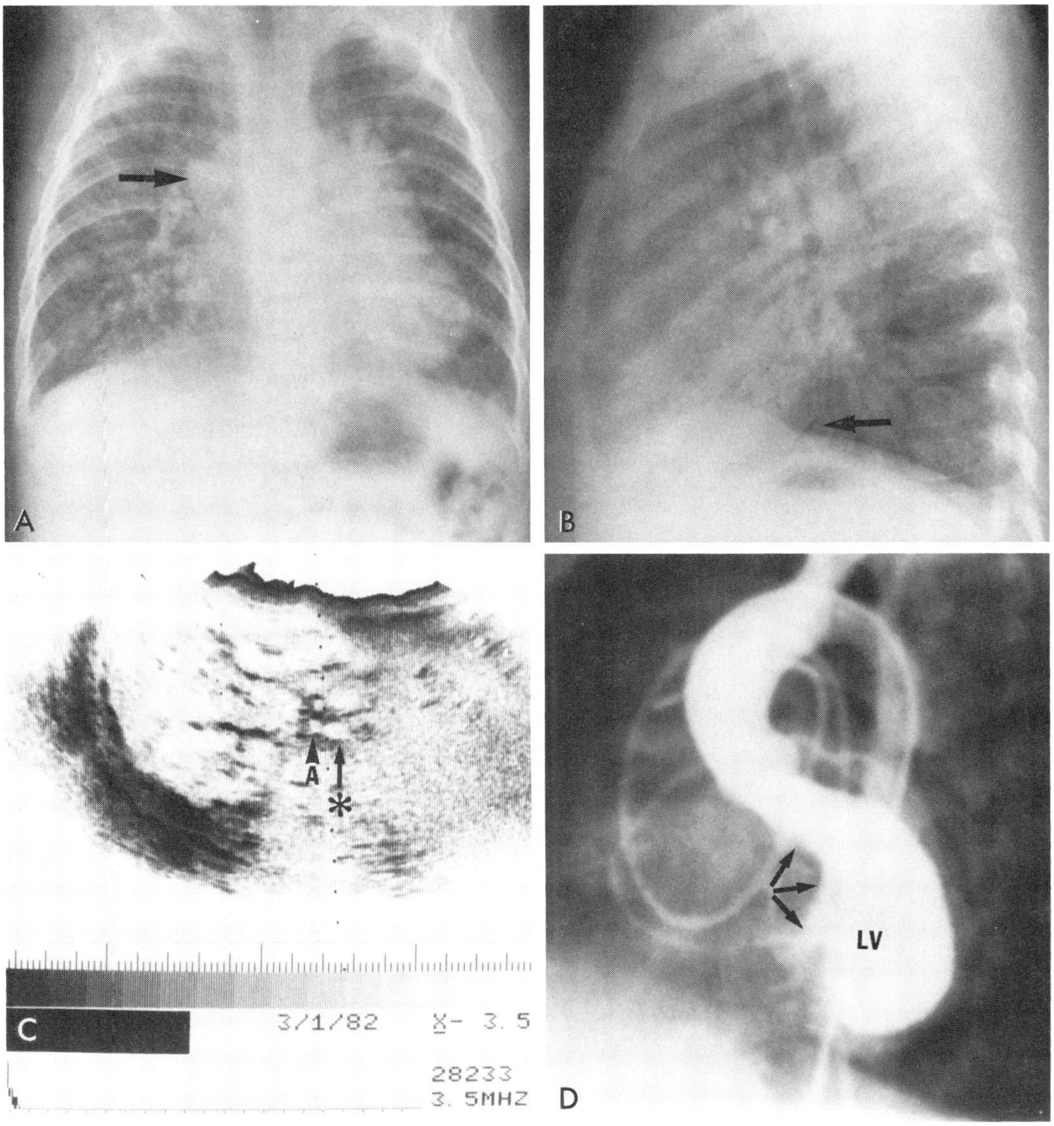

Figure 11. *A*, The PA chest radiograph of an 11-month-old girl, patient no. 17, showed evidence of increased vascularity with congestive heart failure. There is levocardia with a left-sided aortic arch and a left-sided stomach. However, the bronchial anatomy indicates probable hyparterial bronchi, and there is a right paratracheal density (arrow) that may represent an azygos vein. *B*, The chest radiograph shows no evidence of an inferior vena cava shadow (arrow). *C*, A transverse abdominal ultrasonogram at 13.5 cm below the xiphoid process demonstrates the aorta with the superior mesenteric artery (A, arrowhead) and the vascular structure now to the left of the aorta, which represents the azygos vein (asterisk, arrow). There was no inferior vena cava–right atrial continuity on the longitudinal ultrasonogram. *D*, At cardiac catheterization, a left ventriculogram (LV) was performed in the long axial oblique projection; it shows evidence of a partial endocardial cushion defect with an abnormal mitral valve (arrows) and opacification of the aorta, which is a left-sided structure. The venous catheter is looped into the azygos vein, superior vena cava, right atrium, and right ventricle. The catheter's tip in the right pulmonary artery again confirms the ultrasonographic findings of interruption of the inferior vena cava with azygos continuation. This patient has had successful total cardiac correction.

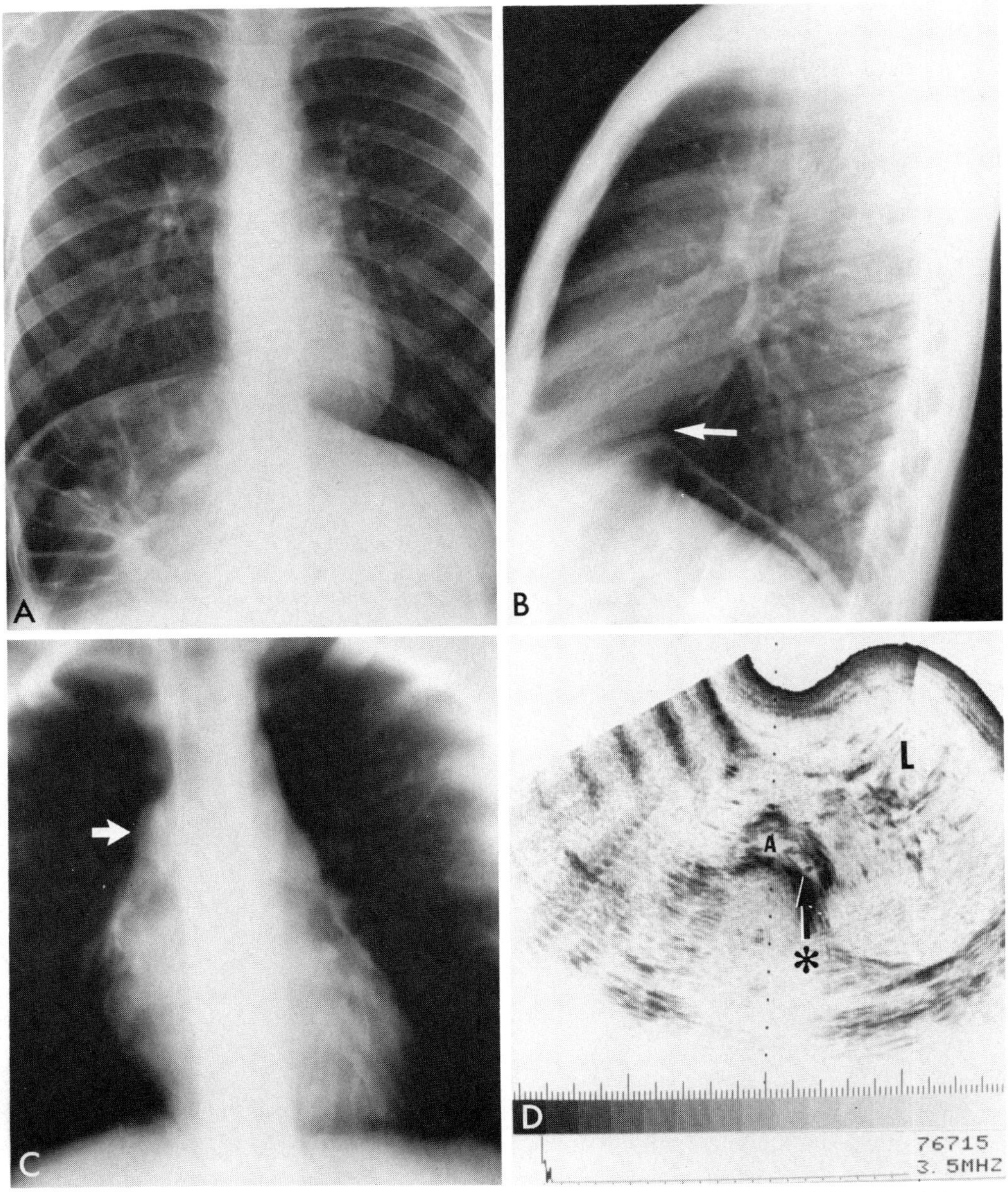

Figure 12. *A*, The PA chest radiograph of a 10-year-old girl, patient no. 19, showed probable hyparterial bronchi with a left aortic arch and levocardia. The stomach is not well demonstrated, but it is probably on the right. The pulmonary vascular anatomy is now normal, and this patient may have azygos continuation, but the diagnosis is not certain from the PA chest radiograph. *B*, The lateral chest radiograph shows absence of the inferior vena cava shadow (arrow). *C*, A single midline tomographic cut of an additional patient (no. 20) showed bilateral, long, symmetric hyparterial bronchi and an azygos vein (arrow) diagnostic of polysplenia syndrome. This result can also be obtained with the CT scout view of the chest. *D*, The transverse B-mode ultrasonogram of the abdomen demonstrates a left-sided liver (L) with the aorta (A) to the left of the spine and a vascular structure that is retrocrural and to the left of the aorta, representing a hemiazygos vein (asterisk, arrow). The transverse ultrasonogram demonstrated no evidence of a normal inferior vena cava entering an atrial structure. As determined from the chest radiograph and ultrasonogram, this patient has polysplenia syndrome, or left isomerism, with interruption of the inferior vena cava and azygos continuation.

versus) with polysplenia syndrome in a family has been reported. It has been noted recently in the literature that abnormal respiratory cilia may occur with polysplenia syndrome in these patients. There may be a link between abnormal respiratory cilia, polysplenia, and Kartagener's syndrome.[25]

The splenic abnormalities are most easily visualized with CT examination; however, radionuclide venography associated with liver-spleen scanning has been useful in diagnosing the heterotaxic syndromes.[7, 9] In the author's experience, as well as in that of others, however, there have been several false-negative results in using these methods to diagnose the polysplenia syndrome.[8, 21, 30] The polysplenia syndrome can be diagnosed by angiography, which will demonstrate multiple splenules and a common celiacomesenteric artery,[36] which can be detected by abdominal ultrasonography in some patients.

Patients with left isomerism (polysplenia syndrome) have a 5 to 10 per cent incidence of no congenital heart disease (Cases 13 and 20) and have the milder cardiac defects, i.e., ventricular septal defect, double outlet right ventricle, and partial anomalies of the systemic veins and pulmonary veins (Tables 1, 2, and 3).

RIGHT ISOMERISM (ASPLENIA SYNDROME)

Ten patients with right isomerism, or asplenia syndrome, were evaluated during this three-year period. All patients initially presented in the newborn period with cyanosis. Several patients were studied at the time of their second cardiac catheterization after palliation (Table 2). Owing to the occurrence of more severe cardiac anomalies, there is a higher mortality rate with asplenia syndrome than with polysplenia syndrome. Six of the ten patients died; postmortem examination was performed in three of the six patients.

In all cases of asplenia syndrome, the aorta and inferior vena cava were in juxtaposition on the same side of the spine[6, 21, 30, 33] (Fig. 13A–C

Table 3. *Situs Ambiguus*

RIGHT ISOMERISM ASPLENIA SYNDROME	LEFT ISOMERISM POLYSPLENIA SYNDROME
Diagnostic Signs	
Aorta and IVC course on the same side of spine "kissing" or "piggyback" IVC–aorta	Interruption of IVC with azygos or hemiazygos continuation (a large azygos vein may appear as a mediastinal mass)
Normal IVC–atrial communication	Absence of IVC at level of liver with independent drainage of hepatic veins into right atrium
Bilateral eparterial bronchi with pulmonary arteries below bronchi on anterior view and projecting anterior to trachea on lateral view	Bilateral hyparterial bronchi with arteries projecting over bronchi on anterior view and posterior to tracheobronchial tree on lateral view
Bilateral, broad-based right atrial appendages	Bilateral, narrow-based, pointed left atrial appendages
Bilateral minor fissures (bilateral, trilobed lungs)	No minor fissures (bilateral, bilobed lungs)
No spleen (CT scan or radionuclide scan)	Multiple spleens (two or more) (CT scan) almost always along greater curvature of stomach with a common celiacomesenteric artery (real-time ultrasound or angiography)
Commonly have cardiac malformations (more serious), i.e., AV canal, single ventricle, pulmonary stenosis or atresia, TGA, anomalous pulmonary venous connections (higher mortality)	Five to 10 per cent have *no* CHD; often see VSD, double outlet right ventricle, or systemic venous anomalies rather than pulmonary venous anomalies
Clinical-Laboratory Findings	
Slight predominance among males	Marked predominance among females
Presents with cyanosis in newborn	Often seen into adulthood
Howell-Jolly and Heinz bodies on blood smear	None
Malrotation of gut, microgastria	Partial or complete rotation of gut common
No characteristic ECG abnormality	Abnormal P-wave vector and complete AV block
Predisposition to sepsis	Abnormal cilia

Note: IVC: inferior vena cava; CT: computed tomography; TGA: transposition of the great arteries; AV: atrioventricular; CHD: congenital heart disease; ECG: electrocardiogram; VSD: ventricular septal defect.

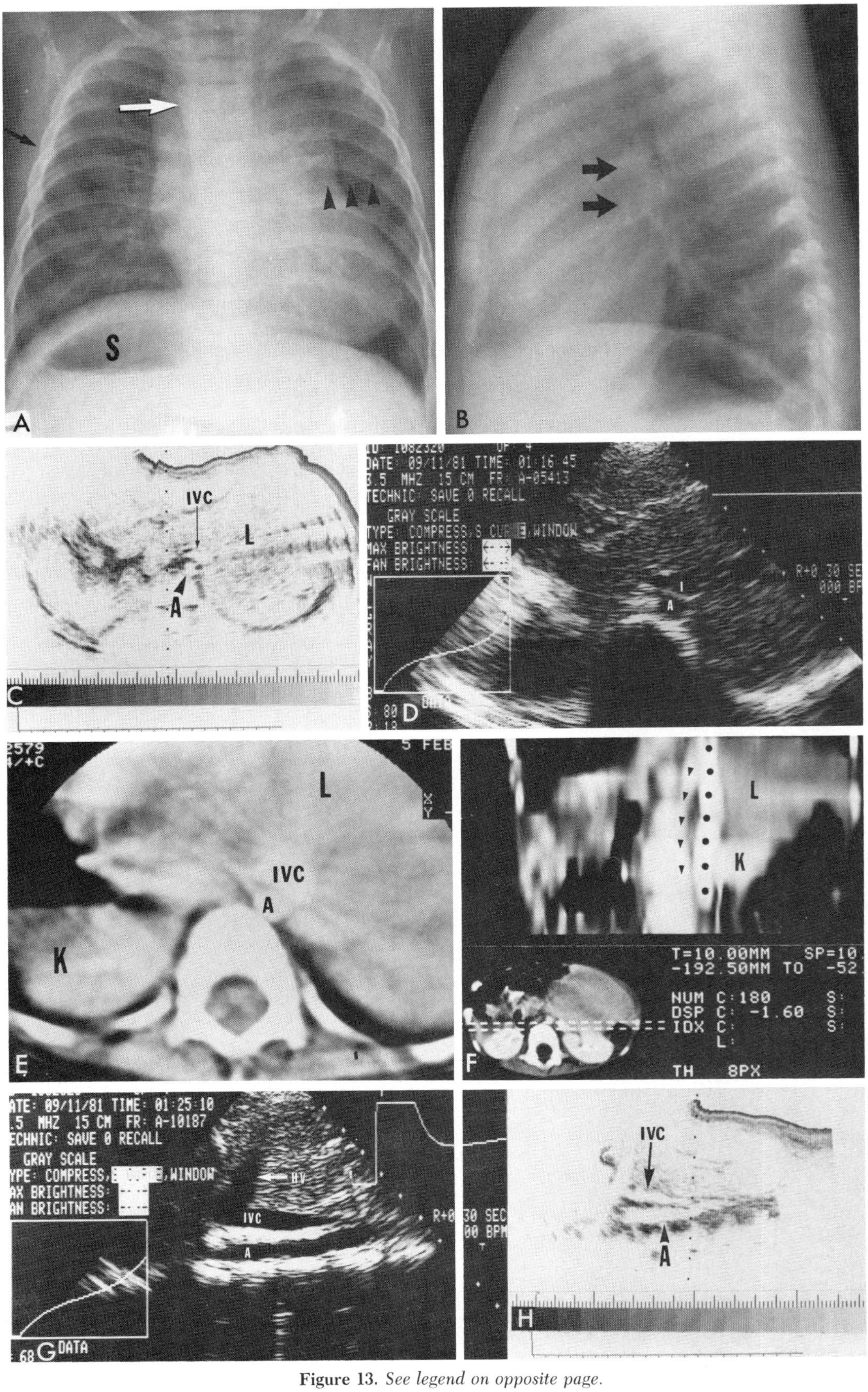

Figure 13. *See legend on opposite page.*

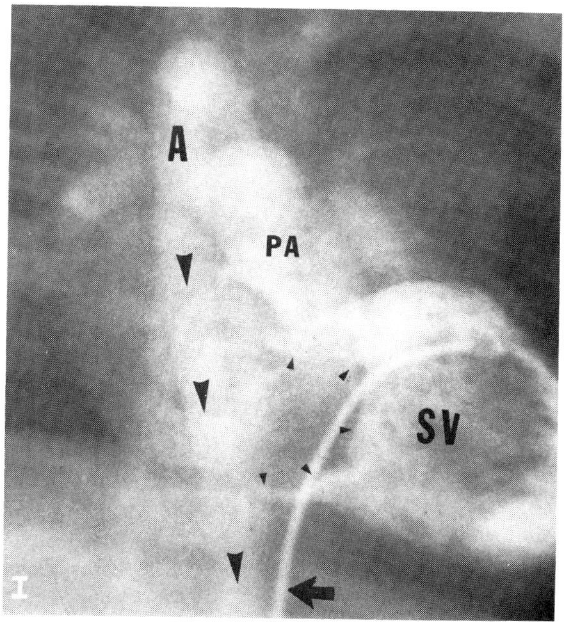

Figure 13. *A*, The PA chest radiograph of a four-year-old girl, patient no. 21, with situs ambiguus with a right-sided aortic arch (white arrow), a right-sided stomach (S), and levocardia. At birth, the vascularity was decreased, indicating obstruction to pulmonary flow; however, now vascularity on the right is slightly increased compared with that of the left secondary to a right Waterston anastomosis (small arrow). There is faint visualization of a minor fissure on the left (arrowheads), indicating probable right isomerism, or asplenia syndrome. The patient subsequently underwent a left Blalock-Taussig anastomosis. *B*, The lateral projection of the same patient does not show evidence of the inferior vena cava entering the right atrium, owing to the degree of inspiration. However, both pulmonary arteries (arrows) appear anterior to the trachea on the lateral projection, indicating probable bilateral right pulmonary arteries with asplenia syndrome. *C*, Right isomerism (asplenia syndrome) in a four-year-old girl (patient no. 21). The transverse ultrasonogram at 0.5 cm below the xiphoid process shows crossing of the inferior vena cava (IVC, arrow) and aorta (A, arrowhead) to the left of the spine. In all cases of asplenia syndrome, the aorta and inferior vena cava cross midline or are located on the same side of the spine. The vascular anatomy can be easily identified with B-mode ultrasonography. The liver (L) is on the left. *D*, The transverse two-dimensional sector scan image of this same patient demonstrates even better the vascular anatomy with the aorta (A) and inferior vena cava (I) located to the left of the spine. With real-time dynamic scanning, the vascular pulsations can be easily identified in the evaluation of the visceroatrial situs. *E*, A CT scan at a comparable level shows the inferior vena cava (IVC) and aorta (A) with contrast enhancement. The kidney (K) on the right is visualized with a left-sided liver (L). No splenic tissue was seen. *F*, Coronal reconstruction in a plane through the inferior vena cava and aorta shows the actual course of the inferior vena cava (dots) and aorta (arrowheads). The aorta and inferior vena cava, contrary to the normal relationship, are on the same side of the upper abdomen and often superimpose or cross in the frontal projection. The liver (L) and left kidney (K) are visualized. *G*, The longitudinal two-dimensional sector scan at 1 cm to the left of the midline shows a large hepatic vein (arrow, HV) and inferior vena cava (IVC) entering an atrial structure with the aorta (A) directly below the caval segment on the same side of the spine. Real-time imaging easily shows the "piggyback" vascular pulsation. *H*, However, the vascular anatomy in this case could also easily be demonstrated with a longitudinal B-mode ultrasonogram at 1 cm to the left of the midline showing the inferior vena cava (arrow, IVC) and aorta (arrowhead, A) overlapping on the same side of the spine. *I*, The initial, AP cineangiocardiogram is illustrated to show the course of the inferior vena cava outlined by the catheter (arrow) as the inferior vena cava courses to the left of the spine, enters an atrial structure, and enters the large single ventricle (SV). An injection is made in this location, and the large common AV valve (small arrowheads) is shown. There is immediate opacification of the pulmonary arteries (PA) and aorta (A), showing a right-sided aortic arch. Note the course of the right-sided, type I right aortic arch in the abdomen as it courses to the right side of the trachea in the chest and to the left of the spine within the abdomen (A, arrowheads). Thus, the diagnosis of right isomerism is confirmed, as identified by the plain chest radiograph, ultrasonography, and CT in this patient.

(*C*, *E*, *F*, and *G* reprinted with permission from Tonkin IL, Tonkin AK: Visceroatrial situs abnormalities: Sonographic and computed tomographic appearance. AJR, *138*:509, 1982. Copyright ©, 1982, The Williams and Wilkins Company.)

and Tables 2 and 3). This juxtaposition can be seen with ultrasonography, two-dimensional echocardiography, or CT of the chest and abdomen (Fig. 13*C–H*). With CT, the scout view of the thorax will excellently demonstrate bronchial anatomy when there are bilateral eparterial bronchi. In addition, with CT, the presence or absence of splenic tissue can be determined (Fig. 13*E* and *F*). Coronal reconstruction of CT images at the level of the major abdominal vessels will depict their course in the abdomen (Fig. 13*F*). These findings can be correlated with the longitudinal or sagittal ultrasonographic examination, which will show the inferior vena cava and aorta on the same side of the spine situated in a "piggyback" fashion, with the inferior vena cava entering the right atrium (Fig. 13*G* and *H*). This inferior vena cava–right atrial communication indicates the location of "right-sided atrium" in patients with right isomerism or asplenia syndrome. The correlative anatomy was demonstrated at catheterization, with the venous catheter in the inferior vena cava to the left of the spine and the right-sided aortic arch crossing to the left of the spine in the abdomen (Fig. 13*I*).

Ultrasonography or echocardiography was performed in all patients, and even in infancy, the position of the aorta and inferior vena cava could be detected on the same side of the spine (Fig. 14). In addition, inferior vena cava–right atrial communication could be identified on the longitudinal ultrasonogram or the two-dimensional echocardiogram (Fig. 14*D*). Abdominal ultrasonographic findings correlated well with the angiographic findings in all cases (Figs. 14*C*,*D–I*, 15, and 16).

Patients with right isomerism frequently have severe congenital heart lesions (Tables 1, 2, and 3). The plain chest radiograph of the very sick and cyanotic newborn is frequently difficult to evaluate. (Figs. 14*A* and *B*, 17, 18, and 19). Occasionally, one may see bilateral minor fissures, indicative of right isomerism (Fig. 18*A* and *B*). Sometimes a newborn may present with a left-sided azygos lobe, which is suggestive of bilateral right isomerism (Fig. 19*A*). One may also be able to demonstrate that both pulmonary arteries are anterior to the tracheobronchial tree, as one would expect with asplenia syndrome[27] (Fig. 19*E* and *F*). In addition, there are various cardiac malpositions usually occur-

Text continued on page 185

Figure 14. *A*, The AP supine chest and abdominal radiograph of a three-day-old boy with cyanosis (patient no. 22). There are no osseous abnormalities with dextrocardia and a right-sided aortic arch, as visualized by the course of the umbilical artery catheter (arrows). The pulmonary vascularity appears decreased, indicating obstruction to pulmonary flow. The stomach is not well visualized but may be located in the midline (arrowheads) with a horizontal upper abdominal configuration to the liver, indicating hepatic symmetry. In addition, there is a density to the left of the spine that may indicate a paraspinal mass or abnormal stomach. *B*, The lateral projection of this same patient shows a radiolucent retrocardiac structure (arrowheads), which most likely represents a midline stomach or some form of hiatal hernia. However, because of this midline abdominal structure, the inferior vena cava cannot be seen entering an atrial structure, which is often the case in sick, newborn infants. *C*, Situs ambiguus, right isomerism (asplenia syndrome) in patient no. 22. The transverse ultrasonogram shows evidence of a midabdominal liver (L). The dense echo complex in the midline represents the stomach. The vascular anatomy in the newborn can be difficult to resolve with confidence, however. The aorta (A, arrowhead) and the inferior vena cava (IVC, arrow) appear to lie to the right of the spine, consistent with asplenia syndrome. *D*, The longitudinal scan, 1 cm to the right of midline, shows the inferior vena cava (IVC, arrow) entering an atrial structure (RA). This allowed the cardiologist to place the catheter from the femoral vein into the right atrium rather than considering a brachial vein approach. From ultrasonograms and radiographs, right isomerism was diagnosed before cardiac catheterization. *E*, At cardiac catheterization, the inferior vena cava was noted as coursing to the right of the spine and entering an atrial structure (white arrow). An injection was made in the straight PA projection, confirming the vascular anatomy and showing the large functional single ventricle in a patient with double outlet right ventricle, small outlet chamber, and a common AV valve (arrows). There is opacification of both the pulmonary arteries (PA) and the aorta (A) with evidence of pulmonic valve stenosis. The aorta (A) descends to the right of the spine, showing the course of the descending thoracic aorta, also to the right of the spine (A, arrows). *F*, The catheter from the femoral vein was then placed from the atrial structure into the ventricular structure and into the aorta, where an aortogram was performed. This procedure also demonstrated the vascular anatomy found in the abdomen with the inferior vena cava (white arrow) outlined by the catheter and descending aorta (A, arrows), both to the right of the spine. *G*, After cardiac catheterization, an upper GI study was performed; it confirmed our suspicions of a midline stomach or microgastria, which may occur with right isomerism, or asplenia syndrome. At least half of the stomach is within the thorax, extending through a diaphragmatic defect slightly to the left of midline. In addition, there is malrotation of the bowel. *H*, In this case, a radionuclide liver-spleen scan was performed; it showed evidence of hepatic symmetry with a large midline liver on the anterior view and no evidence of splenic tissue. The scan also confirmed the diagnosis of asplenia syndrome, or right isomerism. *I*, The postmortem examination of this patient, no. 22, at age nine months, demonstrated right isomerism (asplenia syndrome). There is evidence of situs ambiguus with dextrocardia, with a double outlet right ventricle, pulmonary atresia, and common AV valve (H). The hepatic symmetry, with a large midline liver (L) and gallbladder (g), is noted with absence of the splenic tissue. There is a midline, partially thoracic stomach (S) with bilateral trilobed lungs.

(*A*, *C*, and *D* reproduced with permission from Tonkin IL, Tonkin AK: Visceroatrial situs abnormalities: Sonographic and computed tomographic appearance. AJR, *138*:509, 1982. Copyright ©, 1982, The Williams and Wilkins Company.)

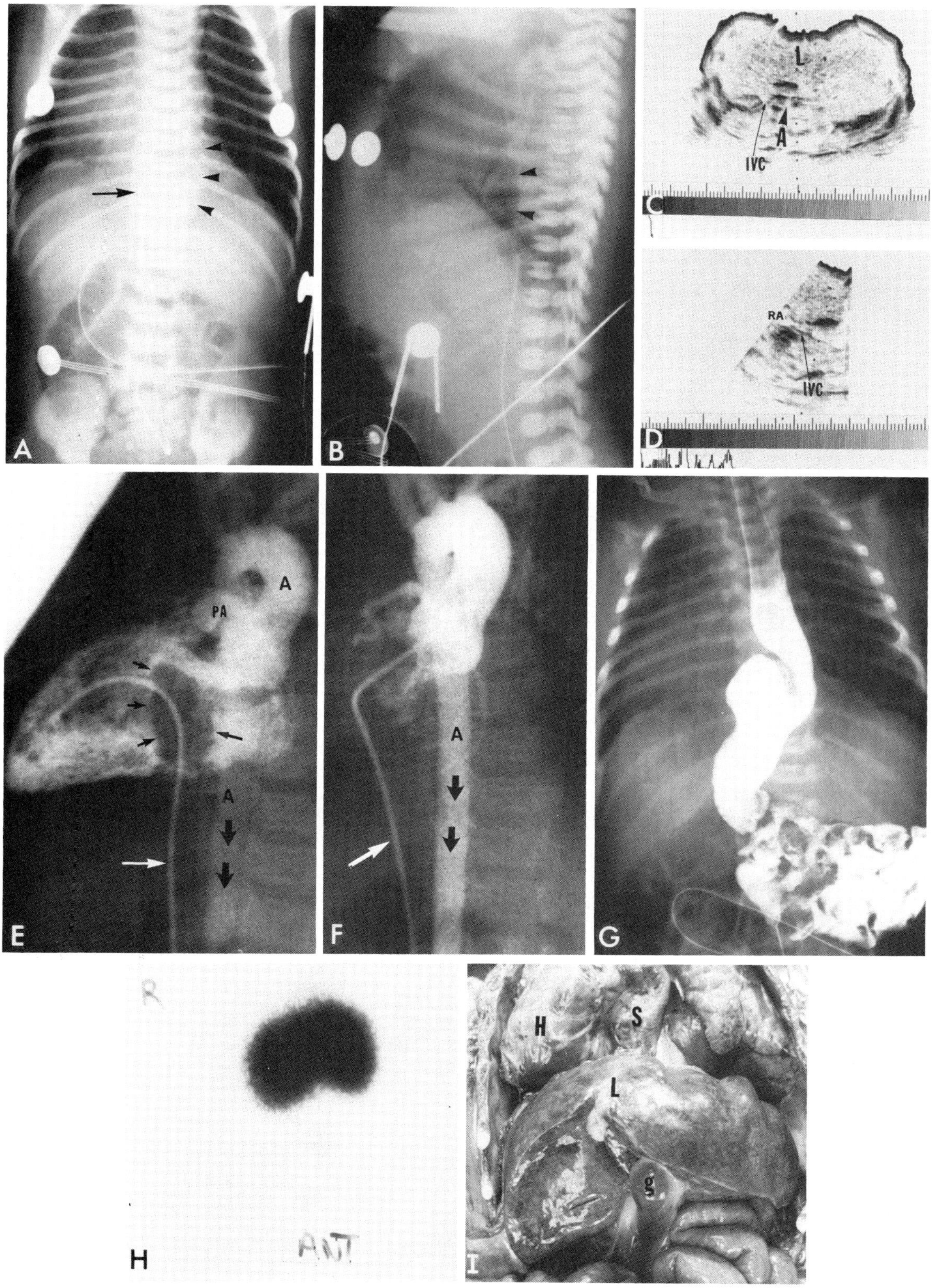

Figure 14. *See legend on opposite page.*

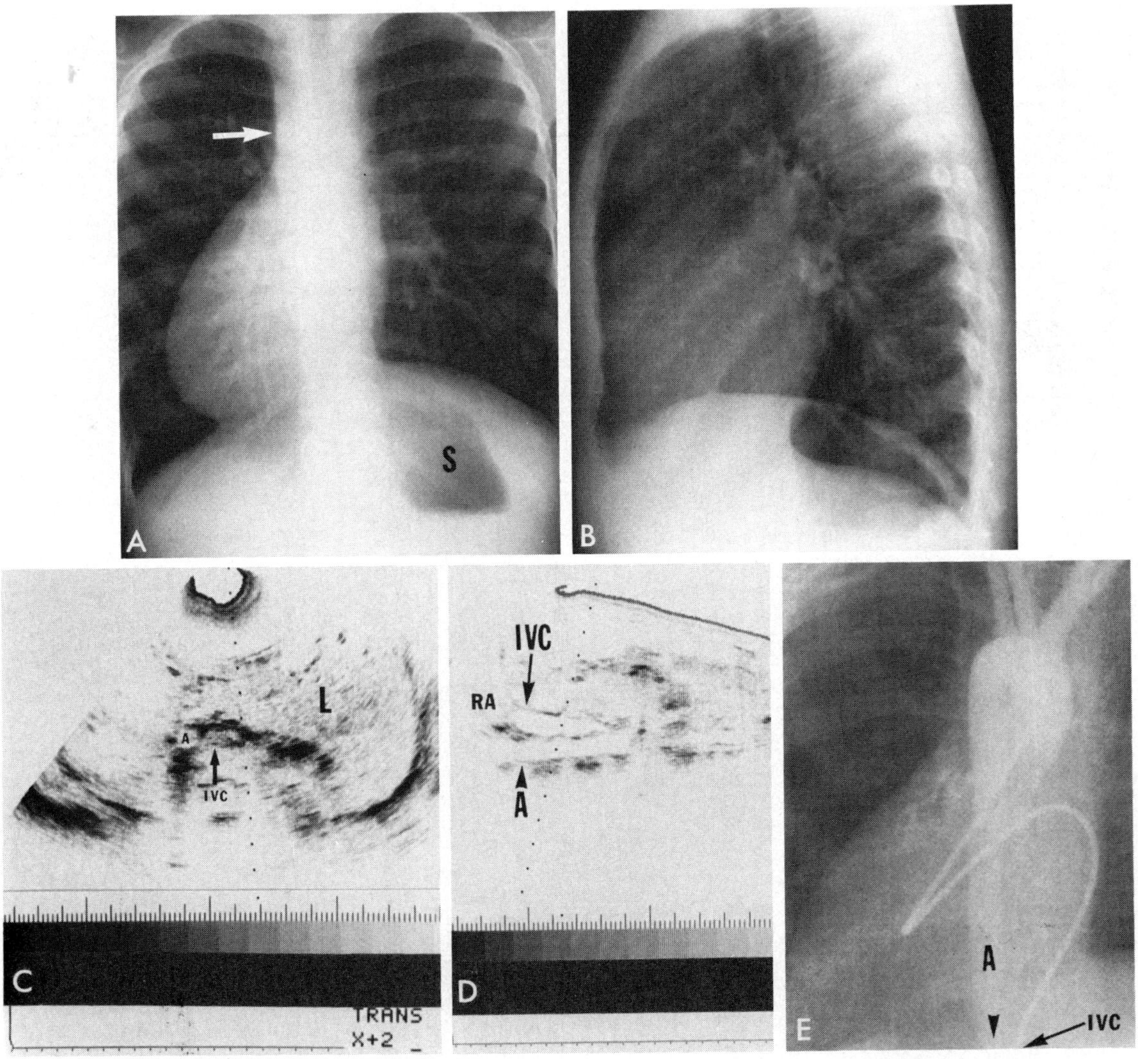

Figure 15. *A*, The PA chest radiograph of this four-year-old boy, patient no. 23, shows situs ambiguus with dextrocardia, a right-sided aortic arch (white arrow), and a left-sided stomach (S). The pulmonary vascularity is normal on the left and diminished on the right, indicating probable obstruction to the pulmonary flow in this patient with cyanosis. *B*, The lateral chest radiograph does not show adequately the inferior vena cava shadow. The pulmonary vascularity suggests pulmonary arteries anterior to the tracheal bronchial tree and probable right isomerism. *C*, Right isomerism (asplenia syndrome) in a four-year-old boy, patient no. 23. The transverse ultrasonogram at 0.5 cm below the xiphoid process shows the aorta (A) and inferior vena cava (IVC, arrow) to the left of the spine. The liver (L) is located primarily to the left. *D*, The longitudinal B-mode ultrasonogram shows the inferior vena cava (IVC, arrow) entering the right atrium (RA) directly on top of the abdominal aorta (A, arrowhead), 1 cm to the right of midline. This shows the "piggyback" vascular anatomy. This anomaly should not be confused with the normally visualized tubular anechoic crus of the diaphragm seen ventral to the abdominal aorta on longitudinal scans in normal patients. Without angulation of the transducer, the inferior vena cava can be seen to cross the aorta or travel on the same side of the spine with the aorta in most cases of right isomerism. Real-time imaging shows the vascular pulsations. *E*, At catheterization, the vascular anatomy was demonstrated by the course of the catheter extending from the femoral vein into the inferior vena cava (IVC, arrow), which is noted just to the right of the spine as it enters a right atrial structure, a single ventricle, and the ascending aorta. The ascending aortogram shows a right-sided aortic arch descending to the right of the spine (A, arrowhead). The findings of right isomerism (asplenia syndrome) were also confirmed at postmortem examination in this patient.

(*D* reproduced with permission from Tonkin IL, Tonkin, AK: Visceroatrial situs abnormalities: Sonographic and computed tomographic appearance. AJR, *138*:509, 1982. Copyright ©, 1982, The Williams and Wilkins Company.)

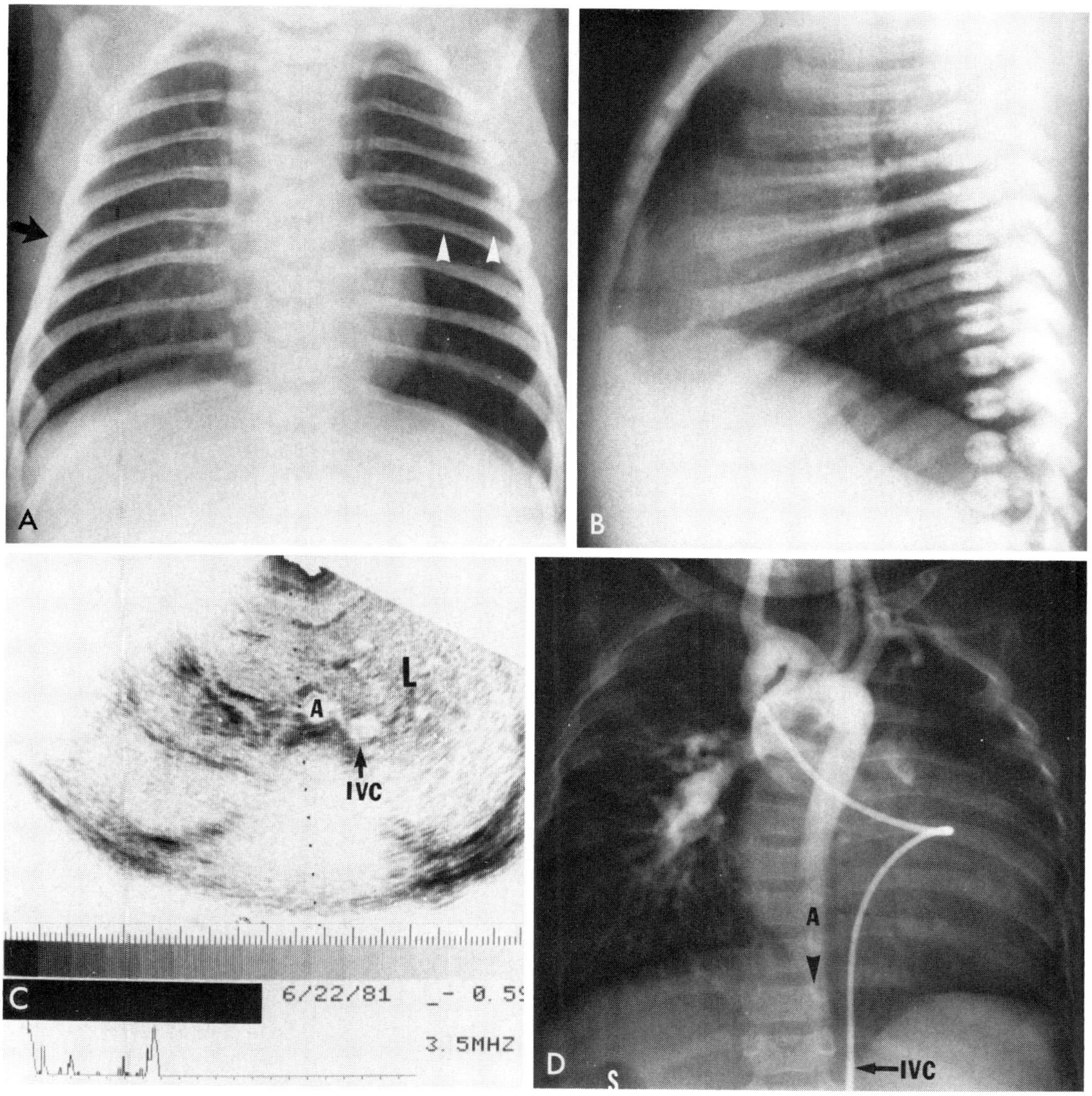

Figure 16. *A*, The PA chest radiograph of a three-month-old infant, patient no. 26, shows evidence of a right thoracotomy (arrow) secondary to a right Blalock-Taussig shunt. The pulmonary vascularity is now slightly increased on the right compared with the left, secondary to the right Blalock-Taussig shunt. There is visualization of a left-sided minor fissure (white arrowheads), indicating probable right isomerism (asplenia syndrome). *B*, The lateral chest radiograph shows poor visualization of the inferior vena cava shadow with the pulmonary arteries anterior to the trachea. *C*, Right isomerism (asplenia syndrome) in a four-year-old boy, patient no. 26. At four years of age, this patient underwent abdominal ultrasonography to better define the type of situs ambiguus. The study demonstrated the aorta (A) and inferior vena cava (arrow, IVC) to be to the right of the spine. The liver in this patient (L) is to the left of the spine primarily. There is a right-sided stomach. Findings are compatible with bilateral right isomerism, or asplenia syndrome. *D*, The vascular anatomy was confirmed with this aortogram. The catheter was placed from the femoral vein into the inferior vena cava (arrow, IVC), which courses to the left of the spine. It was then placed into the large single ventricle and into the ascending aorta to visualize the Blalock-Taussig anastomosis. The right Blalock-Taussig anastomosis is patent, filling the right pulmonary artery. The course of the descending aorta (A, arrowhead) is also visualized to the left of the spine, again confirming right isomerism (asplenia syndrome) with a right-sided stomach (S).

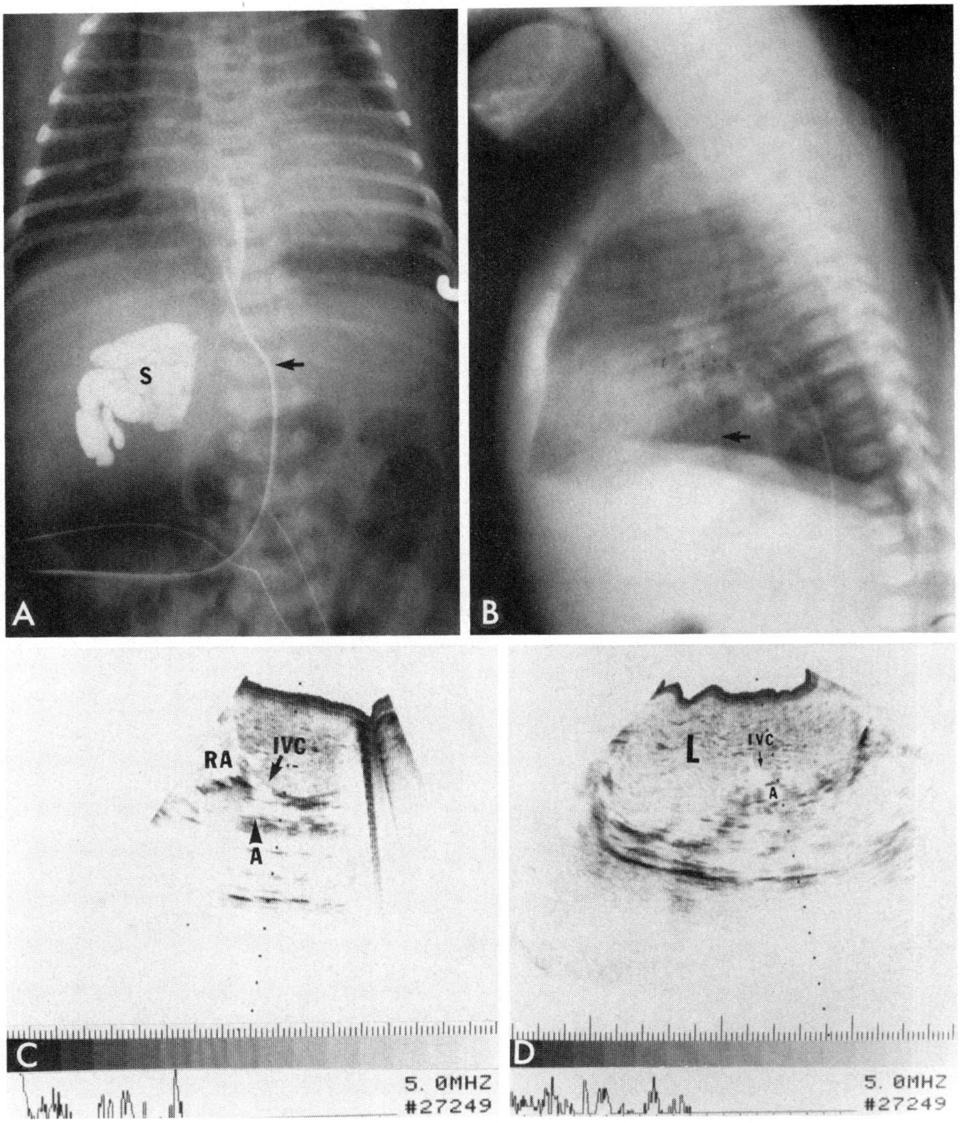

Figure 17. *A*, The AP supine chest radiograph of this one-day-old girl with cyanosis, patient no. 28, shows evidence of situs ambiguus with levocardia and a left-sided aortic arch. Barium in the esophagus confirmed a right-sided stomach (S). There is an umbilical venous catheter that courses slightly to the left of the spine and takes a midline change of direction (arrow), coursing to the right of the spine, and resides within the liver. There appears to be hepatic symmetry with a midline liver. *B*, A lateral upright projection was obtained that showed a probable inferior vena cava (arrow) entering an atrial structure. *C*, Ultrasonography was performed before cardiac catheterization to confirm the inferior vena cava–right atrial communication. The longitudinal transverse ultrasound examination at 1.5 cm to the left of midline shows the inferior vena cava (IVC, arrow) entering a right atrium (RA). In addition, the "piggyback" configuration of the aorta seen posteriorly on the same side of the spine (A, arrowhead) can also be demonstrated. *D*, The transverse ultrasonogram at approximately 3 cm below the xiphoid process again confirms the pulsating vascular anatomy of the inferior vena cava (IVC, arrow) and aorta (A) crossing to the left of the spine at this level. The bulk of the liver (L) is mostly on the right with hepatic symmetry. Cardiac catherization confirmed the vascular anatomy, indicating asplenia syndrome or right isomerism with complex congenital heart disease (patient no. 28, Table 2).

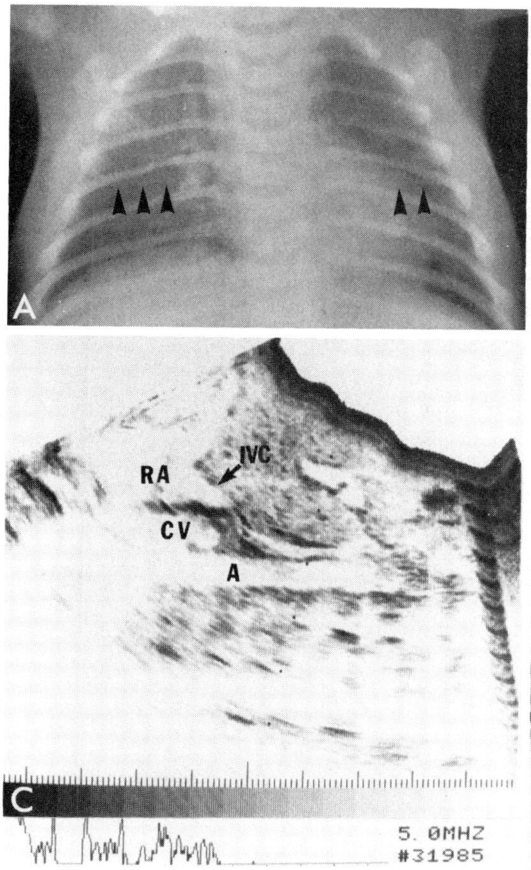

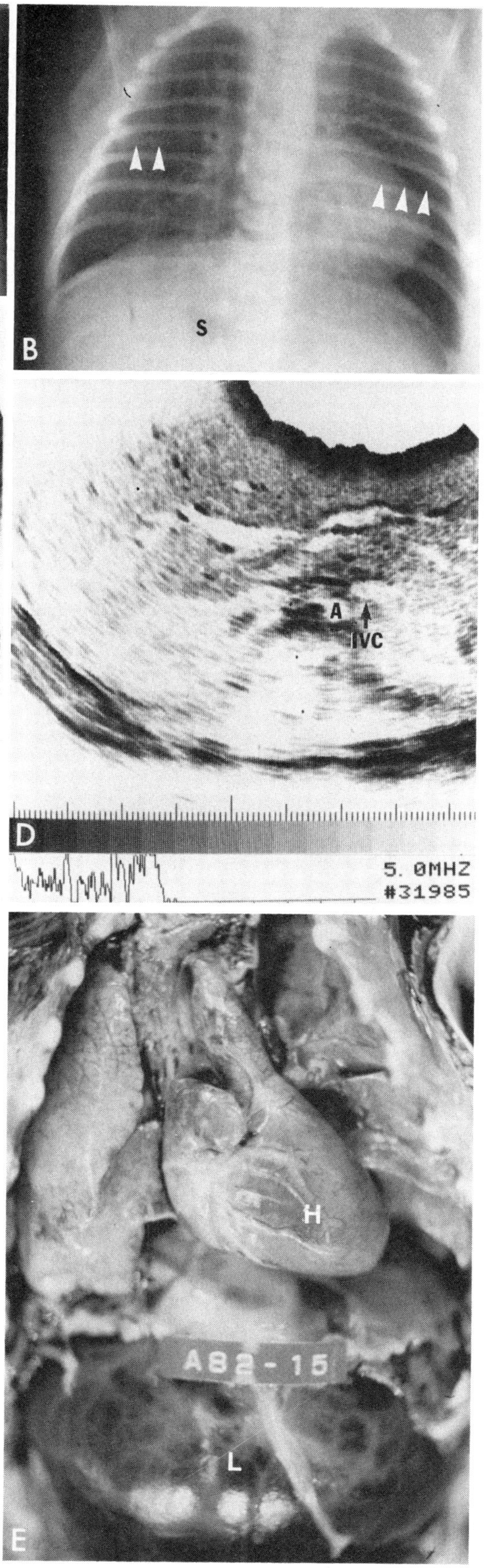

Figure 18. *A*. The AP supine chest radiograph at a few hours of age in this male infant with cyanosis (patient no. 29) shows situs ambiguus with probable bilateral minor fissures (arrowheads), indicating probable right isomerism, or asplenia syndrome. There is levocardia, left-sided aortic arch, and hepatic symmetry demonstrated. *B*, The upright PA chest radiograph at one day of age again faintly demonstrates bilateral minor fissures (arrowheads), with decreased vascularity indicating obstruction to pulmonary flow. There is a definite left-sided aortic arch, levocardia, and a midline stomach (S), which is slightly to the right of the spine. *C*, Right isomerism (asplenia syndrome) in a one-day-old boy, patient no. 29. An ultrasound examination was performed before cardiac catheterization, and the inferior vena cava (IVC, arrow) was noted to enter a right atrium (RA). In addition, the "piggyback" relationship of the inferior vena cava crossing the aorta (A) at 2 cm to the left of the spine is also noted. The sonolucent structure between the atrium may have represented the common pulmonary veins (CV) in this patient, with total anomalous pulmonary venous return to the liver demonstrated partially at catheterization and at postmortem examination at two months of age. *D*, The transverse ultrasonogram at 2.5 cm below the xiphoid process demonstrated the vascular anatomy, with the inferior vena cava (IVC, arrow) and aorta (A) situated to the right of the spine. *E*, Cardiac catheterization confirmed the vascular anatomy. These findings were also confirmed at postmortem examination of the patient, showing evidence of a functional single ventricle of the heart (H), hepatic symmetry of the liver (L), and congenital absence of the spleen, with bilateral, trilobed lungs.

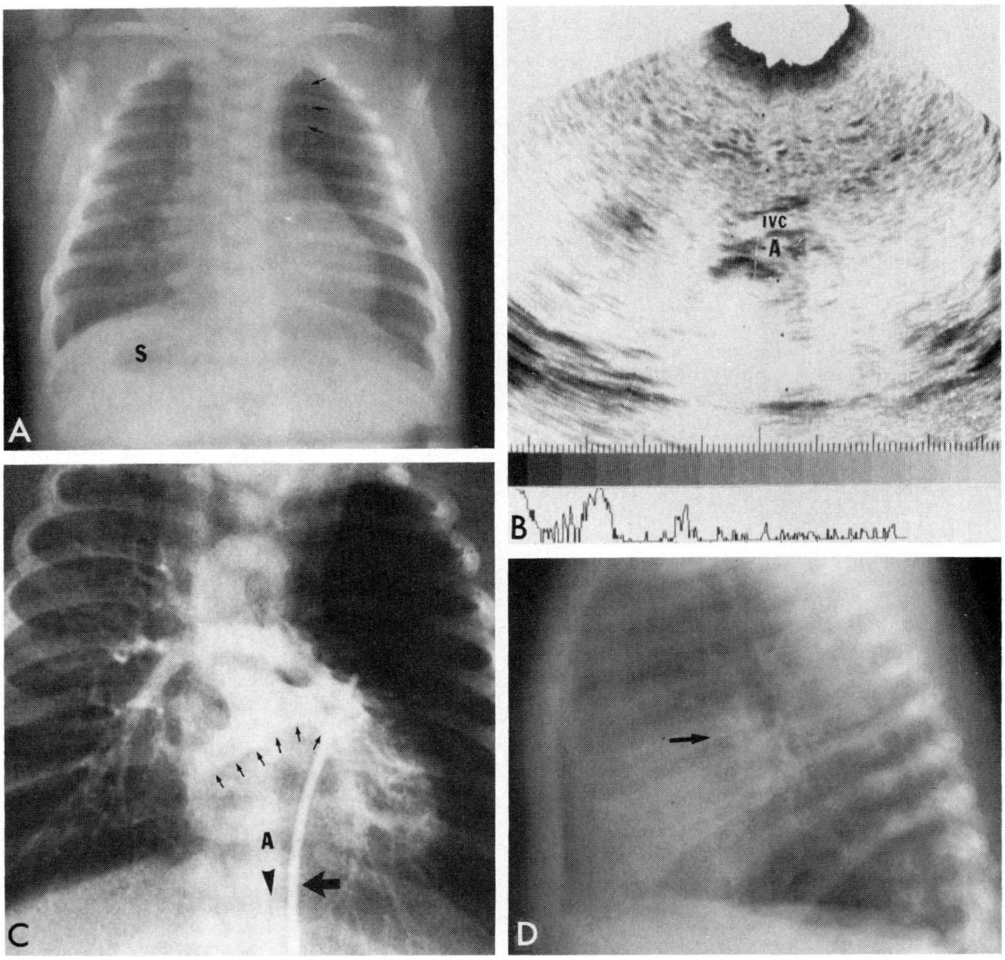

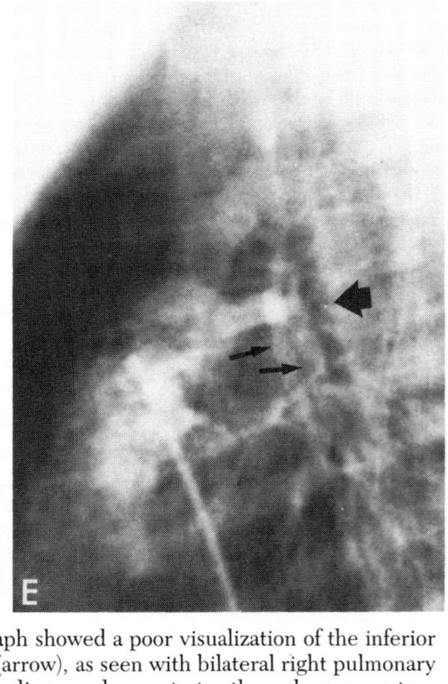

Figure 19. *A*, The PA chest radiograph of a two-week-old girl shows evidence of situs ambiguus with levocardia and a right-sided stomach (S). It was difficult to evaluate the position of the aortic arch in this patient. However, there appeared to be hepatic symmetry with a curvilinear density in the left upper lobe, which probably represents an azygos lobe (small arrows), indicating that the patient may have right isomerism, or asplenia syndrome. *B*, Right isomerism (asplenia syndrome) in a two-week-old girl, patient no. 30. The transverse ultrasonogram also demonstrated that the inferior vena cava (IVC) and aorta (A) were to the left of the spine, indicating right isomerism or asplenia syndrome. The liver is located mostly to the left in this patient. Real-time sector scanning showed that the inferior vena cava was entering an atrial structure to the left of the spine, but there was continuity. Two-dimensional sector scanning also showed probable common AV valve, a single or common ventricle, and common atrium. *C*, At cardiac catheterization, the course of the inferior vena cava is seen to the left of the spine and is outlined by the catheter (arrow). The injection into the single ventricle shows a common AV valve (small arows) with a double outlet right ventricle, pulmonic stenosis, and a large left aortic arch that descends to the left of the spine (A, arrowhead). There is an emphysematous left upper lobe with decreased pulmonary vascularity. *D*, The lateral chest radiograph showed a poor visualization of the inferior vena cava, with the pulmonary arteries anterior to the trachea (arrow), as seen with bilateral right pulmonary arteries and the asplenia syndrome. *E*, The lateral cineangiocardiogram demonstrates the pulmonary artery anatomy with both pulmonary arteries (arrows) anterior to the tracheobronchial tree (large arrow), as would be seen with bilateral right pulmonary arteries or right isomerism (asplenia syndrome).

ring with hepatic symmetry or with the liver extending across the abdomen (Figs. 14*A*, 17*A*, 18*A*, and 19*A*). In the normal newborn infant, the left lobe of the liver is extremely prominent and may give the appearance of hepatic symmetry. Therefore, it is important to identify the abdominal vascular anatomy with real-time ultrasonography to differentiate an extremely prominent left lobe of the liver from hepatic symmetry and the asplenia syndrome. The position of the stomach bubble may vary in the asplenia syndrome, and the stomach may be located on either side or in the midline (Figs. 14*A* and 18*A* and *B*). In addition, patients with the asplenia syndrome may have microgastria[14] or a small, tubular stomach in the midsagittal position (Fig. 14*G*). This finding may obscure the vascular anatomy on the posteroanterior (PA) and lateral chest radiographs (Fig. 14*A* and *B*). Moreover, it is often difficult to see the shadow of the inferior vena cava even with upright PA projection in the very ill or cyanotic newborn infant (Figs. 14*B*, 15*B*, 16*B*, and 19*E*).

Ultrasonography, even in the very ill patient, will show the location of the inferior vena cava and the site of the inferior vena cava–atrial communication[17, 30] (Figs. 14*D*, 15*D*, 17*C*, and 18*C*). It is important to demonstrate this anatomy before cardiac catheterization to ensure that a catheter can be passed via the femoral venous route into the heart. In patients with interruption of the inferior vena cava or with the azygos or hemiazygos continuation, an antecubital venous approach should be used in many cases. The anomalous relationship of the inferior vena cava and abdominal aorta was present in all cases of asplenia syndrome in this series, with both vessels coursing on the same side of the spine. This relationship can be demonstrated on ultrasonography, two-dimensional echocardiography, or CT. There are rare case reports of interruption of the inferior vena cava in asplenia syndrome.[4, 8, 27]

Patients with right isomerism have cardiac malformations commonly including atrioventricular canal, univentricular heart (single ventricle), pulmonic stenosis or atresia, transposition of the great arteries, and anomalous pulmonary venous connections[2, 4, 6, 8, 16, 21–23, 27, 28, 32–35] (Tables 2 and 3; Figs. 14*I* and 18*E*). Patients with visceral heterotaxia and severe obstruction to pulmonary flow may have "silent" obstruction of the pulmonary venous return. In one patient (Case 29) in this series, it was difficult to evaluate the complete course of the pulmonary veins owing to poor visualization of the levophase and severe pulmonic valve atresia. The infusion of prostaglandin E_1 before operation in patients with the asplenia syndrome or similar cardiac disease may create the radiographic appearance of pulmonary edema and aid in unmasking "silent" obstructions of the pulmonary veins. This technique is of value in the preoperative assessment of these patients before palliation or total correction.[10] The incidence and severity of cardiac anomalies are usually greater with the asplenia syndrome than with the polysplenia syndrome (Tables 1, 2, and 3).

The presumptive but not definitive diagnosis of asplenia syndrome can be made by evaluation of the peripheral blood smear, which may show Howell-Jolly and Heinz bodies in the absence of the spleen.[21, 22]

It is important to recognize the visceroatrial situs abnormalities so that the prognosis and possible surgical palliation or correction may be determined. In addition, an accurate diagnosis is vital because patients with the asplenia syndrome are at a greater risk of sepsis; thus prophylactic antibiotics are recommended.[37]

The plain radiographic signs of asplenia have been well defined.[2, 8, 16, 18, 19, 21, 22, 26, 27, 32–35] These signs include bilateral eparterial bronchi with a corresponding pulmonary artery anatomy, like that of a normal right lung.[16] The pulmonary arteries are anterior to the tracheobronchial tree on the lateral projection.[27] Occasionally, one can see bilateral minor fissures, secondary to bilateral, trilobed lungs with right isomerism. (Figs. 13*A*, 16*A*, and 18*A* and *B*) The inferior vena cava can usually be seen on the erect lateral chest radiograph, but it may be difficult to detect in the infant or in those patients with cardiac enlargement; ultrasonography or two-dimensional echocardiography will be helpful in these cases.

Radionuclide venography and liver-spleen scanning have been used to diagnose the heterotaxic syndromes.[7, 9] However, there have been several false-positive diagnoses of the asplenia syndrome reported owing to the extremely large liver, which appears to mask the uptake of a very small but normal spleen in some cases.[9, 21, 30] With an extremely careful examination and adequate equipment, though, radionuclide venography with follow-through arteriography and oblique liver-spleen scanning can be helpful and even diagnostic[7, 9] (Fig. 14*H*).

CONCLUSION

In the author's experience, echocardiography or ultrasonography and CT correlated with chest radiographs are the most accurate means of diagnosing the type of visceroatrial situs before cardiac catheterization, with confirmation by angiocardiography or ultimately by postmortem examination. In our series, the exact diagnosis was made in 29 of 30 patients, with an unusual heterotaxic pattern occurring in one patient (Case 16) in this series. Atypical heterotaxic patterns are occasionally reported in other series as well.[2, 4, 8, 27] However, in general, radiographic evaluation in association with two-dimensional echocardiography or CT will correctly determine the visceroatrial situs. With the definitive repair of complex congenital heart disease now undertaken in early infancy,[1, 15] it is essential to diagnose in complete detail even the most complex lesions in the newborn period. Two-dimensional echocardiography, with contrast material limitations, is currently being used as an excellent and often more complete counterpart of cardiac catheterization in the very sick newborn.

As sonography and, to a lesser extent, CT are used for the initial abdominal evaluation, incidental visceroatrial situs abnormalities will be encountered and should be recognized.

ACKNOWLEDGMENTS

I gratefully acknowledge the secretarial assistance of Ms. Brenda Adkins, with assistance from Ms. Sheila Jones.

REFERENCES

1. Ando F, Shirotani H, Kawai J, et al: Successful total repair of complicated cardiac anomalies with asplenia syndrome. J Thorac Cardiovasc Surg, 72:33, 1976.
2. Brandt PWT, Calder AL: Cardiac connections: The segmental approach to radiologic diagnosis in congenital heart disease. *In* Moseley RD (ed): Current Problems in Diagnostic Radiology. Chicago, Year Book Medical Publishers, 1977, pp. 5–32.
3. Burckart GJ, White TJ III, Siegle RL, et al: Rectal thiopental versus an intramuscular cocktail for sedating children before computerized tomography. Am J Hosp Pharm, *37*:222, 1980.
4. Bussatt PL, Bopp P, Duchosal PW: Congenital heart disease with the Ivemark syndrome and absence of the inferior vena cava. Radiology, *84*:657, 1965.
5. DeMaeyer P, Wilms G, Baert AL: Polysplenia. J Comput Assist Tomgr, 5:104, 1981.
6. Elliott LP, Cramer GG, Amplatz K: The anomalous relationship of the inferior vena cava and abdominal aorta as a specific angiocardiographic sign in asplenia. Radiology, *87*:859, 1966.
7. Fitzer PM: An approach to cardiac malposition and the heterotaxy syndrome using ^{99m}Tc sulfur colloid imaging. AJR, *127*:1021, 1976.
8. Freedom RM, Fellows KE Jr: Radiographic visceral patterns in the asplenia syndrome. Radiology, *106*:387, 1973.
9. Freedom RM, Treves S: Splenic scintigraphy and radionuclide venography in the heterotaxy syndrome. Radiology, *107*:381, 1973.
10. Freedom RM, Olley PM, Coceani F, et al.: The prostaglandin challenge. Test to unmask obstructed total anomalous pulmonary venous connections in asplenia syndrome. Br Heart J, *40*:91, 1978.
11. Garcia OL, Mehta AV, Pickoff AS, et al: Left isomerism and complete atrioventricular block: A report of six cases. Am J Cardiol, *48*:1103, 1981.
12. Garris JB, Kangarloo H, Sample WF: Ultrasonic diagnosis of infrahepatic interruption of the inferior vena cava with azygos (hemiazygos) continuation. Radiology, *134*:179, 1980.
13. Ginaldi S, Chuang VP, Wallace S: Absence of hepatic segment of the inferior vena cava with azygous continuation. J Comput Assist Tomogr, *4*:112, 1980.
14. Kessler H, Smulewicz JJ: Microgastria associated with agenesis of the spleen. Radiology, *107*:393, 1973.
15. Kirklin JW, Pacifico AD, Bargeron LM Jr., et al: Cardiac repair in anatomically corrected malposition of the great arteries. Circulation, *48*:153, 1973.
16. Landing BH, Lawrence TK, Payne VC, et al: Bronchial anatomy in syndromes with abnormal visceral situs, abnormal spleen and congenital heart disease. Am J Cardiol, *28*:456, 1971.
17. Meyer RA, Schwartz DC, Covitz W, et al: Echocardiographic assessment of cardiac malposition. Am J Cardiol, *33*:896, 1974.
18. Partridge, J: The radiological evaluation of atrial situs. Clin Radiol, *30*:95, 1979.
19. Partridge JB, Scott O, Deverall PB, et al: Visualization and measurement of the main bronchi by tomography as an objective indicator of thoracic situs in congenital heart disease. Circulation, *51*:188, 1975.
20. Piekarski, J, Federle MP, Moss AA, et al: Computed tomography of the spleen. Radiology, *135*:683, 1980.
21. Randall PA, Moller JH, Amplatz K: The spleen and congenital heart disease. AJR, *119*:551, 1973.
22. Rose V, Izukawa T, Moes CAF: Syndromes of asplenia and polysplenia. A review of cardiac and non-cardiac malformations in 60 cases with special reference to diagnosis and prognosis. Br Heart J, *37*:840, 1975.
23. Rowe RD, Freedom RM, Mehrizi A, et al: Cardiac malpositions: Dextrocardia; thoracopagus conjoined twins; ectopic cordis; and congenital diverticulum of the left ventricle. *In* Schaffer AJ, Markowitz M (eds): The Neonate with Congenital Heart Disease. Philadelphia, W. B. Saunders, 1981, p. 503.
24. Royal SA, Callen PW: CT evaluation of anomalies of the inferior vena cava and left renal vein. AJR, *132*:759, 1979.
25. Schidlow DV, Katz SM, Turtz MG, et al: Polysplenia and Kartagener syndromes in a sibship: Association with abnormal respiratory cilia. J Pediatr, *100*:401, 1982.
26. Shinebourne EA, Macartney FJ, Anderson RH: Sequential chamber localization—Logical approach to diagnosis in congenital heart disease. Br Heart J, *38*:327, 1976.
27. Soto B, Pacifico AD, Souza AS Jr, et al: Identification of thoracic isomerism from the plain chest radiograph. AJR, *131*:995, 1978.
28. Stanger P, Rudolph AM, Edwards JE: Cardiac malpositions. An overview based on study of sixty-five necropsy specimens. Circulation, *56*:159, 1977.

29. Tegtmeyer CJ, Hust FS, Keats TE: Arteriographic manifestations of abdominal situs inversus. AJR, *125*:427, 1975.
30. Tonkin IL, Tonkin AK: Visceroatrial situs abnormalities: Sonographic and computed tomographic appearance. AJR, *138*:509, 1982.
31. Train JS, Henderson MR, Smith AP: Sonographic demonstration of left-sided inferior vena cava with hemiazygos continuation. AJR, *134*:1057, 1980.
32. Van Mierop, LHS, Eisen S, Schiebler, GL: The radiographic appearance of the tracheobronchial tree as an indicator of visceral situs. Am J Cardiol, *26*:432, 1970.
33. Van Mierop LHS, Gessner IH, Schiebler GL: Asplenia and polysplenia syndrome. Birth Defects, *8*:74, 1972.
34. Van Praagh R, Vlad P: Dextrocardia, mesocardia and levocardia: The segmental approach to diagnosis in congenital heart disease. *In* Keith JD, Rowe RD, Vlad P (eds): Heart Disease in Infancy and Childhood. New York, Macmillan 1978, p. 638.
35. Van Praagh R, Weibert PM, Van Praagh S.: Malposition of the heart. *In* Moss AJ, Adams, FH, Emmanoulides GC (eds): Heart Disease in Infants, Children, and Adolescents. Baltimore, Williams & Wilkins, 1977, p. 410.
36. Vaughan TJ, Hawkins IF Jr, Elliott LP: Diagnosis of polysplenia syndrome. Radiology, *101*:511, 1971.
37. Waldman JD, Rosenthal A, Smith AL, et al: Sepsis and congenital asplenia. J Pediatr, *90*:555, 1977.
38. Weiand VG, Lackner K, Koischwitz D: CT-Nachweis des Venosen umgehungskreislaufs bei verschluss oder Agenesie der Vena Cava. ROEFO, *133*:250, 1980.

11

AN ULTRASONIC APPROACH TO THE DIAGNOSIS OF CARDIAC SITUS, CONNECTIONS, AND MALPOSITIONS

NORMAN H. SILVERMAN, M.D.

By virtue of the ability to display structures spatially, two-dimensional echocardiography offers substantial advantages over M-mode echocardiography for the evaluation of complex congenital cardiac malformations and definition of cardiac situs and connections.[3, 4, 7, 8, 10]

Two-dimensional echocardiography can be combined with simultaneous M-mode echocardiography and contrast echocardiography for structure validation.[7] Although echocardiography can be performed independently of the history, clinical examination, chest roentgenogram, electrocardiogram, and computed tomographic scan, a more rapid and complete evaluation can be achieved when all of these modalities are combined.

The nomenclature of malpositions of the cardiac segments is an unsettled issue; however, if a descriptive approach is used, it could be applied to any of the existing systems of nomenclature.[11, 12, 14]

A sequential approach to the definition of situs and connections has been used for this presentation. In this approach, the cardiac situs is first determined. Because disorders of cardiac situs occur frequently with malposition, the position of the heart must be determined. The atrioventricular connections are then established, and the ventricular morphology defined. Finally, the ventriculoarterial connections and relations are established. This is achieved either by gleaning information from each plane as it is obtained or by examining each of the cardiac segments in sequence using multiple planes. The former approach is more desirable because it uses a step-by-step integration of the information derived from each of the planes as they are routinely acquired. Although the sequence of planes may not be routine, a sequence of examining from each plane ensures that information is not missed by not performing the examinations from any plane or location.

Ultrasonic contrast induced by rapidly injecting intravenously a small bolus of 1 to 2 ml of aerated saline solution is used to define venous drainage patterns, direction of flow, and intracardiac shunting. Finally, after all information is gathered from the study, the diagnosis can usually be established by integrating all the direct information and by inference (Table 1).

SUBCOSTAL PLANES

The subcostal short views of the abdominal vessels through the abdomen are most useful for defining the aortic and vena caval spatial relations (Fig. 1).[1, 2] In splenic syndromes, the inferior vena cava and aorta can be identified as arising from the same side of the vertebral spine (Fig. 2). In addition, the inferior vena cava can be traced to its connection with the anatomic right atrium. Interruption of the inferior vena cava is frequently associated with polysplenia (left isomerism)[6, 11] and can be detected in the subcostal long axis view (Fig. 3). Interruption of the inferior vena cava can only be diagnosed after an extensive search in the

Table 1. *Segmental Analysis of the Heart by Two-dimensional Echocardiography*

	PLANES
Atrial situs	
Connection of superior and inferior venae cavae with anatomic right atrium.	Subcostal long and short axis Contrast echocardiography Suprasternal short axis
Connection of pulmonary veins with anatomic left atrium.	Apical four-chamber Subcostal four-chamber
Inference from pulmonary artery anatomy and bronchial relationships.	Suprasternal long and short axis
Inference from aorta and inferior vena cava positions.	Subcostal long and short axis
Ventricular morphology	
Definition of anatomic left ventricle.	
Two papillary muscles.	Parasternal short axis
"Fish-mouth" valve (mitral valve).	Parasternal short axis
Atrioventricular valve further from cardiac apex.	Apical four-chamber
Definition of anatomic right ventricle.	
Moderator band.	Apical four-chamber
Course trabecular pattern = right ventricle.	Apical and subcostal four-chamber
Atrioventricular valve closer to cardiac apex.	Apical four-chamber
Atrioventricular connections	
Concordant or discordant, double inlet ventricle, absent right or left connections, straddling atrioventricular valve.	Apical four-chamber Subcostal four-chamber
Ventriculoarterial connections	
Presence of one or two semilunar valves.	Parasternal long and short axis
Vessel that bifurcates = pulmonary artery.	Parasternal short axis Subcostal short axis
Relationship of semilunar valves to ventricular septum and ventricles.	Parasternal long and short axis
Position of cardiac apex	
Dextrocardia, mesocardia, levocardia.	Apical four-chamber Subcostal four-chamber
Aortic arch	
Right or left-sided arch.	Suprasternal long axis
Detection of thoracic aorta.	Subcostal long axis Apical long axis Parasternal short axis

long-axis plane for the inferior vena cava below the hepatic veins. In addition, in polysplenia, the interruption of the inferior vena cava can be confirmed by injections of contrast medium into a leg vein and following the bolus into the superior vena caval system via azygous collateral vessels. In situs inversus, the aorta is to the right of and posterior to the inferior vena cava (Fig. 4).

The subcostal four-chamber view yields similar information to the apical four-chamber view, demonstrating atrial anatomy, atrioventricular connections, ventricular morphology, and ventriculoarterial connections (Fig. 5D).[1, 2] The subcostal four-chamber view provides visual display of the position of the cardiac apex. The position of the aortic root, arch, and ventricular connections can be seen (Fig. 6). In mesocardia, for example, the apex points towards the transducer. Imaging the apex in mesocardia can produce circular ventricular outlines lying side-by-side (Fig. 7).

The subcostal views show both the pulmonary and systemic venous connections to the atria (Fig. 8). The tricuspid valve has attachments to the right side of the ventricular septum. The eustachian valve is part of the limbic system of the right atrium. Identifying this valve and the inferior vena cava helps define the right atrium.

APICAL FOUR-CHAMBER PLANE

To obtain the apical four-chamber view, the cardiac apex should be located by palpation or its direction determined from the subcostal plane. When it is difficult to palpate the cardiac apex, the transducer can be moved around in the region where the apex is suspected until a representative image is obtained. When properly obtained, the image of the cardiac apex should be in the apex of the fan. In situs inversus with dextrocardia, the transducer is positioned in a plane that is the mirror image of the standard four-chamber plane, but the left-right orientation of the transducer must be maintained.

The transducer position used to obtain the apical views defines whether there is levocardia with the apex pointing to the left, mesocardia with the apex pointing to the midline, or dextrocardia (Fig. 9) with the apex pointing toward the right. This contribution of the two-dimensional echocardiogram is useful because the frontal chest film may not show the precise position of the cardiac apex.

There are characteristic anatomic features of the left ventricle, the right ventricle, the left atrium, and the right atrium (See Table 1). Identification of these features in the four-chamber view helps to define the atrioventricular connections and allows one to infer the ventriculoarterial connections. The following examples illustrate the use of this plane.

The apical four-chamber view in Figure 10 is from a newborn infant with dextrocardia. The image was obtained from the fourth right intercostal space in the midclavicular line. This confirmed the presence of dextrocardia with the cardiac apex pointing towards the right. The

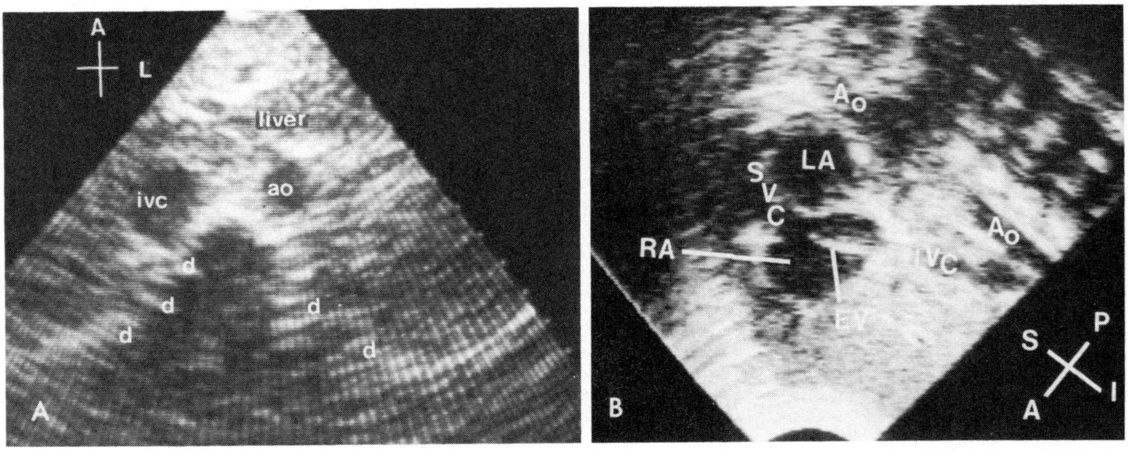

Figure 1. *A*, A subcostal short axis plane taken through the abdomen to demonstrate the normal relationships of the inferior vena cava (ivc) and aorta (ao) in a normal patient. The position of the left and right hemidiaphragms (d) are shown. A: anterior, L: left. Posterior and right are not labeled. *B*, Subcostal plane in the long axis of the body demonstrating the position of the aorta and inferior vena cava in the abdomen. Note the continuity of the inferior vena cava (IVC) and superior vena cava (SVC) with the right atrium (RA). A prominent eustachian valve (EV) is shown. The position of the descending aorta (AO) is seen passing behind the left atrium (LA) and anterior to the inferior vena cava. A: anterior, I: inferior, P: posterior, S: superior.

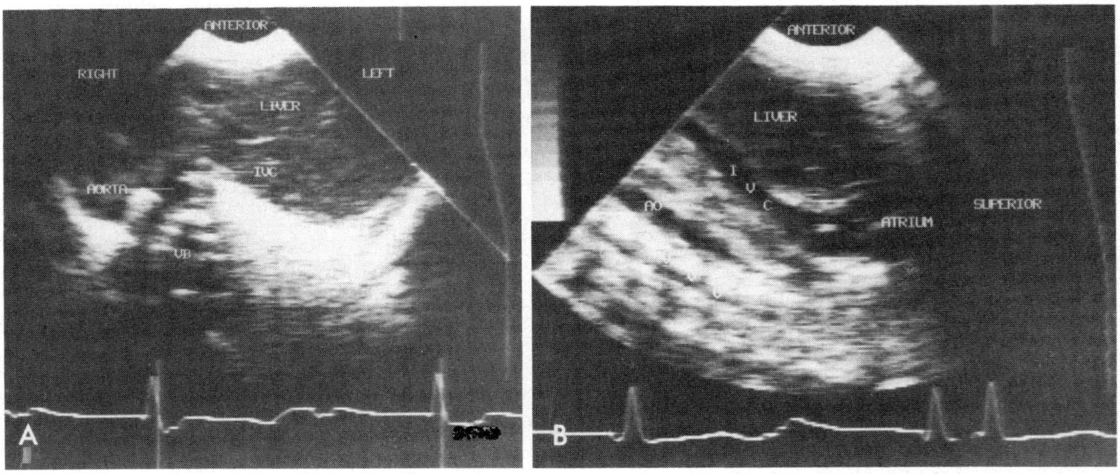

Figure 2. *A*, Transverse plane through the abdominal viscera and abdominal vessels showing the inferior vena cava (IVC) lying anterior to the aorta in a patient with polysplenia. The position of the ventricle body (VB) is shown. Right, left, and anterior positions are defined. *B*, Long axis through the abdominal vessels demonstrating a continuous length of the inferior vena cava and aorta lying anterior to the ventricle bodies (V). This, as shown in *A*, was located in a plane slightly to the right of the ventricle bodies. The anterior and superior directions are demonstrated on the figure.

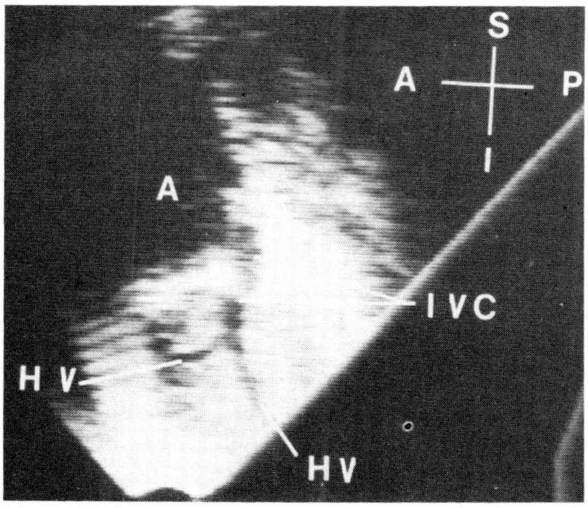

Figure 3. Subcostal long-axis plane through the abdominal and thoracic and inferior vena cava in a patient with polysplenia syndrome. The inferior vena cava (IVC) is continuous with the atrium (A). The hepatic veins (HV) are defined within the substance of the liver and going to the atrium. The portion of the vena cava below the hepatic veins is deficient. A: anterior, I: inferior, P: posterior, and S: superior.

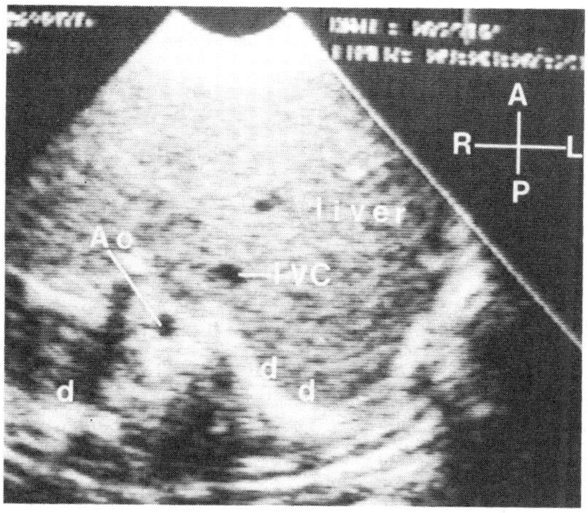

Figure 4. A transverse abdominal view of the aorta (Ao) and inferior vena cava (IVC) in a patient with situs inversus. The aorta is to the right and inferior vena cava to the left. The liver and diaphragms (d) are also labeled. A: anterior, L: left, P: posterior, R: right.

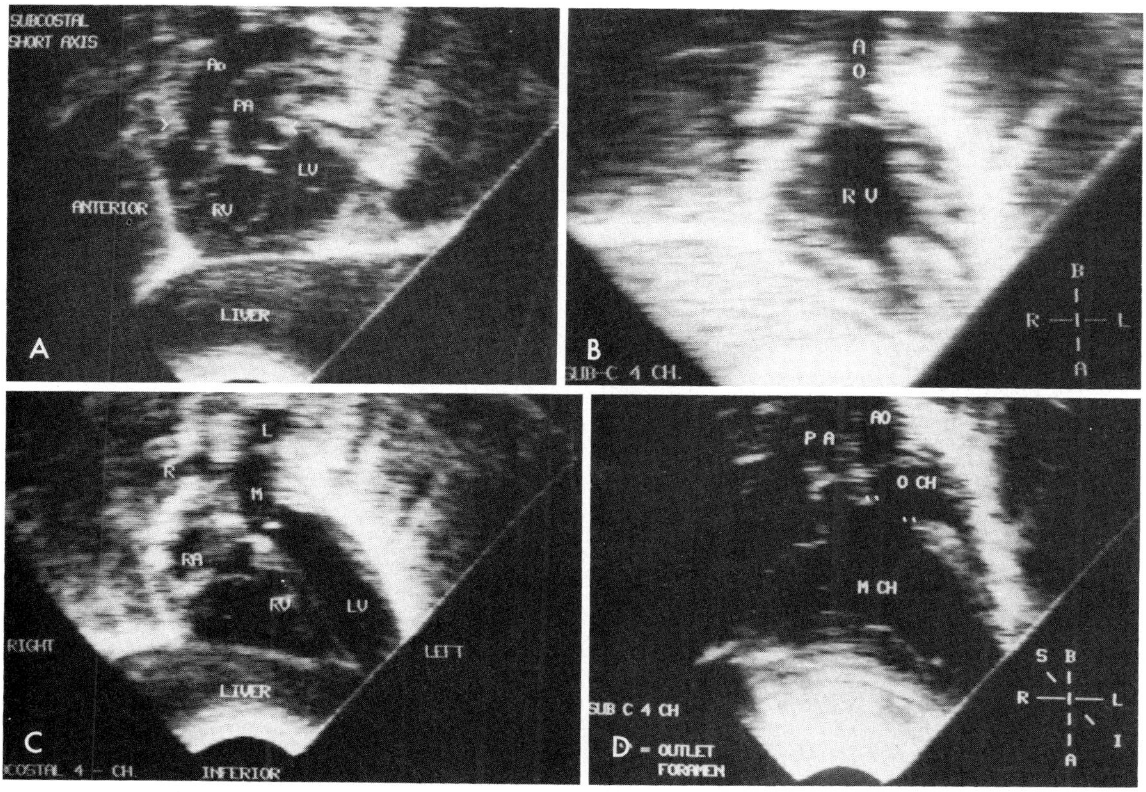

Figure 5. *A*, Subcostal short-axis projection in a patient with transposition of the great vessels. This figure is displayed in anatomic position. The anterior direction is defined, and the liver can be identified below the heart and diaphragm. The ventriculoarterial connections of the aorta (Ao) with the right ventricle (RV) and the pulmonary artery (PA) with the left ventricle (LV) are clearly shown. The position of both semilunar valves is identified by small arrows. *B*, Anteriorly directed subcostal four-chamber view in the previous patient with transposition demonstrating the aorta (Ao) arising from the right ventricle (RV). A: apex, B: base, L: left, R: right. *C*, Posteriorly directed subcostal four-chamber view displayed in anatomic position. The left ventricle (LV) is seen to give rise to the main pulmonary artery (M), which bifurcates into its two branches, R (right) and L (left). The bifurcation of this vessel clearly defines it as a pulmonary artery, and the ventricular arterial connections can be established as they were in Figure 5B. RA: right atrium, RV: right ventricle. *D*, Subcostal four-chamber view in a patient with a univentricular heart and anterior leftward outlet chamber (och). The pulmonary artery (PA) is situated to the right of the aorta (Ao) in transposition. The pulmonary artery arises from the main chamber (M CH) and the aorta from the outlet chamber. The outlet foramen is indicated by " " marks. A: apex, B: base, I: inferior, L: left, R: right, S: superior.

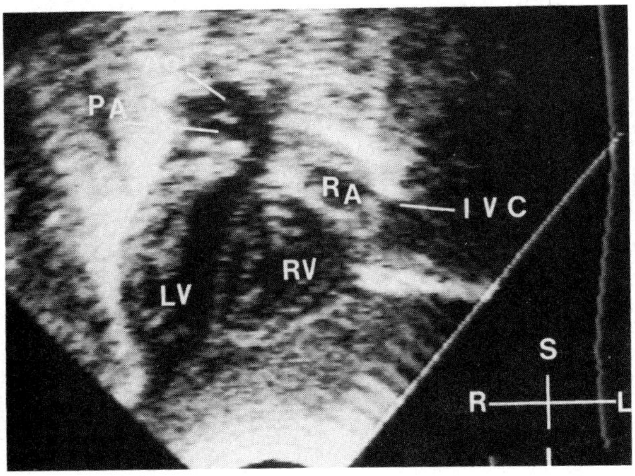

Figure 6. Subcostal four-chamber plane taken in a neonate with situs inversus. The subcostal four-chamber plane is displayed in the anatomic position. I: inferior, L: left, R: right, S: superior. The apex of the heart can clearly be seen pointing towards the right. The left-sided ventricle has the morphologic characteristics of a right ventricle (RV), and the right-sided ventricle, the morphologic characteristics of a left ventricle (LV). The inferior vena cava (IVC) can be seen running into a left-sided atrium, which is a morphologic right atrium (RA). The aortic arch (Ao) can be seen arising from the morphologic left ventricle and is a right aortic arch. The pulmonary artery (PA) can be identified below the aortic arch.

atrioventricular valve on the left is closer to the cardiac apex than that on the right, indicating that the left-sided ventricle is an anatomic right ventricle. On the right side, the mitral valve is located further from the cardiac apex. Also, in the parasternal short-axis view, the right-sided ventricle had features of an anatomic left ventricle. The pulmonary veins are seen draining

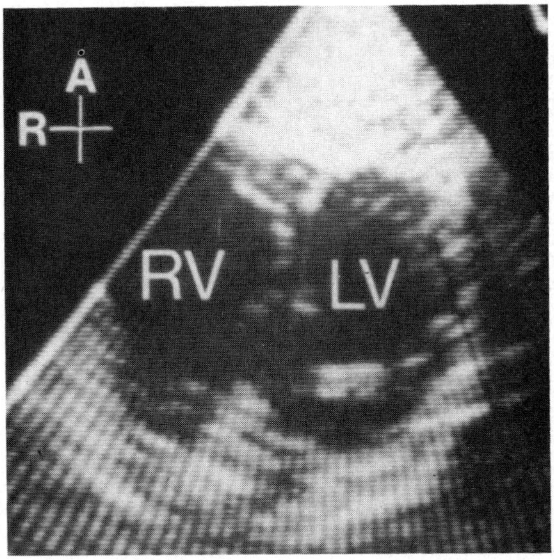

Figure 7. Subcostal four-chamber view in a patient with mesocardia. The right ventricle is right-sided, the left ventricle is left-sided, and a ventricular septal defect can be seen in the posterior portion of the ventricular septum. The cardiac apex is indeterminate, and the septum is directed towards the central part of the transducer fan. The transducer was placed in the subcostal position indicating mesocardia. The liver and diaphragm are situated anterior to the heart. A: anterior, R: right. (*From* Silverman NH, Snider AR: A segmental approach to the diagnosis of cardiac situs and malpositions. *In* Two-dimensional Echocardiography in Congenital Heart Disease. Norwalk, Appleton-Century-Crofts, 1982, pp. 229–245, with permission.)

to the right-sided atrium. This suggests that the atrium is the anatomic left atrium. A contrast echocardiogram in another neonate was performed from an arm vein and demonstrates that the systemic veins are draining to the left-sided anatomic right atrium. The left atrium is connected to the anatomic left ventricle, and the right atrium is connected to the anatomic right ventricle. The atrioventricular connections are normal, and the four chambers are positioned in a mirror image of normal. Situs inversus with dextrocardia, l-loop (anatomic right ventricle on the left), and normally related great vessels can be diagnosed from this plane.

The apical four-chamber views of the next example (Fig. 11*A*) were obtained from the fifth left intercostal space at the midclavicular line, indicating levocardia. The pulmonary veins enter the left-sided atrium, indicating that this is the anatomic left atrium. An injection of contrast medium in this patient (Fig. 11*B*) fills the right-sided atrium, indicating that this is the anatomic right atrium and that there is normal cardiac situs. A small right-to-left ventricular shunt is present. Inspection of the right-sided ventricle (see Fig. 11*A*) shows that it is an anatomic left ventricle because it is smooth-walled and has an atrioventricular valve that is further from the apex. The left-sided ventricle is an anatomic right ventricle because it has coarse trabeculations in its apex, a prominent moderator band, and an atrioventricular valve situated closer to the cardiac apex. The atrioventricular connections are, therefore, discordant. In the parasternal short-axis view, there was l-transposition of the great vessels. The patient's diagnosis is situs solitus, l-loop, l-transposition, and ventricular septal defect.

The apical four-chamber view in Figure 12

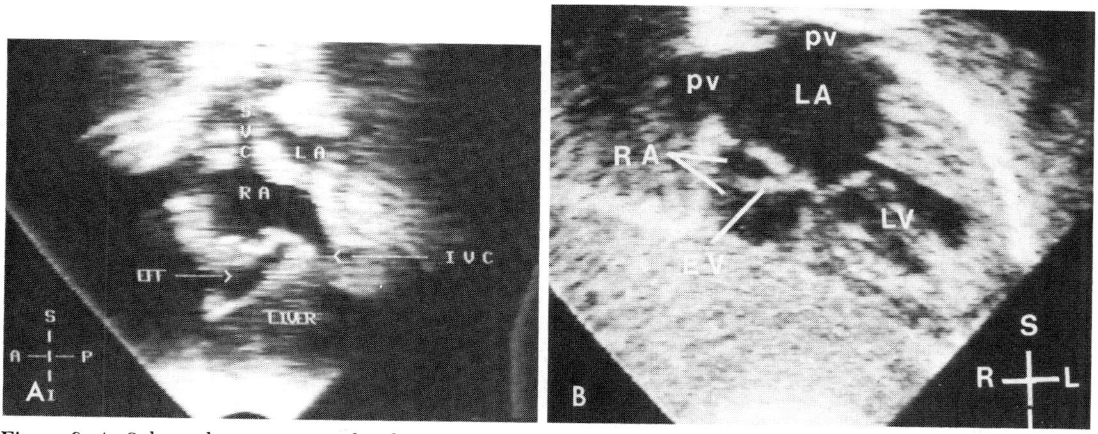

Figure 8. *A*, Subcostal projection in the short-axis plane displayed in the anatomic orientation. The superior vena cava (SVC) and inferior vena cava (IVC) can be seen draining into the right atrium (RA). The atrial septum separates the right atrium from the left atrium. The liver is separated from the floor of the right atrium in this instance by an effusion (EFF). A: anterior, I: inferior, P: posterior, S: superior. *B*, Subcostal four-chamber view demonstrating features of a morphologic right atrium (RA) and left atrium (LA). The pulmonary veins (pv) can be seen draining into the left atrium. In the right atrium, a prominent eustachian valve can be seen inseting into the lower part of the atrial septum and appears to divided the right atrium into two separate segments. I: inferior, L: left, R: right, S: superior.

was obtained from the fifth right intercostal space, indicating dextrocardia. An injection of contrast medium fills the left-sided atrium, indicating that it is an anatomic right atrium and

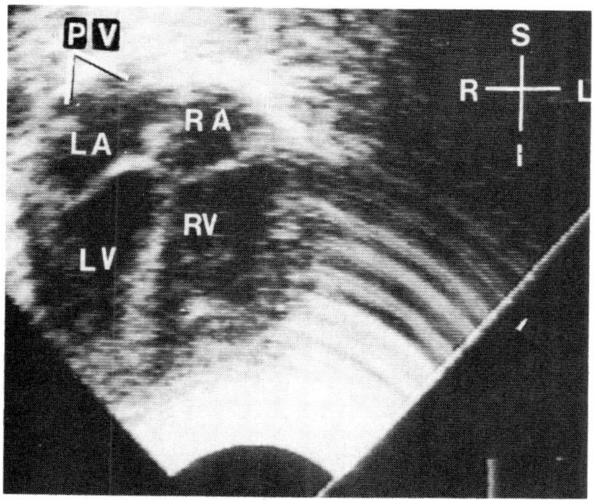

Figure 9. Apical four-chamber plane obtained from the right fourth intercostal space in the midclavicular line in an infant with situs inversus. The apical four-chamber plane is presented in anatomic display. The pulmonary veins (PV) can be seen draining into the right-sided morphologic left atrium (LA). The right ventricle (RV) has a prominent trabecular pattern typical of a normal right ventricle. The right atrioventricular valve is further from the cardiac apex than that on the left, indicating that the ventricles are inverted. There is, therefore, normal atrioventricular connection and situs inversus. I: inferior, L: left, R: right, S: superior.

that, therefore, there is situs inversus. The anatomic right ventricle with its moderator band and atrioventricular valve closer to the cardiac apex is right-sided. The left-sided ventricle is smooth-walled and has an atrioventricular valve further from the apex, defining it as an anatomic left ventricle. In the parasternal short-axis view, the great vessels were situated in the position of d-transposition. The final diagnosis is situs inversus with dextrocardia, d-loop (anatomic right ventricle on the right), d-transposition, and ventricular septal defect. All of these features cannot be defined in every patient, especially when associated intracardiac abnormalities are present.

In situs ambiguus, the definition of atrial anatomy can be difficult, and contrast echocardiography may provide important information about systemic venous drainage. The patient in Figure 13 has polysplenia (left isomerism) and an atrioventricular canal defect. No anatomic features in this view distinguish an anatomic right atrium or an anatomic left atrium. An injection of contrast medium into a vein in the left arm shows that there is a left superior vena cava draining directly to the left-sided atrium. An injection of contrast medium into a vein in the right arm shows a right superior vena cava draining to the right-sided atrium. Patients with situs ambiguus frequently have bilateral superior venae cavae draining directly to both atrial

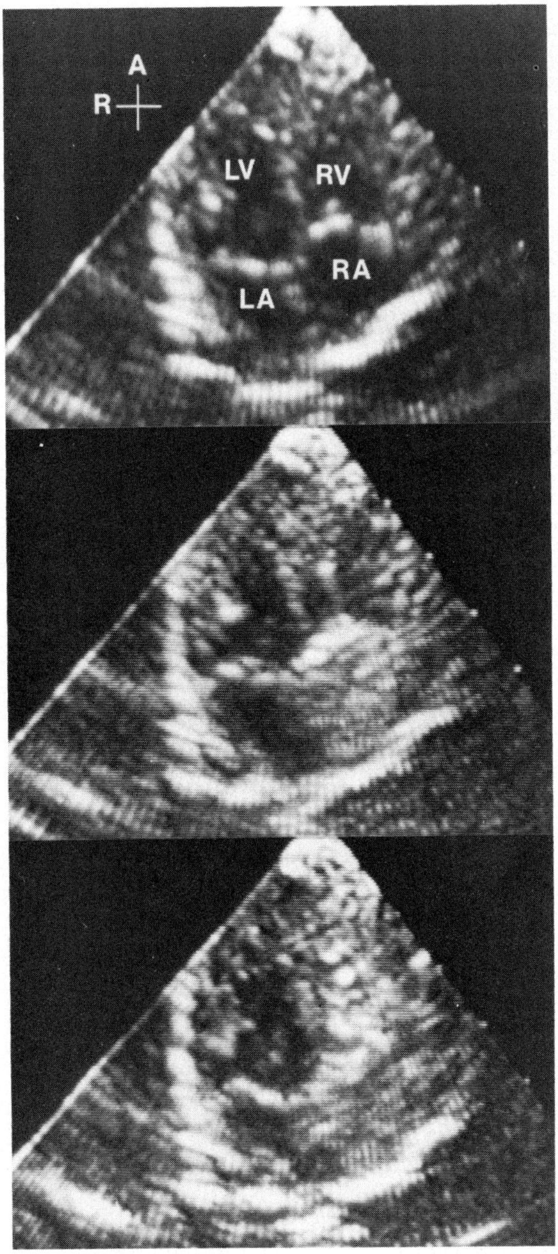

Figure 10. This sequence of frames is part of a peripheral venous injection of contrast medium in another infant with situs inversus. The apical four-chamber plane was obtained from the right fourth intercostal space. The bolus of contrast medium in the middle frame is seen to arise into the left-sided atrium, indicating that this is the systemic venous (right) atrium. The connections are therefore normal. (*From* Silverman NH, Snider AR: A segmental approach to the diagnosis of cardiac situs and malpositions. *In* Two-dimensional Echocardiography in Congenital Heart Disease. Norwalk, Appleton-Century-Crofts, 1982 pp. 229–245, with permission.)

and anomalous pulmonary venous connections, making it impossible to define atrial situs.

THE PARASTERNAL SHORT AXIS PLANE

The parasternal short-axis plane provides important information about the laterality of cardiac structures, the morphology of the ventricles and the atrioventricular valves, the ventriculoarterial connections, and positions of the atrial appendages. Regardless of where on the precordium the short axis is obtained, the examiner must ensure that left-right laterality is maintained for the particular instrument used.

With malpositions, this plane of the parasternal short axis can be altered, depending on the orientation of the major axis of the heart. When the heart is lying behind the sternum, it may not be possible to obtain complete evaluation from this plane.

In situs inversus with dextrocardia, the short-axis plane is the mirror image of the standard short-axis plane and is oriented between the right shoulder and left hip. The direction of the right ventricular outflow tract and pulmonary artery is reversed as they course around the aortic root (Fig. 14).

The short-axis view at the base of the heart is especially useful for defining ventriculoarterial positions in double-outlet right ventricle, truncus arteriosus, or transposition of the great vessels. In transposition, the great vessels are seen as "double circles" in the short-axis view. With cranial angulation of the transducer, the posterior pulmonary artery can be seen bifurcating into its two branches (Figs. 15 and 16). This view helps to define the spatial relations of the two great arteries.

When dextroposition is due to pulmonary disease, diaphragmatic hernia, or other causes that shift the mediastinum to the right, the short-axis view of the great vessels is obtained from the right precordium in a plane parallel to the normal short-axis view, for example, in a plane parallel to one from the left shoulder to the right hip, but with a normal right-left orientation.

The short-axis view through the ventricles shows certain anatomic features that help distinguish the right from the left ventricle (Fig.

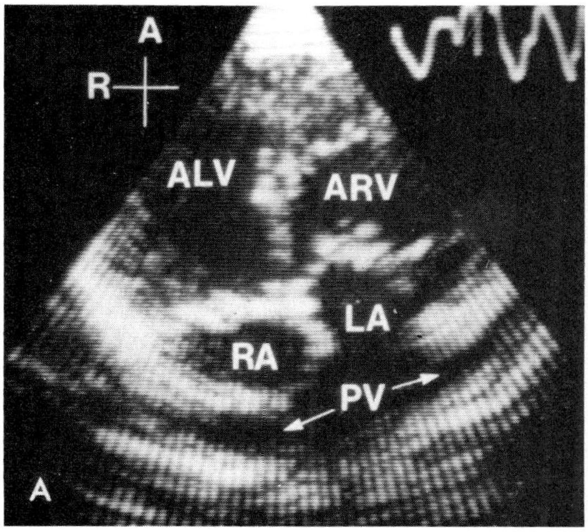

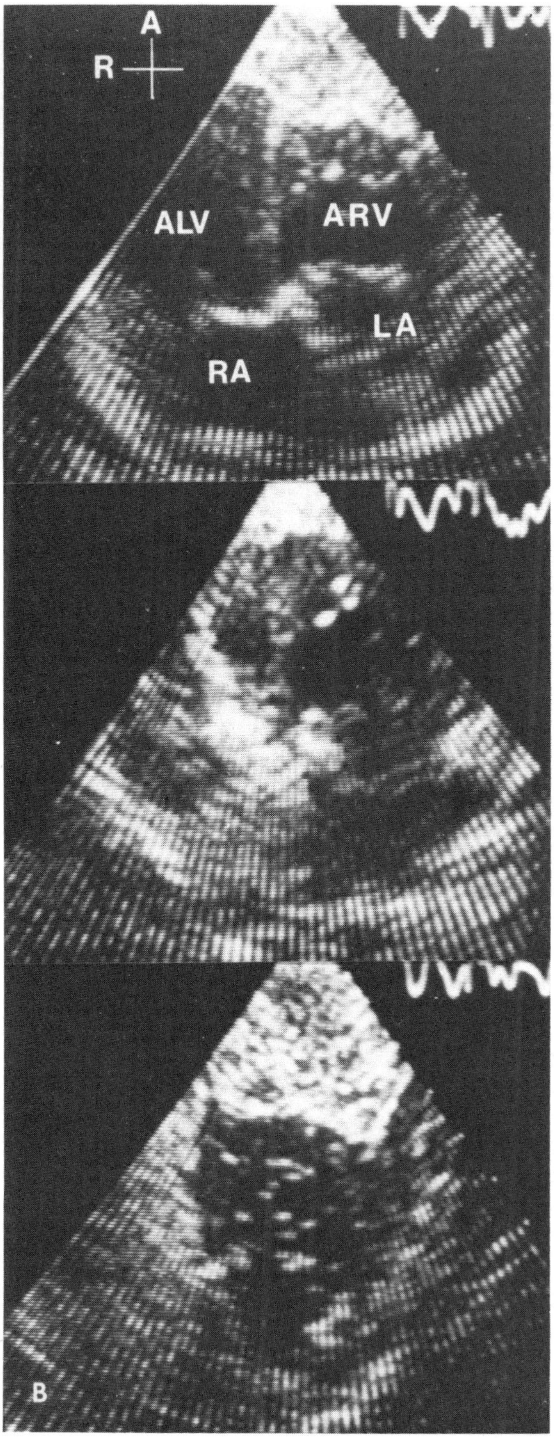

Figure 11. *A*, An apical four-chamber view from the left precordium in the usual position. The pulmonary veins (PV) are seen draining into the left-sided left atrium (LA), indicating situs solitus. The left-sided atrioventricular valve lies closer to the cardiac apex, and a prominent moderator band is present in the left-sided ventricle. The anatomic right ventricle (ARV) is therefore left-sided, and the anatomic left ventricle (ALV) is right-sided. The anatomic left ventricle is a smooth-walled ventricle with the atrioventricular valve being further from the cardiac apex, indicating this is a mitral valve. This patient, therefore, has discordant atrioventricular connections with situs solitus. Further examination of this patient led to the complete diagnosis of situs solitus, l-loop, and l-transposition. A: anterior, R: right, RA: right atrium. *B*, This shows a peripheral venous injection of contrast medium in the same patient. A: apex, ALV: anatomic left ventricle, ARV: anatomic right ventricle, LA: left atrium, R: right, RA: right atrium. In the second frame, contrast echoes fill the right-sided atrium, confirming the presence of situs solitus. In the third frame, a small right-to-left ventricular shunt can be seen.

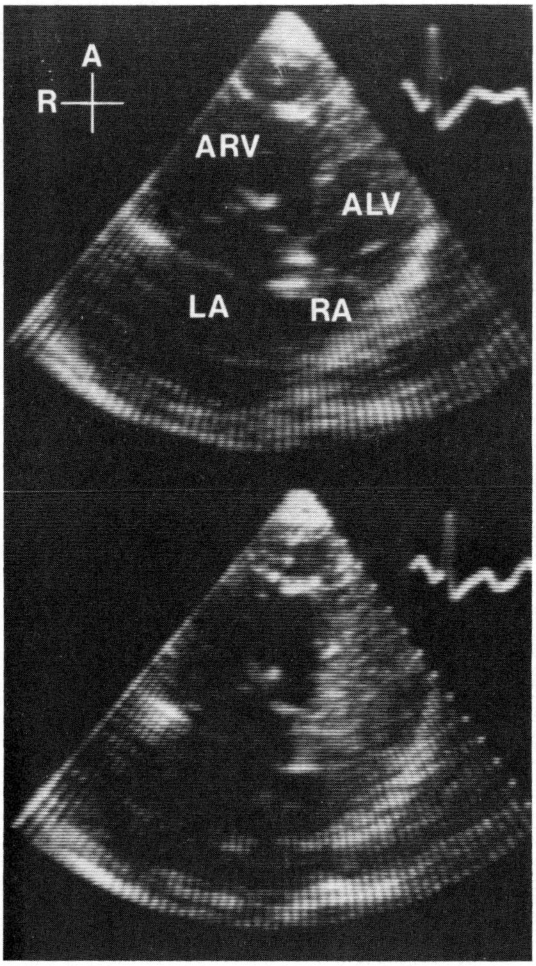

Figure 12. An apical four-chamber view obtained from the right parasternal area in the region of the midclavicular line. Note the left ventricle is smooth-walled, and the atrioventricular valve is further from the cardiac apex, indicating this is the anatomic left ventricle (ALV). The right-sided ventricle has a prominent moderator band and atrioventricular valve closer to the cardiac apex, defining it as the anatomic right ventricle (ARV). Atrial anatomy cannot be clearly defined, and contrast echocardiography was used to define the systemic venous flow patterns from a left-sided morphologic right atrium. Complete study demonstrated situs inversus, d-loop, and d-transposition. A: apex; LA: left atrium, R: right, RA: right atrium. (*From* Silverman NH, Snider AR: A segmental approach to the diagnosis of cardiac situs and malpositions. *In* Two-dimensional Echocardiography in Congenital Heart Disease. Norwalk, Appleton-Century-Crofts, 1982, pp. 229–245, with permission.)

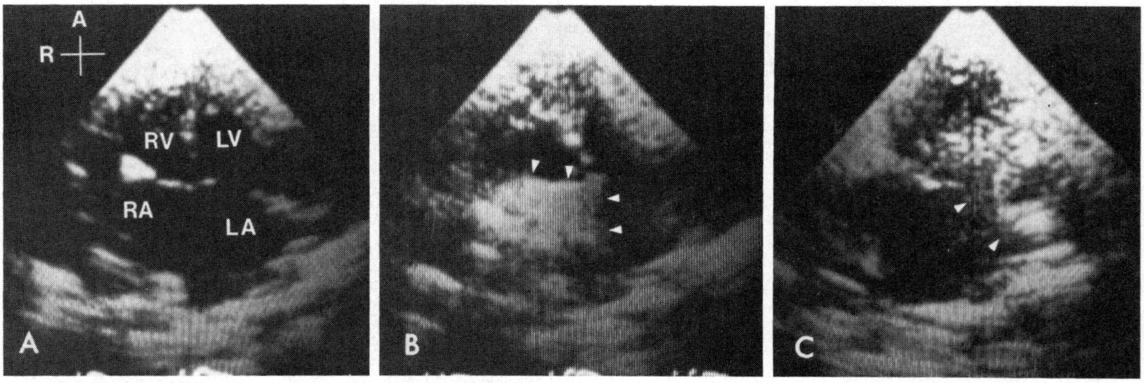

Figure 13. *A*, Apical four-chamber view from a patient with polysplenia syndrome and a common atrium. A: apex, LA: left-sided atrium, LV: left ventricle, R: right, RA: right-sided atrium, RV: right ventricle. *B*, An injection of contrast medium into a vein in the right arm fills the RA, confirming the presence of a right superior vena cava draining to the RA. *C*, An injection of contrast medium into a vein in the left arm fills the LA, confirming the presence of a left superior vena cava draining directly to the LA. (*From* Silverman NH, Snider AR: A segmental approach to the diagnosis of cardiac situs and malpositions. *In* Two-dimensional Echocardiography in Congenital Heart Disease. Norwalk, Appleton-Century-Crofts, 1982, pp. 229–245, with permission.)

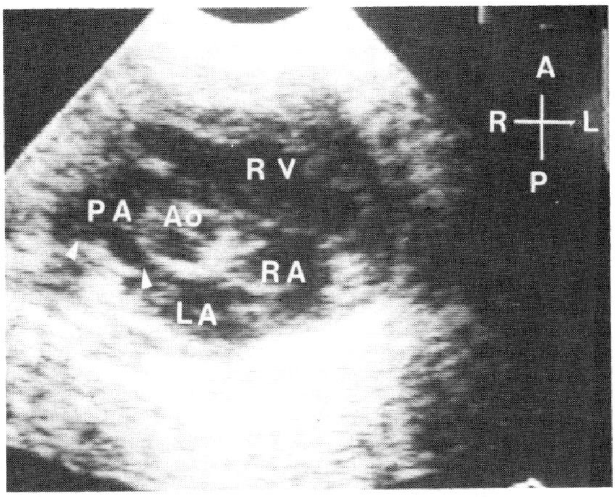

Figure 14. Parasternal short-axis view in a newborn infant with situs inversus. The orientation of the transducer was appropriate, and laterality was not distorted. The right ventricular outflow tract winds from the body of the right ventricle (RV) to a right-sided pulmonary artery (PA), which can be seen to bifurcate. The right atrium is left-sided, and the left atrium is right-sided. A: anterior, L: left, P: posterior, R: right.

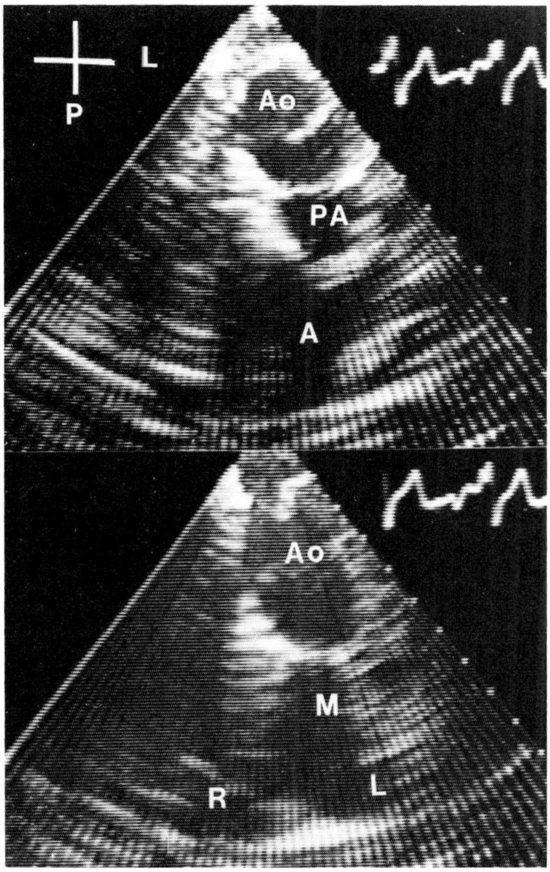

Figure 15. Parasternal short-axis projection in a patient with transposition of the great arteries. The aorta (Ao) is anterior and to the right, the pulmonary artery (PA) posterior and to the left. The left atrium (A) can be seen posterior to the pulmonary artery. With slight cranial angulation, the bifurcation of the posterior vessel from the main pulmonary artery (M) into its right (R) and left (L) branches can be seen. This defines the posterior vessel as a pulmonary artery. L: left, P: posterior.

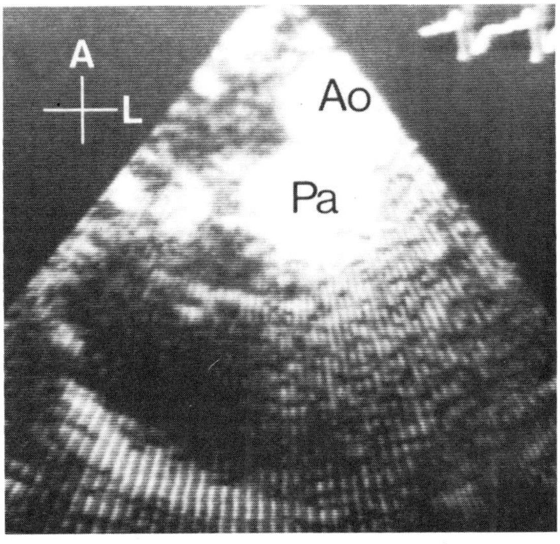

Figure 16. A parasternal short-axis plane taken at the level of the great vessels in a patient with l-transposition and single ventricle. The aorta (Ao) and pulmonary artery (Pa) fill simultaneously from the peripheral venous injection of contrast medium. The position with the aorta anterior and to the left and the pulmonary artery posterior and to the right can be defined. A: anterior, L: left. (*From* Silverman NH, Snider AR: A segmental approach to the diagnosis of cardiac situs and malpositions. *In* Two-dimensional Echocardiography in Congenital Heart Disease. Norwalk, Appleton-Century-Crofts, 1982, pp. 229–245, with permission.)

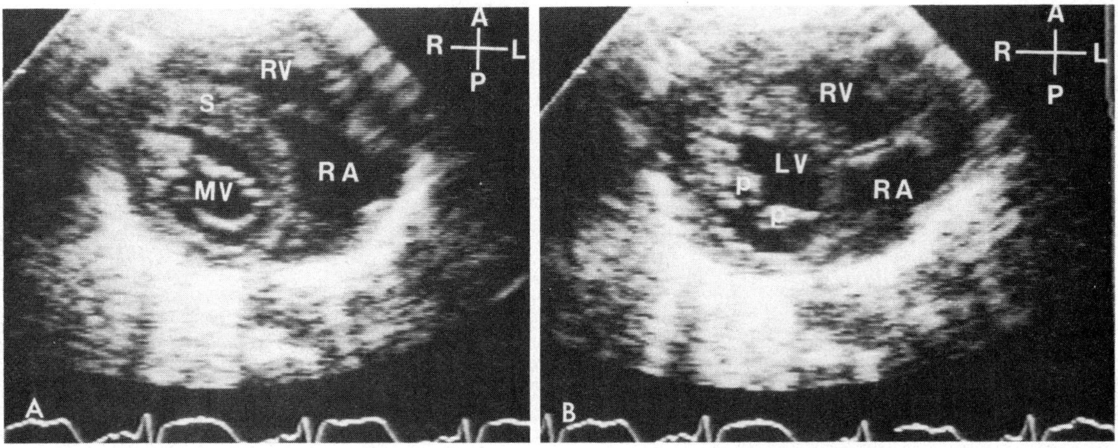

Figure 17. *A* and *B*, Parasternal short-axis planes in a neonate with situs inversus. *A* is at the level of the mitral valve (MV) and *B* at the level of the papillary muscles (p). A: anterior, L: left, P: posterior, R: right. In this patient, the right ventricle is left-sided, and the morphologic left ventricle, which has the characteristic morphologic features of the left ventricle, is a right-sided structure. RA: right atrium, RV: right ventricle.

17). The two papillary muscles of the left ventricle are readily defined. In addition, the mitral valve is a bicommissural valve with a characteristic "fish-mouth" appearance. These two features characterize the left ventricle whether it is found to the left or right of the right ventricle. In complex anomalies, the characteristic features of the ventricles may be difficult to define in this view.

THE PARASTERNAL LONG-AXIS PLANE

This plane provides little information about cardiac situs but establishes ventriculoarterial connections and relations. An attempt should first be made to obtain the standard parasternal long-axis view with the plane oriented between the left hip and right shoulder. If the parasternal long-axis view cannot be obtained in this plane, there may be some form of malposition.

Several other transducer positions should be tried in an attempt to image the long-axis view. The transducer can be placed in the right side of the chest in a plane parallel to the standard long-axis plane. This technique is useful in patients with dextroposition (heart shifted to the right because of pulmonary disease), where the long axis of the heart lies parallel to the normal long axis with the plane oriented from the right shoulder to the left hip but found at the right of the sternum. In patients with situs inversus and dextrocardia, the long-axis view is obtained from the right side of the sternum in a plane oriented between the right hip and left shoulder (the mirror image of the standard long-axis plane). Under this circumstance, it is helpful to examine the patient in a right lateral decubitus position. In transposition of the great arteries, the long-axis plane is oriented slightly more vertically than usual because the pulmonary artery is positioned more leftward than in the normal heart.

In malpositions in which the heart is retrosternal or the ventricles and great vessels have a complex arrangement, it may not be possible to obtain a recognizable long-axis view. These complex spatial arrangements may lead to unusual appearances of the cardiac chambers in this view.

THE SUPRASTERNAL PLANES

The suprasternal long-axis view defines the ascending, transverse, and descending aorta. The usual plane runs from the right nipple to the tip of the angle of the left scapula. When the aortic arch is right-sided, the examiner has to rotate the plane counterclockwise until the entire aortic arch can be imaged.[9] The degree of rotation can range between 30 to 90°. The plane in which the aortic arch is imaged should be noted because it cannot be determined by viewing the recorded image. Occasionally, the suprasternal long-axis view of the aortic arch can be obtained from the infraclavicular area from the lateral cardiac margin. This frequently occurs in transposition complexes.

In the suprasternal long-axis plane, the bronchial-pulmonary artery relationships help define the body situs (Fig. 18).[5, 9, 13] The right pulmonary artery is circular, and the right mainstem bronchus, an eparterial bronchus, intercedes

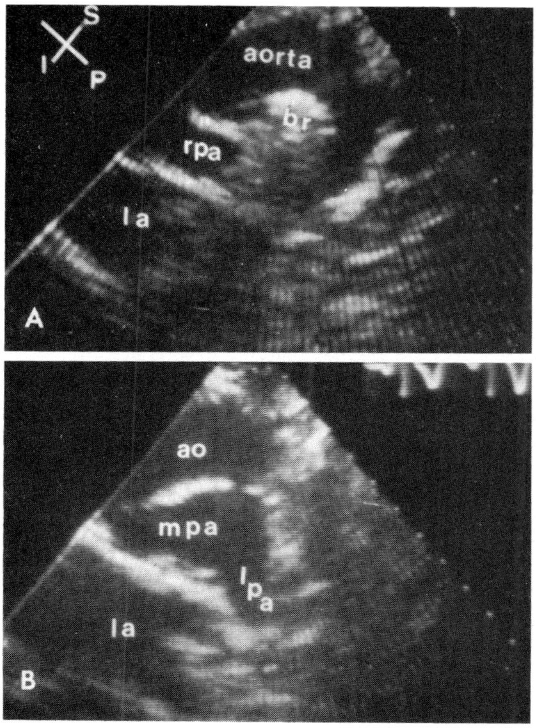

Figure 18. Suprasternal notch, long-axis plane in a normal patient. *A*, The transducer is in the standard position, oriented from the angle of the left scapula to the right nipple. The aorta can be seen arching over the right pulmonary artery (rpa) and bronchus (br). The left atrium can be seen posteriorly. When the transducer is tilted to the left, part of the aorta, the main pulmonary artery (mpa) and left pulmonary artery (lpa) can be seen. The right pulmonary artery has the bronchus in an eparterial position, whereas in *B*, the left pulmonary artery demonstrates no interposition of the bronchus between it and the aorta. These features define the morphologic right and left pulmonary arteries.

between the pulmonary artery and the aortic arch.[9] When the transducer is oriented towards the left from the suprasternal long-axis view, the pulmonary artery appears as a comma-shaped structure. The circular portion is the main pulmonary artery, and the tail is the left pulmonary artery (see Fig. 18). No bronchial tissue intercedes between the left pulmonary artery and the aorta because the left bronchus is a hyparterial structure. In conditions with abnormal situs, diminished pulmonary blood flow, and distortion of the pulmonary artery anatomy, these bronchial-pulmonary artery relations are less helpful for defining the atrial situs.

In the suprasternal short-axis plane (Fig. 19), the spatial position of the superior vena cava can be established, and its connection to the anatomic right atrium defined. This connection can be confirmed by contrast echocardiography.

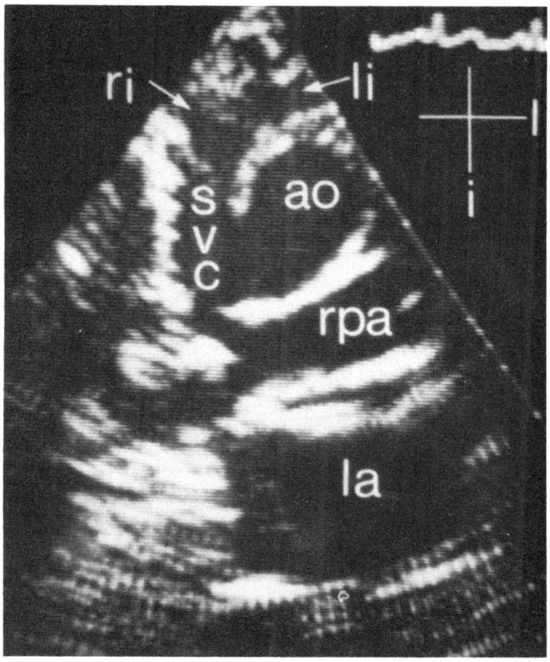

Figure 19. A normal example of the anatomic relationships in the suprasternal notch short-axis plane. i: inferior, l: left. Note that the left innominate (li) courses anterior to the aorta to join with the right innominate vein (ri) to form the superior vena cava (svc), which courses inferiorly to the right of the aorta (ao). The right pulmonary artery (rpa) can be seen to bifurcate into its main branches from a left-sided main pulmonary artery. The left atrium is defined posterior to the pulmonary artery.

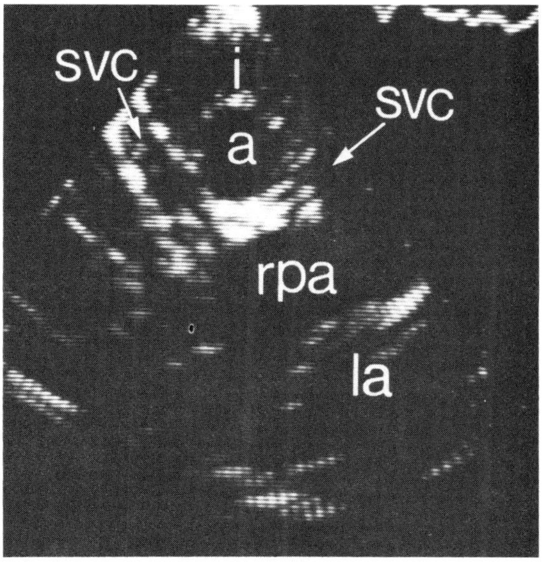

Figure 20. Suprasternal short-axis view from a patient with situs ambiguus and bilateral superior venae cavae (svc). Note the innominate vein joining the venae cavae. a: aorta, la: left atrium, rpa: right pulmonary artery. (*From* Silverman NH, Snider AR: A segmental approach to the diagnosis of cardiac situs and malpositions. *In* Two-dimensional Echocardiography in Congenital Heart Disease. Norwalk, Appleton-Century-Crofts, 1982, pp. 229–245, with permission.)

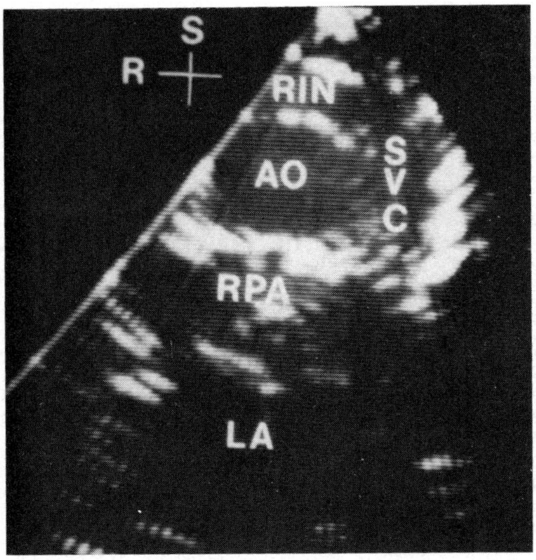

Figure 21. Suprasternal short-axis plane from a patient with situs inversus. The right innominate vein (RIN) can be seen joining the superior vena cava (SVC) to the left of the aorta (AO). The pulmonary artery can be identified posterior to the aorta. The right pulmonary artery (RPA) arises from the main pulmonary artery on the right and passes toward the left. The left atrium (LA) can be observed posterior to the pulmonary artery. R, right; S, superior. (*From* Silverman NH, Snider AR: A segmental approach to the diagnosis of cardiac situs and malpositions. *In* Two-dimensional Echocardiography in Congenital Heart Disease. Norwalk, Appleton-Century-Crofts, 1982, pp. 229–245, with permission.)

Table 2. *Step-by-Step Approach to Situs and Malposition Problems*

NORMAL SITUS	SITUS AMBIGUUS	SITUS INVERSUS
Subcostal abdominal views		
Abdominal aorta left, inferior vena cava right.	Aorta and inferior vena cava on same side. Inferior vena cava interrupted = polysplenial left isomerism.	Abdominal aorta right, inferior vena cava left.
Subostal four-chamber view		
Apex left and proceed with left apical and parasternal examination. Pulmonary veins to left atrium.	Apex central, continue subcostal examination or right parasternal examination of cardiac chambers and great vessels. Anomalous or indeterminate pulmonary venous drainage. Associated defects.	Apex right, proceed with right-sided apical and parasternal examination Pulmonary veins to right-sided atrium.
Subcostal short-axis view		
Eustachian valve in right-sided atrium, define right atrium as right-sided structure. Superior vena cava and inferior vena cava to right-sided atrium.		Eustachian valve in left-sided atrium, define right atrium as left-sided structure. Superior vena cava and inferior vena cava to left-sided atrium.
Apical four-chamber view		
Moderator band in right-sided ventricle. Tricuspid valve closed to apex, then mitral valve, trabeculations.	Associated defects	Reversed: Moderator band in left-sided ventricle, tricuspid valve closer to apex than mitral valve.
Suprasternal—long-axis view		
Aortic arch to left, identify pulmonary artery, bronchial relationships. Pulmonary artery separated from aorta by bronchus, right = right pulmonary artery.	Indeterminate pulmonary artery anatomy	Aortic arch to right. Pulmonary artery separated from aorta by bronchus on left = right pulmonary artery = situs inversus.
Suprasternal notch—short-axis view		
Pulmonary artery horizontal to right from a left-sided main pulmonary artery. Super vena cava on right from left innominate vein.	Double superior vena cava. Pulmonary anatomy difficult to define.	Pulmonary artery horizontal to left from a right-sided main pulmonary artery. Superior vena cava on left from right innominate vein.
Atrial situs by contrast echocardiography		
Contrast study defines systemic atrium (right-sided).	Injections of contrast medium into veins of left and right arm draining to each atrium.	Defines systemic venous atrium (left-sided).

Bilateral superior venae cavae, especially common in patients with situs ambiguus, can be identified from the suprasternal short-axis view (Fig. 20). In the normal patient, the right pulmonary artery in the suprasternal short-axis plane can be seen from its junction with the main pulmonary artery to its branches in the right lung. In situs inversus, the longitudinal course of the right pulmonary artery from the main pulmonary artery to the right hilum is reversed. Also, the innominate veins join to form the superior vena cava on the left side of the aorta (Fig. 21).

SUGGESTED ECHOCARDIOGRAPHIC APPROACH TO SITUS PROBLEMS

When the echocardiographic examination suggests ectopic position or possibly abnormal situs (Table 2), it is suggested that the examination proceed directly to the subcostal position because the cardiac position can be best defined from this position. The position of the cardiac apex can be seen from the chamber plane, the position of the inferior vena cavan and aorta can be defined, and the inferior vena cava can be traced to the morphologic right atrium. From this plane, the examination can proceed to the apical, parasternal, and suprasternal locations.

REFERENCES

1. Bierman FZ, Williams RG: Subxyphoid two-dimensional imaging of the interatrial septum in infants and neonates with congenital heart disease. Circulation, 60:80–90, 1979.
2. Lange LW, Sahn DJ, Allen HD, et al: Subxyphoid cross-sectional echocardiography in infant's and children with congenital heart disease. Circulation, 59:513–524, 1979.
3. Meyer RA, Schwartz DC, Covitz W, et al: Echocardiographic assessment of cardiac malposition. Am J Cardiol, *33*:896–903, 1974.
4. Mortera C, Hunter S, Terry G, et al: Echocardiography of primitive ventricle. Br Heart J, *39*:847–855, 1977.
5. Partridge JB, Scott O, Deverall PB, et al: Visualization and measurement of the main bronchi by tomography as an objective indicator of thoracic situs in congenital heart disease. Circulation, *51*:188–196, 1975.
6. Rose V, Izukawa T, Moes CAF: Syndromes of asplenia and polysplenia. Br Heart J, *37*:840–852, 1975.
7. Silverman NH, Snider AR: A segmental approach to the diagnosis of cardiac situs and malpositions. *In* Two-dimensional Echocardiography in Congenital Heart Disease. Norwalk, Appleton-Century-Crofts, 1982, pp. 229–245.
8. Silverman NH, Snider AR, Colo J: A segmental approach to the diagnosis of congenital heart disease: The usefulness of two-dimensional echocardiography. *In* Hunter S, Hall R (eds): Echocardiography. I. Edinburgh, Churchill Livingstone, 1982, pp. 165–191.
9. Snider AR, Silverman NH: Suprasternal notch echocardiography: A two-dimensional technique for evaluating congenital heart disease. Circulation, *63*:165–173, 1981.
10. Solinger R, Elbl F, Minhas K: Deductive echocardiographic analysis in infants with congenital heart disease. Circulation, *50*:1072–1096, 1974.
11. Stanger P, Rudolph AM, Edwards JE: Cardiac malpositions: An overview based on a study of sixty-five necropsy specimens. Circulation, *52*:159–172, 1977.
12. Tynan J, Becker AE, Macartney FJ, et al: Nomenclature and classification of congenital heart disease. Br Heart J, *41*:544–553, 1979.
13. Van Mierop LHS, Eisen S, Schiebler GL: The radiologic appearance of the tracheobronchial tree as an indicator of visceral situs. Am J Cardiol, *26*:432–436, 1970.
14. Van Praagh R, Weinberg PW, Van Praach S: Malpositions of the heart. *In* Moss AJ, Adams FH, Emmanouilides GC (eds): Heart Disease in Infants, Children, and Adolescents. Baltimore, Williams and Wilkins, 1977, pp. 394–417.

12

FETAL ECHOCARDIOGRAPHY

A Technique and its Applications

NORMAN H. SILVERMAN, M.D.

INTRODUCTION

Several recent papers on fetal echocardiography attest to its usefulness in prenatal diagnosis.[1–3, 9–11, 14, 16, 18] Two-dimensional echocardiography, M-mode echocardiography, and pulsed Doppler ultrasound all can be used for defining structural heart defects, for following cardiac development in utero, for defining fetal cardiac arrhythmias, and for determining blood flow patterns. The state-of-the-art instrument for fetal echocardiographic diagnosis, therefore, is one that combines all these ultrasound modalities.

MODALITIES OF ULTRASOUND USED FOR FETAL CARDIAC EXAMINATION

Two-Dimensional Echocardiography

Sector-shaped and linear (rectangular) formats each offer their own particular advantages and disadvantages. The sector format shows larger fields of view as the distance from the transducer increases. Unfortunately, as the scan lines diverge with the increasing depth, there is also less actual ultrasound information available for analysis, regardless of the addition of electronic smoothing techniques. The sector format is useful for examining the fetus when there is a limited ultrasound field of view because of the fetal lie within the pelvis or lower abdomen. It is also advantageous when images are generated from the abdomen and are not obscured by rib or vertebral shadows. The linear array systems, which use a rectangular format, offer the same resolution throughout the field of view. In our experience, the linear array transducer is slightly easier to manipulate than the sector transducer, but adequate information can be obtained with either type of apparatus.

The transducer frequency is best centered at 3.5 mHz, as the lower frequencies lead to poorer resolution of structures and the higher frequency transducers do not have adequate powers of penetration for any but the very smallest of fetuses.

M-Mode Echocardiography

Although M-mode echocardiography has been performed as an isolated technique with a single-crystal apparatus, we have abandoned it in favor of performing M-mode recordings directly from a two-dimensional sector scanner. The M-mode must be of high resolution in order to yield diagnostic information. The simultaneous use of M-mode and two-dimensional echocardiography diminishes the amount of time spent with each technique, as structures can be more accurately validated (Fig. 1).

Doppler Ultrasound

When range-gated pulsed Doppler ultrasound with full spectral output is displayed with simultaneous two-dimensional and M-mode images, it further augments diagnostic ability by providing data on blood flow velocity, direction, and turbulence (Figs. 2 and 3). For quantitative analysis, a pulsed Doppler system with a spec-

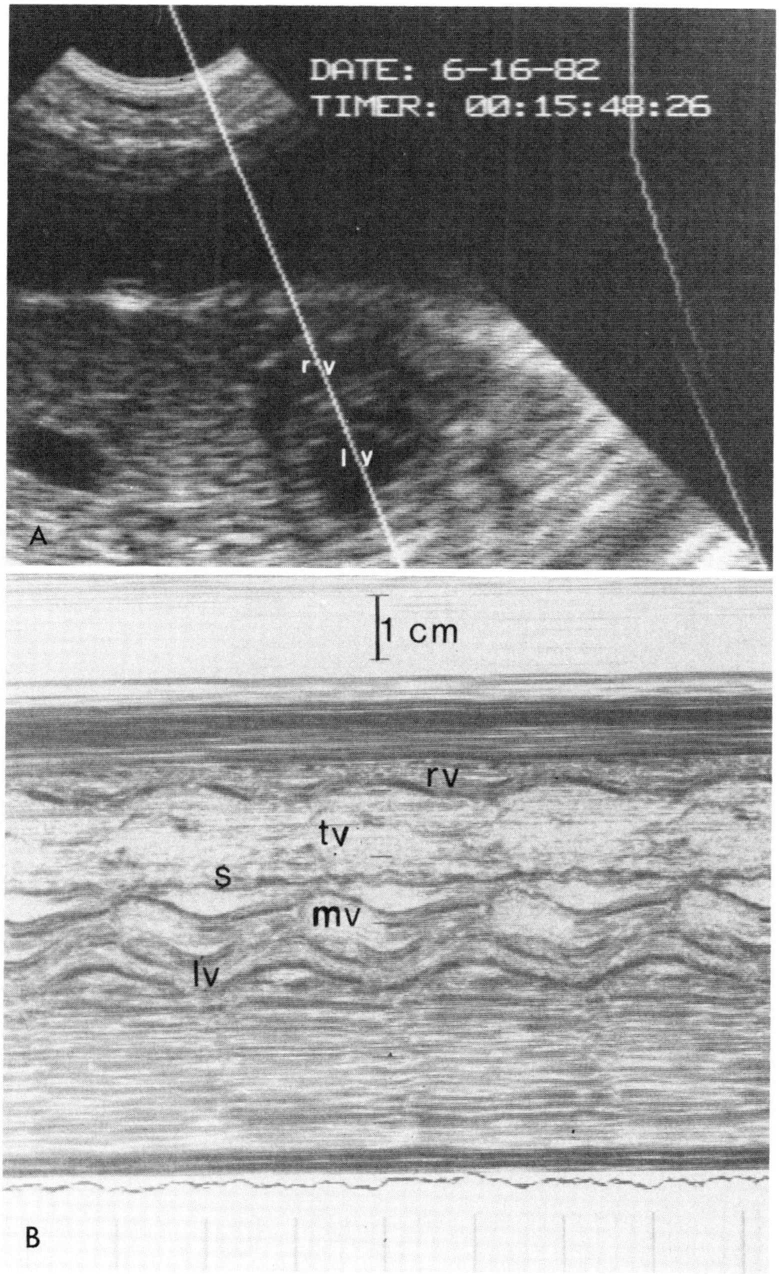

Figure 1. *A*, A short-axis projection through the fetal right ventricle (rv) and left ventricle (lv) in a fetus of 30 weeks' gestation. The M-mode line is passing through the center of the ventricles in the position suitable for recording an M-mode echocardiogram. The scale marker with centimeter and half-centimeter marks is indicated on the right. *B*, The M-mode showing the resulting M-mode echocardiogram from this normal 30-week-old fetus. The 1-cm marker is displayed, and the paper speed markers are 0.2 sec apart for the large markers and 0.04 sec apart for the small markers. The paper speed was run at 100 mm per sec.

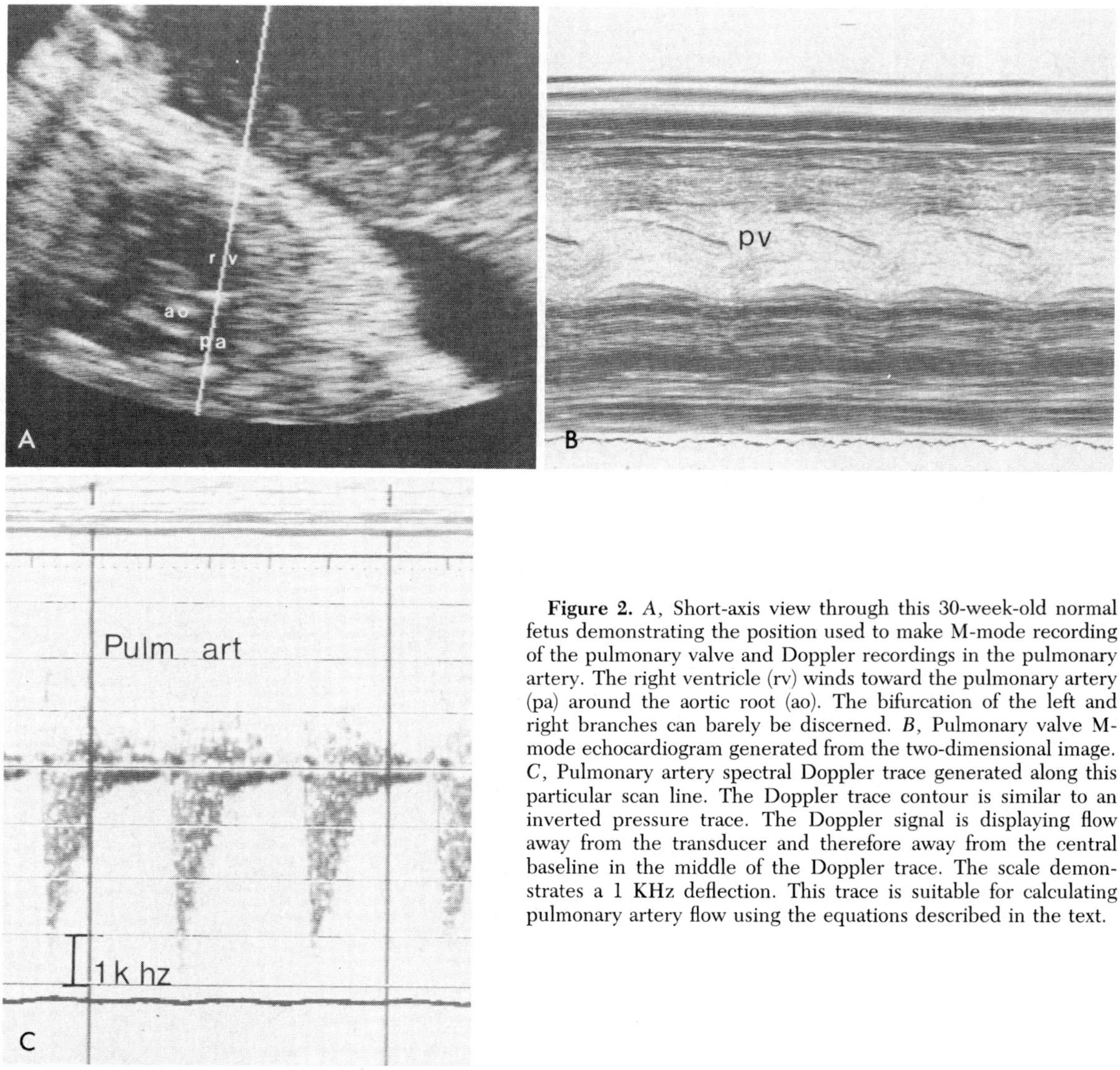

Figure 2. *A*, Short-axis view through this 30-week-old normal fetus demonstrating the position used to make M-mode recording of the pulmonary valve and Doppler recordings in the pulmonary artery. The right ventricle (rv) winds toward the pulmonary artery (pa) around the aortic root (ao). The bifurcation of the left and right branches can barely be discerned. *B*, Pulmonary valve M-mode echocardiogram generated from the two-dimensional image. *C*, Pulmonary artery spectral Doppler trace generated along this particular scan line. The Doppler trace contour is similar to an inverted pressure trace. The Doppler signal is displaying flow away from the transducer and therefore away from the central baseline in the middle of the Doppler trace. The scale demonstrates a 1 KHz deflection. This trace is suitable for calculating pulmonary artery flow using the equations described in the text.

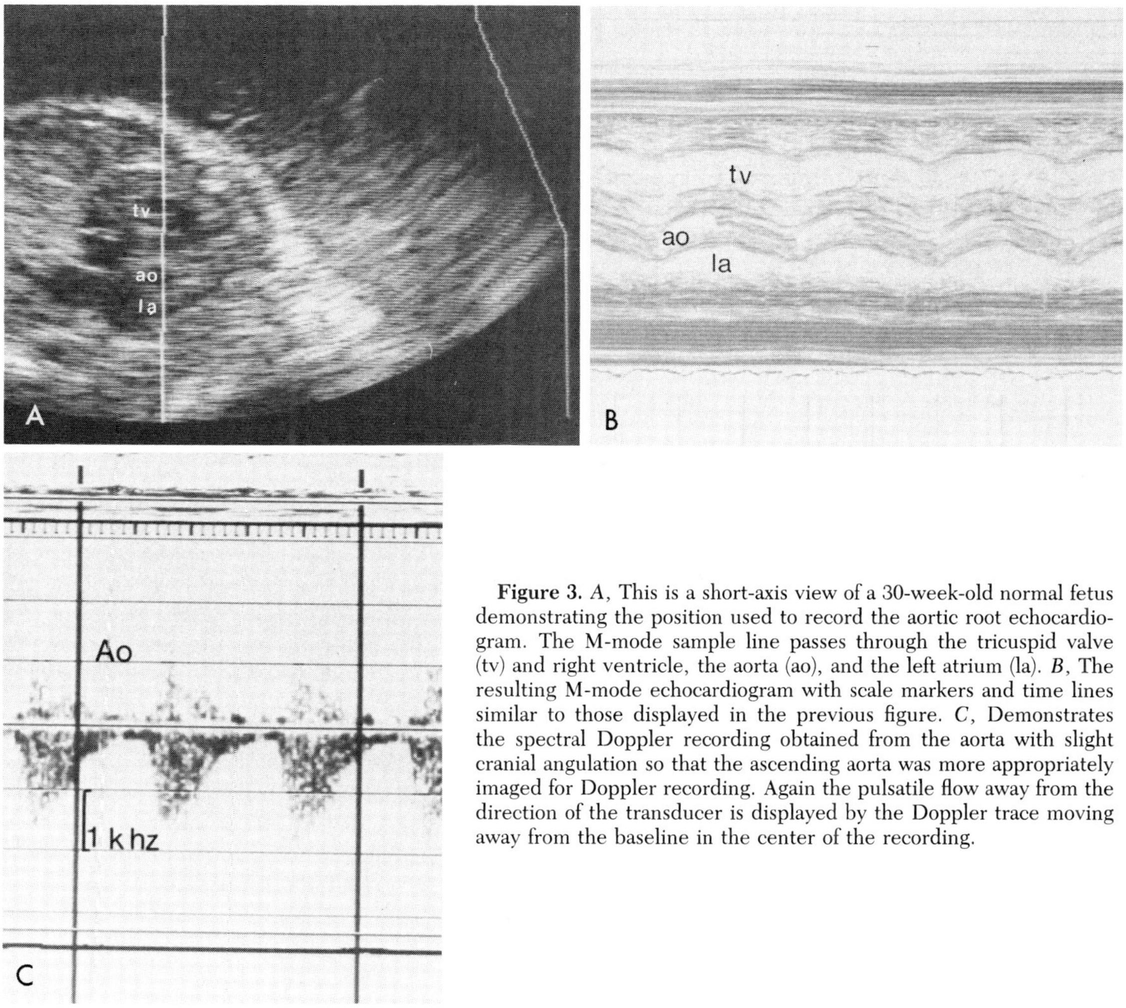

Figure 3. *A*, This is a short-axis view of a 30-week-old normal fetus demonstrating the position used to record the aortic root echocardiogram. The M-mode sample line passes through the tricuspid valve (tv) and right ventricle, the aorta (ao), and the left atrium (la). *B*, The resulting M-mode echocardiogram with scale markers and time lines similar to those displayed in the previous figure. *C*, Demonstrates the spectral Doppler recording obtained from the aorta with slight cranial angulation so that the ascending aorta was more appropriately imaged for Doppler recording. Again the pulsatile flow away from the direction of the transducer is displayed by the Doppler trace moving away from the baseline in the center of the recording.

tral output generated from a fast Fourier transform is preferable. To date there are two different techniques for generating pulsed Doppler with two-dimensional echocardiograms. The first uses a pulsed Doppler generated from a transducer within the sector fan; the second employs an offset Doppler mounted at the side of a linear array. This offset creates an angle that can be calculated between the Doppler transducer and the array so that accurate velocity measurements can be derived by using the Doppler equation. Flow can be calculated from Doppler flow signals from the following equation:

$$V = \frac{Fc}{2FoCos\ \theta}$$

where F is ultrasound frequency shift, Fo is frequency of the transmitted ultrasound (e.g., 3.0 MHz), c is that velocity of the sound medium (1540 m/sec) and θ is the angle of incidence between the Doppler sound beam and the direction of flow. Doppler flow measurements ($\dot{Q}$) are derived from the equation

$$\dot{Q}\ \text{ml/min} = V \times A\ \text{cm}^2 \times 60$$

where V is the mean velocity per cycle and A is the cross sectional area of the aorta derived from measurement of vessel diameter.

TECHNIQUE FOR ECHOCARDIOGRAPHIC IMAGING IN UTERO

The initial part of the examination is performed to localize the fetal position. The head and body are defined, and the gestational age is assessed by biparietal and chest circumferential measurements. The fetal lie and position are noted. If the fetus is lying with its back situated closer to the maternal abdominal wall, it may be necessary to rotate the mother onto either side so that the vertebral column and ribs are not directly in front of the heart because they absorb a considerable amount of the sound energy, thereby diminishing the acuity of the cardiac image. If this maneuver fails, the mother is asked to walk around for a few minutes in order to attempt to change the fetal position. It is best to obtain images of the heart through the fetal abdomen because they are of much higher quality than those obtained either through the precordium or from the back, where rib and bone shadows obscure the image. The echocardiographic "window" for examining the fetal heart is rather limited if these criteria are accepted. Because the transducer is some distance away from the heart, even slight transducer movements of a few degrees are likely to cause the scan field to pass out of the area where the heart is located. The examiner must exercise care to maintain the transducer position. It is, however, possible to perform examinations from the posterior aspect of the fetus. The images are then situated in an inverted position from those normally seen when ultrasound images are generated either in utero or postnatally. When recordings are obtained through the back, the M-mode is displayed upside down relative to conventional display. These can be oriented in a normal position by holding the paper upside down and viewing the image in a mirror. When one is accustomed to reviewing the image in the upside-down orientation, it becomes as easy to read as the conventional M-mode image.

Satisfactory diagnostic ultrasound images of the fetal heart are possible from as early as 14 to 16 weeks of gestation, but in our experience reasonable accuracy is possible only after this time. The preferred time for examination is from 18 weeks of gestational age onward. We have concentrated on fetuses of this age in the hope of determining cardiac defects for the purpose of genetic counseling. Generally, the most satisfactory resolution is achieved at 20 or more weeks of gestation; we attempt to perform at least one examination in this gestational period. It is important that, when studies are of substandard quality, they be repeated within two to three weeks to ensure adequate examination.

A number of echocardiographic views can be obtained in the fetus. The planes of examination described further on refer to the axis of the heart and not to the axis of the plane relative to the body planes. We attempt to obtain equivalents of four-chamber, short-axis, and long-axis views in each fetal study. To obtain the four-chamber view, we attempt primarily to identify the abdomen and liver. The umbilical cord is traced to the area of the umbilical vein and then from the liver toward the heart (Fig. 4). This allows a reference point from which the transducer is angled and moved slightly toward the heart in a cranial direction until the four-chamber view is displayed (Fig. 5). The four-chamber view is situated in a more horizontal plane than during the postnatal period because of the large liver.[2] In the four-chamber view, the two atrioventricular valves can be identified. The moderator band frequently can be identified within the right ventricular cavity. The right ventricle is usually slightly larger than

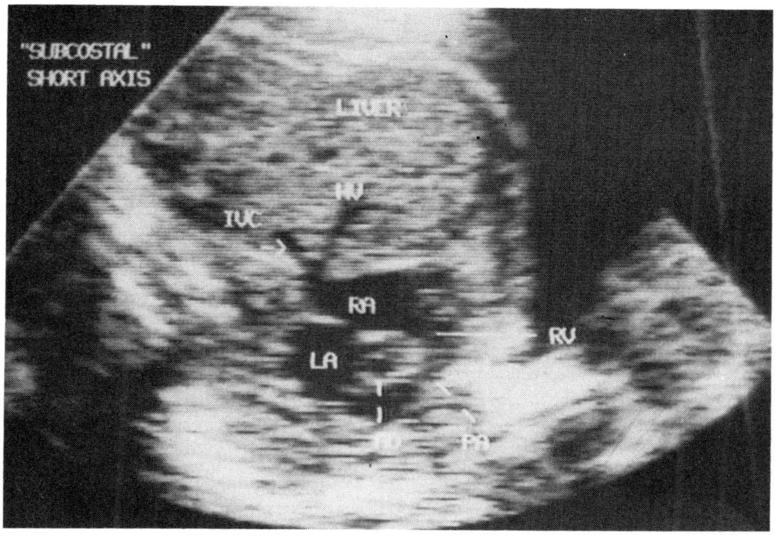

Figure 4. Subcostal short-axis view of a 22-week-old fetus demonstrating the fetus lying with its abdomen toward the transducer. The transducer plane passes from the liver through the heart. The hepatic vein (HV) and inferior vena cava (IVC) can be identified and are seen to enter the right atrium (RA). The right ventricle can be traced around the aorta (AO) and into the pulmonary artery (PA). The aortic valve can also be identified. The right atrium is separated from the left atrium by the atrial septum. The atrial septum appears to be open, with its flaplike motion.

the left ventricle.[16] The tricuspid valve is positioned slightly closer to the cardiac apex than is the mitral valve. The inferior vena cava usually can be traced to the right atrium by cephalad manipulation of the transducer (Fig. 4). The eustachian valve, which is prominent in the fetus, can often be identified within the right atrium. In addition, the valve of the foramen ovale is usually seen in the atrium toward the left side. The motion of the flap valve represents the phasic separation between the secundum and primum atrial septa (Fig. 6). Slight cephalad angulation and rotation from this plane bring the connection of the aortic valve and the left ventricle into view. The four-chamber view is useful for imaging ventricular septal defects, atrioventricular valve atresia, ventricular hypoplasia, univentricular hearts,

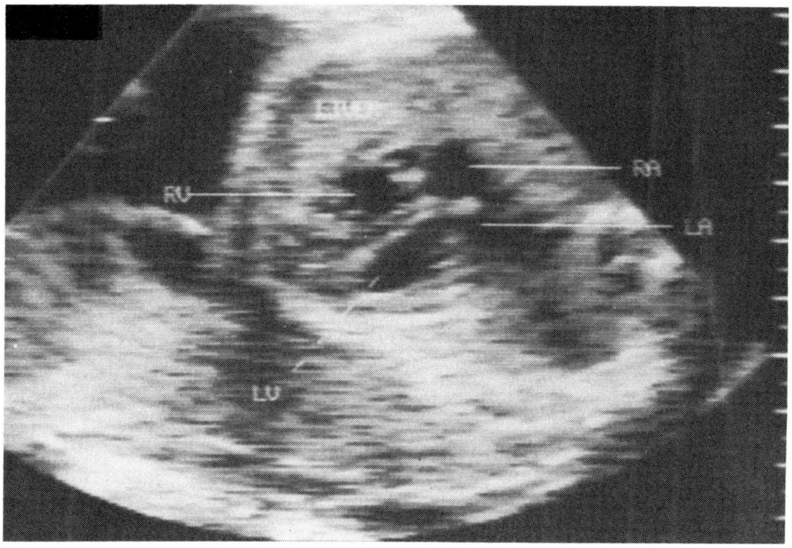

Figure 5. Four-chamber view of the same fetus shown in Figure 4 demonstrating the normal intracardiac anatomy. The beam is passed inferiorly through a portion of the liver through the right ventricle (RV) anteriorly and the left ventricle (LV) posteriorly. The moderator band echoes can be identified within the right ventricle underneath the arrow marker. Posteriorly the right and left atria (RA, LA) can be identified, and an area of drop-out can be identified in the region of the foramen ovale representing the patency present in utero.

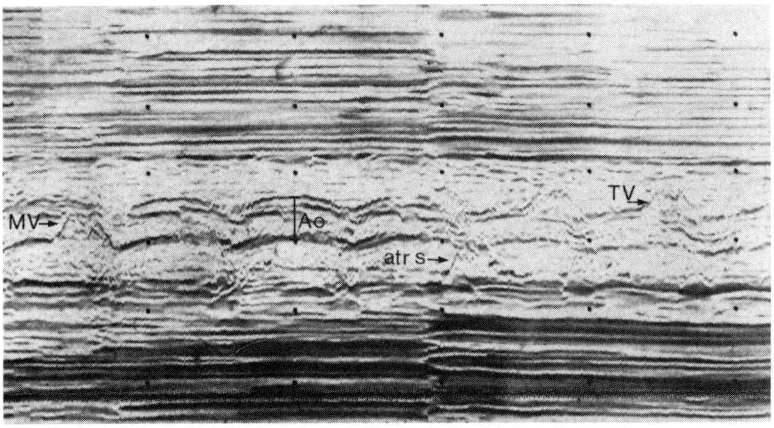

Figure 6. An M-mode scan in a 20-week-old fetus from the mitral valve (MV) through the aortic root (Ao) and toward the tricuspid valve (TV). When passing through the area of the atrial septum (atr s), a similar phasic motion representing the phasic flow across the atrial septum can be seen.

atrioventricular canal defects (Fig. 7), Ebstein's anomaly, and pericardial effusion (Fig. 8). In addition, this is an excellent view for performing M-mode echocardiography to define arrhythmias because a simultaneous M-mode produced from one of the scan lines can generate information regarding atrioventricular valve motion and atrial and ventricular contraction.

After a four-chamber view has been obtained, the transducer can be rotated and moved to obtain long-axis views. This is similar to the long-axis view obtained after birth except that a larger area can be seen because the heart is at a greater distance from the transducer than it is after birth (Fig. 9). This view shows the aortic valve and ascending aorta. Mitral aortic continuity and the size of the aortic root, left ventricle, and left atrium can be assessed. The view is useful for demonstrating pericardial effusion as well (Fig. 10).

With slight rotation toward the pulmonary valve, it is often possible to obtain long-axis projections of both the aorta and the pulmonary artery as they leave the heart and to define ventriculoarterial connections (Fig. 11). It is also possible with slight manipulation to define the entire aortic arch (Fig. 12). Potentially, coarctation and aortic atresia can be defined from this plane. It is important to bear in mind that normal isthmic narrowing, a prominent feature in utero, not be confused with coarctation of the aorta.[15]

With most patients the short-axis views, analogous to parasternal or subcostal plane images, can be obtained with slight manipulation of the transducer. The short-axis views are a series of

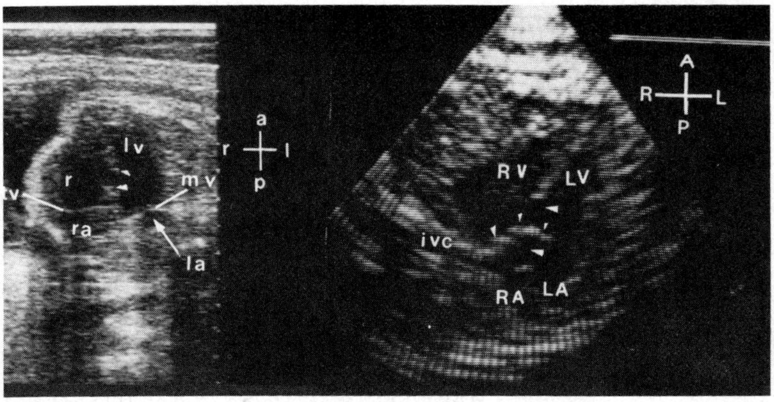

Figure 7. A linear scan on the left and a sector scan on the right demonstrating a ventricular septal defect. In the scan on the left-hand side, which was referred for opinion, a ventricular septal defect (arrowheads) can be identified. The right ventricle (r) and right atrium (ra) are much larger than the left ventricle (lv) and left atrium (la). The mitral valve (mv) and tricuspid valve (tv) can be seen. a: anterior; 1: left; p: posterior; r: right. The right panel demonstrates a sector scan performed in our division showing a fetus with a complete atrioventricular canal defect. A common atrioventricular leaflet (arrows) can be seen spanning the left ventricle (LV) and right ventricle (RV). A primum atrial septal defect (arrowhead) can be seen between the lower portions of the right atrium (RA) and the left atrium (LA). The right atrium is further identified by the presence of the inferior vena cava (ivc) draining into it. The ventricular septal defect is defined by an arrowhead.

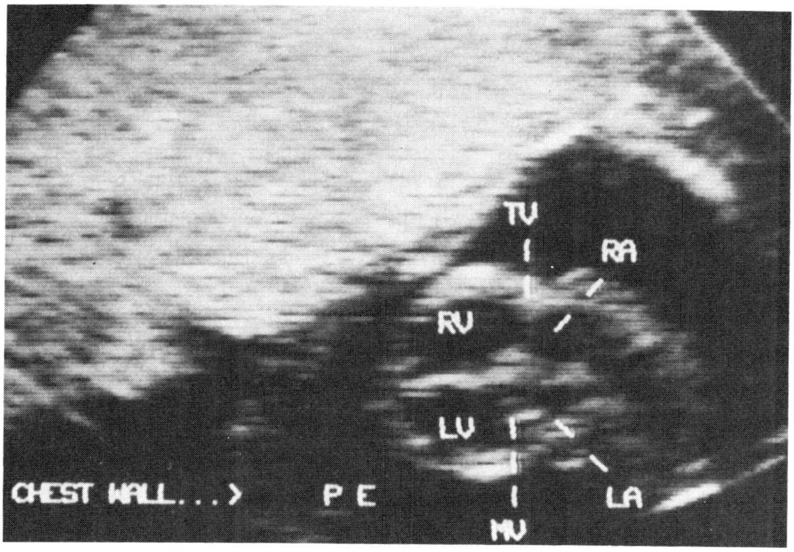

Figure 8. A four-chamber view in a fetus with nonimmune hydrops demonstrating normal intracardiac anatomy but with a massive pericardial effusion (PE) and pleural effusions surrounding the heart. The chest wall echo can be identified surrounding the heart effusions. LA: left atrium; LV: left ventricle; MV: mitral valve; RA: right atrium; RV: right ventricle; TV: tricuspid valve.

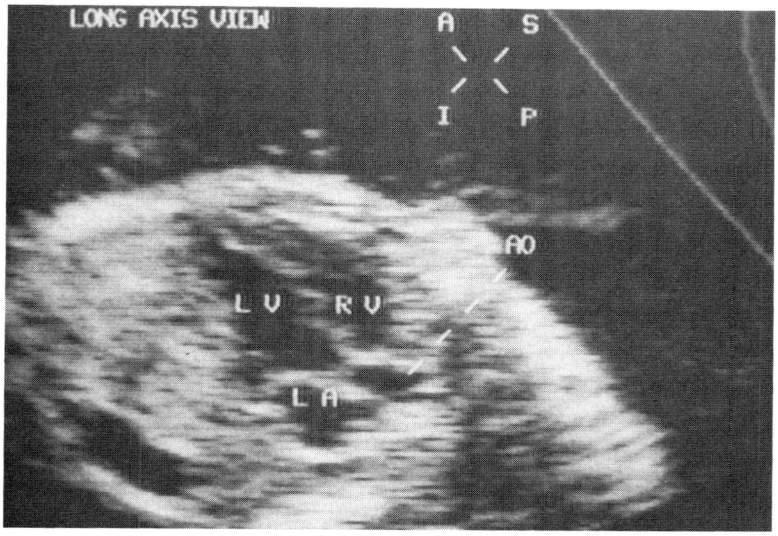

Figure 9. A long-axis view in a normal 22-week-old fetus demonstrating intracardiac anatomy. The left ventricle (LV) is separated from the left atrium (LA) by the mitral valve, and outflow can be traced into the aorta (AO) through the aortic valve. The right ventricle (RV) is situated anteriorly. A: anterior; I: inferior; P: posterior; S: superior.

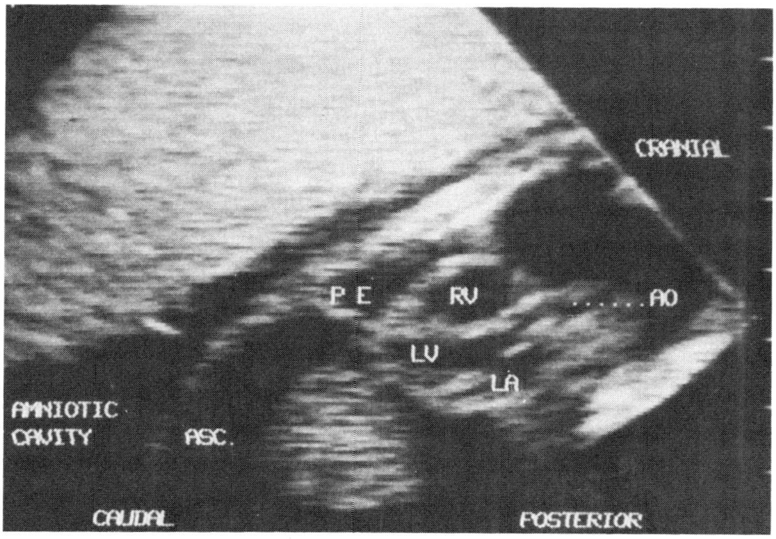

Figure 10. Pericardial effusion and ascites demonstrated in the same patient as shown in Figure 8. The fetus is noted to be hydropic with ascites (ASC) and a pericardial effusion (PE). The same anatomy as defined in the previous patient can be seen with a long section of a posterior sweeping aorta (AO).

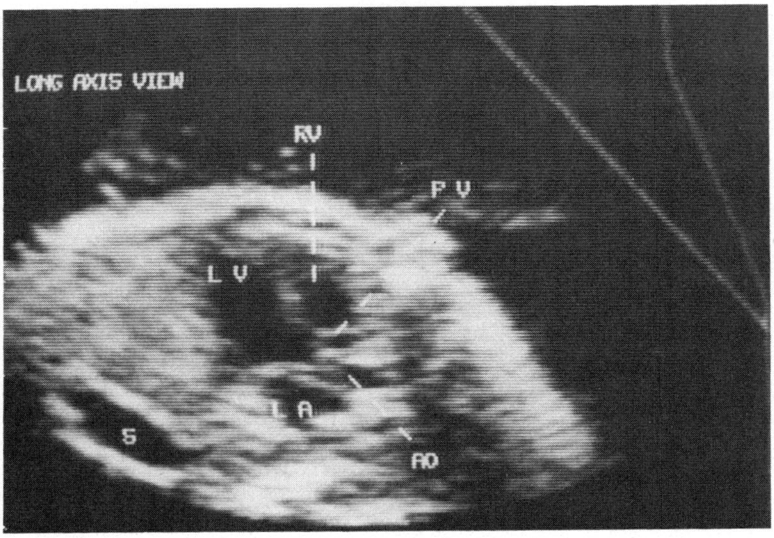

Figure 11. This is a long-axis scan from the same patient as demonstrated in Figure 9. Here the transducer was angled toward the left, demonstrating the pulmonic valve and a small portion of the pulmonary artery anteriorly. AO: aorta; LA: left atrium; LV: left ventricle; PV: pulmonic valve; RV: right ventricle; S: stomach.

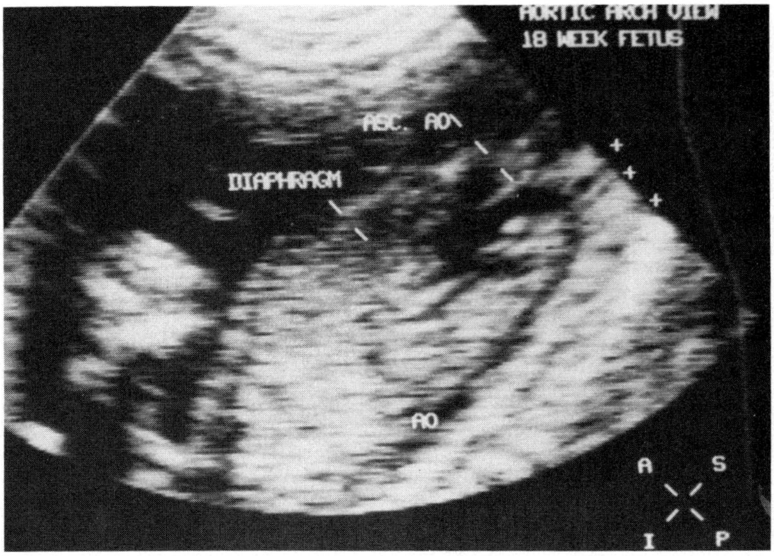

Figure 12. View of the aortic arch obtained from a long-axis plane in an 18-week-old fetus. In this example, the aortic arch from the ascending aorta (ASC AO) through to the descending aorta (AO) can be traced in its entirety to below the level of the diaphragm. The plus signs indicate the origin of the three vessels to the head and neck in normal sequence. A: anterior; I: inferior; P: posterior; S: superior.

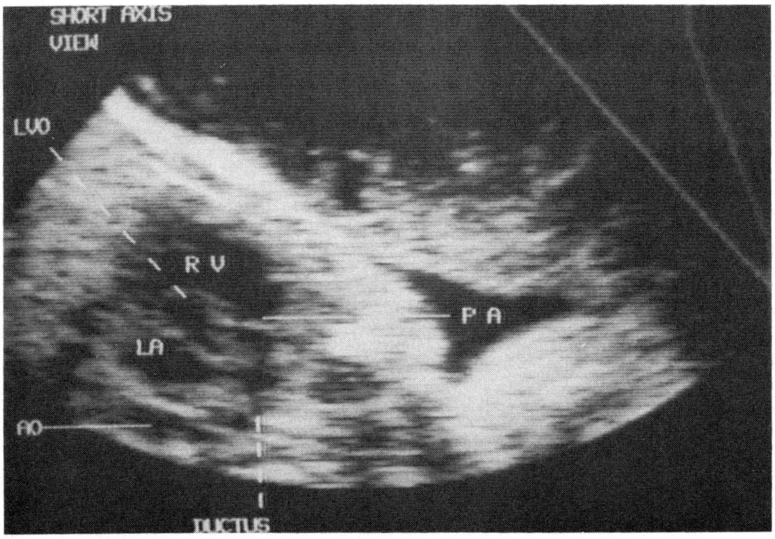

Figure 13. A parasternal short-axis view in the same patient as displayed in Figures 9 and 11 demonstrating the anatomy typically seen in the short-axis view. The circular left ventricle (LVO) can be seen in the center of the figure. The left atrium (LA) is situated posteriorly and the right ventricle (RV) anteriorly. The pulmonary artery (PA) is continuous with the ductus ateriosus and the descending aorta (AO).

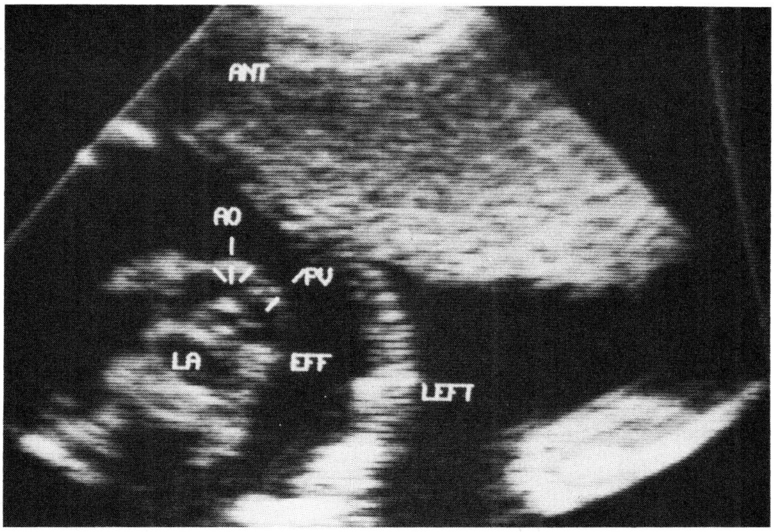

Figure 14. Short-axis view in the same fetus as shown in Figures 8 and 10 demonstrating a large pericardial effusion (EFF). The circular aorta (AO) can be seen toward the center of the field, and the pulmonic valve (PV) is situated to the left. The left atrium (LA) is defined behind the heart. Ant: anterior.

tomographic planes passing from the diaphragmatic surface of the heart from the apex of the ventricles through to the base of the heart. The most cephalad view shows the pulmonary artery and right ventricular outflow tract as they course around the aorta (Fig. 2*A*). The bifurcation of the pulmonary artery can be identified, although in the fetus the pulmonary branches are small. The ductus arteriosus and descending aorta can be seen (Fig. 13) and can be traced into the descending aorta. The aortic and pulmonic valves can be identified from this plane (Fig. 14). Theoretically, this tomographic plane affords the potential for differentiating transposition of the great arteries, pulmonic atresia, aortic atresia, double outlet right ventricle, and truncus arteriosus from normal anatomy. With caudad angulation from this plane, the ventricles and their respective atrioventricular valves can be identified (Fig. 1*A*).

INDICATIONS FOR FETAL ECHOCARDIOGRAPHY

Because the incidence of cardiac abnormalities in utero is quite low, routine examinations would be time-consuming and would result in a very small yield of pathologic findings. For these reasons we have used certain guidelines to increase the likelihood of detecting affected fetuses (Table 1).

RESULTS

Several lesions have been detected successfully by echocardiography (Table 2), and the number of correctly diagnosed cases is increasing. We have studied 116 fetuses one or more times. One source of these patients, who have had previous children with congenital heart disease, has been from the genetics and cardiology divisions. Another source of referral has been from the obstetrical department where nonimmune fetal hydrops or in utero heart rate problems have been detected and referred for further study. Interested hospital personnel have volunteered to act as "normal" controls (Table 3).

Detection of Congenital Heart Disease

Most fetuses, even in high-risk populations, will be normal. The impact of reassuring the parents that the current fetus does not have a significant cardiac abnormality cannot be assessed in purely statistical terms. It is in this "normal" group, in which the ultrasound test is easiest to interpret, that we have had the most success (Table 3). Such studies have excluded

Table 1. *Lesions Successfully Diagnosed In Utero by Two-Dimensional Echocardiography*

Pulmonary atresia and right ventricular hypoplasia
Univentricular heart
Premature closure of foramen ovale
Tetralogy of Fallot
Coarctation of the aorta
Septal rhabdomyoma
Hypoplastic left ventricle
Diabetic cardiomyopathy
Atrioventricular canal defect
Myocardial infarction
Cardiomyopathy

Table 2. *Guidelines for Detection of Heart Disease In Utero*

1. Family history of congenital cardiac abnormalities or hereditary disease affecting the heart.
2. Chromsomal abnormalities detected by amniocentesis.
3. Abnormalities of other organ systems detected by amnioscopy or ultrasound.
4. Fetal cardiac arrhythmia.
5. Polyhydramnios or oligohydramnios.
6. Maternal ingestion of substances known to be associated with production of congenital heart disease.
7. Maternal disease known to affect the fetal cardiac status.
8. Intrauterine growth retardation.

hypoplastic left and right heart, single ventricle, transposition (ventriculoarterial discordance) and Ebstein's anomaly (see Table 3).

We have examined six fetuses with congenital heart disease, in three of which a ventricular septal defect was identified. Two instances of congenital heart disease were confirmed by postmortem examination after therapeutic abortion and two during postnatal examination. Figure 7 shows the different techniques for defining the same lesion, one by linear scanner and one by phased-array sector scanner. In this particular patient, the mitral orifice was small, and there was a primum atrial septal defect. Although there is some difference in the display, both techniques defined the dominant lesion. The postnatal echocardiographic examination with a sector scanner confirmed the findings detected prenatally. Because the infant had multiple congenital defects, the parents refused all further treatment.

In a 23-week fetus whose mother presented with polyhydramnios and fetal ascites and pleural effusions, classic aortic atresia was found (Fig. 15). The parents elected to have a therapeutic abortion. At postmortem examination the diagnosis was confirmed.

In one patient an atrioventricular canal defect was recognized in association with complete heart block and hydrops fetalis. At birth, the full spectrum of abnormalities included polysplenia, ventricular arterial discordance (corrected transposition), and complete atrioventricular canal defect. Nonimmune hydrops has been found to be associated with a high incidence of congenital disease. We have encountered nonimmune hydrops in eight infants, in 4 of whom (50 per cent) there was cardiac disease. Two of the three had associated arrhythmias, and one had structural heart disease.

Table 3. *Fetal Two-Dimensional Echocardiographic Studies*

ARRHYTHMIAS	
Congenital heart block	2
Supraventricular premature beats	8
Ventricular premature beats	1
Paroxysmal atrial tachycardia	2
Sinus bradycardia	1
	14
CONGENITAL HEART DEFECTS	
Ventricular septal defects	3
Cardiomyopathy	2
Atrioventricular canal	1
Hypoplastic left ventricle and aortic stenosis	1
	7
FETUSES WITH RELATIVES HAVING CONGENITAL HEART DISEASE	
Tetralogy of Fallot	3
Aortic atresia	3
Transposition	3
Ebstein's anomaly	1
Cardiomyopathy	1
Left-sided Ebstein's anomaly	1
Single ventricle	4
Aortic stenosis	1
Pulmonary atresia	1
Atrioventricular canal	1
	19
LESIONS UNDETECTED BY ECHOCARDIOGRAPHY AND CONFIRMED AT POSTMORTEM EXAMINATION	
Pulmonary atresia	1
Bicuspid aortic and pulmonic valves	3
Secundum atrial septal defect	1
Double outlet right ventricle	2
Corrected transposition	1
	8
PERICARDIAL AND OTHER EFFUSIONS	9
STRUCTURALLY NORMAL HEARTS (random studies)	67
INCORRECT ASSESSMENT	
Tetralogy of Fallot	1
Atrioventricular canal defect	1
	2

Arrhythmia Interpretation

Because fetal electrocardiographic monitoring is not practical unless an electrode can be applied directly to the scalp, it cannot be done until the membranes have been ruptured. Arrhythmia detection has been accomplished by inference and by echocardiography both in utero and after birth.[6–13, 17] The echocardiogram has the ability to define more than just the heart rate. It can evaluate, in sequence, atrial and ventricular contractions and atrioventricular valve response to atrial contractions, and it can define the responses of these structures to ectopic contractions.[5] The echocardiogram has limitations because the diagnosis of arrhythmias relies on mechanical rather than true electrical activity. In order to evaluate the arrhythmia, the sequence of atrial contraction, atrioventricular contraction, and ventricular contraction is determined by constructing a ladder diagram.

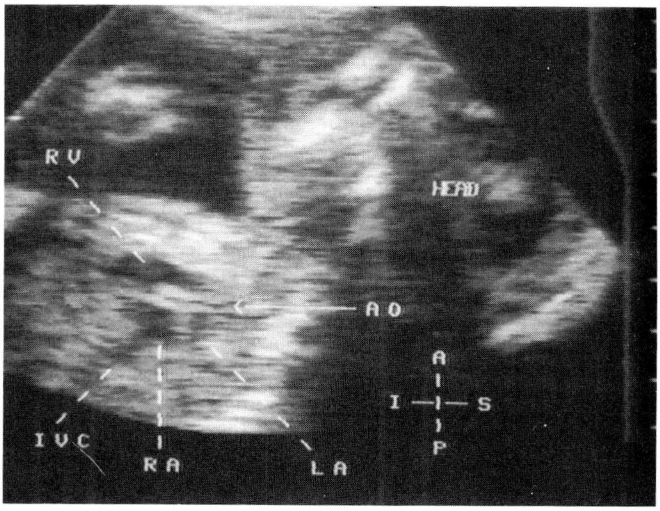

Figure 15. This scan demonstrates a long-axis view in a fetus with hypoplastic ascending aorta (Ao). The right ventricle (RV) is seen anteriorly, and the left and right atria (LA,RA) are seen posteriorly. A: anterior; I: inferior; P: posterior; S: superior.

The atrial contraction is defined by the onset of the A wave on the atrioventricular valve or by observing atrial contraction directly. Ventricular contraction is determined by closure of the atrioventricular valve, by the C-D slope of the mitral valve, and/or by noting the onset of atrial and ventricular contraction. Care must be taken to differentiate between the response of the atrioventricular valve opening (the D point) and a subsequent atrial contraction. These may be very close together in tachycardia. The echocardiographic technique also provides an opportunity for continuous monitoring of the fetus during the time of the echocardiographic study. Because these studies last approximately 30 to 60 minutes, the number of ectopic beats can be recorded and counted so that one can determine whether the rhythm is predominantly sinus or ectopic. We have been able to evaluate 14 infants with in utero arrhythmias using this technique (Table 3). The echocardiogram can also be used to monitor response to pharmacologic interventions.

In utero, complete heart block can be suspected when the heart rate is 40 to 80 beats per min and can be subsequently confirmed by echocardiography, which demonstrates ventricular rate and multiple atrial contractions that map out at regular intervals. Figure 16 is an echocardiogram obtained from a fetus at 32 weeks of gestation whose mother had serologic evidence of lupus erythematosus.[4] In a subsequent pregnancy another infant who also had congenital heart block was born. The serologic evidence of lupus erythematosus persisted in this mother.

We have examined eight patients with premature atrial contractions. The reason for referral in each case was the recognition of an irregular heart rate by the obstetrician. This has been the most frequent finding and in our experience appears to be of no prognostic significance. Delineation of arrhythmia has been performed by M-mode echocardiography. The construction of a ladder diagram helps define the type of arrhythmia (Fig. 17).

We have identified one 30-week fetus with premature ventricular contractions (Fig. 18). As these were infrequent, no intervention was undertaken. Postnatally, unifocal isolated ventricular premature contractions were demonstrated on electrocardiography. The arrhythmia disappeared within one week of postnatal life.

We have seen one fetus of 29 weeks' gestational age in whom supraventricular tachycardia was identified by echocardiography (Fig. 19). There was an atrial rate of 220 beats per min, as judged by the D and A points on the echo, and 1:1 ventricular responses, as indicated by the ventricular wall motion. Since the fetus demonstrated cardiac failure with ascites and pericardial effusion, the mother was given digitalis, and when there was no response, propranolol was given, with no effect. The fetus responded when an intravenous infusion of procainamide was given to the mother, and sinus rhythm occurred in the fetus after 340 mg had been infused into the mother. The fetus was maintained in sinus rhythm for 5 weeks by oral digitalis and procainamide administered to the mother, but it then relapsed into supraventricular arrhythmia. A hydropic 34-week female infant was delivered and successfully treated with antiarrhythmic agents, with resolution of the hydrops. With these agents, the child is maintained on sinus rhythm at 10 months of age.

On echocardiographic examination, we also

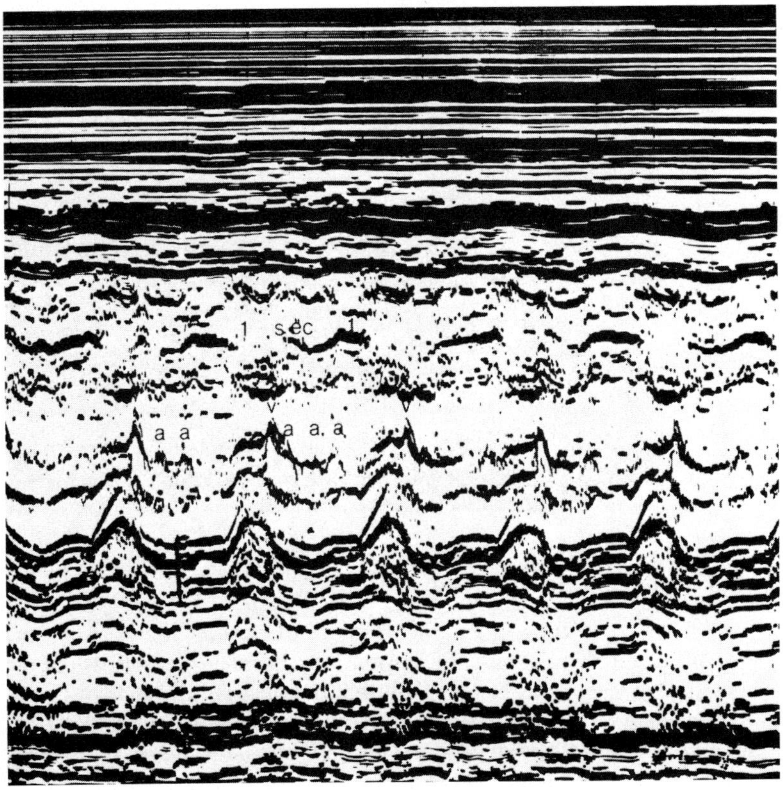

Figure 16. Taken from a 32-week fetus with congenital heart block. A 1-sec interval is shown in the right ventricular cavity. The ventricular rate is judged from mitral valve opening and ventricular contractions at 53 per min, whereas the atrial rate is judged from the a waves of the mitral valve at 180 beats per min. The a waves cannot be seen during ventricular contraction.

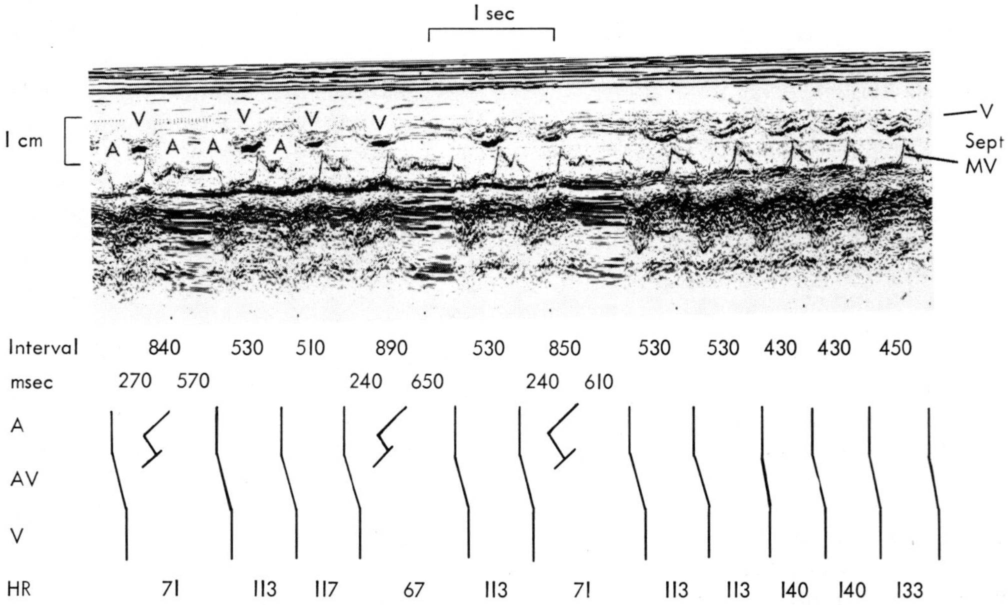

Figure 17. M-mode recording generated from a two-dimensional sector scan in a 30-week-old fetus with irregular rhythm detected by auscultation. Atrial contraction is defined by the onset of the A wave on the mitral valve and ventricular contraction by the D point of the mitral valve or the onset of ventricular contraction, as defined on the ventricular septum. A ladder diagram that shows the intervals in milliseconds of the atrial contraction is constructed. The block beats are defined as the second, seventh, and tenth beats; as can be seen from the length of the interval, they are followed by an incomplete compensatory pause. These findings are those of premature atrial contractions. V Sept: ventricular septum; MV: mitral valve.

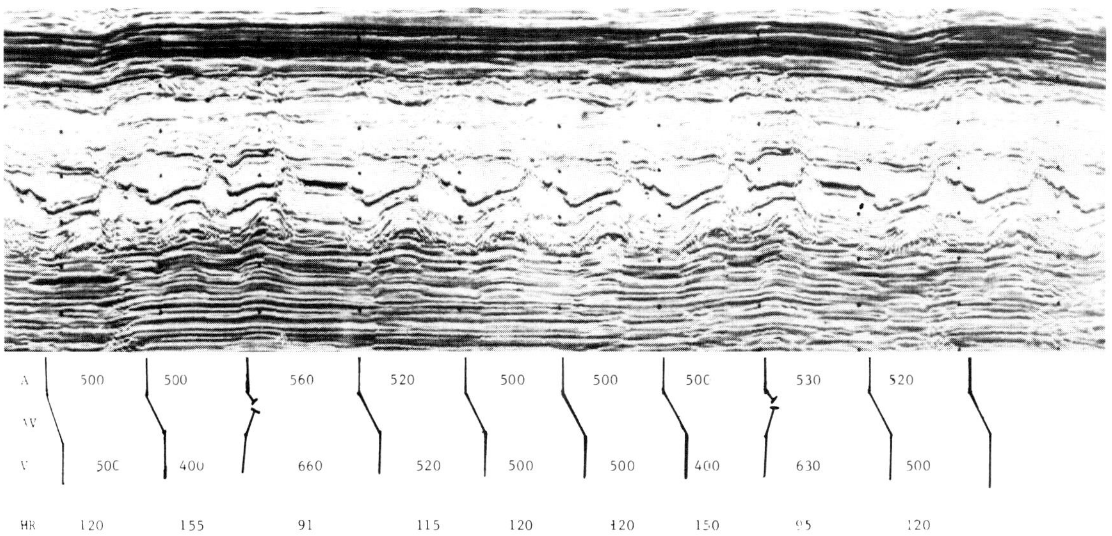

Figure 18. M-mode echocardiogram generated from a two-dimensional sector scanner in an infant with irregular rhythm. In this infant the mitral valve can clearly be seen within the left ventricular cavity. Premature ventricular contractions can be noted particularly well on the posterior left ventricular wall echo. There is obviously an irregularity, with beats 3 and 8 demonstrating slower contraction. It can be seen that the following contraction is preceded by an atrial tick on the mitral valve echocardiogram. When the arrhythmia is charted as for the previous example, it can be seen that there is premature ventricular contraction.

noted one fetus at 38 weeks of gestation with atrial flutter and pericardial effusion (Fig. 20). There was a 2:1 block, with occasional higher grade block being noted. Since small pericardial effusions suggesting incipient cardiac failure were observed, the infant was delivered immediately by cesarean section. The arrhythmia was confirmed postnatally, responded well to standard digitalis therapy, and converted to normal sinus rhythm.

Lesions Undetected by Two-Dimensional Echocardiography

In our postmortem examination of 19 fetuses who were therapeutically aborted because of a demonstrated chromosomal abnormality, there were a number of lesions that were not detected (see Table 3). We believe that with the resolution of current systems it is not possible to diagnose (in utero) bicuspid semilunar valves and atrial septal defects of the secundum type. In one patient with pulmonic atresia and ventricular septal defect, we were unable to define the pulmonic valve and pulmonary artery and were therefore unable to comment on this part of the lesion. The ventricular septal defect, however, was identified in this patient. In another patient with an omphalocele detected in utero, we were unable to diagnose double outlet right ventricle.

A second type of error we have made was the incorrect diagnosis of defects that were not present on postmortem examination after birth. One patient thought to have tetralogy of Fallot was found to have no cardiac defect at birth. In this patient the aorta was seen to be coursing anteriorly from the left ventricle, and artificial echo dropout from the outlet septum was interpreted as being a septal defect. On review of the videotape, the pulmonary artery in this patient was identified and no evidence of pulmonary artery narrowing was noted. In another patient who had trisomy 21 detected by amniocentesis, an atrioventricular canal defect was suspected. Review of the videotape showed that the drop-out of the ventricular septum was artifactual. These diagnostic errors reflect our earlier experience with less sophisticated equipment and our learning errors. These cases underline the importance of careful analysis in which not only the anatomic recognition of structures is important but also the technical considerations of the overall quality of the echocardiographic record are taken into account. This is especially important because accurate prenatal diagnosis of congenital heart disease is necessary for the planning of future care for these infants.

DEFINITION OF AN ADEQUATE ECHOCARDIOGRAPHIC STUDY BY TWO-DIMENSIONAL ECHO

Attempts to establish criteria for adequate studies have been based on recording each

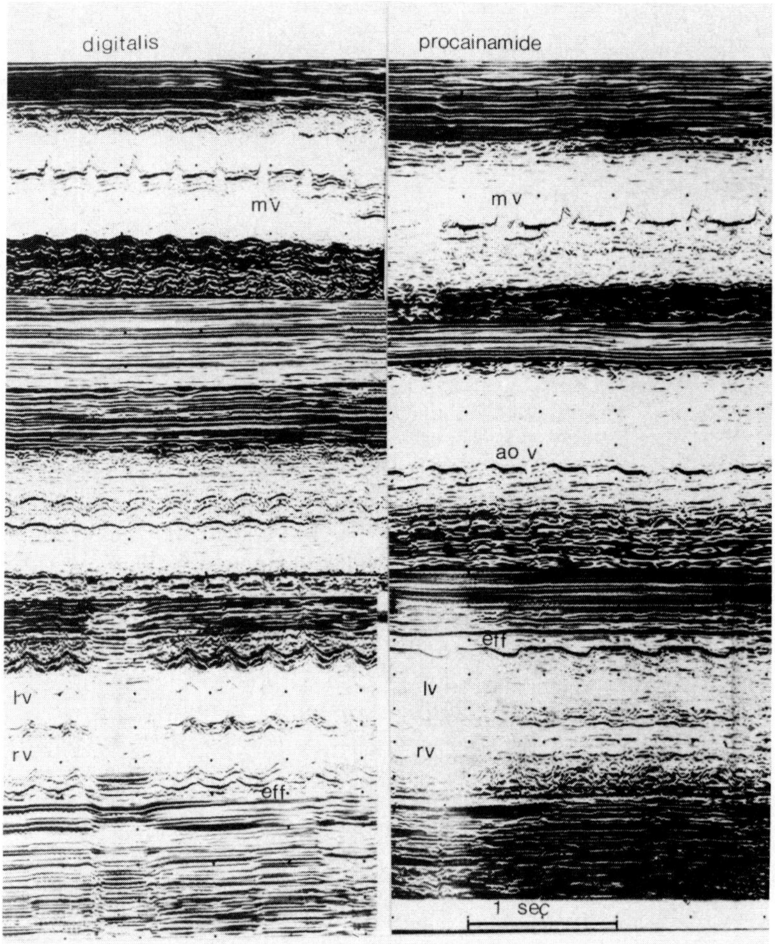

Figure 19. An example of fetal tachycardia. The time line dots occur every half a second and are 1 cm apart. The top panels demonstrate mitral valve motion, the middle panels demonstrate aortic root motion, and the bottom panels demonstrate ventricular wall motion. The left-hand panels were obtained to determine the result of digitalis being administered to the mother. The right-hand panels demonstrate the response of the arrhythmia to an intravenous infusion of procainamide into the mother's circulation. The time dots occur every half a second and are 1 cm apart. As judged by mitral valve opening, the heart rate is approximately 240 beats per min. There appears to be 1:1 ventricular response, as indicated by the opening of the aortic valve and the ventricular contractions demonstrated on the left ventricle, the right ventricle, and the ventricular septum. The right-hand panels demonstrate the abrupt onset of normal fetal heart rate after administration of 340 mg of procainamide to the mother, with the A wave now being visible on the mitral echogram and 1:1 atrioventricular conduction, defined by the normal rate, shown on the aortic valve (ao v) and the left and right ventricles in the bottom panel. Thus, procainamide was effective in restoring this fetus to normal sinus rhythm. Note that an effusion (eff) can be identified around the ventricular walls on this M-mode echogram, reflecting the effect of cardiac failure. This effusion disappeared within 48 hours. A 1-sec indicator is displayed at the bottom of the figure.

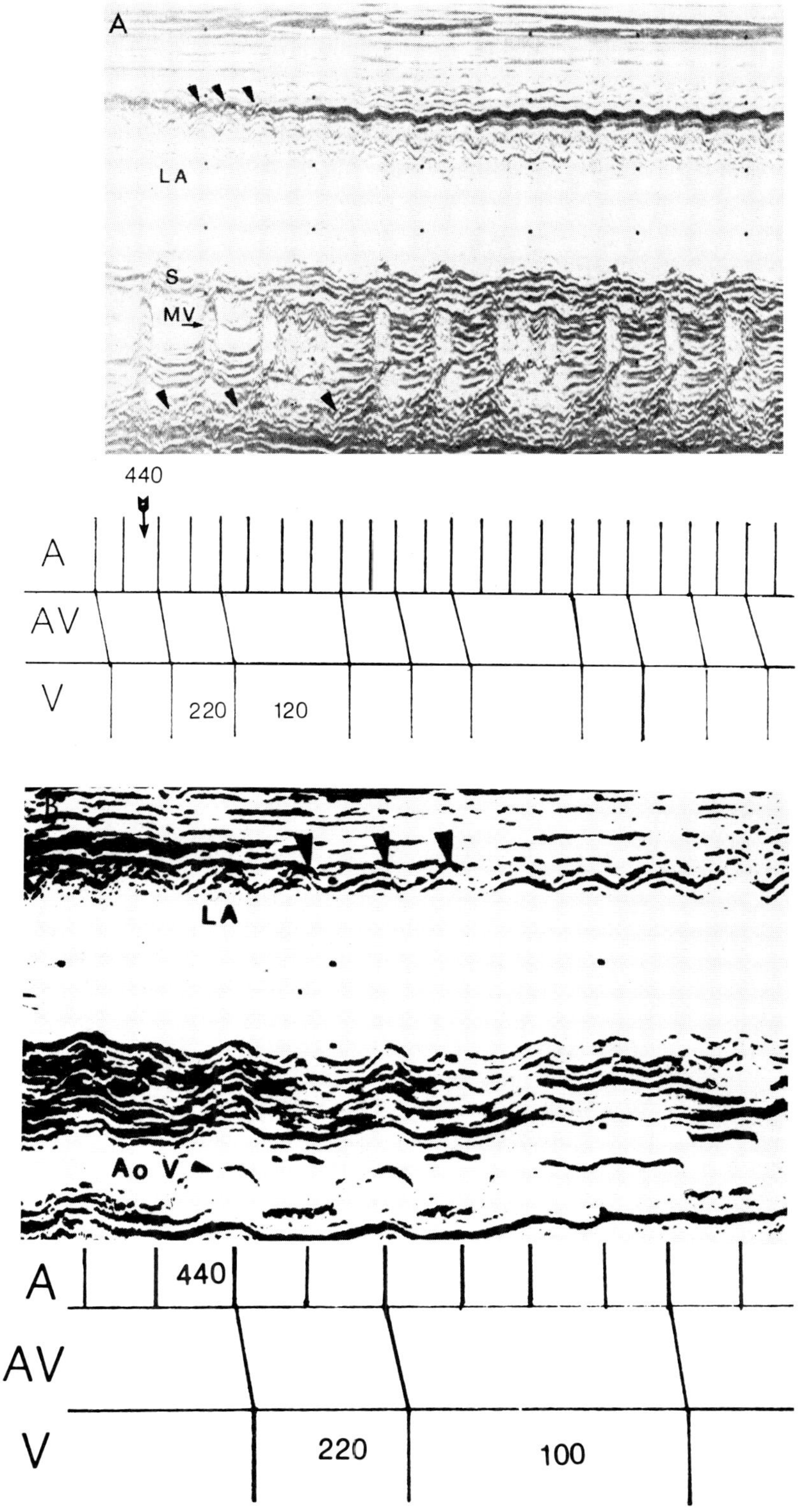

Figure 20. *A*, Ladder diagram in a fetus of 38 weeks gestation who presented with a very rapid heart rate. On auscultation the heart rate was approximately 220 beats per min, although there were some episodes of slowing. The atrial trace (LA), top panel, shows a ventricular response occurring 4 to 6 beats every half a second as defined by the time dots. The ventricular response is demonstrated by the ventricular wall contractions at the base of the left ventricle (bottom arrows). Mitral valve motion is noted in response to atrial and ventricular filling. A ladder diagram is constructed from atrial beats and ventricular response and demonstrates an atrial rate of 440 beats per min and a prevailing rate of 220 beats per min with occasional pauses. Thus, this fetus demonstrates a rate consistent with atrial flutter, predominantly 2:1 block, but often with a higher grade 4:1 atrioventricular block. *B*, Another view in the same fetus demonstrating a recording made at rapid speeds of the aortic valve (Ao V) and left atrial wall (LA). Again the rapid contractions at approximately 440 beats per min can be identified with a prevailing rate of ventricular response of 220 beats per min, but with occasional higher grade block—in this instance, with a rate of 100 beats per min.

view. It seems logical to ask whether an adequate study is one in which all cardiac structures have been imaged. Because the echocardiographic window in the fetus may be limited, a less than complete number of views may be accepted as being complete if all structures have been identified. It may be necessary to reexamine the patient at a subsequent examination in order to obtain a complete study, although this is not common practice in our laboratory.

WHO SHOULD PERFORM ULTRASOUND EXAMINATIONS?

The scope of fetal cardiac ultrasound encompasses the disciplines of obstetrics, perinatology, radiology, and cardiology, and persons involved in all these areas are interested in this technique. Pediatric cardiologists with expertise in cardiac development and electrophysiology and with postnatal experience with congenital heart lesions would seem to be most suited to perform ultrasound examinations. Obstetricians or radiologists, on the other hand, perform ultrasound studies on other fetal organs and, by scanning the heart as well, are in the position to comment on cardiac anatomy. It seems reasonable that, by a combined effort rather than by competition, the patient and the art of fetal cardiac echocardiography stand to benefit most.

CONCLUSION

The accurate recognition of cardiac lesions such as aortic atresia incompatible with life may facilitate counseling with regard to therapeutic abortion. For the mother who has an infant with the Down syndrome, the additional recognition of serious cardiac abnormalities such as a complete atrioventricular canal defect or the detection of hypoplastic left heart may make genetic counseling more complete. Since intrauterine surgery is now being performed, it is possible that serious cardiac defects may be palliated and treated in utero. Arrhythmias and possibly cardiac failure may also be managed in utero. Decisions on when and where to deliver infants with cardiac defects may be made, and delivery can be planned to take place in a center competent to handle infants with heart disease, thereby increasing the infant's chance of survival.

ACKNOWLEDGMENTS

The author is indebted to Ms. Martha Prince for assistance with preparation of this manuscript.

REFERENCES

1. Allan LD, Joseph MC, Boyd GCAE, et al: M-mode echocardiography in the developing human fetus. Br Heart J, *47*:573–583, 1982.
2. Allan LD, Tynan M, Campbell S, et al: Fetal echocardiography. *In* Hunter S, Hall R (eds): Echocardiography 1. Edinburgh, Churchill-Livingston, 1982.
3. Allan LD, Tynan M, Campbell S, et al: Identification of congenital cardiac malformations by echocardiography in midtrimester fetus. Br Heart J, *46*:358–362, 1981.
4. Chameides L, Treux RC, Vetter V, et al: Association of maternal systemic lupus erythematosus with complete heart block. N Engl J Med, *297*:1204–1207, 1977.
5. Hagan AD, Disessa TG: Echocardiographic features of sinus rhythm, arrhythmias, and conduction abnormalities. *In* Linhart JW, Joyner CR (eds): Diagnostic Echocardiography. St. Louis, C. V. Mosby, 1982, pp. 144–157.
6. Harrigan JT, Kangos JJ, Sikka A, et al: Successful treatment of fetal congestive heart failure secondary to tachycardia. N Engl J Med, *304*:1527–1529, 1981.
7. Kesson CW: Foetal paroxysmal auricular tachycardia. Br Heart J, *20*:552–556, 1958.
8. Klein AM, Holzman IR, Austin EM: Fetal tachycardia prior to the development of hydrops—Attempted pharmacologic cardioversion: Case Report. Am. J Obstet Gynecol, *134*:347–348, 1979.
9. Kleinman CS, Hobbins JC, Jaffe CC, et al: Echocardiographic studies on the human fetus: Prenatal diagnosis of congenital heart disease and cardiac dysrhythmias. Pediatrics, *65*:1059–1067, 1980.
10. Kleinman CS, Hobbins CC, Lynch DC, et al: The use of fetal echocardiography in the diagnosis and management of antenatal arrhythmias. Am J Cardiol, *47*:457, 1981.
11. Lange LW, Sahn DJ, Allen HD, et al: Quantitative real-time cross-sectional echocardiographic imaging of the human fetus during the second half of pregnancy. Circulation, *62*:799–806, 1980.
12. Lingman G, Ohrlander S, Ohlin P: Intrauterine digoxin treatment of fetal paroxysmal tachycardia. Br J Obstet Gynecol, *87*:340–342, 1980.
13. Newburger JW, Keane JF: Intrauterine supraventricular tachycardia. J Pediatr, *95*:780–786, 1979.
14. Redel DA, Hansman H: Fetal obstruction of the foramen ovale detected by two-dimensional Doppler echocardiography. *In* Rijsterborgh H (ed): Echocardiography. Proceedings of the 4th Symposium on Echocardiology. The Hague, Martinus Nijhoff, 1981, pp. 425–429.
15. Rudolph AM: Congenital Diseases of the Heart. Chicago, Year Book Medical Publishers, 1974, pp. 329–354.
16. Sahn DJ, Lange LW, Allen HD, et al: Quantitative real-time cross-sectional echocardiography in the developing human fetus and newborn. Circulation, *62*:588–597, 1980.
17. Teuscher A, Bossi E, Imhof P, et al: Effect of propranolol on fetal tachycardia in diabetic pregnancy. Am J Cardiol, *42*:304–307, 1978.
18. Wladimiroff JW, McGrie J, Fosters R: Fetal cardiac activity. *In* Rijsterbourgh H (ed): Echocardiography. Proceedings of the 4th Symposium on Echocardiology. The Hague, Martinus Nijhoff, 1981, pp. 417–429.

13

ECHOCARDIOGRAPHIC EVALUATION OF CARDIAC PERFORMANCE

THOMAS G. DISESSA, M.D., and WILLIAM F. FRIEDMAN, M.D.

A valuable clinical application of echocardiography is the noninvasive assessment of cardiac performance. To achieve an accurate determination of cardiac function, a clear understanding of its determinants and their effects on the echocardiogram is necessary. In addition, knowledge of the relative merits of M-mode, two-dimensional, and Doppler echocardiography in the evaluation of function is important. Thus, the purpose of this discussion will be to define the role of each echocardiographic method in the evaluation of cardiac performance.

LEFT VENTRICULAR FUNCTION

The variables that influence left ventricular function are the contractile state of the myocardium, preload, afterload, and heart rate. In the intact heart, these variables are closely interdependent. Thus, it is important to be aware of the clinical setting in which the echocardiogram is placed. For example, patients with a ventricular septal defect, patent ductus arteriosus, or anemia may have increased ejection phase indices due to increased preload. Subjects with thyrotoxicosis would have increased indices of function due to increased heart rate and inotropic state.

MEAN VcF

The M-mode echocardiogram was employed initially in the evaluation of cardiac function. Early reports in adults found a close correlation between mean VcF derived from echocardiography and angiography (Fig. 1).[6, 25]

$$\text{Mean VcF} = \frac{\text{LVEDD} - \text{LVESD}}{\text{LVET} \times \text{LVEDD}}$$

where VcF is velocity of circumferential fiber shortening, LVEDD is left ventricular end-diastolic dimension, LVESD is left ventricular end-systolic dimension, and LVET is left ventricular ejection time.

Subsequent studies in children demonstrated mean VcF to be a valuable means of measuring left ventricular performance.[15, 27] Since VcF is heart-rate dependent, it must be remembered that this index of contractility will be higher in young children and infants. Gutgesell et al.[15] derived a formula for the accurate estimation of normal mean VcF in children.

$$\text{Mean VcF} = 1.075 + 0.005\,(\text{HR}) - 0.02\ \text{Age}$$

where VcF is velocity of circumferential fiber shortening and HR is heart rate.

FRACTIONAL SHORTENING

An equally useful index of left ventricular function is the per cent change with systole of the left ventricular end-diastolic dimension (per cent fractional shortening). This short axis dimensional change measured at the level of the

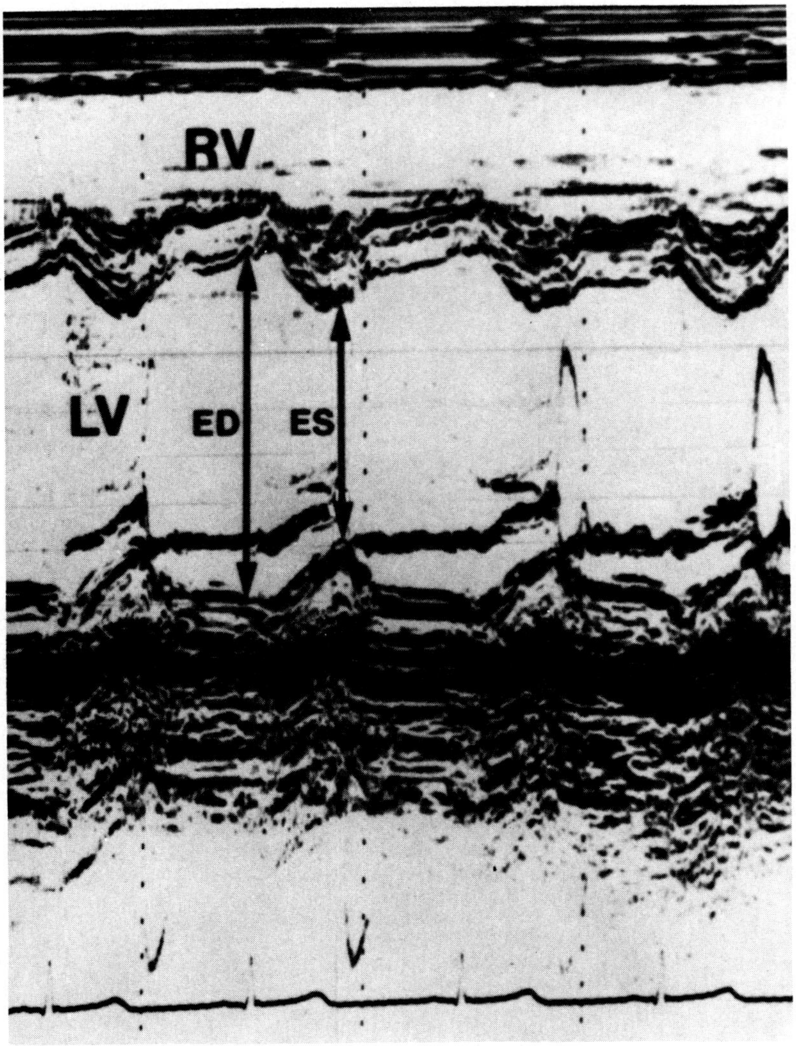

Figure 1. M-mode echocardiogram recorded below the level of the mitral valve demonstrates the method for measuring end-diastolic dimension (ED) and end-systolic dimension (ES) of the left ventricle (LV). RV: right ventricle. (*From* Hagan AD, DiSessa TG: Two-dimensional Echocardiography. Boston Little, Brown and Co., (in press), with permission.)

chordae tendineae is calculated in the same manner as mean VcF.

$$\%FS = \frac{LVEDD - LVESD}{LVEDD} \times 100\%$$

where %FS is per cent fractional shortening, LVEDD is left ventricular end-diastolic dimension, and LVESD is left ventricular end-systolic dimension.

In contrast to mean VcF, fractional shortening does not depend upon ejection time and heart rate. Both fractional shortening and mean VcF are inaccurate in the presence of segmental wall motion abnormalities. The most frequent cause of abnormal wall motion in children is paradoxic septal motion from right ventricular volume overload.

E-POINT-SEPTAL SEPARATION

The mitral valve E-point-septal separation (EPSS) is a very useful indicator of left ventricular performance (Fig. 2).[8, 19] Studies in adults have demonstrated a good linear correlation between EPSS and either angiographic or radionuclide ejection fraction.[8, 19] Since EPSS does not depend on left ventricular size, is not influenced by segmental wall motion disturbances, does not rely on mathematic formulae or geometric assumptions, and is recorded easily in almost all patients, it may be more useful than fractional shortening or mean VcF in the evaluation of left ventricular function. We have established the utility of normal valves for EPSS in children. A mitral valve EPSS greater than 6 mm indicates reduced ventricular function in both children and adults.

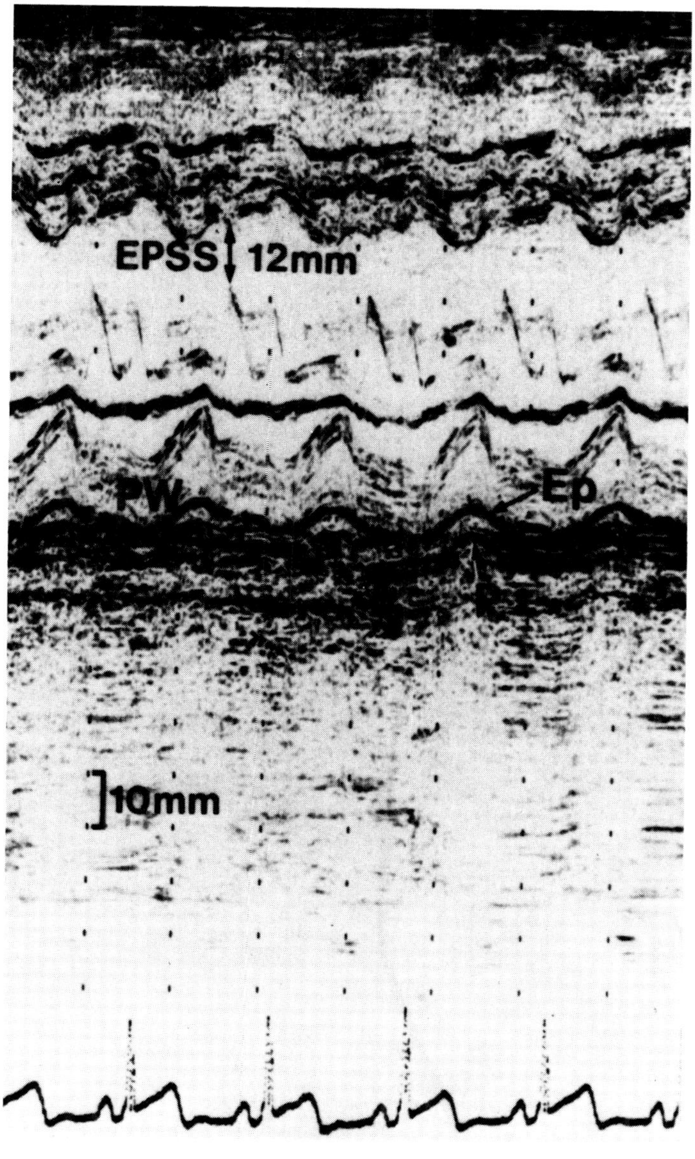

Figure 2. M-mode echocardiogram shows reduced ventricular function and increased mitral valve, E point-septal separation (EPSS) EP: epicardium, PW: posterior wall, S: septum (*From* Hagan AD, DiSessa TG: Two-dimensional Echocardiography. Boston Little, Brown and Co., (in press), with permission.)

LEFT VENTRICULAR VOLUMES AND EJECTION FRACTION

Initial M-mode attempts at estimation of left ventricular volume was based on the assumption that the ventricle is a prolate ellipse and that the minor axis length equals twice the long axis length.[2, 24] Thus, estimation of left ventricular volume could be made from the cube of the minor axis dimension.[24] Left ventricular ejection fraction was calculated from the following equation:

$$\text{LVEF} = \frac{(\text{LVEDD})^3 - (\text{LVESD})^3}{(\text{LVEDD})^3}$$

where LVEF is left ventricular ejection fraction, LVEDD is left ventricular end-diastolic dimension, and LVESD is left ventricular end-systolic dimension.

The cube method of calculation of left ventricular volumes proved inaccurate when compared with angiographic volume determination. Subsequently, Teichholz[33] in adults and Meyer[22] in children developed regression equations for the more accurate estimation of left ventricular volumes by M-mode echocardiography. Despite these more precise methods, it became apparent that the estimation of left ventricular volumes and ejection fraction is compromised severely by segmental wall motion disturbances and volume overload. Recently, studies in adults[5, 11, 29] and children[21, 30] have demonstrated the superiority of two-dimensional images over M-mode traces in the estimation of left ventricular volumes and ejection fraction. This superiority lies in the ability of two-dimensional echocardiography to image the heart from multiple tomographic planes (Fig. 3). Thus, estimation of volume by this latter technique is not affected by abnormal wall motion or volume overload.[5, 11, 21, 29, 30] However, the ability to produce multiple cardiac cross-sections has created numerous methodologies for the determination of volumes and ejection fraction. Either single plane or biplane methods have been employed. Multiple algorithms applied to different geometric assumptions have been tested (Fig. 4). It appears that Simpson's rule using multiple, short-axis cross-sections and the apical four-chamber view provides the most accurate assessment of left ventricular volume and ejection fraction in adults[5, 11, 29] and children (Figs. 5 and 6).[21, 30]

Left ventricular volume derived from two-dimensional echocardiography routinely underestimates an angiographically determined volume (see Fig. 5). The degree of systolic and diastolic volume underestimation is the same. Therefore, ejection fraction derived from two-dimensional images correlates well with ejection fraction derived from cineangiocardiography (see Fig. 6) or nuclear angiography.

LEFT VENTRICULAR WALL STRESS

The determination of left ventricular wall stress by echocardiography in conjunction with an intracardiac left ventricular pressure tracing (Fig. 7) or cuff blood pressure has been validated.[20, 26] The force per unit area, or stress, acting along the circumference of the left ventricle at its minor axis depends directly on intracavity pressure and the radius of curvature and inversely depends on wall thickness.[26] Therefore, conditions leading to either chronic pressure or volume overload result in an increase in wall stress. Angiographic studies analyzing wall dynamics and its directional components revealed three components of cardiac work or power: meridional (longitudinal), equatorial (circumferential), and radial.[13] The per cent contribution of the directional components to total cardiac work developed by the mid wall equatorial element of the myocardium is the following: longitudinal, 14 per cent in normal and diseased ventricles; circumferential, 45 per cent in normal, increasing to 55 per cent in dilated ventricles; radial, 40 per cent in normal and 31 per cent in dilated ventricles.[13] Circumferential wall stress can be calculated from the M-mode echocardiogram and cuff blood pressure at end systole by use of the following equation:[20]

$$\text{End-systolic wall stress index} = \frac{\text{systolic arterial pressure} \times \text{radius}}{\text{end-systolic wall thickness}}$$

Meridional wall stress may be similarly calculated by using the following equation:[4]

$$\text{Meridional wall stress} = PD/4h\,(1 + h/d)$$

where P is pressure, D equals 2 (left ventricular radius), h is left ventricular wall thickness.

Since end-systolic meridional wall stress is a quantitative index of true myocardial afterload that can be plotted against left ventricular end-systolic diameter, an index of contractility independent of loading conditions can be achieved.[26] Echocardiography can be used in conjunction with cardiac catheterization to determine wall stress throughout the cardiac cycle (Fig. 7.)[4, 20] Such information provides greater insights into left ventricular performance.

LEFT VENTRICULAR CAVITY SIZE, WALL THICKNESS, AND MASS

Noninvasive measurement of cavity size and wall thickness provides further insights into cardiac hemodynamics. Normal values for left ventricular dimensions and wall thickness in infants and children have been investigated thoroughly.[15, 27] The effects of intracardiac shunt, mitral valve and aortic valve insufficiency, and reduced myocardial function on left ventricular cavity size have been well established.[28] In addition, the effects of an obstruction of the left ventricular outflow tract on the thickness of the left ventricular wall can be determined easily by M-mode echocardiography. A formula of the systolic wall thickness-dimension ratio has proved useful in the noninvasive estimation of peak systolic left ventricular pressure and aortic valve pressure gradient in children with aortic stenosis.[1]

$$LVPSP = 225 \times \frac{LVESD}{LVWT_s}$$

where LVPSP is left ventricular peak systolic pressure, LVESD is left ventricular end-systolic dimension, and $LVWT_s$ is left ventricular end-systolic wall thickness.

Left ventricular mass is best estimated by two-dimensional echocardiography that is not

Text continued on page 227

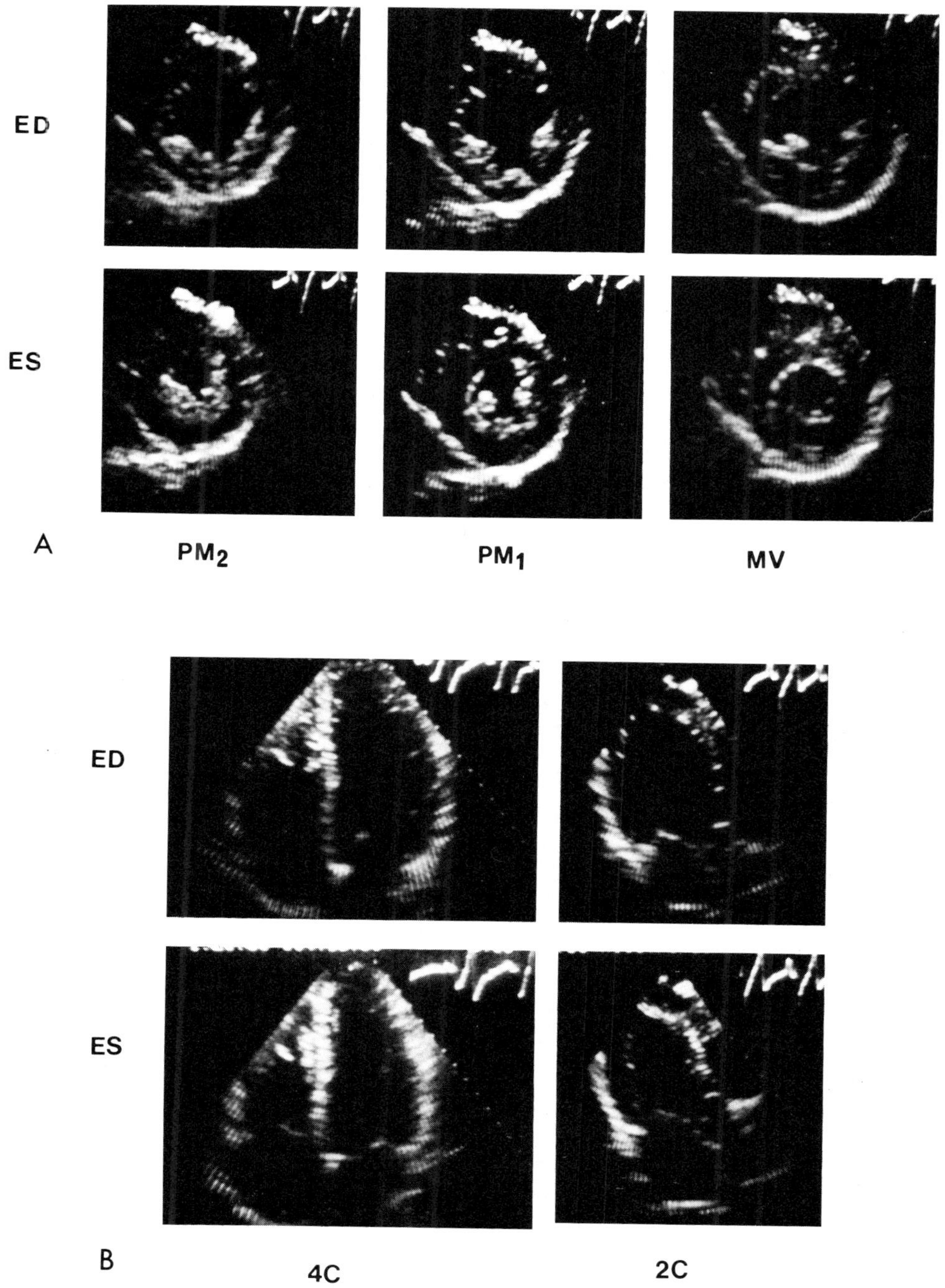

Figure 3. *A*, Short axis and *(B)* apical views used for the calculation of left ventricular volume from two-dimensional echocardiography. (*From* Mercier JC, DiSessa TG, Jarmakani JM, et al: Two-dimensional echocardiographic assessment of left ventricular volumes and ejection fractions in children. Circulation, 65:962, 1982, with permission of the American Heart Association, Inc.)

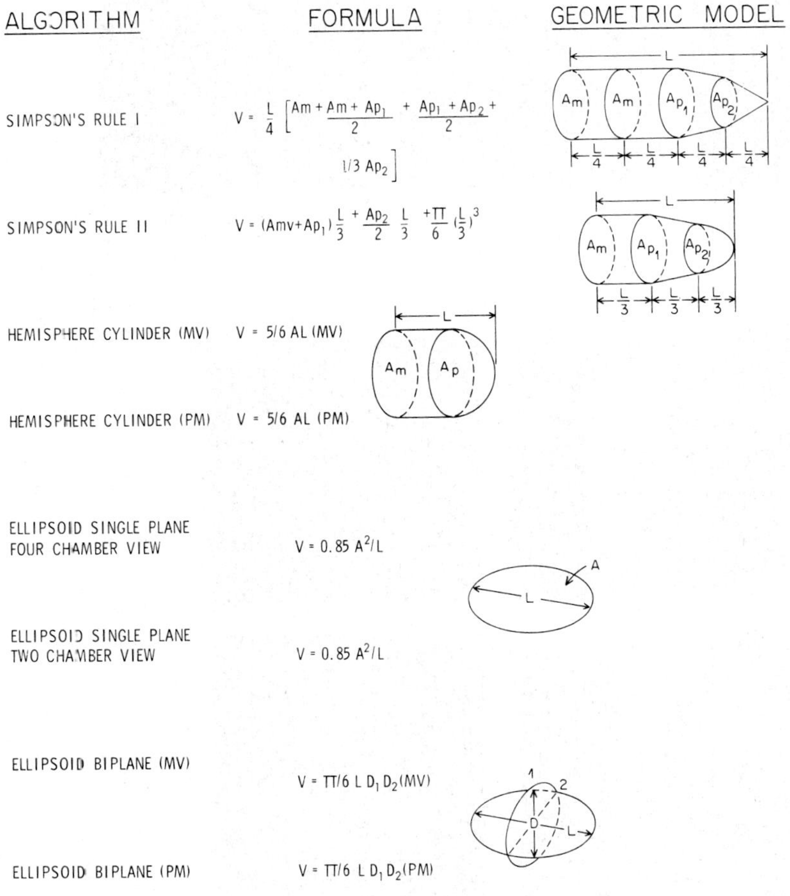

Figure 4. Formulae and geometric models used to calculate left ventricular volumes by two-dimensional echocardiography. A: area, Am: area of short axis at mitral valve level, Ap and Ap_1: area of short axis at high papillary muscle level, Ap_2: area of short axis at low papillary muscle level, D_1: minor axis diameter (right-left), D_2: minor axis diameter (anterior-posterior), L: longest length from the apical four-chamber view, MV: mitral valve, PM: papillary muscle, V: volume. (*From* Mercier JC, DiSessa TG, Jarmakani JM, et al: Two-dimensional echocardiographic assessment of left ventricular volumes and ejection fractions in children. Circulation, 65:962, 1982, with permission of the American Heart Association, Inc.)

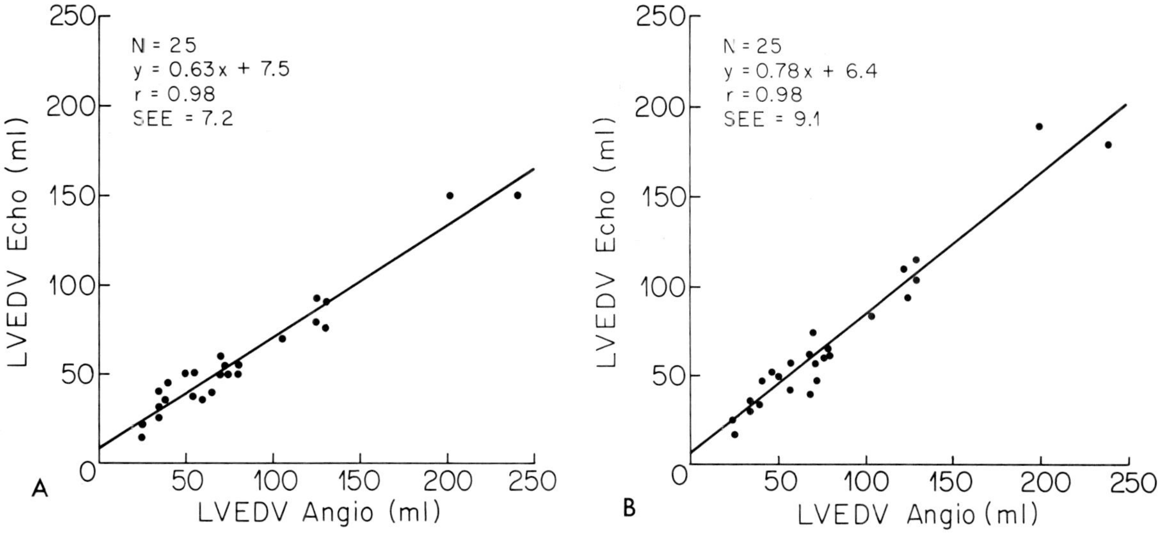

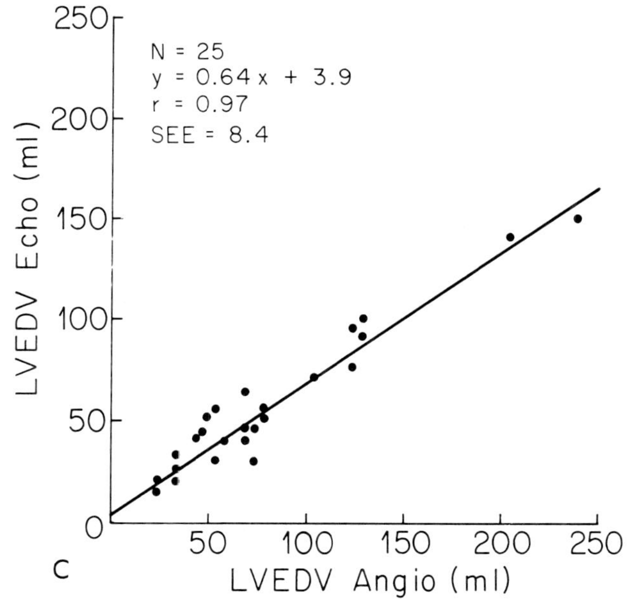

Figure 5. Correlation between left ventricular end-diastolic volume (LVEDV) calculated from two-dimensional echocardiography (echo) and angiography (angio). *A*, Simpson's rule I. Assuming the ventricle to be a truncated cone. *B*, Simpson's rule II. Assuming the ventricle to be a truncated ellipse. *C*, Ellipsoid biplane area-length using the papillary muscle level in short axis. PM: papillary muscle, SEE: standard error of the estimate. (*From* Mercier JC, DiSessa TG, Jarmakani JM, et al: Two-dimensional echocardiographic assessment of left ventricular volumes and ejection fractions in children. Circulation, 65:962, 1982, with permission of the American Heart Association, Inc.)

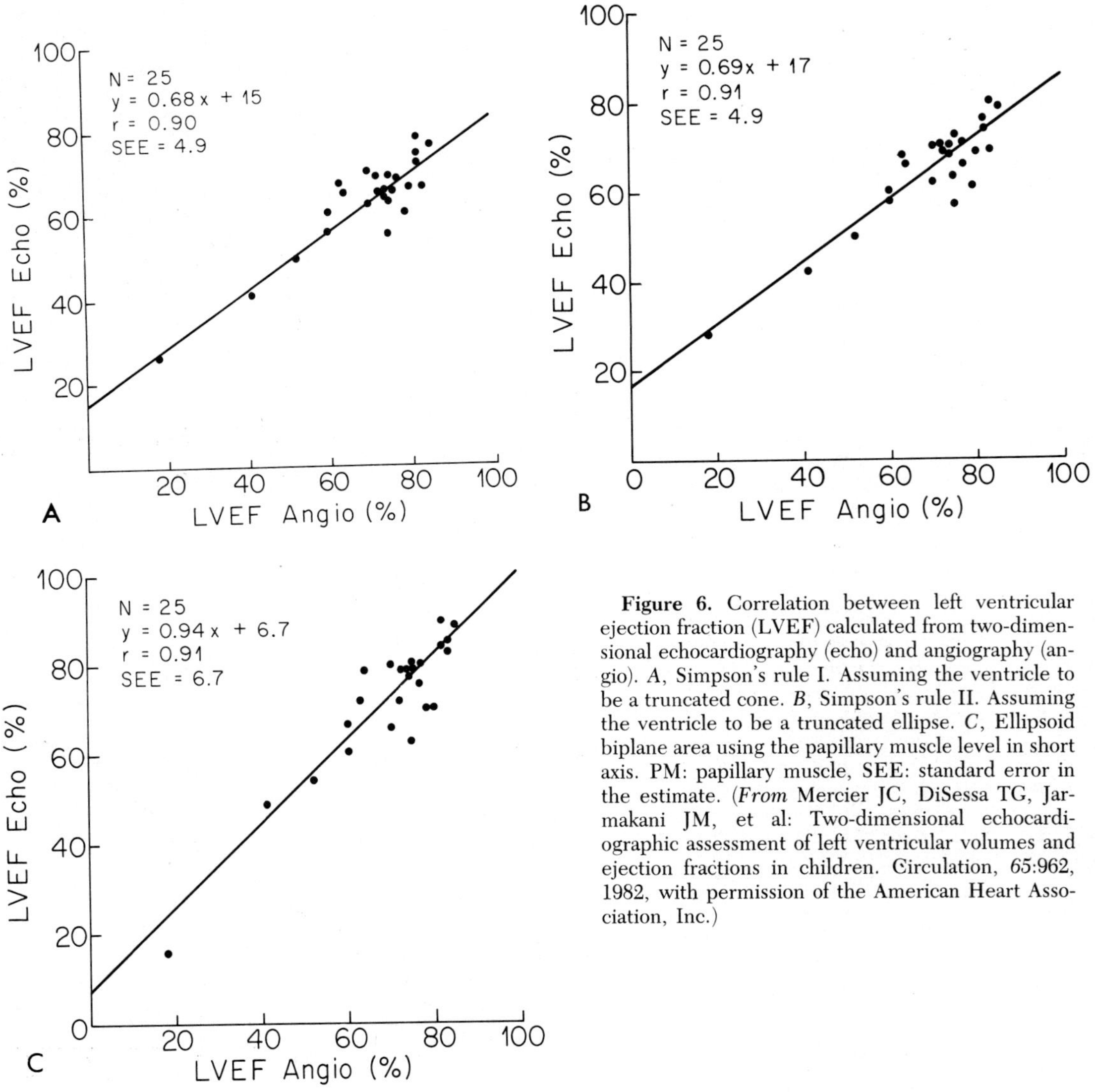

Figure 6. Correlation between left ventricular ejection fraction (LVEF) calculated from two-dimensional echocardiography (echo) and angiography (angio). *A*, Simpson's rule I. Assuming the ventricle to be a truncated cone. *B*, Simpson's rule II. Assuming the ventricle to be a truncated ellipse. *C*, Ellipsoid biplane area using the papillary muscle level in short axis. PM: papillary muscle, SEE: standard error in the estimate. (*From* Mercier JC, DiSessa TG, Jarmakani JM, et al: Two-dimensional echocardiographic assessment of left ventricular volumes and ejection fractions in children. Circulation, 65:962, 1982, with permission of the American Heart Association, Inc.)

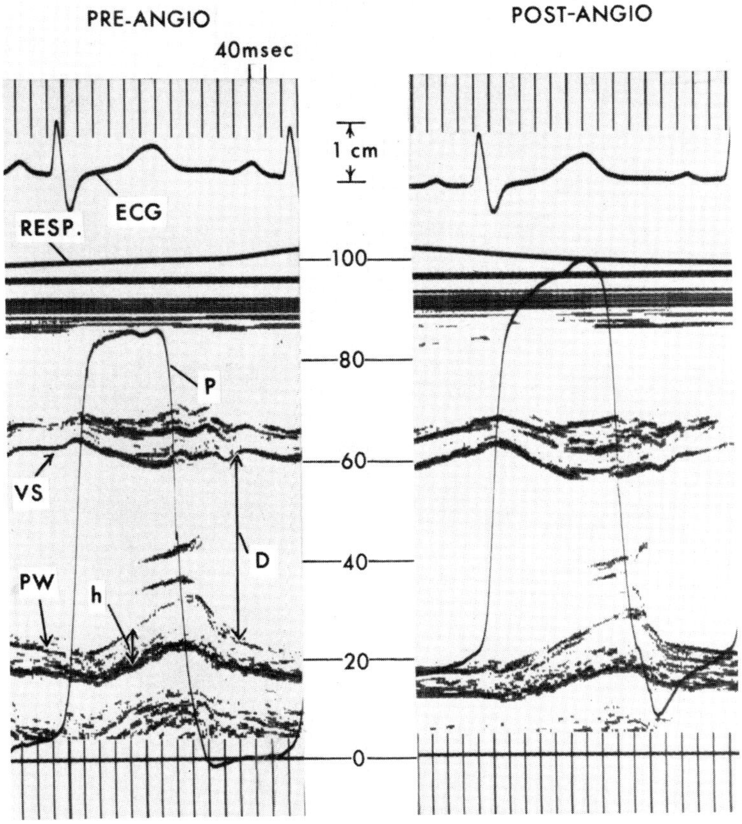

Figure 7. M-mode echocardiogram recorded simultaneously with a left ventricular pressure tracing to calculate wall stress. D: dimension, ECG: electrocardiogram, h: wall thickness, P: pressure, PW: posterior wall, RESP: respiration, VS: ventricular septum (Courtesy of Leland Benson, M.D.).

affected by asymmetric or segmental hypertrophy, localized thinning, or altered geometry.[34] Two-dimensional echocardiography has proved accurate in the assessment of left ventricular mass in vitro in dogs[34] and in adults.[34] Its application to the estimation of mass in children has yet to be explored.

DOPPLER ESTIMATES OF CARDIAC OUTPUT

Recently, Doppler echocardiography has been utilized to measure intracardiac flows.[14] The Doppler principle relies on the property of blood flow in vessels to reflect emitted sound waves with a frequency shift. A sound wave emitted at a known frequency will be reflected back to the sound source with a change in frequency if it strikes fluid in motion at an angle θ. Measurement of this frequency shift allows estimation of blood flow velocity.[7]

Blood flow velocity =

$$\frac{(f_1 - f_0) \times \text{velocity of sound in blood}}{2fo \times \cos\theta}$$

where the velocity of sound in blood equals 1580 m/sec, f_1 equals the received backscattered frequency, f_0 equals emitted frequency, and θ equals the angle of incidence of the volume of blood.

Blood velocity thus determined allows the estimation of stroke volume and cardiac output.

Stroke volume =

$$\frac{\text{mean flow velocity} \times \text{vessel area} \times \text{ejection time}}{\cos\theta}$$

The cos θ should be included in only one of the two above equations. The combination of Doppler techniques with two-dimensional imaging has allowed accurate placement of the Doppler sample volume (range gating) and correction of the angle θ. Initial studies using this method estimated cardiac output by placing the sample volume in the ascending aorta using the subcostal or suprasternal notch window and main pulmonary artery using the left parasternal window (Fig. 8). Although a good correlation between Doppler-estimated cardiac output and thermodilution-determined cardiac output has been reported,[14] several limitations of this ap-

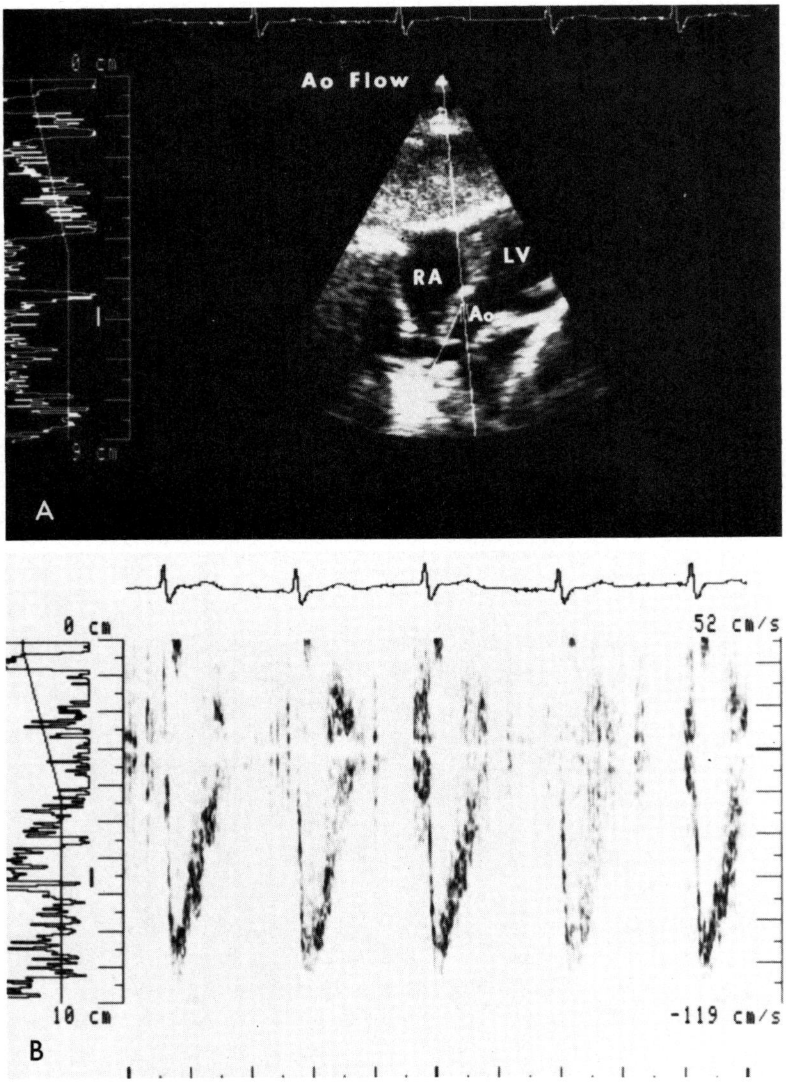

Figure 8. *A*, Two-dimensional echocardiogram recorded from the subcostal window demonstrating the Doppler sample volume in the ascending aorta (Ao). *B*, Doppler flow pattern used to calculate aortic flow (cardiac output). LV: left ventricle, RA: right atrium (Courtesy of David Sahn, M.D.).

proach are apparent: (1) potential error in angle measurement, (2) potential error in measuring the diameter of the vessel, (3) potential for a nonuniform flow profile at the sample site, (4) variations in cardiac output with transducer location, which are presumably caused by errors associated with the angle, attenuation of signal, and acoustic noise caused by rib reflections, and (5) high flow velocities.

LEFT VENTRICULAR DIASTOLIC FILLING AND COMPLIANCE

The term "ventricular compliance" refers to the distensibility of the ventricle in diastole. M-mode echocardiography is particularly well suited for evaluating early diastolic filling (mitral valve E to F slope),[9] left atrial emptying,[10] left ventricular end-diastolic pressure (abnormal PR-AC interval),[18] and a delay in opening of the mitral valve after closure of the aortic valve.[31] These indices of left ventricular diastolic function are used widely in the adult and pediatric population. Goldberg et al.[12] measured incremental posterior wall thickening and thinning from the M-mode echocardiogram in children with Duchenne's muscular dystrophy. In these children and in children who had received large doses of Adriamycin, a decreased rate of posterior wall thinning was observed. These authors assumed that this decreased rate of relaxation was related to myocardial fibrosis. Moreover, in the detection of left ventricular dysfunction, the alteration in the rate of diastolic thinning may be more sensitive than mean VcF or fractional shortening.

RIGHT VENTRICULAR FUNCTION

M-mode echocardiographic estimation of right ventricular function relies on the measurement of systolic time intervals.[17] The inaccessible intrathoracic position of the right ventricle precludes measurement of right ventricular volumes and ejection fraction by M-mode echocardiography. Until recently, nuclear angiography provided the only noninvasive means of estimating right ventricular ejection fraction.

RIGHT VENTRICULAR SYSTOLIC TIME INTERVALS

The right ventricular systolic time intervals include the preejection period and ejection time measured from the pulmonic valve echogram. The preejection period is measured from the onset of the QRS complex to the onset of pulmonic valve opening. Ejection time is measured from valve opening to valve closure. These ejection phase indices are affected by heart rate, preload, afterload, and contractility. A preejection period-ejection time ratio has been used to remove heart rate as a modifier of the systolic time intervals. Initial studies evaluated the use of right ventricular systolic time intervals in the determination of pulmonary hypertension. However, the extreme variability of these echo indices with the loading conditions of the heart had led many echocardiographers away from their use.

RIGHT VENTRICULAR VOLUMES AND EJECTION FRACTION

Two-dimensional echocardiography has provided multiple windows from the parasternal border, apex, and subcostal area for imaging of the right ventricle. Bommer et al.[3] demonstrated that the short-axis diameter and planimetered area of the right ventricle measured from the apical four-chamber view correlated well with the volume of the ventricle. The subcostal view has been employed in adults with chronic obstructive lung disease for the estimation of right ventricular volume and ejection fraction.[32] Simpson's rule has been applied to the short axis and apical four-chamber view in patients with complete transposition of the great arteries for the estimation of right ventricular volume and ejection fraction.[23]

$$RVV = \frac{\pi H}{3} \times \frac{1}{4}$$

$$[(XoYo + X_{20}Y_{20}) + \underset{N}{\overset{\text{Odd segments}}{\Sigma}} XnYn + \underset{N}{\overset{\text{Even segments}}{\Sigma}} \tfrac{1}{2}\, XmYm]$$

where RVV is right ventricular volume, Xn is the minor axis in the apical four-chamber view,

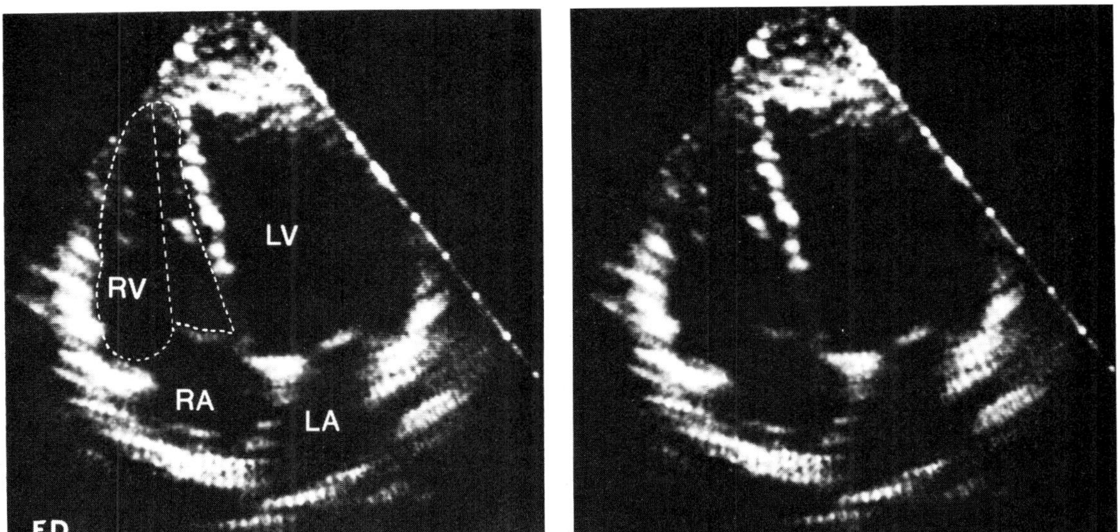

Figure 9. Apical four-chamber view demonstrates the method for planimetering the right ventricular area and measuring the length of the right ventricle for volume calculation (*From* Hiraishi S, DiSessa TG, Jarmakani, JM, et al: Two-dimensional echocardiographic assessment of right ventricular volume in children with congenital heart disease. Am J Cardiol, *50*:1368, 1982, with permission.)

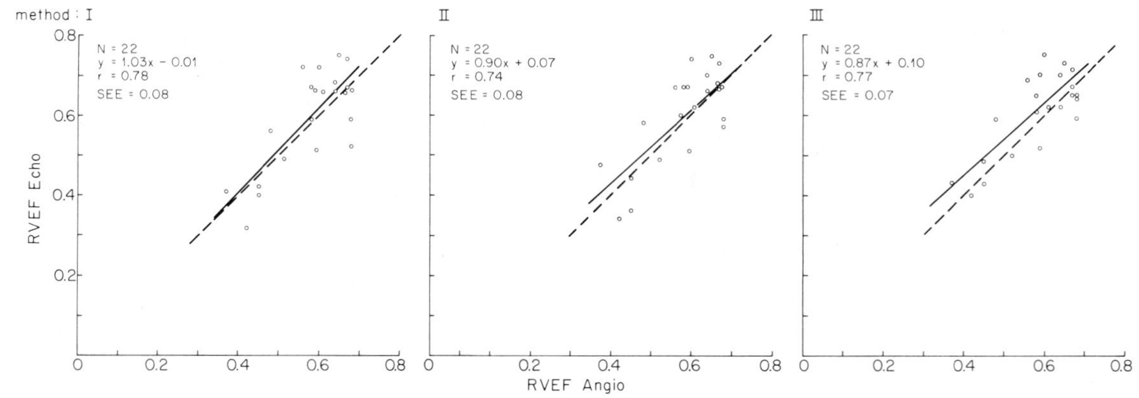

Figure 10. Correlation between right ventricular ejection fraction (RVEF) obtained from two-dimensional echocardiography and angiography using three area-length methods. Solid line: the regression line, dashed line: the line of identity. (*From* Hiraishi S, DiSessa TG, Jarmakani JM, et al: Two-dimensional echocardiographic assessment of right ventricular volume in children with congenital heart disease. Am J Cardiol, *50*:1368, 1982, with permission.)

Yn is the minor axis in the short axis view, and H is the thickness of the segment.

Recent experience in our laboratory has demonstrated that right ventricular volumes can be determined from the apical four-chamber view (Fig. 9) and that ejection fraction derived from these volumes correlated well with angiographically determined ejection fraction (Fig. 10).[16] We have shown that the long-axis length and the planimetered area measured from the apical four-chamber view correlate closely with the longest length and planimetered area and volume of the right ventricular sinus measured from the anterioposterior and lateral angiogram. Thus, we used the echo length and area measurements to predict the angiographic parameters and calculated right ventricular volumes from three area-length formulae.

Method I

$$RVV = 1.061 \times \frac{CEA_{Ap} \times CEA_{Lat}}{CELL_{Ap}}$$

Method II

$$RVV = 0.849 \times \frac{CEA_{Ap} \times CEA_{Lat}}{CELL_{Lat}}$$

Method III

$$RVV = 1.316 \times \frac{(CEA_{Lat})^2}{CELL_{Lat}}$$

where Ap is anterioposterior, CEA is corrected echo area, CELL is corrected echo long-axis length, Lat is lateral, and RVV is right ventricular volume.

CONCLUSION

Echocardiography provides a noninvasive reproducible means of evaluating cardiac function. M-mode echocardiography can readily evaluate ejection phase indices, wall stress, and diastolic left ventricular function, whereas two-dimensional imaging allows optimal assessment of right and left ventricular ejection fraction. A blood velocity profile obtained by Doppler methods allows direct estimation of cardiac output.

REFERENCES

1. Bennett, DH, Evans DW, Raj MUJ: Echocardiographic left ventricular dimensions in pressure and volume overload: Their use in assessing aortic stenosis. Br Heart J, *37*:971, 1975.
2. Bennett DH, Rowlands DJ: Test of reliability of echocardiographic estimation of left ventricular dimensions and volumes. Br Heart J, *38*:1133, 1976.
3. Bommer W, Weiner L, Neumann A, et al.: Determination of right atrial and right ventricular size by two-dimensional echocardiography. Circulation, *60*:91, 1979.
4. Brodie BR, McLaurin LP, Grossman W: Combined hemodynamic-ultrasonic method for studying left ventricular wall stress. Am J Cardiol, *37*:864, 1976.
5. Carr KW, Engler RL, Forsythe JR, et al: Measurement of left ventricular ejection by mechanical cross-sectional echocardiography. Circulation, *59*:1196, 1979.
6. Cooper RH, O'Rourke RA, Karliner JS, et al: Comparison of ultrasound and cineangiographic measurements of the mean rate of circumferential fiber shortening in man. Circulation, *46*:914, 1972.
7. Darsee JR, Walter PF, Nutter DO: Transcutaneous Doppler method of measuring cardiac output. II. Non-invasive measurement by transcutaneous Doppler aortic blood velocity integration and M-mode echocardiography. Am J Cardiol, *46*:613, 1980.

8. D'Cruz IA, Lalmali GG, Sambasivan V, et al: The superiority of mitral E point-ventricular septum separation to other echocardiographic indicators of left ventricular performance. Clin Cardiol., 2:140, 1979.
9. DeMaria AN, Miller RR, Amsterdam EA, et al: Mitral valve early diastolic closing velocity in the echocardiogram: Relation to sequential diastolic flow and ventricular compliance. Am J Cardiol, 37:693, 1976.
10. Dreslinski GR, Frohlich ED, Dunn FG, et al: Echocardiographic diastolic ventricular abnormality in hypertensive heart disease: Atrial emptying index. Am J Cardiol, 47:1087, 1981.
11. Folland ED, Parisi AF, Moynihan PF, et al: Assessment of left ventricular ejection fraction and volumes by real time two-dimensional echocardiography. A comparison of cineangiographic and radionuclide techniques. Circulation, 60:760, 1979.
12. Goldberg SJ, Feldman L, Reinecke C, et al: Echocardiographic determination of contraction and relaxation measurements of the left ventricular wall in normal subjects and patients with muscular dystrophy. Circulation, 62:1061, 1980.
13. Gould RL, Kennedy JW, Frimer M, et al: Analysis of wall dynamics and directional components of left ventricular contraction in man. Am J Cardiol, 38:322, 1976.
14. Griffith JM, Henry WL: An ultrasound system for combined cardiac imaging and Doppler blood flow measurement in man. Circulation, 57:925, 1978.
15. Gutgesell HP, Paquet M, Duff DF, et al: Evaluation of left ventricular size and function by echocardiography. Results in normal children. Circulation, 56:457, 1977.
16. Hiraishi S, DiSessa TG, Jarmakani JM, et al: Two-dimensional echocardiographic assessment of right ventricular volume in children with congenital heart disease. Am J Cardiol, 50:1368, 1982.
17. Hirschfeld S, Meyer R, Schwartz DC, et al: Measurement of right and left ventricular systolic time intervals by echocardiography. Circulation, 51:304, 1975.
18. Lewis JR, Parker JO, Burggraf GW: Mitral valve motion and changes in left ventricular end-diastolic pressure: A correlative study of the PR-AC interval. Am J Cardiol, 42:383, 1978.
19. Massie BM, Schiller NB, Ratshin RA, et al: Mitral-septal separation: New echocardiographic index of left ventricular function. Am J Cardiol, 39:1008, 1977.
20. McLaurin LP, Grossman W, Stefadouras MA, et al: A new technique for the study of left ventricular pressure volume relations in man. Circulation, 48:56, 1973.
21. Mercier JC, DiSessa TG, Jarmakani JM, et al: Two-dimensional echocardiographic assessment of left ventricular volumes and ejection fractions in children. Circulation, 65:962, 1982.
22. Meyer RA, Stockert J, Kaplan S: Echocardiographic determinations of left ventricular volumes in pediatric patients. Circulation, 51:297, 1975.
23. Ninomia K, Duncan WJ, Cook DH, et al: Right ventricular ejection fraction and volumes after Mustard repair: Correlation of two-dimension echocardiograms and cineangiograms. Am J Cardiol, 48:317, 1981.
24. Pombo JF, Troy BC, Russell RO: Left ventricular volumes and ejection fraction by echocardiography. Circulation, 43:480, 1971.
25. Quinones MA, Gaasch WH, Alexander JK: Echocardiographic assessment of left ventricular function, with special reference to normalized velocities. Circulation, 50:42, 1974.
26. Quinones MA, Mokotoff DM, Nouri S, et al: Noninvasive quantification of left ventricular wall stress. Validation of method and application to assessment of chronic pressure overload. Am J Cardiol, 45:782, 1980.
27. Sahn DJ, Deely WJ, Hagan AD, et al: Echocardiographic assessment of left ventricular performance in normal newborns. Circulation, 49:232, 1974.
28. Sahn DJ, Vaucher Y, Williams DE, et al: Echocardiographic detection of large left to right shunts and cardiomyopathies in infants and children. Am J Cardiol, 38:73, 1976.
29. Schiller NB, Acquatella H, Ports TA, et al: Left ventricular volume from paired biplane two-dimensional echocardiography. Circulation, 60:547, 1979.
30. Silverman NH, Ports TA, Snider AR, et al: Determination of left ventricular volume in children: Echocardiographic and angiographic comparisons. Circulation, 62:548, 1980.
31. Stacks RS, Lee CC, Reddy BP, et al: Left ventricular performance in coronary artery disease evaluated with systolic time intervals and echocardiography. Am J Cardiol, 37:331, 1976.
32. Starling M, Sorenson S, Crawford M, et al: Cross-sectional echocardiographic assessment of right ventricular size and performance in obstructive pulmonary disease. Circulation, 60:II-202, 1979.
33. Teichholz LE, Kreulen T, Herman MV, et al: Problems in echocardiographic volume determinations: Echocardiographic-angiographic correlations in the presence or absence of asynergy. Am J Cardiol, 37:7, 1976.
34. Wyatt HL, Heng MK, Meerbaum S, et al: Cross-sectional echocardiography. I. Analysis of mathematical models for quantifying mass of the left ventricle in dogs. Circulation, 60:1104, 1979.

14

POSITRON EMISSION TOMOGRAPHY

The Technique and Its Applications to the Study of the Cardiovascular System

HEINRICH R. SCHELBERT, M.D., LEE BENSON, M.D., MARKUS SCHWAIGER, M.D., and JOSEPH PERLOFF, M.D.

Morphology, perfusion, and mechanical function of the heart can be accurately evaluated with invasive and noninvasive techniques. The information gained through these diagnostic modalities is physiologically and clinically relevant and has improved our capability for diagnosing and managing cardiac disease. Direct evaluation of the heart's biochemistry and metabolism as the link between flow and mechanical function, however, has remained limited. Because disease originates at the biochemical or metabolic level, probing myocardial chemistry serves to identify abnormalities at an early stage and leads to early therapeutic intervention. Such capability is of particular importance in the pediatric population. Also, metabolic causes of myocardiopathies could be elucidated and treatment instituted.

With positron computed tomography (positron-CT), the evaluation of tissue chemistry and metabolism has become available. As a unique feature, positron-CT offers the capability of recording in vivo autoradiographic-like cross-sectional images of regional concentrations of tracers of flow and, more important, metabolism. With this modality, measurements of local organ function can be communicated in terms of milliliters of blood flowing through or mass substrate utilized or metabolized per gram tissue per minute. In this regard, positron-CT is no longer an imaging device but a technique for studying regional organ physiology; the images are used for selecting the site of measurement for retrieval of tissue tracer concentrations. In the following discussion, we will briefly review technical features of positron-CT and describe positron emitting-tracers of flow and metabolism and their relation to physiologic processes. We report some of our clinical experience with this new modality and emphasize areas of pediatric disorders of the heart that are likely to benefit from positron-CT. Finally, we discuss some observations with this technique in a pediatric patient population.

TECHNICAL CONSIDERATIONS

In vivo measurement of local physiologic processes with positron-CT depends on several conditions: (1) In vivo quantification of local tissue tracer concentrations; (2) appropriate tracers of flow and metabolism; and (3) formulation of tracer kinetic models and operational equations. These three major requirements are then combined for physiologic measurements.

In Vivo Quantification of Tissue Tracer Concentrations. Positron-CT takes advantage of the radioactive decay specific for positron emitters. Positrons are particles with a mass of an electron but a positive charge. When losing kinetic energy, the positron combines with an electron and "annihilates," that is, the mass converts to energy, and two 511 kev photons are emitted in diametrically opposed directions. The "annihilation" event is detected when the two photons strike simultaneously two opposing scintillation detectors (Fig. 1*A*). This is called annihilation coincidence detection (ACD).[58] The location of an annihilation event in a given plane is determined by multiple scintillation detectors connected by coincidence circuitries and arranged in circular or hexagonal arrays (Fig. 1*B*). Earlier tomographs were equipped with only one detector plane and thus only had single slice capabilities with each contiguous cross-sectional image recorded at a time. Newer tomographs contain several detector arrays and hence have a multislice capability with simultaneous recording of several cross-sectional images.

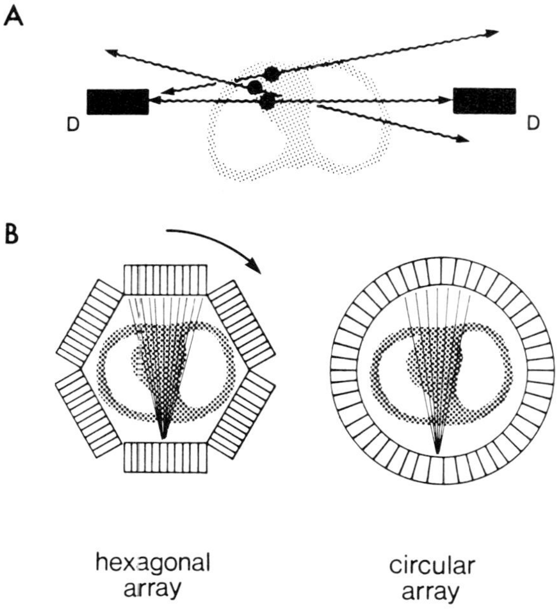

Figure 1. Annihilation coincidence detection. *A*, Schematic drawing of a cross-section of the chest with three annihilation events in the region of the heart. During each annihilation, two photons are emitted in diametrically opposed directions. Of the three, only the one occurring between the two opposing detectors (D) is recorded; the detectors are struck simultaneously by the two photons. *B*, Example of single-plane positron computed tomographs with multiple annihilation coincidence detection between opposing detectors in the same detector ring or hexagon. Lines between detectors represent the detection of the two 511 kev photons leaving the site of annihilation in diametrically opposed directions. Detectors having a fan beam response are shown in the two figures.

ACD provides uniform and high spatial resolution, high detection efficiency, and simultaneous collection of linear and angular data.[56] This represents a considerable advantage over conventional imaging with lead collimators in which spatial resolution and detection efficiency deteriorate as the distance between camera and object increases. Spatial resolution and efficiency are therefore a function of depth with these conventional cameras.

Adequate or near adequate correction for photon attenuation is possible with ACD. Photon attenuation is measured appropriately and corrected for during reconstruction of emission images. The combination of near uniform spatial resolution and adequate correction for photon attenuation, both a result of the unique electronic collimation with ACD, forms the basis for the quantitative imaging capability of positron-CT. The cross-sectional images are recorded in a transaxial orientation (perpendicular to the long axis of the body) (Fig. 2). A commercially available tomograph and a typical set of contiguous cross-sectional images of the heart are shown in Figure 3 and 4. Evaluation of the diaphragmatic portion of the left ventricle is limited when images are recorded in a transaxial orientation. Newer tomographs can therefore be tilted laterally and vertically, and the imaging plane positioned perpendicular to the long axis of the left ventricle.

Positron Emitting Tracers of Flow and Metabolism. A second advantage of positron-CT is the use of positron-emitting isotopes of elements like oxygen, carbon, or nitrogen. With conventional radionuclide techniques, the large atomic size of commonly used radioisotopes, for example, technetium-99m, modifies the biologic properties of the labeled compound. This is not the case with positron emitters. Substrates or metabolites are tagged, for example, with carbon-11 or nitrogen-13 without modifying their biochemical properties. When administered in tracer amounts, these radiopharmaceuticals enter and proceed through physiologic processes in a manner indistinguishable from that of unlabeled metabolic substrates or metabolites. Hence, these positron-emitting radiopharmaceuticals are true tracers of metabolism. Many of these tracers have been developed to date. For example, C-11-labeled palmitate, N-13- or C-11-labeled amino acids, C-11-labeled pyruvate and acetate, and O-15-labeled water are now available for routine use. The physical half-life of these radioactive tracers range from 2 to 120 min, which results not only in a lower radiation burden to the patient but

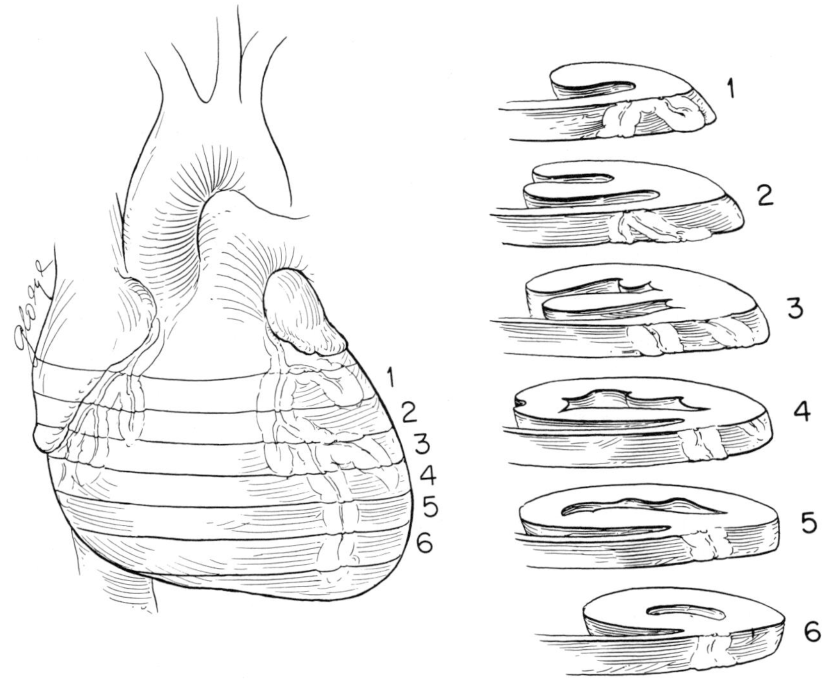

Figure 2. Transaxial cross-sectional imaging of the heart. Schematic representation of the tomographic cross-sectional images in relation to cardiac anatomy. Each slice is approximately 1.5 cm thick. (*From* Schelbert HR, Henze E, Phelps ME: Emission tomography of the heart. Semin. Nucl. Med., *10*:355–373, 1980, with permission.)

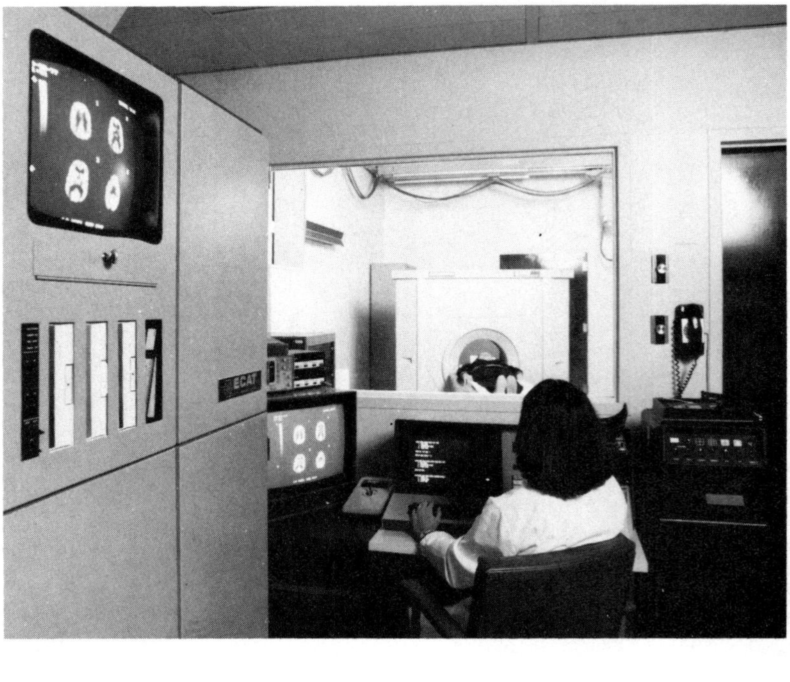

Figure 3. Whole body positron emission tomograph in the UCLA Nuclear Medicine Clinic.

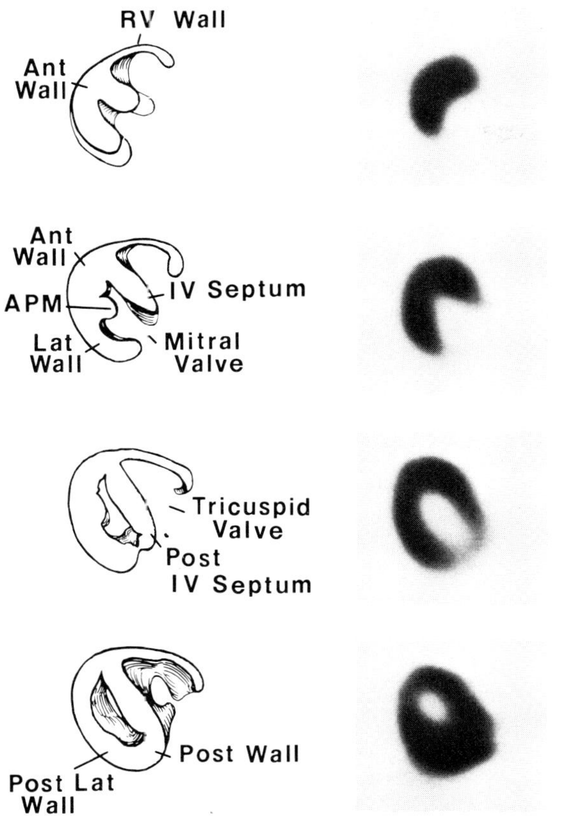

Figure 4. Four contiguous cross-sectional positron CT images of left ventricular myocardium in a normal subject after intravenous infusion of N-13 ammonia and schematic representation of the various anatomic landmarks (i.v.: interventricular septum, APM: anterior papillary muscle, RV: right ventricular wall). The thin right ventricular wall is not visualized because of the disproportionately lower blood flow and less indicator uptake and the object size-related loss in count recovery. (*From* Schelbert HR, Henze E, Phelps ME, et al: Emission tomography of the heart. Semin Nucl Med, *10*:355–373, 1980, with permission.)

also allows rapid repeat studies. This advantage, however, also limits the use of positron-CT. The ultrashort physical half-life requires on-site isotope production. On-site cyclotrons and on-site radiochemistry are therefore needed.

Positron-emitting tracers are suitable for positron-CT only if they meet several criteria: their residence time in myocardium must be sufficiently long to permit statistically adequate imaging; the chemical form in which the radioactive label is contained must be known; the kinetics, that is, extraction, transport, distribution, and clearance must be defined and their relation to the process under study established; finally, the tracer kinetics must be amenable to tracer kinetic modeling.

Tracer Kinetic Models. These models are derived from the tissue response to an input function. They describe uptake or initial transmembraneous exchange, tissue distribution, and tracer clearance from tissue as the exchange of tracer between compartments. A typical example of such a compartmental model and its metabolic correlate is shown in Figure 5 for F-18 2-fluoro 2-deoxyglucose (FDG) used for measurements of exogenous glucose utilization. Sokoloff and colleagues established this model initially for measuring metabolic rates of glucose in the brain with C-14 deoxyglucose and autoradiography.[78] To apply this technique to in vivo measurements, Reivich et al. developed the positron-emitting glucose analog FDG.[63] FDG traces only the transmembraneous transport and initial metabolic step of glucose. It

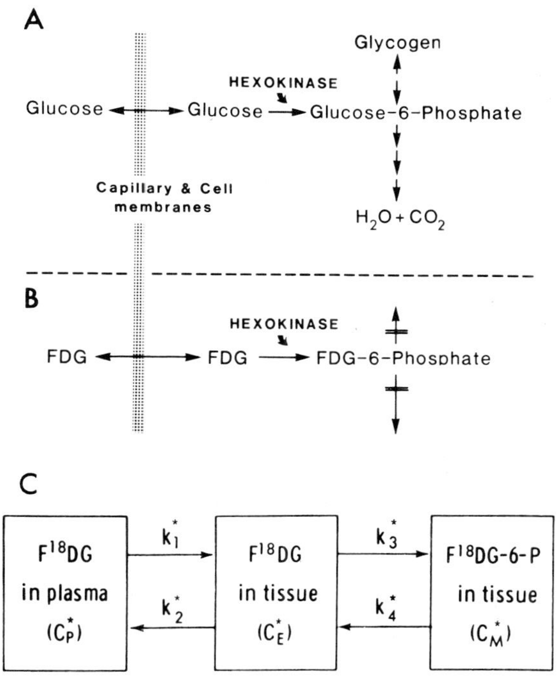

Figure 5. Metabolism of glucose (A) and of FDG (B) and FDG tracer kinetic model (C). *A*, Glucose enters the cell through facilitated transport and is metabolized to glucose-6-phosphate, a metabolic step mediated by the enzyme hexokinase. Glucose-6-phosphate can then be used for formation of glycogen or enters glycolytic pathways and is catabolized to water and carbon dioxide. *B*, FDG exchanges across the capillary and cell membranes in proportion to glucose and is converted to FDG-6-phosphate via the action of hexokinase. However, FDG-6-phosphate is not a substrate for glycogen synthesis or for glycolysis and therefore is trapped in tissue. *C*, Three-compartmental model for FDG. Compartment 1 represents FDG in plasma (C_P*), compartment 2 FDG in tissue (C_E*), and compartment 3 FDG-6-phosphate in tissue (C_M*). The rate constants k_1 and k_2 describe the forward and reverse transport of FDG between plasma and tissue, and k_3 and k_4 describe the exchange between FDG in tissue and phosphorylation to FDG-6-phosphate. Because k_4 is very small, this exchange is virtually unidirectional.

accumulates in tissue in form of FDG-6-phosphate because it is not a substrate for glycolysis or for glycogen synthesis. In organs like the brain where glucose is not converted to glycogen, the rate of the initial metabolic step is representative for the entire glycolytic flux. Hence, the local metabolic rate of glucose in the brain can be calculated.[35, 60, 63]

Each compartment of the tracer kinetic model represents a functional unit and does not necessarily correspond to morphologic structures. The functional units usually represent a series or chains of metabolic reactions. Through these models, operational equations are formulated and used for calculating the metabolic rates, for example, of glucose from the FDG tissue concentrations, the arterial input function, and the concentrations of arterial plasma glucose.

Physiologic Measurements with Positron-CT. These measurements are performed after positioning the patient in the whole body positron computed tomograph (Fig. 3) with the transaxial image plane traversing the heart. Transmission images are acquired for correction of photon attenuation of the cross-sectional emission images. The radiotracer is then administered either intravenously or, in some instances, by inhalation. Emission images are recorded either immediately beginning with tracer administration or after steady state conditions are reached. Statistically adequate images can be obtained within less than 1 min. Image acquisition can also be synchronized with the patient's electrocardiogram to minimize the blurring effects of cardiac motion. Serial arterial blood samples are drawn for determining the arterial input function or arterial substrate plasma levels.

Regional indicator concentrations in myocardial tissue are derived from regions-of-interest assigned to the left ventricular myocardium on the positron-CT images. The size of the region-of-interest corresponds to a given imaged volume, and regional activities are therefore expressed as activity per gram of tissue.

The arterial input function is derived from serial blood samples or from regions-of-interest assigned to arterial blood in the left ventricular chamber on serial positron-CT images. The arterial input function is obtained by integrating serial measurements of concentrations of indicator blood over time. Activity concentrations derived from regions-of-interest and defined as positron-CT units are converted to activity concentrations determined in a well counter. This is accomplished by imaging a cylindrical phantom, which contains a solution of the radiopharmaceutical. The activity per cm^3 is derived from a region-of-interest on the imaged phantom encompassing a known volume and related to the activity concentration measured from an aliquot of the same solution by well counting.

ASSESSMENT OF MYOCARDIAL BLOOD FLOW

Several techniques for evaluating regional myocardial perfusion with positron-CT are available or will be available in the near future. These techniques employ radioactive microspheres, N-13 ammonia, rubidium-82, and more recently, O-15-labeled water.

Regional organ perfusion is measured most accurately with radioactive microspheres and the arterial reference sampling technique.[33, 85] The approach requires determination of concentrations of tissue microsphere activity, which is accomplished by in vitro counting of tissue samples, and which precludes the use of this method in man. Such measurements, however, are possible in vivo with positron-CT. In our laboratory, Wisenberg and colleagues[85] employed this technique in animals. Gallium-68 albumin microspheres were delivered into the left atrium. Regional myocardial blood flow was calculated in vivo, analogous to the arterial reference sampling technique[33] from the withdrawal rate of arterial blood, the Ga-68 activity in the arterial reference sample, and the regional myocardial Ga-68 concentrations derived from cross-sectional positron-CT images of the left ventricular myocardium. Compared with simultaneous in vitro measurements, the in vivo measurements by positron-CT were highly accurate (Fig. 6).

The need of administering microspheres into the left side of the heart renders this approach invasive and limits its clinical applicability. We therefore explored the utility of N-13 ammonia as a diffusible tracer of perfusion that can be used intravenously. N-13 ammonia rapidly clears from blood into myocardium, where it is extracted and retained in proportion to blood flow.[66, 67] Yet, unlike microspheres which are 100 per cent trapped during a single capillary transit, the extraction fraction of N-13 ammonia is less than 100 per cent and inversely related to flow. Consequently, tissue ammonia concentrations of N-13 as the product of flow and extraction fraction are a nonlinear function of flow.[68] For flows from near zero to about 250 to 300 ml per min per 100 gm, however, flow

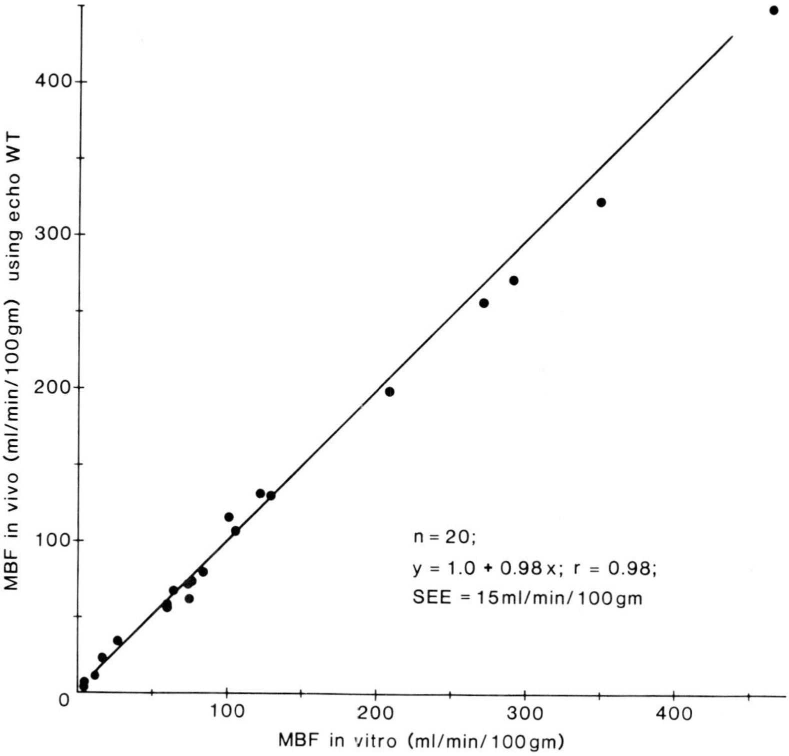

Figure 6. In vivo measurements of regional myocardial blood flow with Ga-68 labeled albumin microspheres, the arterial reference sampling technique, and positron CT. The myocardial indicator concentrations derived from regions-of-interest on the cross-sectional images were corrected for partial volume effect by determining regional thickness of the myocardial wall echocardiographically. The measurements were obtained from experiments with dogs and are compared with in vitro measurements using gamma-emitting, carbonized microspheres and in vitro tissue counting. (*From* Wisenberg G, Schelbert HR, Hoffman EJ, et al: In vivo quantitation of regional myocardial blood flow by positron emission computed tomography. Circulation, *63*:1248–1258, 1981, with permission.)

increases are associated with proportionate increases in N-13 ammonia concentrations.[66, 67] This response plateaus at higher flows when large flow increases cause only small increases in N-13 concentrations.

Nevertheless, N-13 ammonia together with positron-CT allowed detection of mild coronary stenoses during pharmacologically induced vasodilation in intact and awake dogs.[25] More recently, this technique was employed in man and demonstrated a high sensitivity and accuracy in identifying coronary artery disease and its extent (Fig. 7).[68]

With properties like rapid clearance from the blood, trapping in myocardium in proportion to flow, and long myocardial retention times, N-13 ammonia can be compared with radioactive microspheres with a rapidly completed input function, a linear response of microsphere concentrations to flow, and fixation of microspheres in myocardium through capillary trapping.[33] These similarities raise the possibility of quantitative measurements with N-13 ammonia and the arterial reference sampling technique. Studies of dogs provided initial evidence in support of such a possibility.[76] Myocardial blood flow was calculated from the arterial withdrawal rate, the N-13 activity in the arterial reference sample, and the myocardial tissue concentrations of N-13 measured by positron-CT. For flows from near zero to about 250 ml per min per 100 gm, the approach provided reasonably accurate measurements of regional myocardial perfusion in comparison to the standard in vitro microsphere technique (Fig. 8).

Other investigators employed Rb-82 or Rb-81 for evaluating regional myocardial perfusion.[4, 9] Rubidium-82 is generator produced and can be used independently of an on-site cyclotron. Initially evaluated at several institutions, Selwyn et al. used Rb-82 for studying patients with ischemic heart disease.[73] The 2 min physical half-life permits rapid repeat injections and hence the study of rapidly changing physiologic conditions. Segmental decreases in Rb-82 activity and presumably in perfusion were noted not only during episodes of chest pain or electrocardiographic changes but also in their absence. Decreases in segmental activity persisted long after clinical signs of ischemia

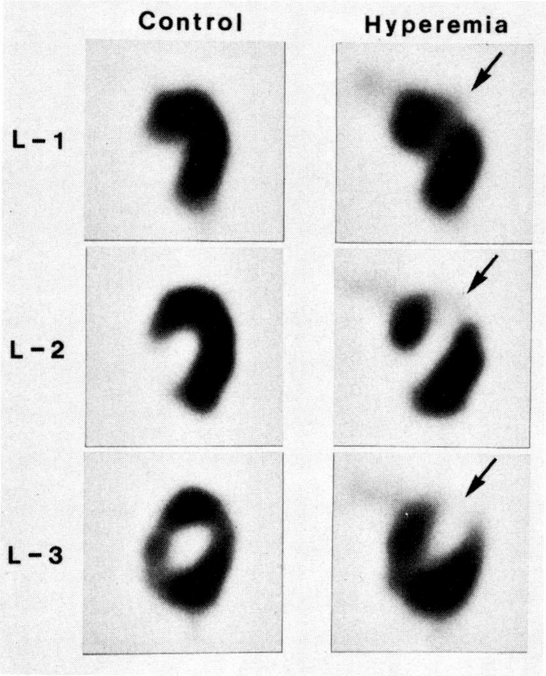

Figure 7. Detection of coronary artery disease by using N-13 ammonia and positron CT during coronary vasodilation pharmacologically induced. Three contiguous cross-sectional images of the left ventricular myocardium are shown. L-1 is recorded through the high, L-2 through the mid- and L-3 through the lower part of the left ventricle. The control study reveals homogeneous perfusion in this patient, with complete occlusion of the left anterior descending coronary artery indicating adequate collateral blood flow to the anterior wall at rest. Coronary vasodilation was induced by infusion of dipyridamole and the N-13 ammonia injection repeated at peak response. The arrows indicate perfusion defects in all three levels in the anterior wall. Quantitative image analysis indicated that tissue concentrations of N-13 failed to increase in the anterior wall from control to hyperemia, whereas N-13 concentrations in the septum and the lateral wall increased by more than 50 per cent. (*From* Schelbert HR, Wisenberg G, Phelps ME, et al: Noninvasive assessment of coronary stenoses by myocardial imaging during pharmacologic vasodilation. VI. Detection of coronary artery disease in man with intravenous N-13 ammonia and positron computed tomography. Am J Cardiol, *49*:1197–1207, 1982, with permission.)

had subsided. This raised the question whether such defects were related not only to diminished perfusion but also to disturbances in transmembraneous exchange of cations. Hence, with this agent, the study of electrolyte kinetics may indeed become possible. In the same context is an earlier study of patients with asymmetric septal hypertrophy in which Rb-82 uptake was increased in the hypertrophied segment. Although technical reasons could to some extent account for the observations, they also could suggest abnormal exchange of cations in the hypertrophic segment.[42]

Selwyn's findings[73] indicate some limitations of diffusible tracers of blood flow. Their net extraction is the product of flow and extraction fraction, that is, the amount of tracer delivered and the fraction of tracer leaving the vascular space and retained in the myocardium. If transmembranous exchange or the trapping mechanism is altered in disease, regional myocardial extraction fractions could change. Accordingly, the relation between flow and tissue response in tracer concentrations could be altered, and the value of these flow tracers limited. As noted by Selwyn, such limitation cannot be ruled out entirely for Rb-82 and is also possible for N-13 ammonia.

Such limitation does not appear to apply to O-15-labeled water for measurements of blood flow. The tracer is almost 100 per cent extracted and is chemically inert. The myocardium-blood partition coefficient is known and not expected to be altered in abnormal metabolic states. The indicator is inhaled as O-15-labeled CO_2, which is immediately converted in the lungs to O-15 water through carbonic anhydrase or is administered as an intravenous bolus. Measurements of organ blood flow require acquisition of sequential positron-CT images from which curves for local tissue clearance are determined and deconvolved for the input function. Local tissue perfusion is calculated by using the same tissue-partition coefficient, and an image of regional perfusion is formed.

This technique for measurements of local cerebral blood flow has recently been reviewed by Phelps et al.[61] Preliminary studies in animals and in man suggest that it also can be applied to the heart, although its use is complicated by considerable O-15 activity in the large cardiac blood pools and lungs with substantial spillover of activity into the myocardium.[1, 5, 36] Techniques to remove this contamination from myocardial activity as well as correction for partial volume effects are therefore required and are under development. Many of these limitations are likely to be resolved with newer tomographs with improved spatial and temporal resolution. Once these current difficulties are overcome, it is possible to combine this technique with measurements of the local extraction fraction of oxygen used already in the brain.[37] Again, this technique has recently been reviewed by Phelps et al.[61] and together with measurements of blood flow will allow determination of the regional myocardial oxygen consumption.

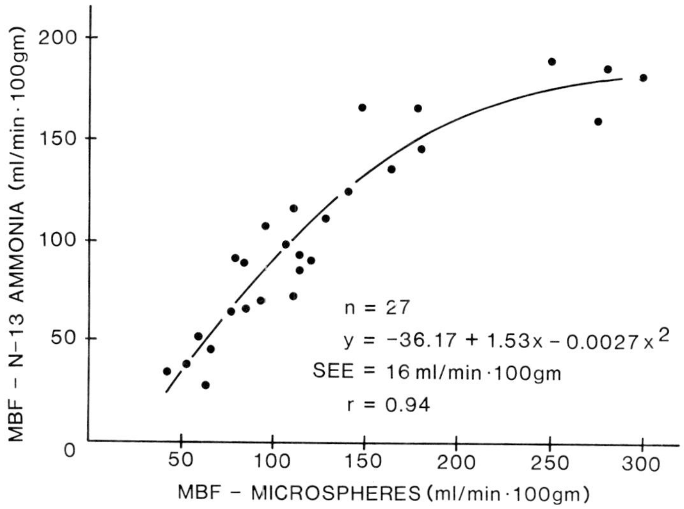

Figure 8. In vivo measurement of regional myocardial blood flow (MBF) with N-13 ammonia and positron CT in chronically instrumented dogs compared with simultaneous in vitro measurements with gamma-emitting microspheres and in vitro tissue counting. Note the linear relationship for flows up to about 200 ml/min/100 gm (Courtesy of A. Shah, M.D., UCLA).

ASSESSMENT OF MYOCARDIAL METABOLISM

Positron-CT's most unique feature is the potential of probing regional myocardial metabolism. This aspect of myocardial function has remained relatively inaccessible to conventional study techniques. Although estimates of metabolic rates have been obtained by blood sampling across the heart, such measurements are not regional and provide limited information on the subsequent turnover of subtrates like glucose, free fatty acids, or lactate. Their value is further limited under specific conditions. For example, myocardial ischemia is identified through production of lactate. Yet, despite the presence of ischemia, production of lactate may cease when ischemia becomes more severe and anaerobic glycolysis is inhibited.

Lipid Metabolism. Free fatty acids (FFA) have long been considered the preferred fuel substrate of myocardium. Several reports presented experimental evidence for the use of C-11 palmitate as a tracer of myocardial FFA metabolism.[23, 34, 39, 65, 70, 71, 84] In isolated perfused hearts, uptake of this tracer by myocardium is quantitatively related to FFA use.[46] Although these findings remain to be tested in vivo, such a relationship has at least been qualitatively observed in in vivo experiments with dogs.[65] Once sequestered into myocardium, C-11 activity typically clears from myocardium biexponentially, which indicates that C-11 palmitate in tissue is distributed between at least two pools that turnover at different rates. The fractional distribution is consistent with findings after infusions of C-14-labeled palmitate or by microautoradiography. According to these observations, a fraction of the labeled palmitate immediately enters oxidative pathways while the remainder is initially deposited in a slow turnover pool probably in the form of triglycerides and phospholipids. The relative size of the early rapid clearance phase on the myocardial C-11 time-activity curve and its clearance rates are related to production of C-11 CO_2.[65, 71] Therefore, this curve component corresponds to oxidation of C-11 palmitate to C-11 CO_2 and reflects the fraction of FFA that becomes immediately oxidized (Fig. 9). From our findings, we formulated a tracer kinetic model that eventually will permit the measurement of exogenous utilization of FFA, its fractional distribution, and rate of beta-oxidation.

For the study of regional myocardial FFA metabolism, C-11 palmitate is administered intravenously. Rapid sequential cross-sectional positron-CT images are recorded for at least 60 min (Fig. 10). After image reconstruction, regions-of-interest are assigned to the left ventricular myocardium and blood pool. The observed tissue concentrations of C-11 activity are corrected for activity spillover, and time-activity curves are constructed. From time-activity curves, the arterial input function, net extraction of C-11 palmitate, and fractional distribution of C-11 palmitate between oxidation and storage pools and the turnover rates are derived (see Fig. 9).

Glucose Utilization. F-18 2-fluoro 2-deoxyglucose (FDG) was mentioned earlier as a tracer of exogenous glucose uptake. FDG is an analog of glucose, which, once phosphorylated to FDG-6-phosphate, is not catabolized and becomes trapped in tissue (see Fig. 5). FDG has been extensively used for measurements of the

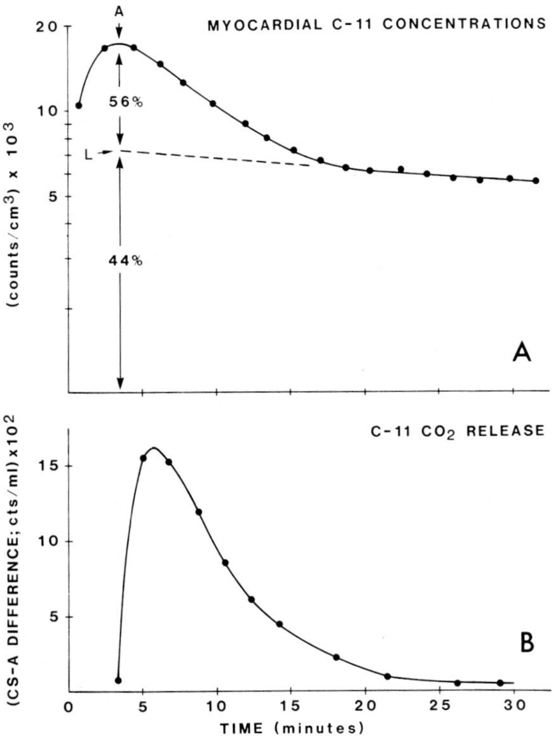

Figure 9. Myocardial C-11 time activity. Curve derived from sequential positron CT images after intravenous infusion of C-11 palmitate in a dog's open chest. Note the initial uptake of C-11 palmitate in the myocardium and the subsequent biexponential clearance of C-11 activity from the myocardium. Extrapolation of the late slow phase to the time of peak activity *(A)* provides an estimate of the fractional distribution of C-11 palmitate in the myocardium. In this dog, 44 per cent of the C-11 palmitate entered the slow turnover pool; the remaining 56 per cent entered the rapid turnover pool. *B*, Serial measurements of the coronary sinus arterial C-11 CO_2 differences. Note that peak release of C-11 CO_2 occurs during the early rapid clearance phase of the time activity curve shown in *A*. (*From* Schelbert HR, Henze E, Schon HR, et al: C-11 labeled palmitic acid for the noninvasive evaluation of regional myocardial fatty acid metabolism with positron computed tomography. III. In vivo demonstration of the effects of substrate availability on myocardial metabolism. Am Heart J, *105*:492–502, 1983, with permission.)

local metabolic rate of glucose in the brain.[35, 60, 61, 63] A tracer kinetic model for FDG is available, and cerebral metabolic rates are calculated through an operational equation from tissue concentrations of FDG, the arterial input function, and plasma concentrations of arterial glucose. More recently, this technique has been successfully employed in the heart.[59] Initially used only qualitatively, variations in myocardial uptake of FDG accurately reflected variations in myocardial substrate utilization such as preferential glucose or FFA utilization (Fig. 11). Subsequent studies in dogs have confirmed the utility of the tracer kinetic model for measurements of myocardial utilization of exogenous glucose. In our laboratory, Ratib and coworkers[62] found an excellent agreement between noninvasive measurements with FDG and positron-CT and glucose utilization calculated from the differences in glucose concentrations in arterial and coronary sinus blood and myocardial blood flow (Fig. 12).

FDG traces only the transport and initial step of glucose metabolism. When glucose is not converted to glycogen as in the brain, the rate of the single initial metabolic step is representative of the entire glycolytic flux.[35, 60, 63] Hence, the local metabolic rate of glucose can be calculated by related tissue concentrations of FDG and arterial input function to glucose concentrations in capillary blood. Unfortunately, glucose metabolism in myocardium is more complex. The metabolic pathway for glucose is branched with a fraction directly entering glycolysis and a fraction synthesized to glycogen. Conversely, intracellular glycogen stores can be mobilized and serve as an endogenous source of glucose. Accordingly, rates of exogenous glucose utilization measured with the FDG technique are not always a true reflection of the glycolytic rate.

Alternate Substrate Utilization. In the above study, glucose utilization rates varied from 1.7 to 21.2 mg per min per 100 gm myocardium. Different cardiac workloads with different MVO_2s and accordingly substrate demand partly account for this wide range. Other factors are differences in substrate availability. The dependency of myocardial substrate utilization on plasma substrate concentrations has long been established.[10, 38] For example, after moderate fasting, plasma FFA levels are in the upper range of normal and glucose and insulin levels are low. Accordingly, the myocardium's energy demands are met mainly through FFA oxidation. Conversely, after carbohydrate intake, glucose and insulin levels rise while FFA levels decline. In response, the myocardium uses less FFA but more glucose.[10] Another example is physical exercise. Lactate levels are known to increase with strenuous exercise, and lactate thus can provide for as much as 60 per cent of the total MVO_2.[38]

Thus, normal myocardium exhibits a remarkable ability to adjust to altered conditions of substrate availability in order to meet its energy demands. In fact, this ability may represent a property characteristic for normal myocardium. It may be impaired in myocardial disease as evidenced by observations in acute myocardial

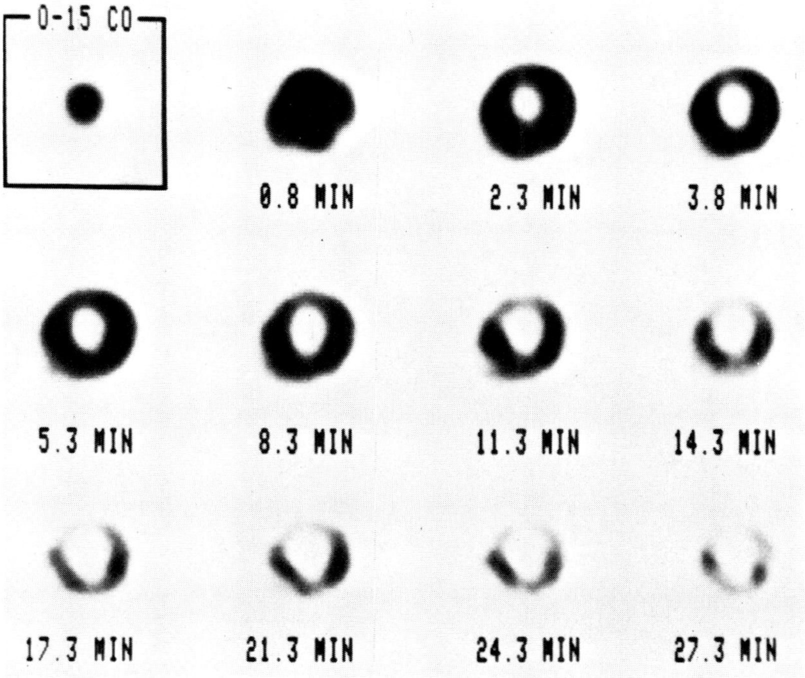

Figure 10. Serial cross-sectional positron CT images of the left ventricular myocardium after intravenous infusion of C-11 palmitate. For comparison, a blood pool image recorded after inhalation of O-15 labeled CO is shown in the left upper corner. Acquisition of image was begun simultaneously with administration of C-11 palmitate. On the initial cross-sectional image, most of the activity is present in blood. As C-11 activity clears from blood into the myocardium, the left ventricular myocardium is well visualized. Maximum activities are reached between 2.3 and 3.8 min. As indicated by the subsequently decreasing intensity, C-11 activity clears from the myocardium as shown in the time activity curve in Figure 9. (*From* Schelbert HR, Henze E, Schon HR, et al: C-11 palmitic acid for the noninvasive evaluation of regional myocardial fatty acid metabolism with positron computed tomography. III. In vivo demonstration of the effects of substrate availability on myocardial metabolism. Am Heart J, *105*:492–502, 1983, with permission.)

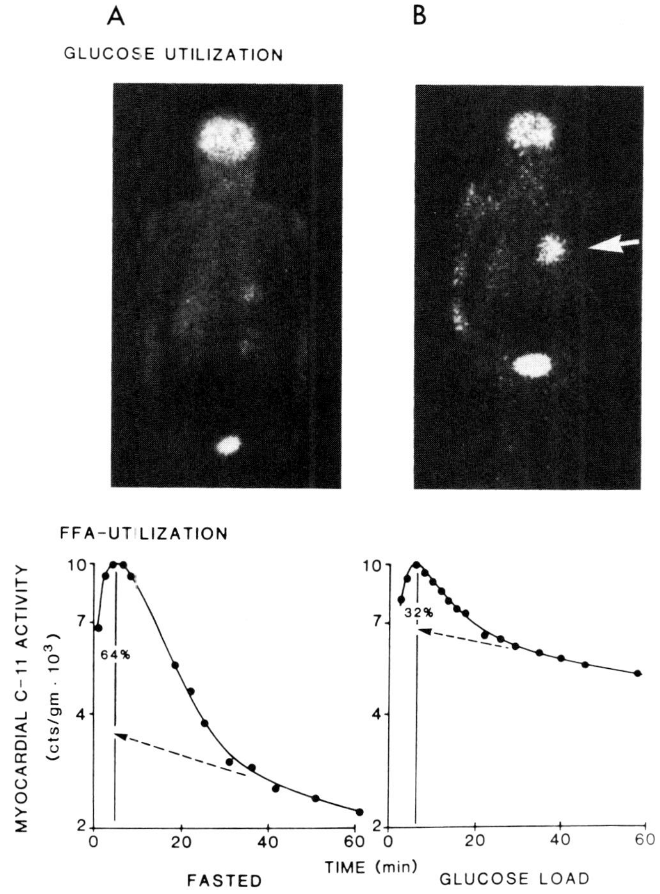

Figure 11. Noninvasive evaluation of myocardial substrate utilization as a function of substrate levels in arterial plasma of two volunteers. The upper panel indicates the glucose utilization assessed with intravenous FDG, the lower panel the free fatty acid (FFA) utilization evaluated with intravenous C-11 palmitate. The rectilinear whole body scan shown in the upper left corner was obtained in a patient after an overnight fast. Note the intense FDG uptake in the brain but the lack of FDG uptake in the myocardium, indicating absent glucose utilization. The time activity below was obtained in another volunteer after an overnight fast when plasma FFA levels were high. Note that 64 per cent of the C-11 palmitate extracted by the myocardium enters the rapid turnover "oxidation" pool, indicating that in this state the myocardium derived energy primarily from free fatty acids. The patient in the upper right panel was studied after administration of an oral glucose load with an increase in plasma glucose levels and a decline in plasma FFA levels. Again, there is intense FDG uptake in the brain but also in the myocardium. In the panel below, the time activity curve markedly differs from that obtained in the fasting state. Only 32 per cent of the C-11 palmitate extracted by the myocardium enters the rapid turnover "oxidation" pool, indicating that after glucose loading the heart primarily meets its energy demands through oxidation of glucose rather than FFA.

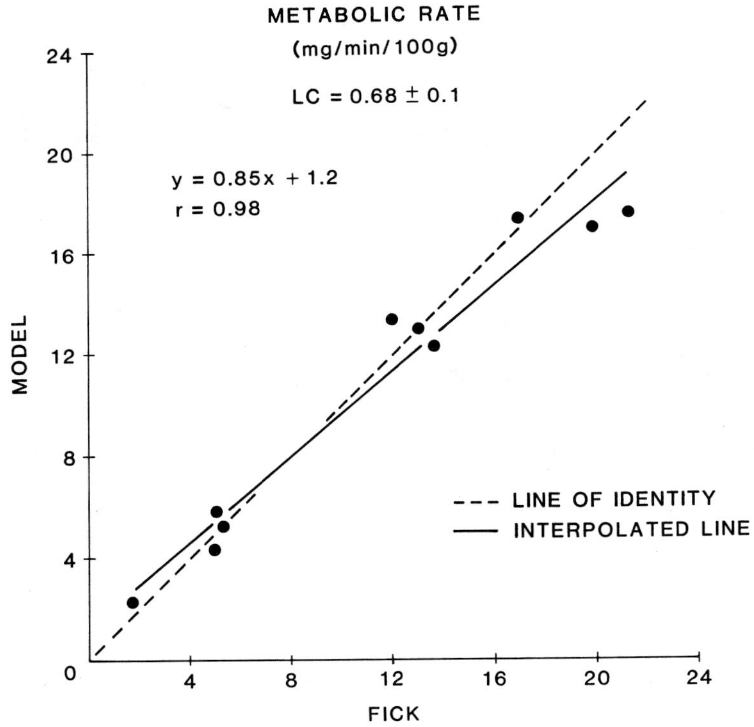

Figure 12. In vivo measurements of regional myocardial glucose utilization with FDG and positron CT compared with invasive glucose utilization measurements with the Fick method. Note the close agreement between the noninvasive and the invasive measurements. (*From* Ratib O, Phelps ME, Huang SC, et al: Positron tomography with deoxyglucose for estimating local myocardial glucose metabolism. J Nucl Med, 23:577–586, 1982, with permission.)

ischemia[41, 50] or, more recently, in cardiomyopathies (see below). Accordingly, myocardial disease could be identified by testing the heart's ability to alternate between substrates in response to changes in substrate plasma levels.

We have examined this possibility in both animals and in man.[29, 65] Patients were studied after an overnight fast and again after an oral glucose load. In the fasted state, there is little if any glucose utilization, which is reflected accurately by a lack of FDG uptake. Conversely, C-11 palmitate uptake is high, with a fractional tissue distribution indicating that a major fraction of the C-11 palmitate is turned immediately into oxidative pathways as reflected by the large size of the early rapid time-activity curve component and its rapid clearance rate. Therefore, after a glucose load, a disproportionately smaller fraction of extracted C-11 palmitate enters the rapid turnover oxidation pool while there is considerable trapping of FDG in myocardium (Fig. 11).

Manipulation of substrate metabolism in acutely ischemic myocardium, for example, was no longer possible to the same extent. While C-11 palmitate uptake and turnover and FDG accumulation could be influenced in normal myocardium, this was not possible in the ischemic segment. Substrate utilization by acutely ischemic myocardium therefore appeared fixed, and this abnormality could be demonstrated by changing plasma substrate levels (Fig. 13). When compared with myocardial perfusion, FDG uptake was in excess of blood flow. Hence, in the glucose preferential uptake, there was a relative and in the preferential FFA utilization an absolute increase in FDG uptake. These observations are consistent with Opie's observations of an increased glycolytic flux and impaired oxidation as a metabolic consequence of acute myocardial ischemia in animals.[50] Similar observations were recently made by Marshall and colleagues in our laboratory in patients with clinical evidence of myocardial ischemia (Fig. 14).[41]

Lactate and Acetate Metabolism. Both substances are normally present in blood, although at relatively low concentrations. They can be labeled with carbon-11. Goldstein et al. used C-11 lactate in acute experimental myocardial ischemia.[22] The tracer cleared rapidly from normal myocardium but was retained in the acutely ischemic segment. Selwyn's findings with C-11-labeled acetic acid in canine experiments and human patients are similar.[74] After being sequestered in myocardium, C-11 activity rapidly cleared from normal myocardium but was retained in ischemic myocardium, which therefore was visualized on late sequential positron-CT images as an area of increased activity.

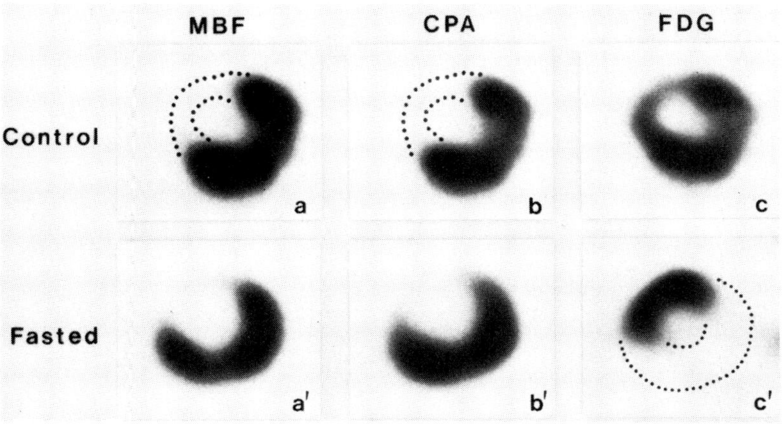

Figure 13. Limited alternate substrate utilization in acute myocardial ischemia. Two canine studies with pacing-induced ischemia are shown. The canine study in the upper panel was performed in the control state, the one in the lower panel after a 36 hr fast. As indicated on the cross-sectional perfusion images (MBF), flow in the ischemic anterior wall is markedly decreased in both studies. Similarly, there was a proportional reduction in C-11 palmitate uptake in the ischemic segment in both experiments (CPA). However, FDG uptake as a reflection of exogenous glucose utilization was decreased in the control animal during pacing-induced ischemia, although disproportionately less than flow or C-11 palmitate uptake. Hence, FDG uptake was in excess of flow. In the dog that fasted, normal myocardium shifted to FFA utilization. Consequently, no FDG uptake is noted in normal myocardium. However, this shift in substrate utilization did not occur in the acutely ischemic segment, which accumulated FDG and hence utilized exogenous glucose. The study further indicates the relative or absolute increases in exogenous glucose utilization in ischemic myocardium.

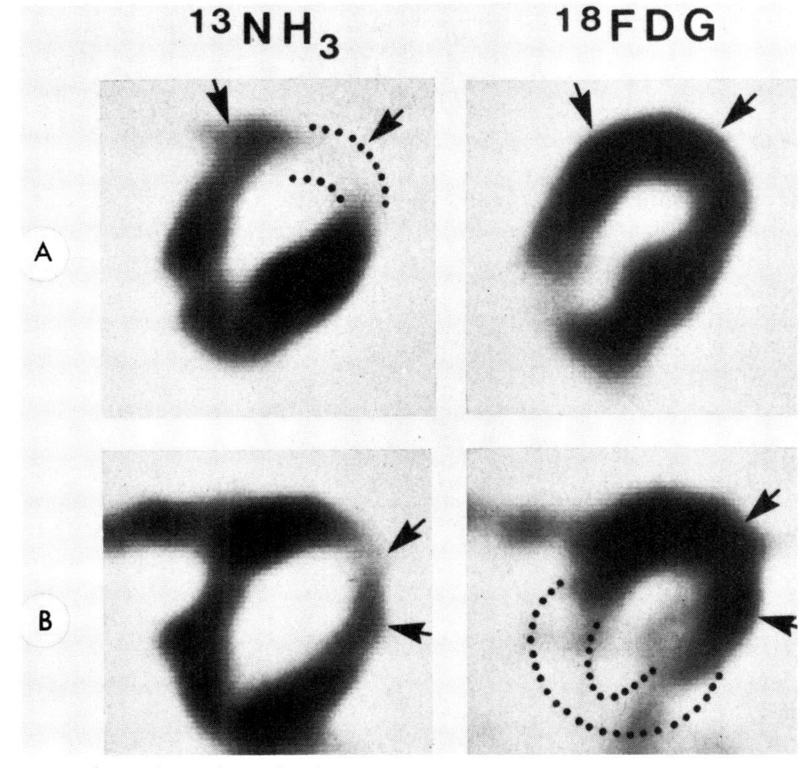

Figure 14. Examples of preferential glucose utilization in chronically ischemic myocardium in two patients. The patient in the upper panel (A) was studied after an overnight fast, the patient in panel B after an oral glucose load. Myocardial perfusion was assessed with intravenous infusion of N-13 ammonia. The positron CT cross-sectional images of the left ventricular myocardium depict segments with markedly decreased concentrations of N-13 and, hence, decreased perfusion (arrows). Regional glucose utilization as shown by the corresponding FDG images on the right was discordant. In patient A, there was FDG in the normal myocardium as well as FDG uptake in the ischemic segment. Hence, as in the dog study shown in Figure 13, FDG uptake and, therefore, utilization of exogenous glucose were markedly in excess of perfusion. In patient B, there was little FDG uptake and hence, exogenous glucose utilization in the normal myocardium. However, utilization of exogenous glucose is markedly increased in the ischemic segment as shown by the markedly increased FDG uptake in the underperfused anterior wall (Courtesy of M. Mandelkern, M.D., UCLA).

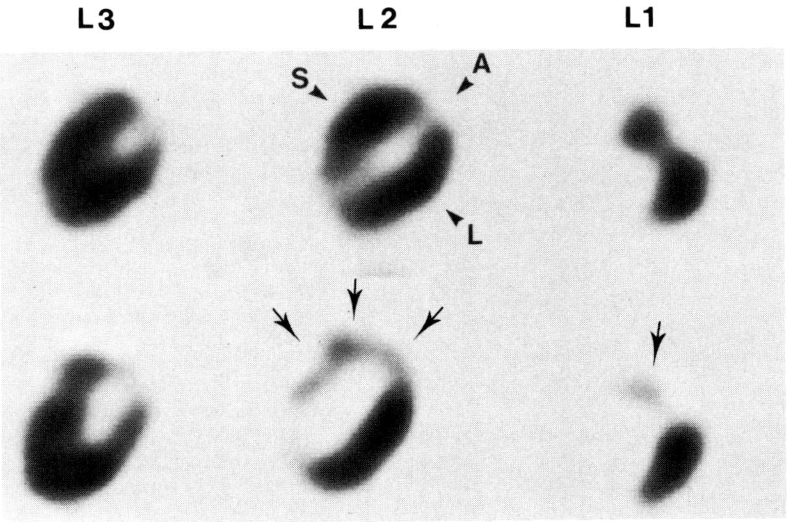

Figure 15. Regional myocardial perfusion and N-13 glutamate uptake in a patient with fibrosarcoma of the anterior wall, impeding left anterior descending (LAD) coronary flow and after a selective administration of Adriamycin into the LAD artery. The three contiguous cross-sectional images (L1 to L3) show the area of decreased perfusion of the anterior wall (A) as a result of the LAD stenosis. Yet, despite normal perfusion of the anterior septum shown on the N-13 ammonia images, trapping of N-13 glutamate in the LAD territory is markedly depressed (arrows). This segmental decrease in N-13 ammonia is likely to reflect the decreased rate of protein synthesis as a consequence of the intracoronary infusion of Adriamycin (Courtesy of E. Henze et al., UCLA).

Selwyn also provided evidence for oxidation of C-11 acetate to C-11 CO_2. Acetate probably more directly enters the citric acid cycle. Hence, although more confirmatory evidence is needed, it is conceivable that the rate of citric cycle activity can be evaluated noninvasively with these tracers.

Amino Acid Metabolism and Protein Synthesis. Several amino acids have been labeled with nitrogen-13 and carbon-11.[3] In fact, Gelbard and co-workers recently demonstrated a high extraction of N-13 glutamate by human myocardium.[20] In our laboratory, Henze and co-workers evaluated the kinetics of C-11 and N-13-labeled amino acids in canine myocardium.[31] From the bi- and triexponential clearance patterns of these compounds and appearance of the C-11 activity in CO_2 in coronary sinus blood, these authors concluded thát the labeled amino acids were distributed between a pool of intermediate metabolism related to citric cycle activity and a pool of protein synthesis. These findings raised the possibility of in vivo studies of intermediary energy metabolism and protein synthesis with labeled amino acids (Fig. 15).

Progress has been made for measuring the rate of protein synthesis in the brain. Smith et al. recently proposed a tracer kinetic model for measuring autoradiographic measurements of protein synthesis with C-14 leucine.[77] This model was adapted to in vivo measurements with C-11 leucine. Indeed, in our laboratory, Phelps et al. developed a method for in vivo measurements of cerebral protein synthesis.[57] The same model and technique can conceivably be used for determining myocardial protein synthesis.

CLINICAL APPLICATIONS

Positron-CT can be used to investigate metabolic pathways noninvasively in patients with a variety of cardiac diseases. Our attention will focus on evaluating myocardial perfusion and, specifically, potential use in the characterization of a variety of cardiac disorders whose origins are believed to be metabolic. Finally, we will describe our observations in patients with Duchenne's dystrophy and dilated cardiomyopathies.

Evaluation of Myocardial Perfusion. The evaluation of myocardial perfusion, both qualitatively and quantitatively, yields important information about coronary artery disease. In the pediatric population, this technique will add to the evaluation of management alternatives in those children suffering from abnormalities such as anomalous origin of the left coronary artery from the pulmonary artery. Moreover, the technique can be applied in the evaluation of children with myocardial injury sustained during ventriculotomies for correction of congenital defects[6] or in patients with Kawasaki's disease for the noninvasive assessment of the structural integrity of the distal coronary artery system and longitudinal follow-up.

The main application of blood flow markers may be in combination with metabolic tracers, allowing for independent analysis of perfusion and metabolism. This is demonstrated by the use of O-15-labeled water and FDG in brain tumors documenting the uncoupling of regional perfusion and metabolism (Frackowiak, personal communication; and reference 61). Hence, the evaluation of tumor metabolism and its response to treatment could be assessed more accurately.

Myocardial Metabolism. If radioactive-labeled tracers are to be used to elucidate pathologic processes in myocardial disease, one must first be familiar with the normal metabolic pathways. Cellular integrity is maintained through energy-dependent processes requiring substrates for high-energy phosphate production. A critical reduction in oxygen delivery, substrate availability, or utilization leads to myocardial dysfunction. Thus, detection of alterations in substrate uptake and utilization form the basis for the application of radiotracers. The following discussion of myocardial metabolism will focus on normal pathways of energy production beginning with the three basic substrates: lipids, carbohydrates, and amino acids. Figure 16 summarizes the entry of these three substrates into myocardial metabolism and subsequent adenosine triphosphate (ATP) production. ATP is produced anaerobically through the glycolytic pathway and aerobically through the tricarboxylic acid cycle and electron transport system. Adult cardiac cells are predominantly oxidative, have large numbers of mitochondria, and mainly exhibit oxidative metabolism of fatty acids.[47, 49] In contrast, the conduction system and the entire neonatal myocardium are predominantly glycolytic.[48] If adequate substrates are available, critical defects limiting ATP production could be caused by partial or complete absence of enzymes catalyzing metabolic steps or inadequate oxygenation of tissue.

Lipid Metabolism. Considerable research has centered on cardiac lipid metabolism, the main energy source of the heart.[47–49] A broad outline is presented in Figure 17. Serum triglycerides can be hydrolyzed to short-, medium-, or long-chain fatty acids that are freely permeable across the cardiac sarcolemma. Also, FFA bound to albumin in blood enter the cell via passive diffusion. In cytosol, only the long-chain fatty acids (palmitate, see Fig. 17) require a complex mechanism for transport through the mitochondrial membrane for beta-oxidation. Palmitate CoA, formed on the outer surface of the mitochondrial membrane, is transported to the inner surface by carnitine palmityl transferase I (Enzyme 6, see Fig. 17), where a second carnitine palmityl transferase II removes the carnitine, allowing beta-oxidation to proceed. In the mitochondrial matrix, FFA undergoes beta-oxidation to two-carbon fragments, which enter the TCA cycle for complete metabolism in the form of acetyl CoA. If acetyl CoA is not required as a substrate, or if its entry to the TCA cycle is blocked, ketone bodies (acetyl acetate and beta-hydroxybuterate) are formed. This pathway is reversible, allowing ketone bodies to be utilized as an important second energy resource in cardiac muscle metabolism.[8, 47–49]

The potential value of C-11 palmitate and positron-CT in evaluating patients with a suspected defect in lipid metabolism as the cause

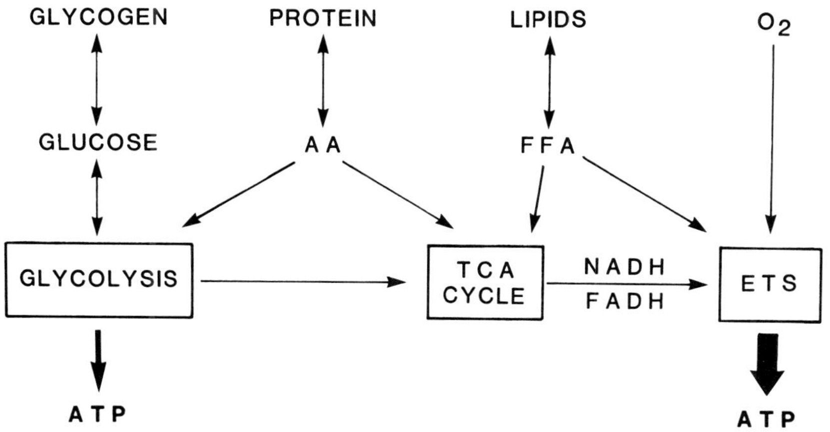

Figure 16. Outline of major sources of high-energy phosphate production in muscle. ATP: adenosine triphosphate, AA: amino acids, TCA: carboxylic acid (Krebs) cycle, FFA: free fatty acids, NADH: nicotine adenine dinucleotide (reduced), FADH: flavin adenine dinucleotide (reduced), ETS: intramitochondrial electron transport system. Carbohydrates, proteins, and lipids generate ATP via the outlined pathways.

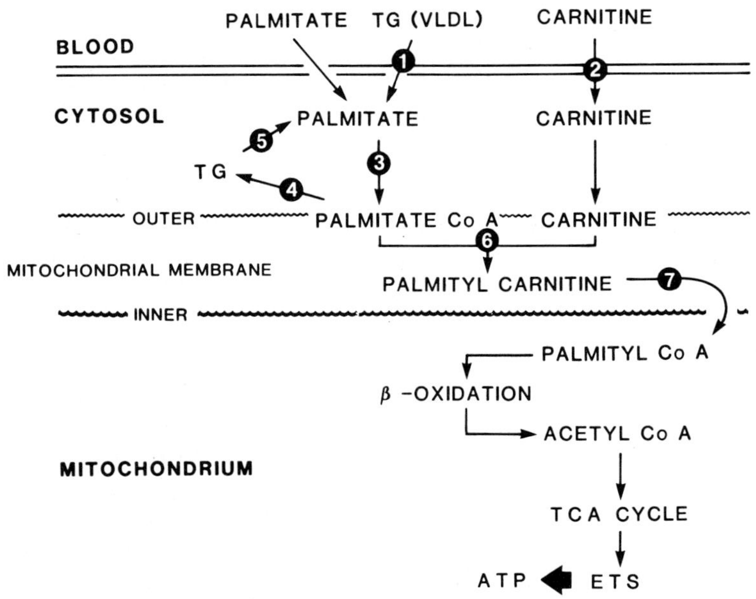

Figure 17. Schematics of the major pathways of FFA in cardiac muscle. Palmitate is used as the typical long-chain fatty acid. Exogenous, blood-borne substrates are represented by fatty acids bound to albumin and triglycerides (TG) as very low density lipoproteins (VLDL). Endogenous stores are in lipid droplets. 1: lipoprotein lipase, 2: active transport of carnitine into muscle, 3: palmityl CoA synthetase, 4: enzyme complex resulting in synthesis of triglycerides from long chain Acetyl-CoA, 5: tri-, di- and monoglyceride lipase, 6: carnitine palmityl transferase (CPT) I, and 7: CPT II.

of cardiac dysfunction is illustrated by the cardiomyopathy of carnitine deficiency. First described by Engel and Angelini in 1973,[17] carnitine deficiency has been found to present cardiac involvement in a number of documented studies.[11, 16, 81, 82] Clinical improvement in congestive failure and cardiomegaly has been demonstrated when L-carnitine was supplemented.[11, 81, 82] Carnitine depletion results in depressed mitochondrial oxidation of fatty acids (see Fig. 17) and myoplasmic accumulation of lipids.[49] Accordingly, C-11 palmitate would not be transported into mitochondria and not be oxidized. The myocardial C-11 time-activity curve would therefore lack an early rapid component because of an absence of beta-oxidation of FFA. Therefore, in these patients the efficacy of carnitine-replacement therapy could be tested by evaluating the fractional tissue distribution of C-11 palmitate.

Furthermore, a variety of known lipid-related myopathies (lipid storage in mitochondrial myopathies, carnitine palmityl transferase deficiency) with early skeletal muscle involvement may find application with C-11 palmitate when the extent of cardiac involvement before clinical evidence of heart failure is being evaluated,[14, 75] as would the cardiomyopathy associated with uremia.[15] In these patients, abnormally low carnitine levels and dyslipidemia have been documented when they were maintained on a chronic hemodialysis program.[28] Thus, evaluation of cardiac involvement at a metabolic level may be possible with positron-CT.

Carbohydrates. An alternate substrate of myocardial energy production, carbohydrates enter the myocyte for immediate utilization and ATP production via the glycolytic pathway or for storage as glycogen.[13] Gluconeogenesis does not occur to any appreciable extent in myocardium. There are two additional entry points for substrates to enter the glycolytic pathway. Triglyceride hydrolysis releases free fatty acids and glycerol. After phosphorylation and reduction, glycerol can enter the pathway as dihydroxyacetone phosphate.[13] ATP is first formed when 1,3 diphosphoglyceric acid is converted to 3-phosphoglyceric acid (Fig. 18). Substrate limitation or enzyme defects above this site will inhibit formation of glycolytically derived ATP.

In contrast to the adult's heart, the neonatal heart depends on glycolytic metabolism with glucose as the major substrate.[19] In this regard, FDG may be utilized to characterize the time course of this metabolic adaptation and become useful for elucidating pathologic processes that alter this natural history. Furthermore, in the mature heart, certain diseases compromise FFA metabolism, and it has been shown that glucose may become the major substrate.[41, 50]

Because FDG is phosphorylated by the hexokinase reaction to FDG-6-phosphate and becomes metabolically inert, it traces only exogenous utilization of glucose. Accordingly, its application in delineating disturbances in glycogen utilization is limited (Pompe's disease) (Fig. 18). However, the availability and application of carbon-labeled glucose will allow tracking of the glucose moiety into the glycolytic and glycogen pathways.

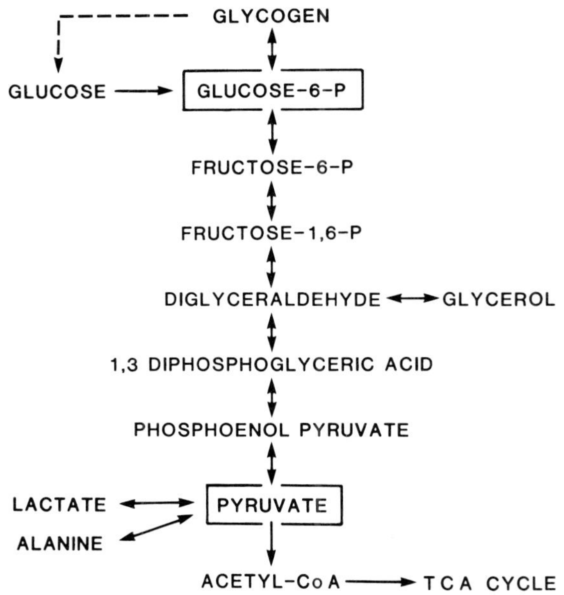

Figure 18. Pathways of glucose metabolism. The broken line indicates the defect in Pompe's disease.

Amino Acid Metabolism. While generally considered the basic elements for protein synthesis, several amino acids are linked through intermediary metabolism to carbohydrate metabolism, participate in maintaining the cytosolic and mitochondrial redox balances, and can play an important role in removing ammonia from myocardium.[64, 79, 80, 83] Although not a major source of energy in myocardium, amino acids may become important during stress, being incorporated into both the glycolytic and TCA pathways after deamination. Many amino acids theoretically enter the cycle to metabolic conversions.[13]

The link between protein synthesis and cardiac hypertrophy in the afterloaded, ischemic, and/or failing ventricle has been established in animal studies.[2, 12, 24, 27, 43, 45, 51, 72] In these ventricles, the space in myocytes occupied by myofilaments increases to a greater extent than in other components.[21, 40, 51] Although there is hypertrophy in various cardiomyopathies, the biochemical background or origin is not well described.[32] Positron-CT with labeled amino acids may substantially increase our knowledge in the pathophysiologic processes involved in the emergence of such diseases.

A large metabolic pool compromises the applicability of single radiolabeled amino acids for the elucidation of specific pathway kinetics. However, early results with C-11 leucine in the brain for the evaluation of protein synthesis have indicated that this tracer may become applicable to cardiac studies in the future.[57] Hence, substantial information about pathophysiologic processes involving hypertrophy of cardiac cells (hypertrophic cardiomyopathies, hypertension, and valvular disease) could be gained. Furthermore, identification of these cardiomyopathies resulting from enzyme defects (beta-ketothiolase deficiency)[32] or the effects of currently administered antimetabolites (Adriamycin) on cardiac protein synthesis may be diagnosed early and monitored clinically (Ref. 24; see also Fig. 15).

Applications in Cyanotic Congenital Heart Disease. In patients with congenital cyanotic heart disease, the heart is perfused by hypoxic blood. Little information is available on the effect of chronic hypoxia on cardiac metabolism and its possible role in affecting ventricular function.[18] A question has arisen whether hypoxia in these patients induces alterations in myocardial metabolism similar to those seen in ischemic coronary heart disease with decreased extraction of lactate and release of phosphate and potassium in the coronary venous effluent. Invasive studies in experimental animals with surgically induced cyanotic lesions or in patients with admixture lesions have revealed that resting myocardial metabolism is normal compared with that of control subjects. However, under stress interventions (atrial pacing, isoproterenol infusions), shifts toward anaerobic metabolism occur with a fall in systemic arterial oxygen saturation.[18, 26, 69] Ongoing investigations in our laboratory have substantiated the conclusions of these early workers in the normalcy of myocardial metabolism during the resting state, as exemplified by normal C-11 palmitate kinetics. The application of this technique in evaluating myocardial metabolic performance in the stressed state is now being investigated before and after surgical intervention. The information from such derived studies may be useful in assessing the timing and efficacy of surgical interventions.

INITIAL CLINICAL EXPERIENCE

Duchenne's Muscular Dystrophy. This disease is unique in genetically targeting specific regions of the myocardium for disease.[53] Postmortem examinations have revealed regional fibrotic degeneration in the posterobasal and contiguous lateral segments of the left ventricular wall, while the coronary arteries supplying these regions have been found to be normal.[53] A predystrophic metabolic fault has been postulated for this region.[52, 55] To test this hypothesis, we used positron-CT with N-13 ammonia and FDG in 15 subjects with Duchenne's dystrophy.[30, 54] Ninety-three per cent of the patients had distinctive electrocardiograms. In only 25 per cent of the patients did conventional Thallium-201 scintigraphy and/or gated radionuclide ventriculography demonstrate regional perfusion or visually detectable regional wall motion abnormalities. Positron-CT revealed regionally decreased uptake of N-13 ammonia in 86 per cent of the patients. In six of the nine patients, the decreased uptake of N-13 ammonia was accompanied by an increased uptake of 18-FDG in the same regions (Fig. 19). This study identified regional myocardial involvement in patients with Duchenne's muscular dystrophy and established the sensitivity of this imaging modality compared with that of conventional noninvasive scintigraphy. Most important, it gives new insights into the metabolic pathophysiology of myocardial involvement and illustrates a potential value of positron-CT for follow-up and monitoring therapeutic interventions.

In another study, we used C-11 palmitate in patients with idiopathic cardiomyopathies and different degrees of left ventricular dysfunction.[29] Myocardial C-11 turnover kinetics were studied in the fasting state and after an oral glucose load. In normal volunteers, glucose administration decreased the turnover of C-11 palmitate during the early rapid phase, suggesting a shift in myocardial metabolism away from fatty acids (see Figs. 11 and 20). In patients with only moderately impaired left ventricular function, the C-11 palmitate kinetics did not significantly differ from normal persons. However, in patients with severely depressed function, the turnover of C-11 palmitate was decreased in the fasting state. Size and clearance rate of the early rapid phase increased after glucose, in contrast to the control population. Plasma substrate levels and hemodynamic findings were similar in both patient subsets. Although the reasons for the observed findings in the fasting state after glucose loading await further clarification, they give rise to some interesting speculations about the enhancement of glycolytic rate or back diffusion of C-11 palmitate into the plasma compartment. These questions and others have been addressed by further studies in our laboratory and provide a working hypothesis through which the study of metabolic derangements in cardiomyopathies can be approached.

A great deal is known about the causes of dilated cardiomyopathy—inflammatory (infectious or noninfectious), toxic (alcohol, adriamycin, and so on), nutritional (beri-beri), and metabolic (hemochromatosis). Among restrictive cardiomyopathies (increased wall thickness type), amyloid is the front runner. Other causes can be metabolic, such as glycogen storage disease or Hunter-Hurler syndrome. In this context, positron-CT as a probe of myocardial biochemistry is likely to be of value in defining or elucidating metabolic derangements, to provide working hypotheses for clarifying mechanisms of disease, and, as we have seen with carnitine deficiencies, for selecting the most appropriate treatment as well as for monitoring its effects.

CONCLUSIONS

Despite its unique potential, positron-CT is still in its infancy. Its widespread use as a powerful and innovative tool for research and

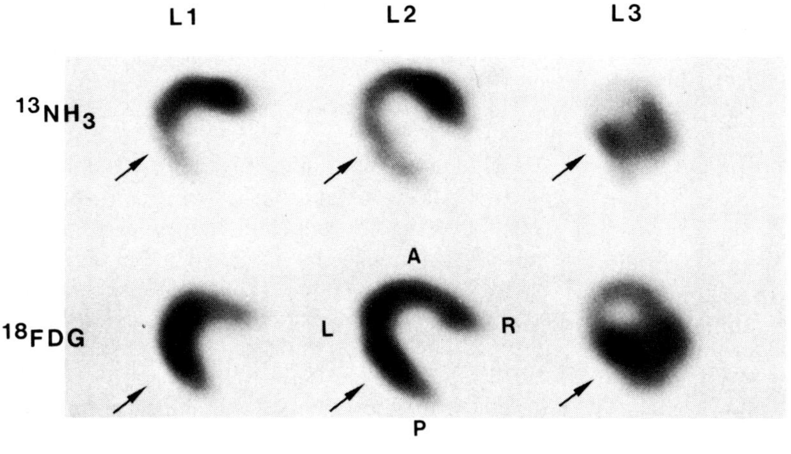

Figure 19. Cross-sectional positron CT images of the left ventricular myocardium obtained after intravenous infusion of N-13 ammonia and intravenous FDG and positron CT in a patient with Duchenne's muscle dystrophy. Note the segmental decrease in N-13 activity on the N-13 ammonia images with the discordant increase in FDG uptake in the same segment (arrows). (A: anterior, L: left lateral, P: posterior, and R: right) (Courtesy of J. K. Perloff et al., UCLA).

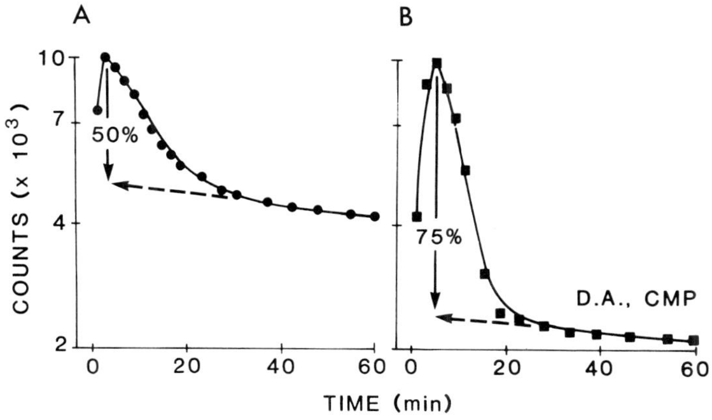

Figure 20. Myocardial uptake, fractional distribution, and clearance of C-11 palmitate in a patient with congestive cardiomyopathy after an overnight fast and after oral glucose loading. *A*, Note on the time activity curve obtained from serial positron CT images after intravenous infusion of C-11 palmitate in the fasted state the relatively small fraction of C-11 palmitate entering the rapid turnover "oxidation" phase. *B*, However, after oral glucose loading with a substantial increase in plasma glucose levels and decline in plasma FFA levels, the fractional distribution of C-11 palmitate changes considerably. A substantially greater fraction enters the rapid turnover pool and clears more rapidly. This response in patients with cardiomyopathy and markedly impaired left ventricular function is contrasted with the normal response as shown in Figure 11*B* (Courtesy of E. Henze et al, UCLA).

evaluation of disease has been limited because of technical complexities with the requirements of on-site isotope and radiopharmaceutical production and hence an on-site cyclotron in chemistry facilities. Although positron-CT is suited for studying all aspects of local myocardial function such as metabolism, flow, and mechanical function, clinically adequate information on flow and mechanical function can be obtained noninvasively with conventional and less costly techniques. The capability unique to positron-CT is the evaluation of the local biochemistry and metabolism of the myocardium. A powerful tool for the study of the metabolic consequences of disease and more important the biochemical identification of disease has become available. We hope this discussion of state of the art applications and speculations stimulates further interest in applying this technique for the elucidation of biochemical processes involved in a variety of myocardial diseases that occur in both the pediatric and adult patient population.

REFERENCES

1. Allan RM, Jones T, Rhodes CCC, et al: Quantitation of myocardial perfusion in man using oxygen-15 and positron tomography. (Abstr.) Am J Cardiol, *47*:481, 1981.
2. Alpert NR (ed): Cardiac Hypertrophy. New York, Academic Press, Inc., 1971.
3. Baumgartner FJ, Barrio JR, Henze E, et al: N-13 labeled L-amino acids for in vivo assessment of local myocardial metabolism. J Med Chem, *24*:764–766, 1981.
4. Beller GA, Cochavi S, Smith TW, et al: Positron tomographic imaging of the myocardium with ^{81}Rb. J Comp Assist Tomogr, *6*:341–349, 1982.
5. Bergmann SR, Fox KAA, Rand AL, et al: Noninvasive measurement of regional myocardial perfusion by positron tomography. (Abstr.). Circulation, *66*:II–148, 1982.
6. Bharati S, Lev M: Sequelae of atriotomy and ventriculotomy on the endocardium, conduction system and coronary arteries. Am J Cardiol, *50*:580, 1982.
7. Braunwald E (ed): Heart Disease: A Textbook of Cardiovascular Medicine, Philadelphia, W. B. Saunders, 1981, p. 1437.
8. Bressler R: Fatty acid oxidation. *In* Florkin M, Stotz EM (eds): Lipid Metabolism: Comprehension Biochemistry. New York, Elsevier EM, *18*:331, 1970.
9. Budinger TF, Yano Y, Derenzo SE, et al: Rb-82 myocardial positron emission tomography. (Abstr.) J Nucl Med, *20*:P603, 1979.
10. Carlsten A, Hallgren B, Jagenburg R, et al: Myocardial metabolism of glucose, lactic acid, amino acids and fatty acids in healthy human individuals at rest and at different work loads. Scand J Clin Lab Invest, *13*:418–428, 1961.
11. Chapoy PR, Angelini C, Brown WJ, et al: Systemic carnitine deficiency—A treatable lipid-storage disease presenting as Page's Syndrome. N Engl J Med, *303*:1389, 1980.
12. Cohen J, Shah P (eds): Cardiac hypertrophy and cardiomyopathy. Circ Res (Suppl.), *35*:1, 1974.
13. Conn EE, Stumpf PK (eds): Outline of Biochemistry. Ed. 3. New York, John Wiley & Sons Inc., 1972.
14. DiMauro S, Trevisah C, Hays A: Disorders of lipid metabolism in muscle. Neuro Muscle, *212*:694, 3533, 1981.
15. Drueke T, LePailleur C, Meilhac B, et al: Congestive cardiomyopathy in uremic patients on long-term hemodialysis. Br. Med J, *1*:350, 1977.
16. Engel AG: Possible causes of effects of carnitine deficiency in man. *In* Frenkel RA, McGarry JD (eds): Carnitine Biosynthesis, Metabolism and Functions. New York, Academic Press, 1980, p. 271.
17. Engel AG, Angelini C: Carnitine deficiency of human skeletal muscle with associated lipid storage myopathy: A new syndrome. Science, *179*:899, 1973.
18. Friedl B, Haennl B, Moret P, et al: Myocardial metabolism in cyanotic congenital heart diseases studied by arteriovenous differences of lactate, phosphate and potassium at rest and during atrial pacing. Circulation, *55*:647, 1977.
19. Friedman WF, Lesch M, Sonnenblick EH: Neonatal Heart Disease. New York, Grune and Stratton, 1973.

20. Gelbard AS, Benua RS, Reiman RE, et al: Imaging of the heart after administration of L-(N-13) glutamate. J. Nucl Med, *21*:988–991, 1980.
21. Goldstein AM, Sordahl L, Schwartz A: Ultrastructural analysis of left ventricular hypertrophy in rabbits. J Mol Cell Cardiol, *6*:265–273, 1974.
22. Goldstein RA, Klein MS, Sobel BE: Detection of myocardial ischemia before infarction, based on accumulation of labeled pyruvate. J Nucl Med, *21*:1101–1104, 1980.
23. Goldstein RA, Klein MS, Welch MJ, et al: External assessment of myocardial metabolism with C-11 palmitate in vivo. J Nucl Med, *21*:342–348, 1980.
24. Goodwyn JF: Daunorubicin cardiomyopathy. *In* Hurst JW (ed): The Heart. New York, McGraw-Hill, 1978, pp. 2573–2574.
25. Gould KL, Schelbert HR, Phelps ME, et al: Noninvasive assessment of coronary stenoses with myocardial perfusion imaging during pharmacological coronary vasodilatation. V. Detection of 47% diameter coronary stenosis with intravenous nitrogen-13 ammonia and emission computed transaxial tomography in intact dogs. Am J Cardiol, *43*:200–208, 1979.
26. Graham TP, Erath HG, Buckspan GS, et al: Myocardial anaerobic metabolism during isoprenaline infusion in a cyanotic animal model: Possible cause of myocardial dysfunction in cyanotic congenital heart disease. Cardiovasc Res, *13*:401, 1979.
27. Gudbjarhanson S, Telerman M, Bing RJ, et al: Protein metabolism in cardiac hypertrophy and heart failure. Am J Physiol, *206*:294–298, 1964.
28. Gusmanor R, Oleggini R, Perfumo F: Plasma carnitine concentrations and dyslipidemia in children on maintenance hemodialysis. J Pediatr, *99*:429, 1981.
29. Henze E, Grossman RG, Najafi A, et al: Measurement of C-11 palmitate kinetics after metabolic interventions in normals and patients with cardiomyopathy using positron emission computed tomography. Am J Cardiol, *49*:1023, 1982.
30. Henze E, Perloff JK, Schelbert HR: Alterations of regional myocardial perfusion and metabolism in Duchenne's muscular dystrophy (DMD) detected by positron computed tomography (PCT). Circulation (Suppl.), *64*:279, 1981.
31. Henze E, Schelbert HR, Barrio JR, et al: Evaluation of myocardial metabolism with N-13 and C-11 labeled amino acids and positron computed tomography. J Nucl Med, *23*:671–681, 1982.
32. Henry CG, Strauss AW, Keating JP, et al: Congestive cardiomyopathy associated with B-ketothiolase deficiency. J. Pediatr, *90*:754, 1981.
33. Heymann MA, Payne BD, Hoffman JIE, et al: Blood flow measurements with radionuclide-labeled particles. *In* Holman BL, Sonnenblick EH, Lesch M (eds): Principles of Cardiovascular Nuclear Medicine. New York, Grune & Stratton, 1979, pp. 135–159.
34. Hoffman EJ, Phelps ME, Weiss ES, et al: Transaxial tomographic imaging of canine myocardium with ^{11}C palmitic acid. J Nucl Med 18:57–61, 1977.
35. Huang SC, Phelps ME, Hoffman EJ, et al: Noninvasive determination of local cerebral metabolic rate of glucose in man with (F-18)-fluoro-2-deoxyglucose and emission computed tomography: Theory and results. Am J Physiol, *238*:E69–E82, 1980.
36. Huang SC, Schwaiger M, Carson RE, et al: An 0-15 water clearance method for quantitative regional myocardial blood flow measurements. (Abstr.). J Nucl Med, *23*:P69, 1982.
37. Jones T, Chesler DA, Ter-Pogossian MM: The continuous inhalation of oxygen-15 for assessing regional oxygen extraction in the brain of man. Br J Radiol, *49*:339–343, 1976.
38. Keul J, Doll E, Steim H, et al: Uber den Stoffwechsel des menschlichen Herzens unter verschiedenen Arbeitsbedingungen. Arch Ges Physiol, *282*:43–53, 1965.
39. Klein MS, Goldstein RA, Welch MJ, et al: External assessment of myocardial metabolism with ^{11}C-palmitate in rabbit hearts. Am J Physiol Heart Circ, *16*:H51–H57, 1979.
40. Legato MJ: Cellular mechanisms of normal growth in the mammalian heart. II. A quantitative and qualitative comparison between the right and left ventricular myocytes in the dog from birth to five months of age. Circ Res, *44*:263–278, 1979.
41. Marshall RC, Tillisch JH, Phelps ME, et al: Identification and differentiation of resting myocardial ischemia and infarction with positron computed tomography, F-18 labeled fluorodeoxyglucose and N-13 ammonia. Circulation, *67*:766–778, 1983.
42. McKenna WJ, Allan RM, Horlock P, et al: Hypertrophic cardiomyopathy: Measurement of cation uptake. (Abstr.). Am J Cardiol, *47*:409, 1981.
43. Meerson FZ: A mechanism of hypertrophy and wear and tear of the myocardium. Am J Cardiol, *15*:755, 1965.
44. Meerson FZ: Role of synthesis of nucleic acids and protein in adaptation to the external environment. Physiol Rev, *55*:79, 1975.
45. Meerson FZ, Aleklua GM, Alexandrov PN, et al: Dynamics of nucleic acid and protein synthesis of the myocardium in compensatory hyperfunction and hypertrophy of the heart. Am J Cardiol, *22*:337–347, 1968.
46. Nomura H, Bergmann SR, Fox KAA, et al: Myocardial fatty acid metabolism quantified externally with ^{11}C-palmitate. (Abstr.). Circulation, *66*:II–147, 1982.
47. Opie LH: Metabolism of the heart in health and disease. I. Am Heart J, *76*:685, 1968.
48. Opie LH: Metabolism of the heart in health and disease. II. Am Heart J, *77*:100, 1969.
49. Opie LH: Metabolism of the heart in health and disease. III. Am Heart J, *77*:383, 1969.
50. Opie LH, Owen P, Riemersma RA: Relative rates of oxidation of glucose and free fatty acids by ischemic and non-ischemic myocardium after coronary ligation in the dog. Eur J Clin Invest, *3*:419–435, 1973.
51. Page E, Polimeni PI, Zak R, et al: Myofibrillar mass in rat and rabbit heart muscle. Circ Res, *30*:430–439, 1972.
52. Perloff JK: Development and regression of increased ventricular mass. Am J Cardiol, *50*:605, 1982.
53. Perloff JK, DeLeon AC, O'Doherty D: The cardiomyopathy of progressive muscular dystrophy. Circulation 33:625, 1966.
54. Perloff JK, Henze E, Schelbert HR: Myocardial metabolism, perfusion, wall motion and electrical activity in Duchenne's muscular dystrophy. Submitted for publication.
55. Perloff JK, Roberts WC, DeLeon AC, et al: The distinction electrocardiogram of Duchenne's progress with muscular dystrophy. Am J Med, *42*:179, 1967.
56. Phelps ME: Emission computed tomography. Semin Nucl Med, *7*:337–365, 1977.
57. Phelps ME, Barrio JR, Huang S-C, et al: The measurement of local cerebral protein synthesis in man with positron computed tomography and L-(1-^{11}C)Leucine. J Nucl Med, *23*:P6, 1982.
58. Phelps ME, Hoffman EJ, Mullani NA, et al: Application of annihilation coincidence detection to transaxial

reconstruction tomography. J Nucl Med, *16*:210–223, 1975.

59. Phelps ME, Hoffman EJ, Selin C, et al: Investigation of ^{18}F-2-fluoro-2-deoxyglucose for the measure of myocardial glucose metabolism. J Nucl Med, *19*:1311–1319, 1978.
60. Phelps ME, Huang SC, Hoffman E, et al: Tomographic measurement of local cerebral metabolic rate in man with 2-(^{18}F)fluoro-2-deoxy-D-glucose: Validation of method. Ann Neurol, *6*:371–388, 1979.
61. Phelps ME, Mazziotta JC, Huang SC: Study of cerebral function with positron computed tomography. J Cerebr Blood Flow Metabol, *2*:113–162, 1982.
62. Ratib O, Phelps ME, Huang SC, et al: Positron tomography with deoxyglucose for estimating local myocardial glucose metabolism. J Nucl Med, *23*:577–586, 1982.
63. Reivich M, Kuhl D, Wolf A, et al: The (^{18}F)-fluorodeoxyglucose method for the measurement of local cerebral glucose utilization in man. Circ Res, *44*:127–137, 1979.
64. Safer B: The metabolic significance of the malate aspartate cycle in heart. Circ Res, *37*:527–533, 1975.
65. Schelbert HR, Henze E, Schon HR, et al: C-11 palmitic acid for the noninvasive evaluation of regional myocardial fatty acid metabolism with positron computed tomography. III. In vivo demonstration of the effects of substrate availability on myocardial metabolism. Am Heart J, *105*:492–504, 1983.
66. Schelbert HR, Phelps ME, Hoffman EJ, et al: Regional myocardial perfusion assessed with N-13 labeled ammonia and positron emission computerized axial tomography. Am J Cardiol, *43*:209–218, 1979.
67. Schelbert HR, Phelps ME, Huang SC, et al: N-13 ammonia as an indicator of myocardial blood flow. Circulation, *63*:1259–1272, 1981.
68. Schelbert HR, Wisenberg G, Phelps ME, et al: Noninvasive assessment of coronary stenoses by myocardial imaging during pharmacologic vasodilation. VI. Detection of coronary artery disease in man with intravenous N-13 ammonia and positron computed tomography. Am J Cardiol, *49*:1197–1207, 1982.
69. Scheuer J, Shaver JA, Kroltz FW, et al: Myocardial metabolism in cyanotic congenital heart disease. Cardiology, *55*:193, 1970.
70. Schon HR, Schelbert HR, Najafi A, et al: C-11 labeled palmitic acid for the noninvasive evaluation of regional myocardial fatty acid metabolism with positron computed tomography. II. Kinetics of C-11 palmitic acid in acutely ischemic myocardium. Am Heart J, *103*:548–561, 1982.
71. Schon HR, Schelbert HR, Najafi A, et al: C-11 labeled palmitic acid for the noninvasive evaluation of regional myocardial fatty acid metabolism with positron computed tomography. I. Kinetics of C-11 palmitic acid in normal myocardium. Am Heart J, *103*:532–547, 1982.
72. Schreiber SS, Ortaz M, Rothschild MA: Post ischemic reperfusion and anoxic perfusion in the isolated heart: Alteration in distribution of radionuclides and in protein synthesis. J Physiol (Paris), *76*:777–784, 1980.
73. Selwyn AP, Allan RM, L'Abbate A, et al: Relation between regional myocardial uptake of rubidium-82 and perfusion: Absolute reduction of cation uptake in ischemia. Am J Cardiol, *50*:112–121, 1982.
74. Selwyn AP, Allan RM, Pike V, et al: Positive labeling of ischemic myocardium: A new approach in patients with coronary disease. (Abstr.). Am J Cardiol, *47*:481, 1981.
75. Sengers RCA, Stadhoriders AV, Jaspar HH, et al: Cardiomyopathy and short stature associated with mitochondrial and/or lipid storage myopathy of skeletal muscle. Neuropaediatrie, *7*:196, 1976.
76. Shah A, Schelbert H, Schwaiger M, et al: Regional myocardial blood flow assessed with N-13 ammonia and positron tomography (PCT) in chronically instrumented dogs. (Abstr.). Circulation, *66*:II–126, 1982.
77. Smith CB, Davidson A, Diebler G, et al: A method for determining the local rates of protein synthesis in brain. Trans Am Soc Neurol Chem, *11*:94, 1980.
78. Sokoloff L, Reivich M, Kennedy C, et al: The (^{14}C) deoxyglucose method for the measurement of local cerebral glucose utilization. Theory, procedure and normal values in conscious and anesthetized rats. J Neurochem, *28*:898–916, 1977.
79. Taegtmeyer H: Metabolic responses to cardiac hypoxia. Increased production of succinate by rabbit papillary muscles. Circ Res, *43*:808–815, 1978.
80. Taegtmeyer H, Peterson MB, Ragavan VV, et al: De novo alanine synthesis in isolated oxygen-deprived rabbit myocardium. J Biol Chem, *252*:5010–5018, 1977.
81. Tripp ME, Katcher ML, Peters HA, et al: Systemic carnitine deficiency presenting as familial endocardial fibroclostoses. N Engl J Med, *305*:385, 1981.
82. Waber LJ, Valle D, Neill C, et al: Carnitine deficiency presenting as familial cardiomyopathy: A treatable defect in carnitine transport. J Pediatr, *101*:700, 1982.
83. Watanabe T: Significance of ammonia in myocardial metabolism. (Abstr.). Jpn Circ J (Suppl.), *32*:1811, 1968.
84. Weiss ES, Hoffman EJ, Phelps ME, et al: External detection and visualization of myocardial ischemia with ^{11}C-substrates in vitro and in vivo. Circ Res, *39*:24–32, 1976.
85. Wisenberg G, Schelbert HR, Hoffman EJ, et al: In vivo quantitation of regional myocardial blood flow by positron emission computed tomography. Circulation, *63*:1248–1258, 1981.

15

NUCLEAR MAGNETIC RESONANCE IMAGING

The Potential for Cardiac Evaluation of the Pediatric Patient

MARK R. GOLDMAN, M.D., and GERALD M. POHOST, M.D.

If one were to imagine the ideal diagnostic instrument for the evaluation of children with heart disease, the following features would come to mind. The device should be noninvasive and harmless, have the ability to depict anatomy and wall motion in either two-dimensional or three-dimensional display, and have the ability to measure flow and oxygen content in the various cardiac chambers. Nuclear magnetic resonance (NMR) imaging, a new form of imaging whose full potential is not yet realized, offers the possibility of providing all the above features in a single instrument. The appeal such a device would have for pediatric cardiologists is obvious. In this article, the technology of NMR imaging and its application to cardiology will be discussed.

PRINCIPLES OF NMR IMAGING

The principles of NMR imaging have been reviewed in several excellent publications[3, 5, 6] but will be presented briefly here. NMR imaging relies on the behavior of the nuclei of certain stable isotopes to align themselves in the direction of an applied magnetic field. The nuclei behave as if they were tiny bar magnets.

In the absence of any applied magnetic field, the orientation of these nuclei are random. Once aligned with an external magnetic field, the nuclei may be "tipped" out of alignment by a short burst of radiofrequency waves (RF) supplied by a coil of wire surrounding the imaging volume. Once tipped from their equilibrium alignment, the nuclei precess in a manner similar to a child's spinning gyroscope when tipped from the vertical position in the earth's gravitational field.

The precessing nuclei emit radio waves that can be detected by the wire coil and analyzed by subjecting the signal to a process known as Fourier transformation. This breaks the radio signal down into its component frequencies. In this manner, a frequency spectrum of the precessional (resonant) frequencies of the sample is obtained.

There is a physical relationship, known as the Larmor principle, which states that the resonant frequency of an NMR sensitive nucleus is proportional to the applied magnetic field at the nucleus,

$$\omega = \gamma H$$

where ω is the resonant frequency, γ is the gyromagnetic ratio (a constant for a given nuclear species), and H is the magnetic field at the nucleus.

If the magnetic field were completely homogeneous (equal at every point in the imaging volume), then the frequency spectrum of the sample would consist of only one peak. In NMR imaging, extra magnetic field gradients are used to exploit the Larmor principle and encode spatial information on the emitted NMR signal. If one performs the NMR experiment with an "extra" magnetic field gradient on, the frequency spectrum obtained is actually a planar distribution of the sensitive nuclei projected onto a line oriented parallel to the field gradient. By repeating the sequence with the magnetic field gradients in different orientations, one obtains a series of plane projections.

Using reconstruction algorithms similar to those used in computed tomography, the NMR image can be reconstructed. NMR imaging may be undertaken as true three-dimensional imaging or may be performed as two-dimensional tomograms using one of several plane selection techniques (which are beyond the scope of this review).

The nuclear species used for NMR imaging is the hydrogen nucleus (protons), ^{1}H. There are two good reasons for this. Protons are the most sensitive nuclei to detection with NMR. This is a physical characteristic of matter and cannot be altered. Protons are also highly abundant in biologic tissue, since they are a component of water and of aliphatic compounds found in tissue. Since water is about 35 M in tissue, proteins are about 70 M. Other NMR sensitive nuclei, such as ^{19}F, ^{31}P, and ^{23}Na, are much less abundant in the body as well as being intrinsically less sensitive to NMR detection. NMR imaging, therefore, has been generally limited to proton imaging, although ^{19}F phantoms have been imaged as well as ^{23}Na images of perfused beating rat hearts.

NMR IMAGES

NMR images, therefore, are images whose brightness is a reflection of proton density in the imaged sample. There is other information, however, incorporated into the NMR image. These data are relaxation times. As the "tipped" nuclei emit radiowaves, they return to their equilibrium alignments by means of a process known as "relaxation." Two time constants describe the exponential time course of relaxation and are known as T_1 and T_2. The T_1 relaxation time describes the rate of return of the longitudinal component of the tipped nuclei to equilibrium; the T_2 relaxation time describes the rate of decay of the emitted signal. Depending on the pulse sequence used to tip the nuclei, more or less T_1 and/or T_2 information may be incorporated into the NMR signal and is translated into image brightness.

Functionally, NMR images are obtained by sliding the patient into the bore of a large magnet until the desired region is in the imaging volume. The magnetic fields used for NMR imaging range from 400 to 15,000 gauss. By comparison, the earth's magnetic field is about 0.5 gauss. Imaging is performed by pulsing the sample with RF radiation as described. The imaging time is variable, depending on the type of image desired, spatial resolution desired, and, in the case of gated heart images, the heart rate. Imaging time varies typically from 2 to 4 min per tomogram for 2-dimensional studies to about 25 to 35 min for 3-dimensional studies. There are no moving parts in the working instrument. The acquisition of the NMR signal can be gated to the cardiac cycle with varying delay times, and the entire cardiac cycle can be displayed sequentially like a radionuclide gated blood scan. The cost and maintenance of these instruments are comparable to that of conventional CT machines.

PEDIATRIC NMR IMAGING

How can NMR imaging help us in the evaluation of the child with heart disease? Both gated and ungated NMR images of the human heart have been published, and the images show impressive detail in the depiction of internal cardiac anatomy.[2, 4] The ventricular walls, septum, atria, large vessels, and occasionally the valves can be identified easily. Because NMR images can be made in 3-dimensional mode, tomograms may then be reconstructed in any desired oblique, offering a unique opportunity to "slice" the heart at levels and angles not possible with other techniques. This could allow examination of the septum at various levels to search for ventricular septal defects, overriding aorta, abnormal placement of the great vessels, and so on. One could conceivably follow the course of a great vessel to observe abnormal placement, stenosis, coarctation, and fistulae, for example (Figs. 1 and 2).

It is conceivable, though not proved, that NMR imaging can be applied to perform noninvasive oximetry. Substances known as paramagnetic materials, whose electron clouds become polarized in magnetic fields, dramatically shorten the T_1 and often the T_2 of nearby protons. These materials can be used to alter NMR signal intensity and image brightness and for this reason are referred to as NMR "contrast agents." Molecular oxygen is a weakly paramagnetic substance, and it has been shown that the NMR image intensity of the blood in the left ventricular cavity is greater than that of the blood in the right ventricular cavity.[1] This effect, presumed to be caused by the oxygen's effect on the T_1 of blood, was enhanced when the NMR images were repeated with the subject breathing 100 per cent O_2. The implication of these findings is that with further refinements in NMR technology it may be possible to perform in vivo oximetry noninvasively. The application for shunt detection and quantification is obvious.

Moving blood purely by virtue of its motion produces little or no NMR signal, which is why

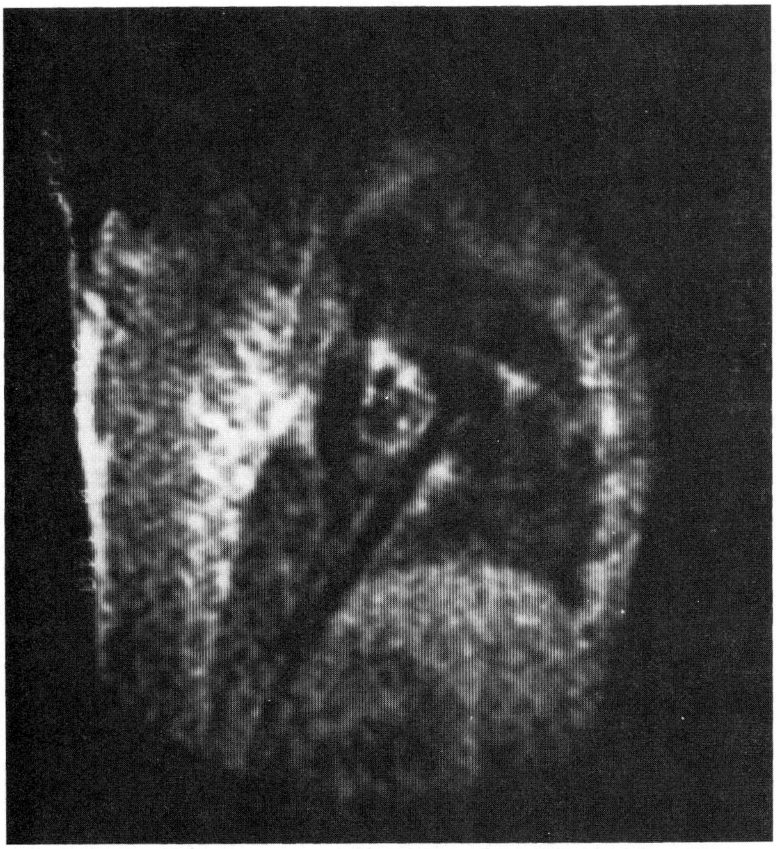

Figure 1. Sagittal section through a dog's chest. This proton saturation-recovery image with image acquisition is gated to the dog's heartbeat. The image was acquired in a 3-dimensional format, allowing reconstruction of planes in any oblique. The slice thickness is about 3 mm. The diaphragm and the inferior vena cava can be clearly seen. Moving blood in a vascular space produces no NMR signal and appears "black."

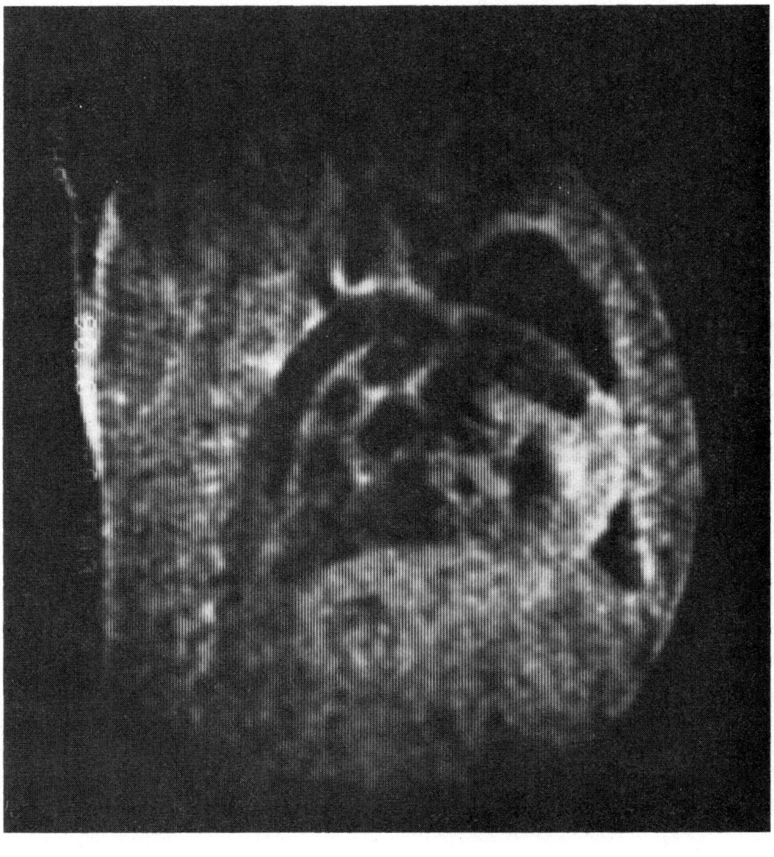

Figure 2. Same animal as in Figure 1. This sagittal slice is a few centimeters to the left of the one in Figure 1. The aorta, aortic arch and arch vessels, pulmonary outflow tract, and some of the pulmonary arterial tree can be identified.

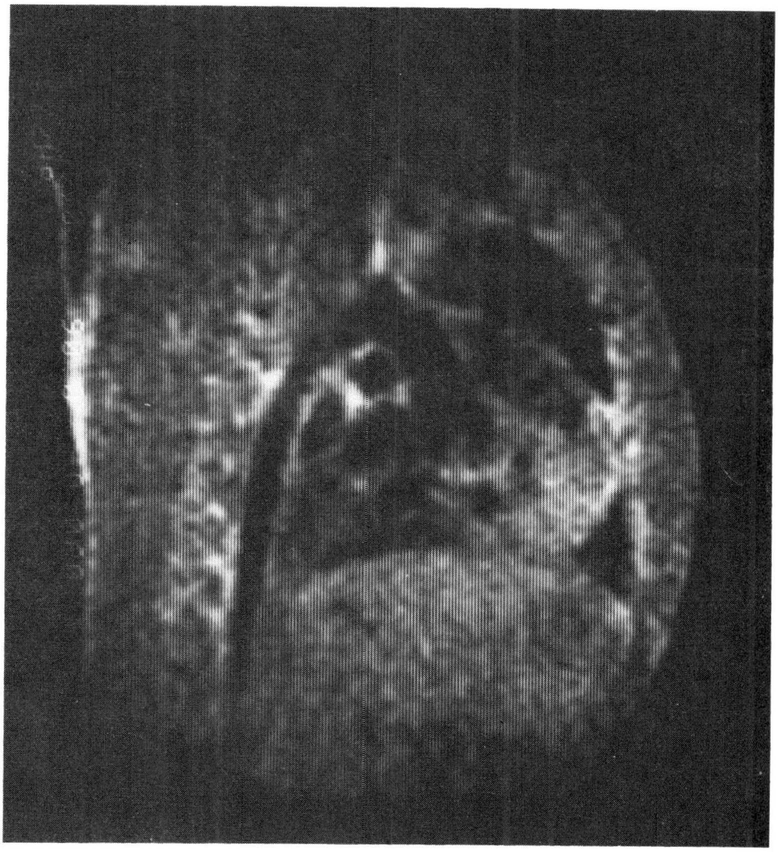

Figure 3. Same animal as in Figures 1 and 2. This sagittal slice is slightly to the left of the one in Figure 2. The descending aorta and parts of the right and left ventricle are shown distinctly.

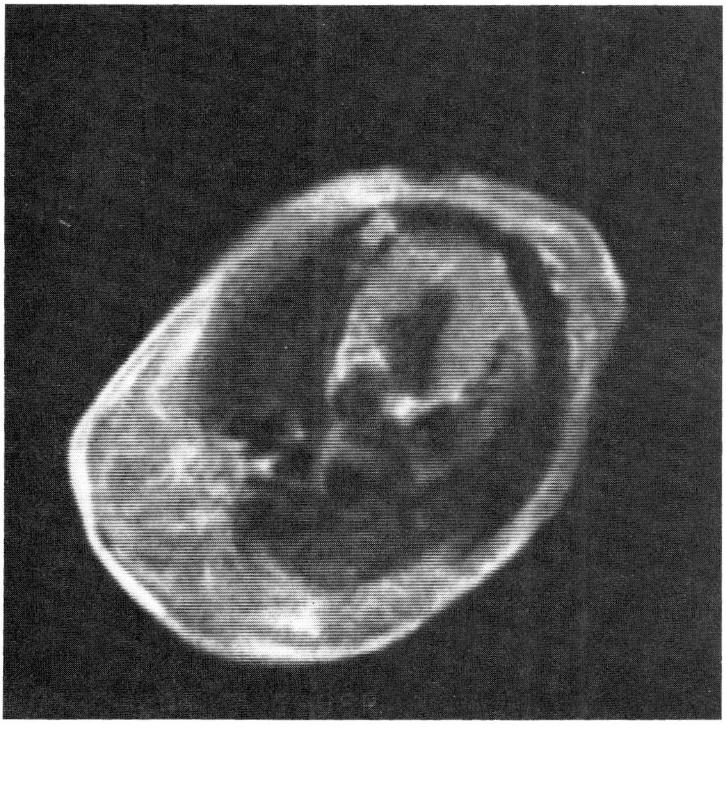

Figure 4. Gated proton saturation-recovery image of a dog's heart, gated to midsystole at the level of the ventricles. This image was acquired as a 2-dimensional Fourier transform image. Slice thickness is about 1 cm. The right and left ventricles, interventricular septum, and atria are distinctly demonstrated.

ventricular cavities and great vessels appear dark on NMR images. Static blood produces a bright intensity on the NMR image and may be indistinguishable from the ventricular wall. Gated NMR images have shown a cyclical variation in the signal intensity of blood in the aorta and probably reflect changes in the blood flow through that vessel. It may be possible to exploit the motion effect and use it to measure a quantitative flow.

Singer has even been able to produce images that depict flow, and it may be possible to produce a quantitative "flow map" by using NMR imaging.[7] These and other approaches are still in their infancy; their ultimate utility remains to be determined.

HAZARDS OF NMR IMAGING

There is no known hazard associated with NMR imaging. Workers exposed for many hours to high-level magnetic fields near particle accelerators have had no ill-effects. Likewise, workers in magnet laboratories also have no known ill-effects. Infants treated for esophageal atresia by electromagnetic bougienage have been exposed for many weeks to high-intensity magnetic fields without adverse effects. Although high-intensity, alternating magnetic field gradients have been reported to produce the perception of flashing lights, called magnetophosphenes, the gradients and frequencies required to produce these effects are much higher than those used for conventional NMR imaging. Patients with cardiac pacemakers, however, present different problems, and these patients should be excluded from NMR imaging. Cardiac pacemakers themselves are affected by the high static magnetic field, and the electrode used in pacing may conduct induced currents caused by gradient changing of the magnetic field.

The radiofrequency pulses used in NMR imaging also have no known hazard. The energy dissipated in tissue samples imaged with NMR is far below the recommended maximum long-term exposure of 10 milliwatts/cm^3. Careful experiments performed with sensitive thermistors have shown no rise in temperature of excised tissue when the radiofrequency power of NMR imaging was used.

The most convincing evidence of the safety of NMR imaging is the experience of many laboratories throughout the world. They have accumulated literally thousands of patient-hours of NMR imaging with no reported untoward effects. Infants have been imaged in Aberdeen, Scotland, as well as at the Hammersmith Hospital in London, England. NMR imaging has proved very useful in the evaluation of children with central nervous system disease in Great Britain. Women about to undergo elective abortion in Aberdeen have undergone NMR imaging, and detailed anatomy of the fetus was demonstrated.

NMR imaging is not mutagenic. It does not interfere with sister chromatid replication, nor does it use ionizing radiation. There is no evidence that there is any long-term delayed harmful effects of NMR imaging.

NMR imaging in the evaluation of the pediatric patient with cardiac disease would therefore appear to offer an entirely new means of diagnosing disease in these children without the need for ionizing radiation or invasive technology. The advent of 2-dimensional echocardiography has significantly improved diagnostic accuracy in the pediatric age group, and in many institutions, surgery is performed without the need for cardiac catheterization, providing the echocardiogram is diagnostic. NMR imaging clearly would not replace, but rather would complement, echocardiography. In addition to depicting internal cardiac anatomy, noninvasive shunt detection and quantification may also be possible as discussed above. The only apparent disadvantage of NMR imaging at the present time is that it is not portable. Patients must be brought to the imaging laboratory rather than having these studies performed at the bedside. Hopefully, with improved technologies, NMR imaging will find a useful application in the evaluation of children with heart disease.

REFERENCES

1. Alfidi RJ, Haaga JR, El Yousef SJ, et al: Preliminary experimental results in humans and animals with a superconducting, whole-body, nuclear magnetic resonance scanner. Radiology, *143*:175–181, 1982.
2. Edelstein WA, Hutchison JMS, Johnson G, et al: Spin-warp NMR imaging and applications to human whole-body imaging. Phys Med Biol, *25*:751–756, 1980.
3. Goldman MR, Pohost GM, Ingwall JS, et al: Nuclear magnetic resonance imaging: Potential cardiac applications. Am J Cardiol, *46*:1278–1283, 1980.
4. Hawkes RC, Holland GN, Moore WS, et al: Nuclear magnetic resonance (NMR) tomography of the normal heart. J Comp Assist Tomogr, *5*:605–612, 1982.
5. Pykett IL: NMR imaging in medicine. Sci Am, *246*:78–88, 1982.
6. Pykett IL, Newhouse JH, Buonanno FS, et al: Principles of nuclear magnetic resonance imaging. Radiology, *143*:157–168, 1982.
7. Singer JR: NMR flow-imaging techniques. Mag Res Med, in press.

16

CARDIOVASCULAR IMAGING WITH NUCLEAR MAGNETIC RESONANCE

CHARLES B. HIGGINS, M.D., ELIAS H. BOTVINICK, M.D.,
PETER LANZER, M.D., ROBERT HERFKENS, M.D.,
MARTIN J. LIPTON, M.D., LAWRENCE E. CROOKS, Ph.D.,
and LEON KAUFMAN, Ph.D.

Nuclear magnetic resonance (NMR) imaging depicts organs and tissues in relation to the interaction of their compositional nuclei with a static magnetic field and fluctuating radiofrequency pulses.[4] Like ultrasound, the technique is completely noninvasive; images of the cardiovascular system are generated without the need for contrast media. Likewise, NMR imaging does not involve ionizing radiation. While NMR imaging does require considerable caution in the immediate environment of the imager, research to date reveals no important genetic or somatic effects.[5] An important consideration for cardiac patients is the effect of NMR imaging on cardiac pacemakers.[5]

Imaging with nuclear magnetic resonance produces clear discrimination between flowing blood and the vascular wall because blood flowing in a laminar fashion at normal velocities produces a low intensity or no NMR signal.[1, 7, 8] On the contrary, the definition of vascular abnormality by x-ray imaging techniques requires the use of contrast medium since the radiodensity of blood and the vascular wall are so similar. The natural contrast between flowing blood and the vascular wall suggests that NMR imaging might be advantageous for defining vascular abnormality, particularly mural lesions that project into the vascular lumen.

An added advantage of NMR imaging is that it can provide at least an estimate of flow velocity and may detect sites of slow or turbulent flow by specific changes in the luminal signal, which can be accentuated by variations in imaging parameters. Thus, NMR imaging seems capable of defining both anatomic and physiologic abnormalities of the cardiovascular system. Through the estimation of hydrogen density, as well as the magnetic relaxation rates of tissues (referred to as T_1 and T_2 values), it seems to be possible to attain discriminate tissue characterization.[9, 12] This latter capability should be particularly important for the diagnosis and investigation of myocardial diseases.

World wide experience with NMR imaging of the cardiovascular system is relatively inchoate. This article is intended to introduce some of the principles of NMR imaging particularly important for imaging of the cardiovascular system and to demonstrate our initial experience with its use in several cardiovascular diseases. There is now virtually no experience with NMR imaging in pediatric cardiovascular disease.

TECHNICAL PRINCIPLES

The basic principles of NMR imaging have been described elsewhere[4] and are beyond the scope of this article. The intensity of any portion of a NMR image using the spin echo technique is governed by the following formula.[4, 6, 7]

$$I = H\, f(v)\, \exp\,(-a/T_2)[1\text{-}\exp(-b/T_1)]$$

where I is the signal intensity, H is the hydrogen density, T_1 is the longitudinal relaxation time, T_2 is the transverse relaxation time, and f(v) is the function that depends on number of hydrogen nuclei in motion and their velocity.

In general, the image intensity depends most upon hydrogen density (H). Hydrogen nuclei are the most abundant nuclei in the body and contain an odd number of protons. Atoms with an odd number of either protons, neutrons, or both within their nuclei have a magnetic moment and can theoretically be utilized for NMR imaging. However, all current imagers use instrument parameters (frequency) that produce hydrogen density images.

As indicated in the above equation, local image intensity depends on the number of resonating nuclei (hydrogen) in the imaged volume, the motion of the nuclei, and the magnetic relaxation time constants T_1 and T_2 of the nuclei. The intensity is also modified by the chemical state of the nuclei, temperature, and electronic noise. The intensity of any structures increases with an increase in hydrogen density, longer T_2 relaxation time, and shorter T_1 relaxation time. Intensity generally decreases markedly or becomes negligible when nuclei flow through an imaged volume at a rate above a cutoff velocity (10 to 15 cm/sec). The signal generated by flowing nuclei (generally blood) can be augmented or attenuated, depending upon the selected imaging parameters of the NMR instrument.

The NMR imager used for our studies has been described in detail previously.[6] Briefly, the imager uses a 3.5 K gauss (0.35 Tesla) superconducting magnet (Oxford Instruments). The magnet and patient couch are contained within a copper mesh room (Faraday cage) that provides shielding against RF sources. Images were obtained at 3.5 K gauss by using the spin echo technique.

IMAGE DISPLAY

The gray scale of the NMR images displays fat as the brightest intensity (white), followed by brain and spinal cord, solid viscera, vessel wall, and muscle in descending order. Air, bone, and calcification produce almost no NMR signal (black). Consequently, lung parenchyma and bowel lumina produce little intensity (nearly black). Fat in the bone marrow produces high signal intensity for the bone marrow. Fluid-filled cavities tend to be low intensity. At normal velocities of blood flow, the lumens of patent vessels produce low or zero signal intensity.[8]

Physiologic Gating for NMR Imaging of the Heart. The full potential of NMR imaging of the heart will require gating. The gated NMR image shown in this article (Fig. 1) and one image published previously[1] reveal excellent detail of the internal topography of the ventricles. In contradistinction to CT scans, motion of the heart does not cause artifacts but does cause loss of signal intensity in the NMR imager. Electrocardiographic gating imposes a technical problem since metallic (ferromagnetic) structures (ECG leads) on the surface of the imaged volume cause electronic noise. Consequently, alternative methods of physiologic gating have been applied by using the arterial pressure pulse detected by a sphygmomanometer sensor, a fiberoptic Doppler flow sensor, and low impedance electrocardiographic leads.

Normal Cardiovascular Morphology. The cross-sectional imaging format displays cardiac and vascular anatomy in a form similar to contrast-enhanced computed tomography (Figs. 1 to 5). In contradistinction to computed tomography, the vascular structures are exquisitely depicted without the use of contrast medium. This enables clear discrimination of solid structures from blood vessels without using a contrast medium. Furthermore, the absence of signal within the vessel lumen enables examination of the vessel wall (see Fig. 5) and displays intimal morphology. Even nongated NMR images in some patients display good detail of the cardiac chambers and great vessels (see Fig. 2).

Gated NMR images of the heart have displayed the internal architecture of the heart (see Fig. 1). The natural sharp interface in contrast between moving blood in the cardiac chamber and the cardiac walls results in clear discrimination of the ventricular and atrial septa. Consequently, it is possible to measure wall thickness at all sites within the ventricles. Even at this early time in the development of NMR imaging, the spatial resolution of the

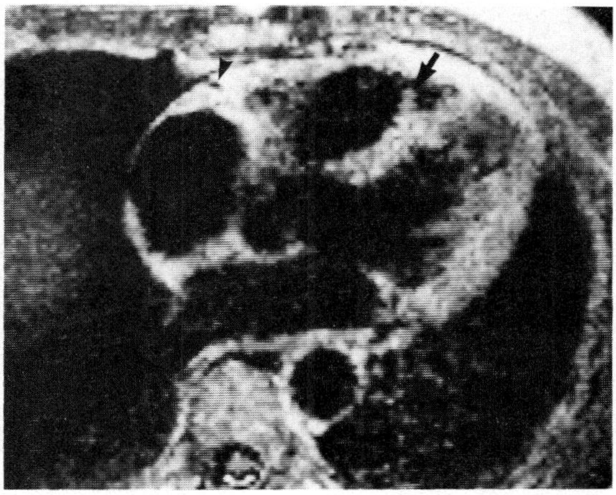

Figure 1. Gated NMR image at the midventricular level of a normal volunteer shows all four cardiac chambers. Internal topography of the ventricles is demonstrated including the moderate band (arrow) of the right ventricle and a papillary muscle of the left ventricle. Note again the right coronary artery in the right atrioventricular groove. (From Herfkens RJ, Higgins CB, Hricak H, et al: Nuclear magnetic resonance imaging of the cardiovascular system: Normal and pathologic findings. Radiology, *147*:749–759, 1983, with permission.)

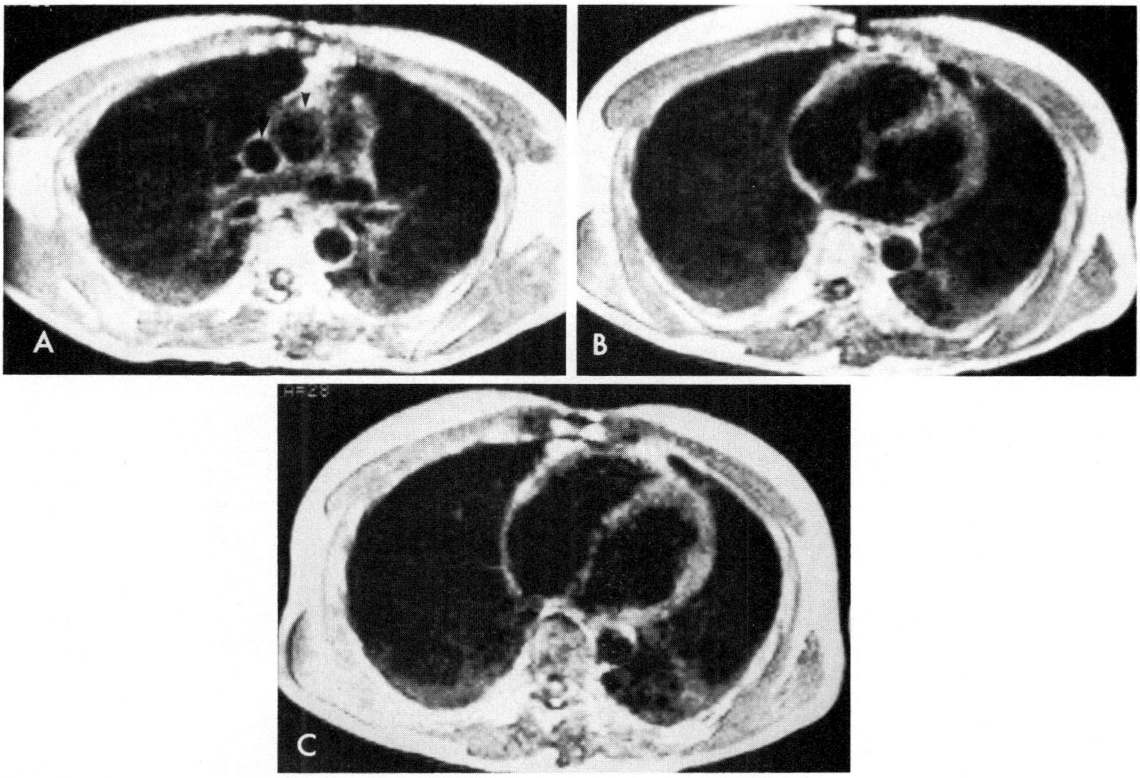

Figure 2. *A* to *C*. Three sequential nongated NMR images of the thorax. There is clear discrimination of the walls of the superior vena cava (arrowhead), aorta (arrowhead), and cardiac chambers.

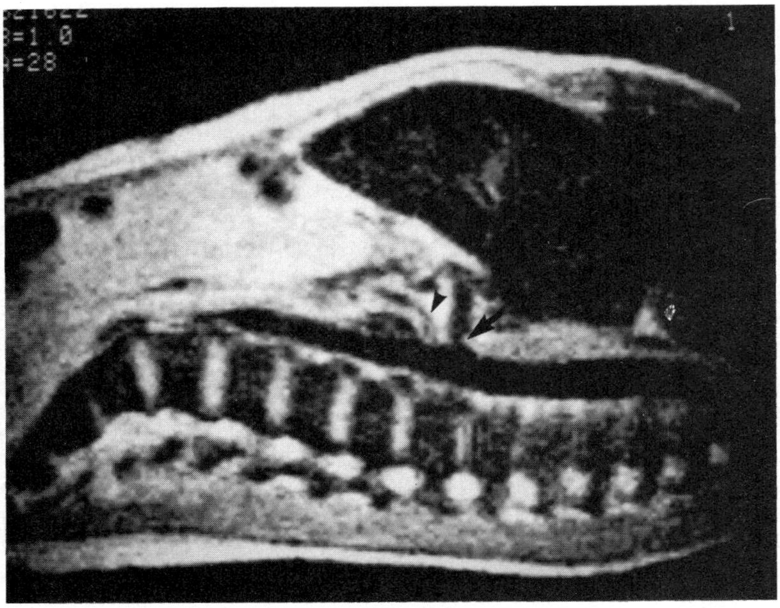

Figure 3. Sagittal image through the abdominal aorta in a child with hemochromatosis due to thalassemia major. Origin of the celiac artery from the aorta is shown (arrow). The origin of the superior mesenteric artery is also seen just caudal to the celiac origin (arrowhead). Note the low intensity of the NMR signal of the liver as a consequence of its high content of iron. (From Higgins CB, Goldberg H, Hricak H, et al: Nuclear magnetic resonance imaging of vasculature of abdominal viscera: Normal and pathologic features. Am J Cardiol, *140*:1217–1226, 1983, with permission.)

imager coupled with the current gating system has permitted visualization of the coronary arteries (see Fig 1). The origin and proximal portions of the coronary arteries have been displayed on NMR axial images at the base of the heart and the right coronary artery has been visualized within the atrioventricular groove on axial images through the middle of the ventricles (see Fig. 1). Resolution of the internal topography of the ventricles has been sufficient to depict the moderator band of the right ventricle (see Fig. 1), the papillary muscles (see Figs. 2 and 3), the junction of the chordae tendineae and papillary muscle (see Fig. 1), the leaflets of the atrioventricular valves (see Fig. 1), and the cusps of the aortic valve.

Sagittal images through the aorta display the smooth anterior and posterior aortic walls (see Fig. 3). In 15 patients and eight normal volunteers less than 30 years of age, the intimal

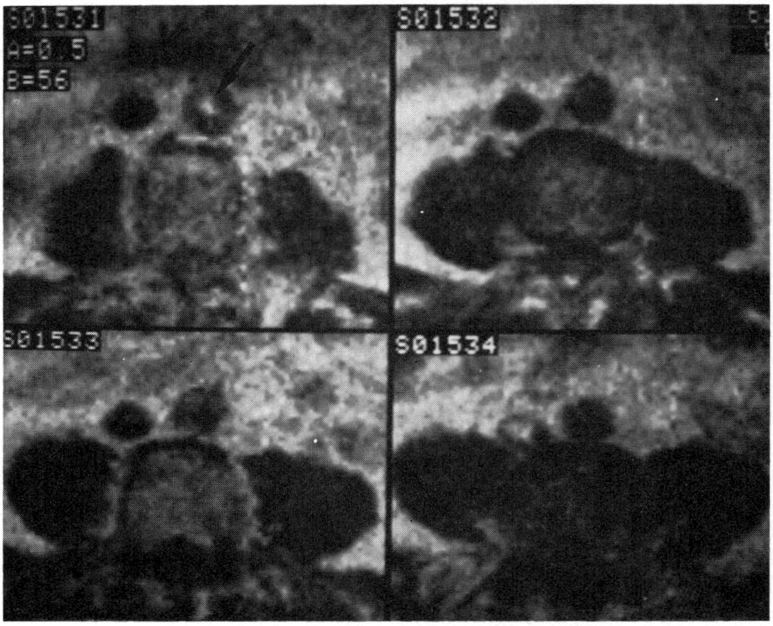

Figure 4. Sequential cross-sectional NMR images of the aorta in an asymptomatic patient reveal a circular contour of the aorta, thin wall, and smooth endocardial surface. Image of the most cranial cross-sectional level is shown in the left upper panel, and images progess to the most caudal cross-sectional level in the right lower panel. Images using the second (A = 56 msec) spin echo at the entrance level of the image volume show an intraluminal flow signal (arrow) in the aortic lumen. Note circumferential separation between the intraluminal flow signal and the vessel wall. Intraluminal flow signal is also in the vena cava at the most caudal level of the imaged volume. (From Herfkens RJ, Higgins CB, Hricak H, et al: Nuclear magnetic resonance imaging of the cardiovascular system: Normal and pathologic findings. Radiology, *147*:749–759, 1983, with permission.)

surface was smooth. However, even in normal patients, intraluminal flow signals (Fig. 4) were observed in images obtained at some instrument imaging parameters.

Within the abdomen, the aorta, vena cava, and visceral vessels, such as the superior mesenteric artery (Fig. 5*A*) and renal vessels (Fig. 5*B*), are clearly distinguished from surrounding parenchymal organs. Likewise, the venous structures within the abdomen such as the splenic vein, portal vein, and inferior vena cava are separable from surrounding organs, such as the pancreas and liver, without the need for contrast medium (Fig. 6).

Effect of Blood Flow on NMR Images. If the hydrogen nuclei flow through the volume being imaged in the time it takes to perform one data acquisition sequence (approximately 50 msec), their signal is lost. The reduction in NMR signal intensity depends on the fraction of hydrogen nuclei that are moving and on their velocity. Concepts about the NMR imaging of flowing blood have been derived from in vitro experiments in which blood was pumped at varying velocities through tubes placed in the NMR imager.[8, 12] The pattern of signals generated from blood flowing at various velocities is shown in Figure 7. The signal intensity from blood is related to the velocity of blood flow (Fig. 8). For any velocity below the cutoff velocity (velocity at which signal intensity of flowing blood approaches background levels), the signal at sequential cross-sectional levels varies in a characteristic manner (see Fig. 6).

With the NMR imaging parameters used in the current study, blood flow at velocities greater than 10 to 15 cm/sec[8] produces a signal intensity approaching the background level. There is little or no signal intensity within the vascular lumina. However, even at normal flow velocities, flow signals are frequently observed on images produced by using the second spin echo (echo delay = 56 msec) (see Fig. 4). In multisection images, paradoxic enhancement may be observed at the initial cross-sectional level into which blood is flowing (see Fig. 4). This is caused by flow into a region of the subject being excited by radiofrequency (RF) pulses.[8, 12] These flowing nuclei have not previously undergone excitations. Consequently, they become fully magnetized at this first cross-sectional level (entrance image) within the imaged volume, and they produce comparatively large signal intensities. The signal intensity is even greater than that expected from stationary blood, and it is considerably greater than the signal from muscle. This phenomenon is recognized as a bright, frequently laminated or solid, high-intensity signal within the lumen (see Figs. 4 and 7). These bright areas within the lumen are frequently separated from the vessel wall by a concentric black ring (decreased or no intensity). In general, paradoxic enhancement and other flow artifacts are most prominent on the second spin echo ("a" = 56 msec) of an imaging sequence. Within the abdomen, the intensity of this flow signal is most prominent at the most cranial level of the imaged volume for arteries and most caudal level for veins corresponding with the direction of flow for these vessels (see Fig. 4). Paradoxic enhancement is greater at lower flow velocities and consequently tends to be most prominent for venous structures.

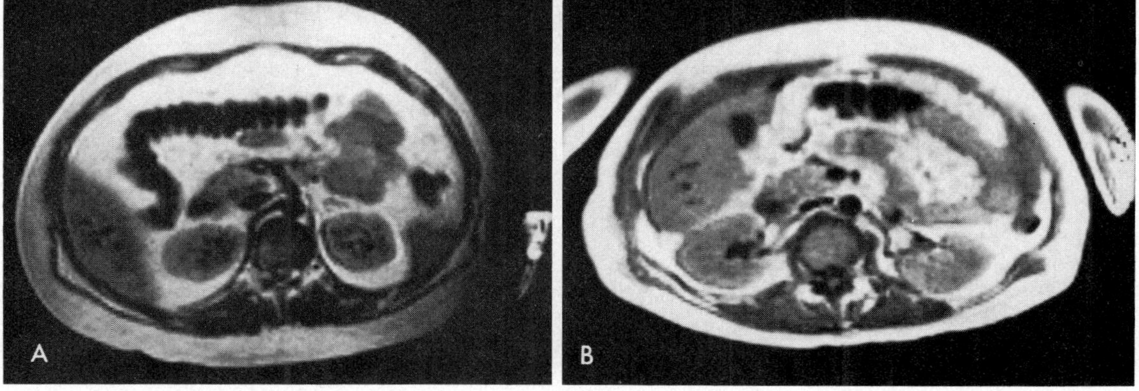

Figure 5. *A*, Cross-sectional NMR image of the abdomen at the level of origin of the superior mesenteric artery from the aorta in a 15-year-old boy with adrenal hyperplasia and another image *(B)* at the level of the renal vessels in a man with pancreatic carcinoma (right). The absence of signal within the superior mesenteric artery and renal vessels clearly distinguishes these vessels from surrounding parenchymal organs.

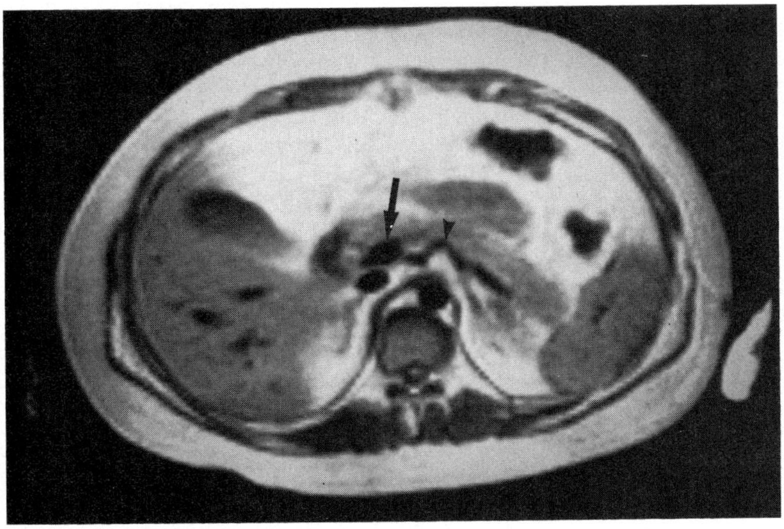

Figure 6. Cross-sectional NMR image of the abdomen at the level of confluence of the portal (arrow) and splenic veins (arrowhead). The absence of signal from the lumina of the portal and splenic veins identifies these structures from the pancreas. The inferior vena cava lies posterior to the portal vein and is clearly distinguished from the liver. (From Herfkens RJ, Higgins CB, Hricak H, et al: Nuclear magnetic resonance imaging of the cardiovascular system: Normal and pathologic findings. Radiology, *147*:749–759, 1983, with permission.)

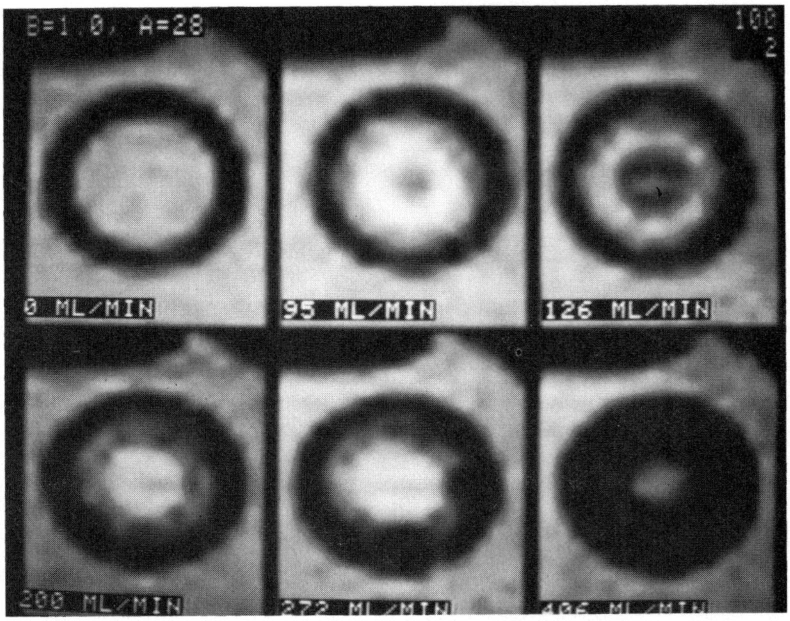

Figure 7. Examples of flow signals produced in 9 mm tubes with blood flowing at various velocities. Note the circumferential lucency separating the laminated flow signal from the wall of the tube. As the flow increases from 0 to 406 ml/min in a tube of 9.6 mm diameter, the average intensity of the signal from moving blood first increases and then decreases to nearly zero. The distribution of signal intensity is not uniform, taking on the pattern of concentric rings. The walls of the tube (Plexiglas) are dark, since this material produces no NMR signal. (From Kaufman L, Crooks LE, Sheldon PE, et al: Evaluation of NMR imaging for detection and quantitation of obstruction in vessels. Invest Radiol, *17*:554–560, 1982, with permission.)

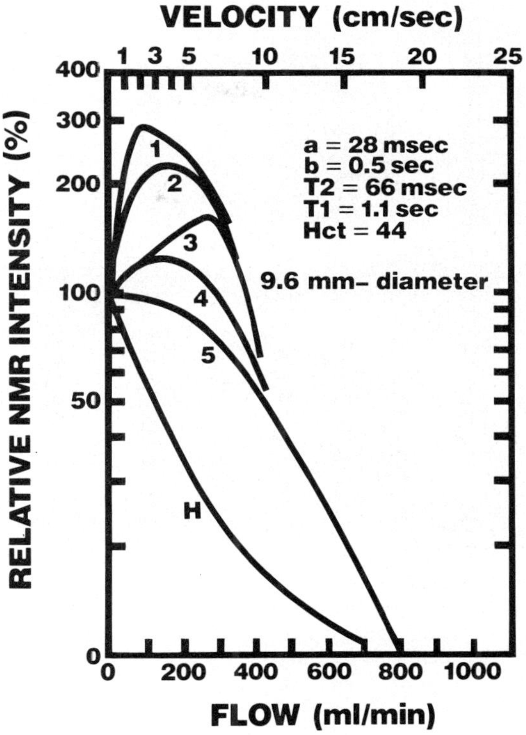

Figure 8. NMR signal intensity versus flow velocity (rate) of flowing blood in Plexiglas tubes of 9.6 mm. Intensity signal is expressed as a percentage of that produced by stationary blood. Curves are displayed for multiple cross-sectional levels within the image volume. The level in which blood flow enters the imaged volume shows the greatest relative intensity of signal. At the entrance section and those near the entrance section, the flow signal at lower velocities is actually higher than that generated from stationary blood. (From Kaufman L, Crooks LE, Sheldon PE, et al: Evaluation of NMR imaging for detection and quantitation of obstruction in vessels. Invest Radiol, *17*:554–560, 1982, with permission.)

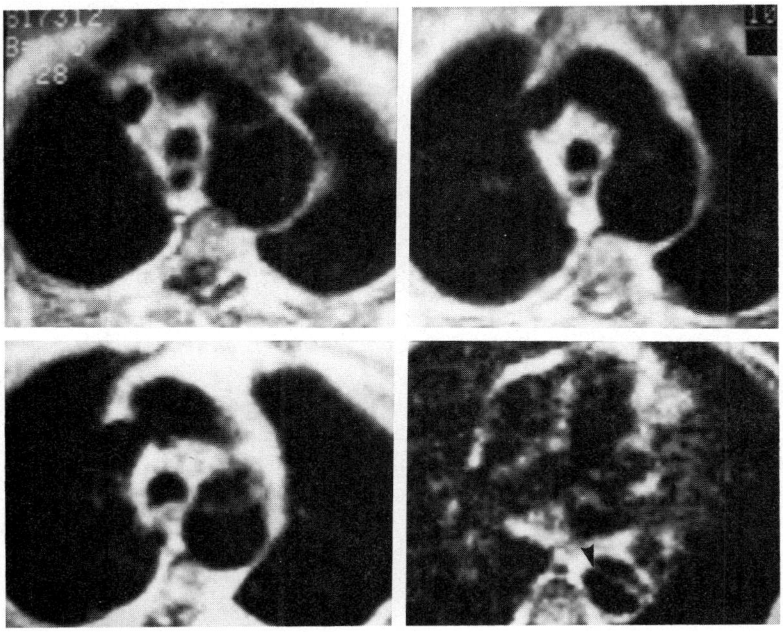

Figure 9. Sequential cross-sectional images in a patient with an aneurysm of the aortic arch and a type B dissection of the descending aorta. Images at the level of the arch display localized dilatation of the aortic arch. Image through the descending aorta shows the intimal flap (arrowhead). (From Herfkens RJ, Higgins CB, Hricak H, et al: Nuclear magnetic resonance imaging of the cardiovascular system: Normal and pathologic findings. Radiology, *147*:749–759, 1983, with permission.)

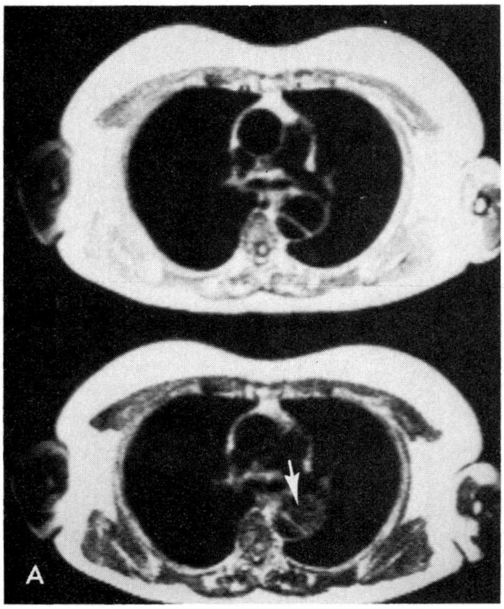

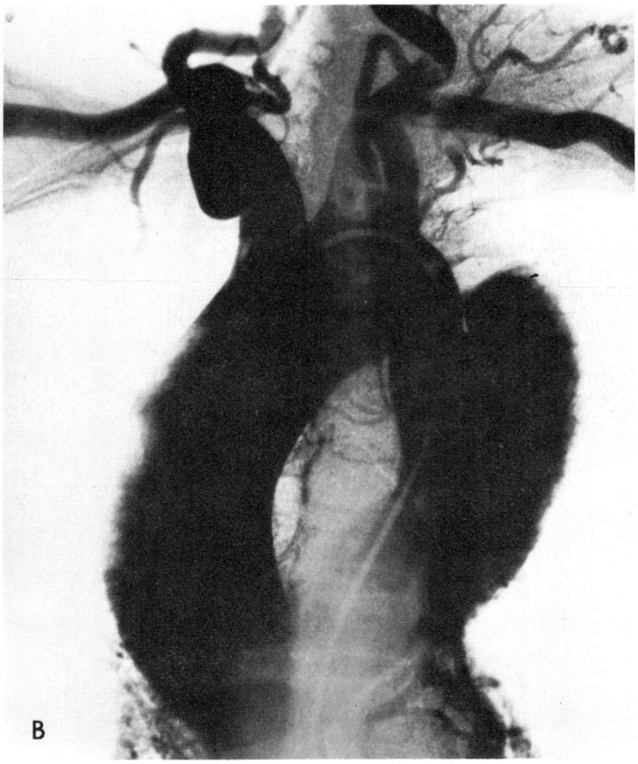

Figure 10. *A*, Series of NMR images and *(B)* angiogram of the descending aorta in a patient with type B aortic dissection reveal the intimal flap and the false and the true lumina of the aorta. At caudal levels (lower panel), the intraluminal signal is detected in the false channel (arrow), but no signal is registered in the true lumen. This finding suggests slow or turbulent flow in the false channel and normal flow in the true channel. (From Herfkens RJ, Higgins CB, Hricak H, et al: Nuclear magnetic resonance imaging of the cardiovascular system: Normal and pathologic findings. Radiology, *147*:749–759, 1983, with permission.)

Pathologic Cardiovascular Morphology. The substantial natural contrast between flowing blood and the vessel wall permits clear demonstration of abnormalities of the vascular wall such as:

1. Intimal flaps of aortic dissections displaced into the aortic lumen (Figs. 9 and 10).
2. Localized dilatation of the lumen and distortion of the contour of the wall of the aorta caused by aneurysms (see Fig. 9).
3. Atherosclerotic plaque protruding into the lumen of the aorta (Figs. 11 and 12).
4. Mural thrombus within the false channel of an aortic dissection (see Fig. 10).

Several abnormal flow patterns have been recognized on NMR images. Abnormal flow patterns are demonstrated better with images produced by the second spin echo ("a" = 56 msec).

Occlusion of a vessel is indicated by obliteration of the vessel lumen by intense NMR signals. In a patient with an aortofemoral bypass graft, there is no signal within the lumen of the patent graft (Fig. 13). On the other hand, the lumen of the occluded native aorta is filled with high-intensity signals.

Slow or turbulent flow causes an increase in the intensity within the lumen of the false channel of an aortic dissection compared with the absence of signal within the true lumen (see Fig. 10). The intensity of the signal from slowly flowing blood was shown best on images obtained with the second spin echo ("a" = 56 msec).

MYOCARDIAL CHARACTERIZATION

Since the NMR signal is exquisitely sensitive to variations in local water content, the edema associated with acute muscle infarction should allow direct visualization of the ischemically damaged area. Acute myocardial ischemia in the dog has been found to cause a prolongation of the T_1 relaxation time of the ischemic tissue, which was directly related to the per cent water content of the myocardium.[17]

We have recently studied the effect of ischemia on the NMR characteristics of muscle. Ischemic injury to muscular tissue was found to cause alterations in the NMR image as well as in the tissue characteristics as reflected by T_1

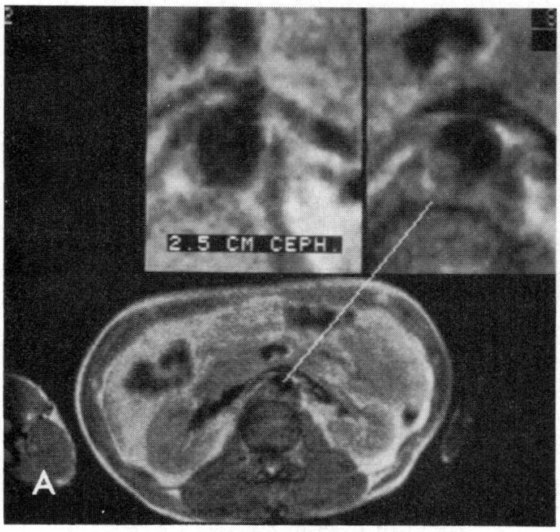

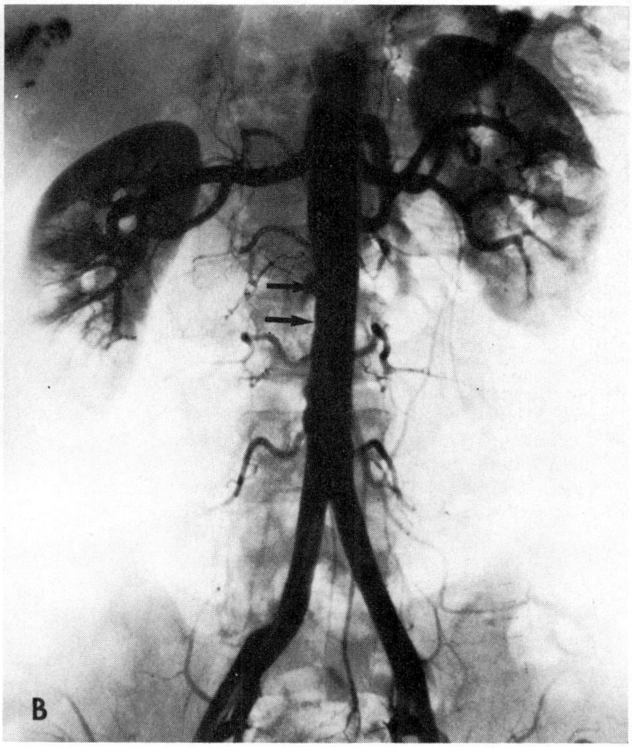

Figure 11. *A*, NMR images reveal atherosclerotic plaque projecting into the aortic lumen in an asymatomatic 48-year-old renal donor. Insets contain magnified views of the aorta at the level of the lesion and at a level 2.6 cm cephalad. *B*, Aortogram confirmed the presence of eccentric atherosclerotic narrowing of the aorta at the site shown on the NMR image (arrows).

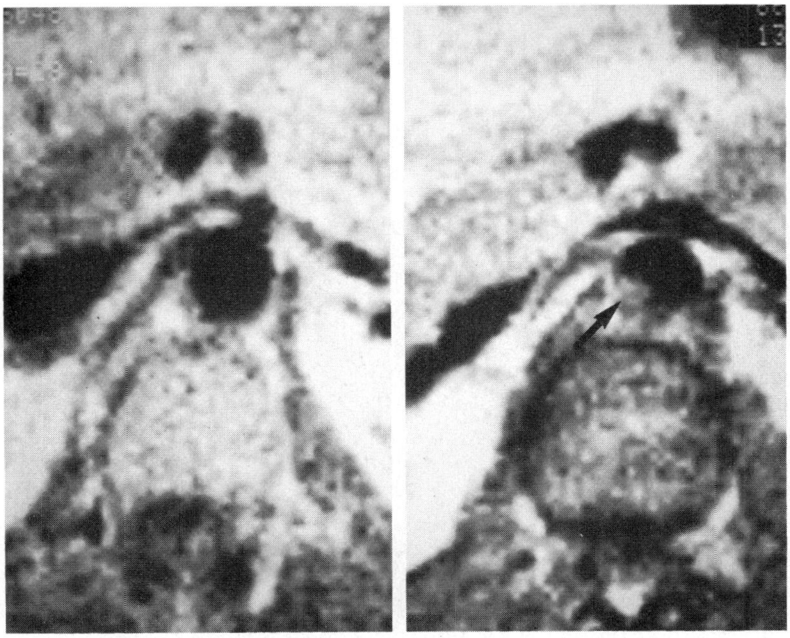

Figure 12. NMR images of the infrarenal abdominal aorta at two cross-sectional levels show eccentric thickening (arrows) of the posterior wall of the aorta by an atherosclerotic plaque projecting into the lumen.

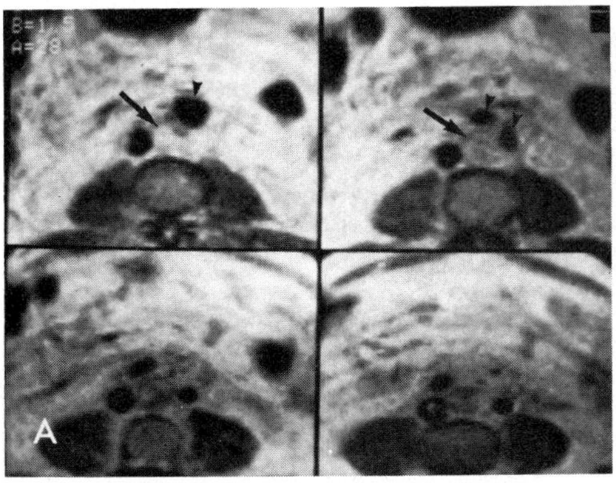

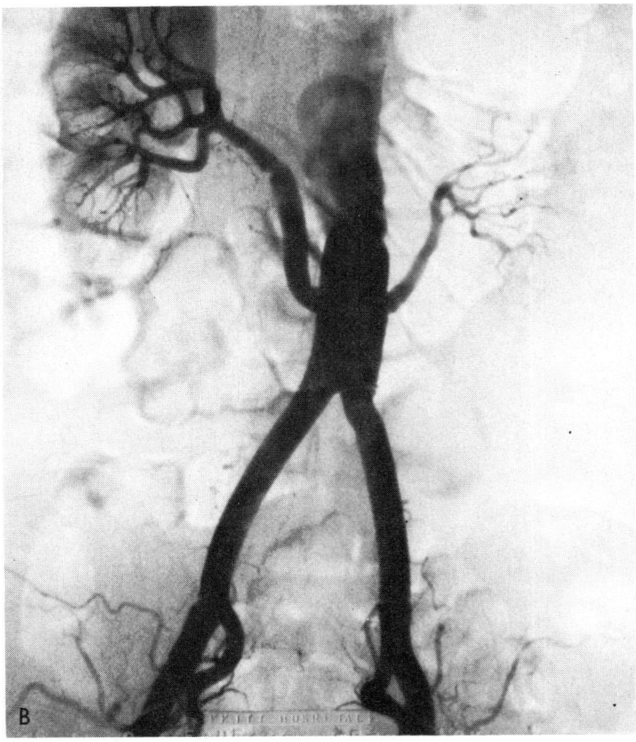

Figure 13. *A*, NMR images at sequential levels of the distal abdominal aorta in a patient with an aortofemoral bypass graft. There is no signal within the patent graft (arrowheads) with presumably normal flow, but a signal fills the lumen of the native aorta, which was occluded (arrows). *B*, Aortogram shows the patent aortofemoral bypass graft and no opacification of the native aorta. There are also side limbs from the graft to the renal arteries. Later sequential radiographs demonstrate no opacification of the distal portion of the aorta. (From Kaufman L, Crooks LE, Sheldon PE, et al: Evaluation of NMR imaging for detection and quantitation of obstruction in vessels. Invest Radiol, *17*:554–560, 1982, with permission.)

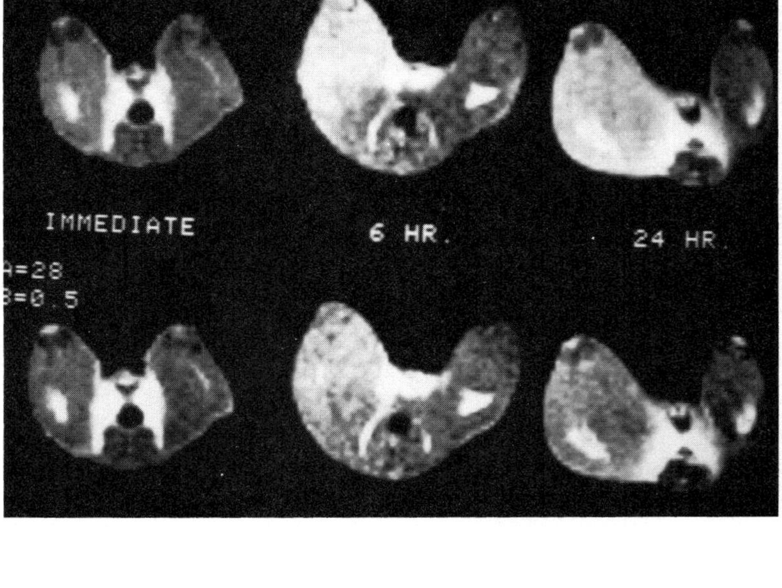

Figure 14. NMR images of the thighs of rats at various time intervals after arterial occlusion of the right limb. There is marked increase in the intensity of the NMR signal (spin echo technique) of the muscle of the infarcted limb at 6 and 24 hr after occlusion. (From Herfkens RJ, Higgins CB, Hricak H, et al: Nuclear magnetic resonance imaging of the cardiovascular system: Normal and pathologic findings. Radiology, *147*:749–759, 1983, with permission.)

to the water content (edema) of the muscle (Fig. 15).[10]

Preliminary experiments using excised canine hearts with 24-hr-old myocardial infarction also demonstrated increased signal intensity from the infarcted area (Fig. 16). Likewise, the measured T_1 and T_2 value and water content were increased in the region of myocardial ischemic and T_2 relaxation times. The effect of ischemia was initially examined in a murine model of limb muscle ischemia. Ischemia caused increase in signal intensity from the ischemically damaged limb musculature (Fig. 14). Both the T_1 and T_2 relaxation times of ischemically damaged

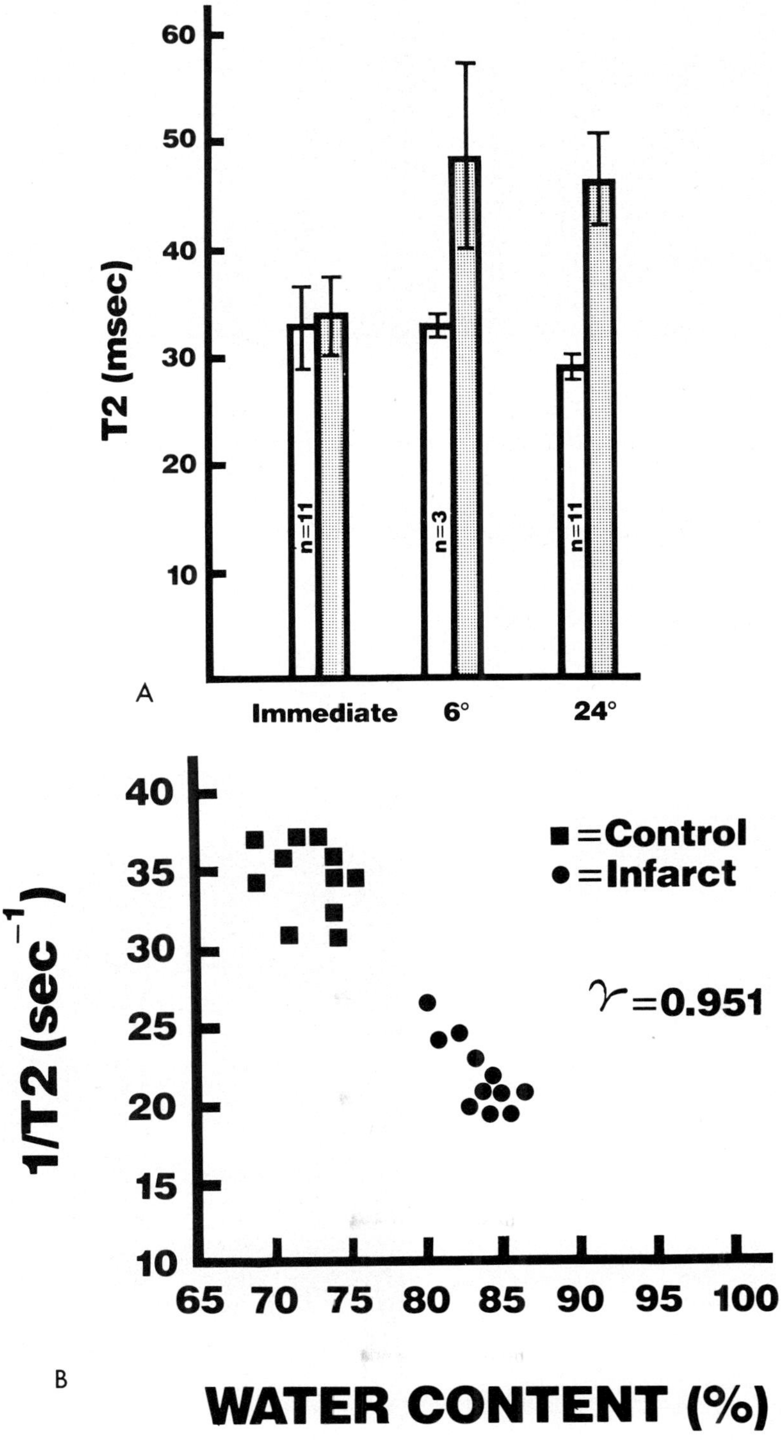

Figure 15. *A*, Block diagram shows the T_2 values of the normal and infarcted limb at various time intervals after vascular occlusion. The T_2 relaxation rate of the infarcted limb was significantly greater at 6 and 24 hr after occlusion. *B*, The T_2 relaxation rates of the control and infarcted limbs correlated with the water content of the muscle at 24 hr after occlusion. (From Herfkens RJ, Higgins CB, Hricak H, et al: NMR imaging of infarcted muscle: A rat model. Radiology, *147*:761–764, 1983, with permission.)

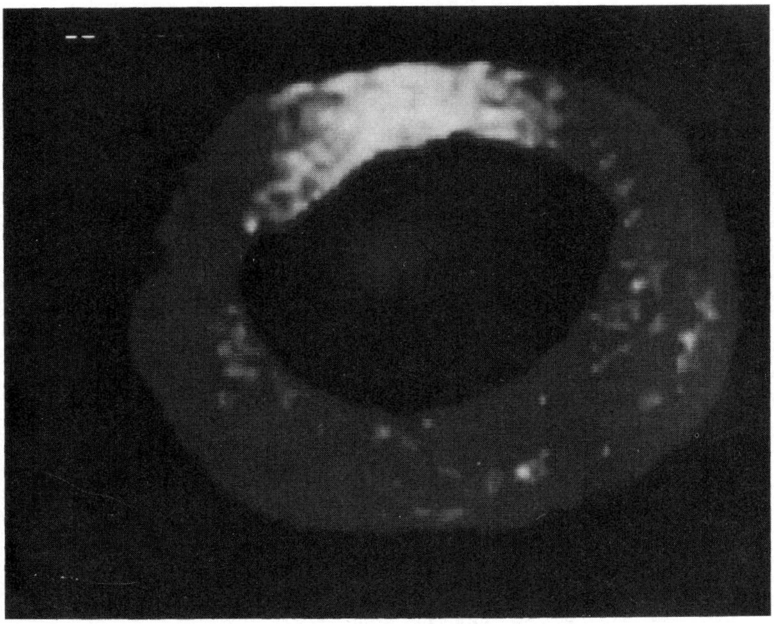

Figure 16. Cross-sectional NMR image through an excised canine heart with a 24-hour-old myocardial infarction. There is increased signal intensity of the anterior region of the left ventricle.

muscle were significantly prolonged. The increase in relaxation times was roughly related injury. In a patient with a transmural myocardial infarction complicated by an anteroapical aneurysm, NMR images displayed localized wall thinning and aneurysmal bulging of the left ventricle (Fig. 17). The images also displayed abnormal signal intensity within this region of the left ventricular chamber, indicating blood stasis and thrombus in the aneurysmal segment.

FUTURE APPLICATIONS

There is currently too little clinical experience with NMR imaging to predict with any

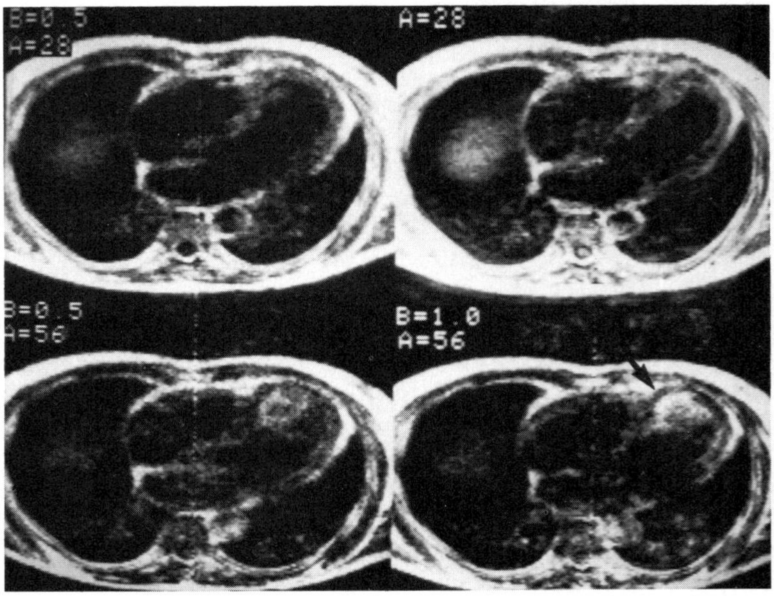

Figure 17. NMR image at different imaging parameters through the same cross-sectional level of the left ventricle in a patient with postinfarctional aneurysm of the anteroapical segment of the left ventricle. The NMR images show good delineation of the left ventricular walls presumably because of decreased myocardial motion. In the area of the infarction, the myocardial wall is thin and displays localized dilatation (aneurysm) (arrow). In addition, the intense NMR signal within the lumen at this site indicates the presence of mural thrombus and stagnant flow (lower panels). The abnormality in intraluminal flow is displayed best on the images produced with the second spin echo (A = 56 msec) (lower panels). (From Kaufman L, Crooks LE, Sheldon PE, et al: Evaluation of NMR imaging for detection and quantitation of obstruction in vessels. Invest Radiol, *17*:554–560, 1982, with permission.)

reliance the eventual role of this technique in cardiovascular diagnosis. However, it offers three intriguing insights into the assessment of cardiovascular disease processes and their response to therapeutic interventions: direct tissue characterization, measurements of noninvasive regional blood flow, and chemical and metabolic imaging.

The magnetic relaxation times (T_1 and T_2 times) of protons in different tissues are currently the basis for tissue characterization. These relaxation times and their diagnostic implications are poorly understood presently. Nevertheless, both normal and abnormal tissues have been shown to have combinations of T_1 and T_2 values that fall in a characteristic range for a specific tissue. These specific relaxation times for various tissues have been estimated in experimental animals[9] and in man.[11] Various disease processes including ischemia have been found to alter the magnetic relaxation times of tissues and organs.[9, 10, 17]

Besides the qualitative identification of abnormal flow patterns discussed in this article, it should be possible to noninvasively quantitate blood flow by using NMR imaging. Several techniques have been suggested for quantitating flow with NMR,[2, 3, 14, 16] including measurement of transit time of excited nuclei[2] and the generation of "flow graphs" that plot the number of nuclei flowing within various velocity intervals.[16]

Perhaps the most promising aspect of NMR imaging is the potential for metabolic imaging. This capability exploits another feature of NMR: the ability to measure chemical shifts. The chemical nuclei (other than hydrogen) that seem most attractive for vivo chemical studies because of a compromise among their NMR sensitivity, abundance in biologic systems, and biochemical interests are sodium-23, carbon-13, and phosphorus-31. Most of the current work on NMR spectroscopy of the myocardium in vivo has involved phosphorus-31. These phosphorus-31 NMR spectroscopic studies have provided a method for monitoring shifts in high-energy phosphate and intracellular pH during myocardial ischemia and interventions intended to attenuate the deleterious myocardial effects of ischemia.[13, 15]

Research into the use of NMR imaging for diagnosing and assessing the severity of cardiovascular disease has just recently begun. Our knowlege of NMR imaging at this time will undoubtedly be shown in the next decade to be quite primitive. The observations presented in this article, gleaned from our initial experience, must be considered tentative.

REFERENCES

1. Alfidi RJ, Haaga JR, El Yousef SJ, et al: Preliminary experimental results in humans and animals with superconducting, whole body, nuclear magnetic resonance scanner. Radiology, *143*:175–181, 1982.
2. Battocletti JH, Halback RE, Salles-Cunha SX, et al: NMR blood flowmeter—theory and history. Med Phys, *8*:435–443, 1980.
3. Battocletti JH, Halback RE, Sances A, Jr, et al: Flat crossed coil detector for blood flow measurement using nuclear magnetic resonance. Med Biol Eng Comput, *17*:183, 1979.
4. Bradley W, Tosteson H: Basic physics of NMR. *In* Nuclear Magnetic Resonance Imaging in Medicine. Tokyo, Igaku-Shoin, 1981, p. 11.
5. Budinger TF: Nuclear magnetic resonance (NMR) in vivo studies: Known threshold for health effects. J Comput Assist Tomogr, *5*:800–811, 1981.
6. Crooks LE, Arakawa M, Hoenninger J, et al: Nuclear magnetic resonance whole body imager operating at 3.5 KGauss. Radiology, *143*:169–174, 1982.
7. Crooks LE, Mills CM, Davis PL, et al: Visualization of cerebral and vascular abnormalities by NMR imaging. The effects of imaging parameters on contrast. Radiology, *144*:843–852, 1982.
8. Crooks L, Sheldon P, Kaufman L, et al: Quantification of obstructions in vessels by nuclear magnetic resonance (NMR). IEEE Trans Nucl Sci, *29*:1181–1185, 1982.
9. Davis PL, Kaufman L, Crooks LE, et al: NMR characteristics of normal and abnormal rat tissue. *In* Nuclear Magnetic Resonance Imaging in Medicine. Tokyo, Igaku-Shoin, 1981, p. 71.
10. Herfkens RJ, Lipton MJ, Crooks LE, et al: NMR imaging of infarcted muscle: A rat model. Radiology, *147*:761–764, 1983.
11. Hutchison JMS, Smith FW: Human NMR imaging. *In* Nuclear Magnetic Resonance Imaging in Medicine. Tokyo, Igaku-Shoin, 1981, p. 101.
12. Kaufman L, Crooks LE, Sheldon PE, et al: Evaluation of NMR imaging for detection and quantification of obstruction in vessels. Invest Radiol, *17*:554–560, 1982.
13. Jacobus WE, Taylor GJ, Hollis DP, et al: Phosphorus nuclear magnetic resonance of perfused working rat hearts. Nature, *265*:756, 1977.
14. Morse OC, Singer IR: Blood velocity measurements in intact subjects. Science, *170*:440–441, 1970.
15. Nunnally RL, Bottomley PA: ^{31}P NMR studies of myocardial ischemia and its response to drug therapies. J Comput Assist Tomogr, *5*:296, 1981.
16. Singer JR: Blood flow measurements by NMR. *In* Nuclear Magnetic Resonance in Medicine. Tokyo, Igaku-Shoin, 1981, p. 11.
17. Williams ES, Kaplan JI, Thatcher F, et al: Prolongation of proton spin lattice relaxation times in regionally ischemic tissue from dog hearts. J Nucl Med, *21*:449–453, 1980.

17

CARDIAC IMAGING WITH NUCLEAR MAGNETIC RESONANCE

Technical Considerations and Potential Clinical Application

THOMAS M. BIANCANIELLO, M.D.,
and MARGERY A. HENEGHAN, M.D.

INTRODUCTION

Block and Purcell won the Nobel Prize in 1952 for their report of the phenomenon of nuclear magnetic resonance (NMR) in bulk materials in 1946.[29, 32] Five years later, in 1957, the NMR spectrum of ribonuclease was demonstrated.[29] In 1973, Lauterbur showed that it was possible to produce images of the spatial distribution of protons in a test object,[27] and NMR body imaging thus became an achievable goal. Since that time, more complex experiments have been described involving imaging of normal organs and neoplastic tissue in cadavers and in living animals and human subjects.[2, 7, 17, 20, 25, 34] Detailed discussions of the physical, chemical, and technical aspects of NMR imaging are available elsewhere.[8, 24, 33]

NMR is a technique that can be applied to biologic tissue and organs to obtain anatomic and physiologic information. The basis of NMR imaging is the emission of electromagnetic signals from atomic nuclei with an odd number of protons or neutrons or both. The creation of an image without the use of ionizing radiation is an attractive advantage of this technique for medical imaging. This feature, as well as the possibility of improved data acquisition, provides the impetus to apply it to the study of congenital heart disease.

NMR IMAGING OF BIOLOGIC MATERIAL

Most elements have at least one isotope in abundance whose nuclei are magnetic and therefore able to emit energy when subjected to radiofrequency (rf) pulses of a specific frequency.

Hydrogen is the most abundant element in the body. Because of the high concentration of hydrogen in tissues, its nuclei, or protons, produce the strongest NMR signal. It is largely for this reason that most biologic NMR imaging is proton-density imaging.

The concentrations of most other significant elements in the body are relatively small. As a result, the NMR signals they emit are weak, and special methods for signal detection and image formation are necessary. Studies of phosphorus spectra in humans and animals have shown that it is possible to apply NMR imaging techniques to the measurement of phosphocreatine, adenosine triphosphate (ATP), and other important enzymes and metabolites in tissues.[1, 5, 16, 37]

DATA ACQUISITION

Several techniques for proton NMR imaging have been described that differ chiefly in the way in which the object is "scanned" for data. In one kind of imaging mode, the effective response to rf excitation is limited to a single point, which is scanned back and forth over the object to create an image.[9, 19] A line of points may be scanned simultaneously, reducing imaging time.[21, 30] A further refinement involves recording NMR signals from an entire plane through an object.[11, 25]

With any of these techniques, the total time required to obtain pictures of sufficiently high spatial resolution and intensity is long, on the order of several minutes. The resulting signal loss due to motion is a potential drawback for cardiovascular imaging. This problem has been partially overcome by exploiting the fact that an image is composed of several hundred projections, for each of which the data collection period is typically 30 to 40 msec. Compared with the duration of the cardiac cycle, this period is very short. By gating or synchronization of the rf pulse to a particular phase of the cardiac cycle, precise images of the heart at a point in the cardiac cycle can be obtained.

IMAGE RECONSTRUCTION

Three-dimensional image reconstruction can be achieved with NMR, as in computerized tomography (CT) scanning, by stacking many contiguous single slices. The limitation of this method is that resolution is good parallel to the plane of section but relatively poor for structures perpendicular to it. A more direct procedure is to detect simultaneously the NMR signals emitted from a sensitive volume and from this information to reconstruct a true three-dimensional map of the object. Isotropic sections, that is, sections having equivalent resolution in all planes, may then be selected in any orientation through the object.[26]

NMR IMAGING OF THE CARDIOVASCULAR SYSTEM

Proton-density NMR images of the normal heart have been obtained in vivo in both animals and humans.[2] Early images of the heart in living subjects were ungated and of relatively coarse quality due to motion artifact. More recently, gated and synchronized images have been obtained, showing superior resolution of cardiac structural detail. Gated studies permit details of structure to be captured in systole and diastole. Since the data collection period is short, multiple images at various phases of the cardiac cycle can be obtained. These images can then be displayed in sequence, and a picture of the heart in motion can be reconstructed. The images of the living human heart shown in Figures 1*A* and *B* were obtained using a 1.5 kilogauss super-conducting magnet, with a 45-msec data collection window.

Blood flow, as well as tissue contrast, may be evaluated by NMR imaging without the use of extraneous contrast media. Fluid flowing within or across the imaging plane may modify the strength of the NMR signal. Under certain conditions, circulating blood is signal-poor, a phenomenon known as "flow void." This phenomenon results in high contrast between vessels and adjacent soft tissue and may even be exploited to measure blood flow rates as well as presence or absence of flow.

A variety of paramagnetic ions, such as manganese, have been used as NMR contrast agents.[28] Compounds containing ^{19}F have similarly been tested in vitro and may be introduced into the body as tracers.[22] In preliminary studies, Alfidi et al. used inhaled 100 per cent oxygen as a vascular contrast agent in human volunteers. They demonstrated increased density of the interventricular septum and blood in the left ventricle after oxygen inhalation.[2]

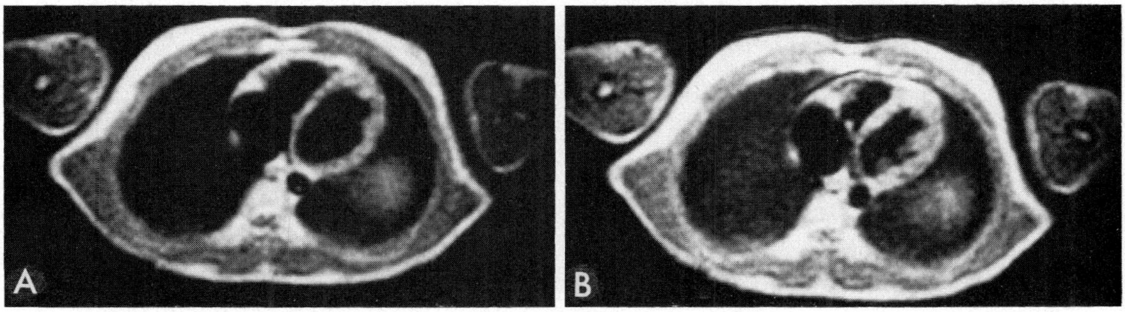

Figure 1. Gated NMR images of the normal heart. Transverse sections of the thorax at the level of the mid ventricles. *A*, Right and left ventricles during diastole. Image obtained 400 msec after peak systolic blood pressure. *B*, Ventricular systole. Gated image acquired at peak blood pressure. Note the thickened ventricular walls, smaller chamber diameters, and contracted papillary muscles. (Courtesy of Technicare Corporation, Solon, OH.)

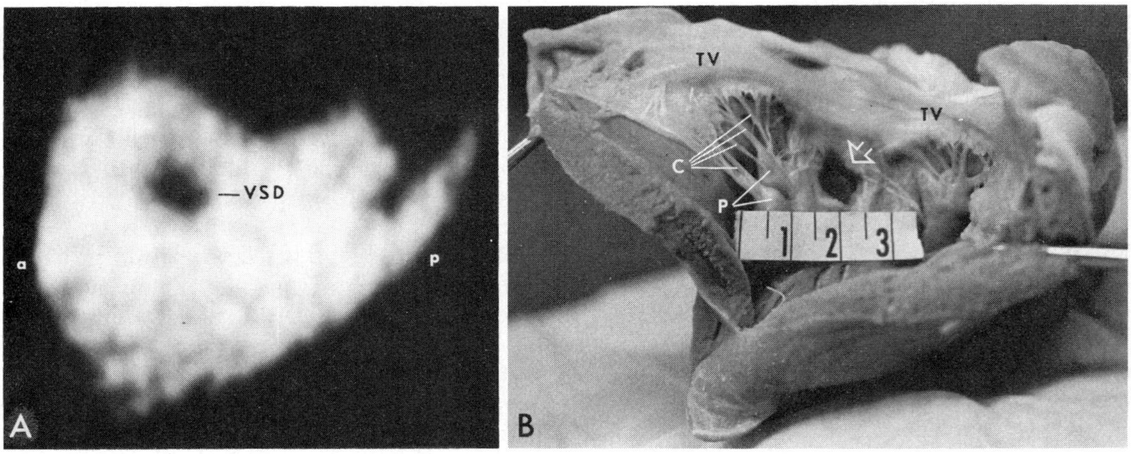

Figure 2. *A*, Sagittal (long-axis) section of a lamb heart with ventricular septal defect, taken from a three-dimensional NMR image. a: anterior; p: posterior. View of the interventricular septum en face shows a 9.0-mm defect (VSD) anterosuperiorly. *B*, Lamb heart specimen with right ventricle incised between papillary muscles. Right ventricular cavity exposed to show 8.5-mm defect in the septum (open arrow), papillary muscles (P) and chordae tendineae (C), and tricuspid valve leaflets (TV).

APPLICATIONS TO CONGENITAL HEART DISEASE

The definition of anatomy is, of course, most important in the study of congenital heart defects. With NMR it is possible to study the often complex anatomy of these defects and the relationships of the cardiac chambers, valves, and great vessels in three dimensions.

Using a 938-gauss–resistive aircore magnet, we recently showed that an artificially created ventricular septal defect (VSD) could be imaged in vitro in a lamb's heart specimen.[18] Figure 2*A* shows a unique en face sagittal view of the ventricular septum, a projection not easily reproduced with other modalities. With this view, it was possible to localize and measure the septal defect precisely. The conventional views used in other sectional imaging techniques such as echocardiography are also obtainable (Fig. 3). We hope to conduct similar studies in vivo in animals with VSD.

Three-dimensional NMR imaging is potentially of great value in the investigation of patients with multiple ventricular septal defects. By cardiac catheterization it is often technically difficult, if not impossible, to delineate the number of defects in the "Swiss cheese" muscular VSD. The abnormalities can be identified only indirectly, by the flow of contrast

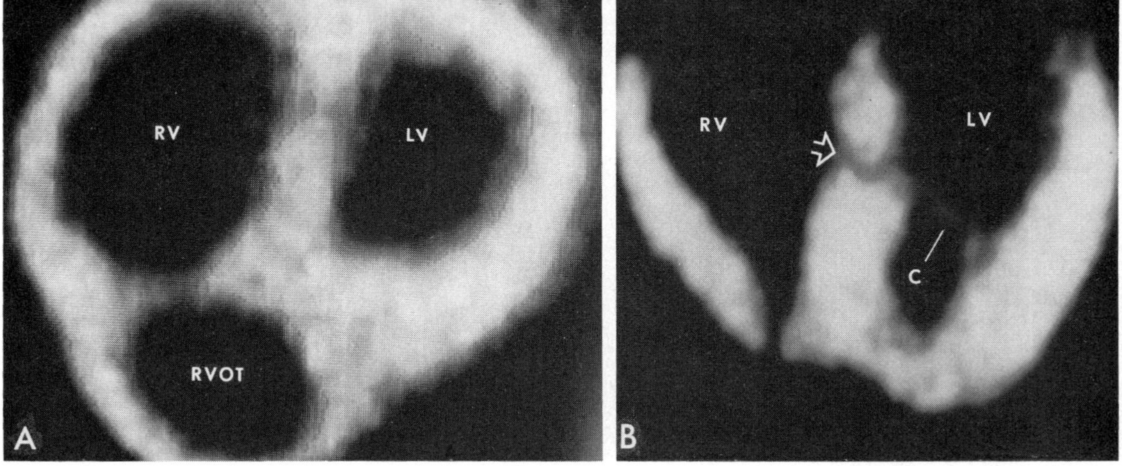

Figure 3. *A*, Transverse (short-axis) section of lamb heart, taken from a three-dimensional NMR image. Section is through the cardiac base above the VSD, at the level of right ventricle (RV), left ventricle (LV), and pulmonary outflow tract (RVOT). *B*, Coronal (four-chamber) section of lamb heart, from three-dimensional NMR image. The ventricular septal defect (open arrow) is demonstrated. Chordae tendineae (C) are seen traversing the left ventricular cavity.

between chambers. The contrast mixes so rapidly, particularly in infants with fast heart rates, that sites of shunting are not clearly delineated. Using NMR, it is theoretically possible to obtain a sagittal (en face) view of the septum and thereby define directly the size, number, and locations of the defects. The preoperative availability of such precise information would allow the cardiac surgeon to avoid extensive incisions and to save valuable operating time searching to ensure that all defects are repaired.

Anomalies of the great vessels, patent ductus arteriosus, and surgically created shunts and conduits lend themselves to study by NMR. Sectional images of this type have already been obtained by conventional and dynamic CT.[15] Since the magnitude of their motion is small compared with the heart, these vessels and shunts can be imaged fairly accurately by CT using a 2½-sec scan time. NMR, with the advantage of its much shorter image time (20 to 40 msec) and the excellent vascular contrast as a result of the "flow void," should also provide high-quality images of these structures. In addition, since the contrast between vessels and conduits and the surrounding soft tissue is intrinsically high, intravascular injection of contrast media is not necessary. The potential applications of NMR in this area are numerous. For example, coarctation of the aorta and interrupted aortic arch could be distinguished and diagnosed. The relationship of the great vessels to each other and other structures can be defined. It may even be possible to evaluate the patency and size of the ductus arteriosus and surgical shunts without iodinated contrast agents, taking advantage of the "flow void" phenomenon. Imaging these vessels and communications is often extremely difficult by other noninvasive means.

Although myocardial ischemia is not the most common problem facing the pediatric patient with heart disease, it may be vitally significant in several instances. Specifically, the presence and extent of myocardial ischemia may have critical importance in infants and children with anomalous left coronary artery, coronary calcinosis, mucocutaneous lymph node syndrome, and transient myocardial ischemia of the newborn and in some patients after cardiac surgery.

In 1977, investigators applied phosphorus-31 NMR imaging to the study of myocardial changes during ischemia.[14, 23] Williams et al.[39] later used proton-density NMR technique to document the effects of ligation of the left anterior descending coronary artery in dogs. They showed that prolongation of the proton spin-lattice relaxation times (T_1) was a reflection of increased water content in ischemic tissue. These studies suggest that NMR may play an important role in defining the extent of damage from myocardial ischemia and also in identifying the areas of irreversibly damaged myocardium. This has important therapeutic as well as prognostic implications.

NMR may be useful in the study of biochemical as well as anatomic changes in both iatrogenic and naturally occurring ischemia. The physiologic effects of cardioplegia on the myocardium in the pediatric surgical patient are of particular interest. ^{31}P NMR imaging techniques have been used to study intracellular pH change, creatinine phosphate content, adenosine triphosphate, and organic phosphate levels in comparing various cardioplegia solutions and hypothermia.[12] Better understanding of the pathophysiology of low output after open heart surgery might improve the management of this complication and reduce the morbidity and mortality associated with it.

EVALUATION OF CARDIAC FUNCTION

True three-dimensional proton-density imaging produces an image of the heart with equivalent resolution in all planes. Direct and precise calculation of chamber volume at different phases of the cardiac cycle therefore becomes feasible, and this would result in greater accuracy of such functional measurements as cardiac output and ejection fraction.

ADVANTAGES OF NMR CARDIOVASCULAR IMAGING

Cardiac catheterization, which still remains the "gold standard" in many ways, is, of course, invasive. Therefore, there are real risks associated with this procedure. In addition, the patient is also subject to discomfort and pain. Imaging requires the use of contrast material and exposure to ionizing radiation. NMR is noninvasive and painless and does not require contrast or the use of ionizing radiation. Contrast agents can cause acidosis, dehydration, and hypernatremia, particularly in small infants. In addition, a positive image is obtained rather than the negative one of a cardiac structure outlined by iodinated contrast media.

Nuclear medicine techniques do not have the risks of cardiac catheterization but do require, in most instances, intravenous isotope injection. They, therefore, are not really noninvasive. In addition, the technique often requires bolus injection, which may be difficult to accomplish in small infants with small-bore needles. The patient is exposed to ionizing radiation, and the resolution of anatomic detail is poor. NMR requires none of this and is capable of much better resolution.

Echocardiography has revolutionized the practice of pediatric cardiology. Most often the diagnosis is made before catheterization. However, in some instances echocardiographic evaluation cannot be completed owing to interference from bone, air, and surgical dressings. NMR is not affected by these. In addition, problems of lateral resolution in two-dimensional studies have limited the use of echocardiography for improved functional evaluation. NMR is inherently three-dimensional and isotropic in all dimensions.

Computerized tomography has had limited usefulness in cardiology because scan time is long compared with the cardiac cycle. This technique also requires a considerable exposure to ionizing radiation. In addition, resolution perpendicular to the imaging plane is poor. NMR can produce images with short scan time and with equal resolution in all planes without ionizing radiation.

DISADVANTAGES OF NMR

Some technical considerations at this stage in the development of NMR for medical use provide some of the obstacles to be overcome. The size of the unit is large, and considerable space must be allocated. The magnets are also quite heavy, and ground floor placement seems most practical. The magnetic fields and induced currents can cause interference with other medical equipment, and adequate insulation must therefore be provided. These same magnetic fields and induced currents interfere with pacemakers and therefore cannot be used to evaluate patients with pacemakers. This last consideration is not of great concern in pediatric cardiac practice.

NMR does not provide "real-time" images, therefore, two-dimensional echocardiography has an advantage here. However, multiple images obtained through the cardiac cycle can be stored and replayed sequentially, resulting in a dynamic display.

BIOLOGIC EFFECTS OF NMR IMAGING

Potential harmful effects to humans from NMR imaging may arise from several sources. These include the effects of strong static magnetic fields (up to 20,000 gauss), the effects of induced currents associated with rapidly varying magnetic fields used for spatial localization in NMR imaging, and the heating effect of radiofrequency magnetic fields.

At high-static magnetic field strengths, electrocardiogram (ECG) abnormalities have been observed in experimental animals. Specifically, alterations in T-wave amplitude may be seen at a threshold of approximately 300 gauss, which increase linearly with field strength up to 20,000 gauss. These are thought to be the result of induced EMF (electromotive force) potentials associated with high-velocity blood flow perpendicular to the static magnetic field. Small EMF potentials may also be induced by changes in thoracic diameter related to diastolic and systolic differences in intravascular volume. Significantly, these potentials have no known physiologic effect. Exposure to strong static magnetic fields has not been shown to cause arrhythmias, changes in heart rate, or alteration in blood chemistry. Moreover, upon cessation of field exposure, the ECG immediately returns to the normal baseline state.[4, 13, 36]

The orientation of most normal human cells is not affected by applied static magnetic fields. However, anisotropic cells, such as sickled erythrocytes, experience alignment changes in fields of 350 gauss.[31] The significance of this phenomenon in patients with sickle cell anemia has not been investigated. Battocletti et al. compared pre– and post–NMR exposure effects on cellular and chemical blood parameters in rhesus monkeys and found no differences.[3]

The biologic effects of rapid magnetic field changes are less well known. No significant threat to human health has been identified under the conditions used for proton NMR imaging. With relatively large field oscillations and resulting high induced current density, ventricular fibrillation is a potential hazard.[34, 38] However, present data are inadequate for establishment of safe limits for exposure to rapidly changing magnetic fields.

The adverse effects of radiofrequency magnetic radiation are mainly related to tissue heating. Davis et al. exposed steel surgical clips, copper wire clips, and metallic hip prostheses to a changing magnetic field created by an aircore magnet and to rf fields created by a standard rf coil. Under their experimental conditions, a heating effect 6 to 42 times that of conventional NMR imaging was produced. They concluded that no significant heating of surgical clips and contiguous soft tissues can be expected during NMR imaging procedures but that the effects on larger metallic implants required further study.[10]

Long-term studies of the effects of NMR on health are not available. At present, there are no reports of chronic or acute illness to workers or volunteers exposed to NMR. In studying the genetic effects of NMR, Wolf et al.[40] exposed Chinese hamster ovary cells and human cells to strong magnetic fields, pulsed field gradients, and radiofrequency energy. They found no chromosomal aberrations or sister chromatid exchanges in the hamster cells and no inhibition of DNA synthesis in the human cells.

In conclusion, no significant adverse physiologic, cellular, biochemical, or genetic consequences have been shown in humans or animals after exposure to magnetic fields up to 20,000 gauss.[6]

CONCLUSION

NMR has the potential for improving acquisition of anatomic and physiologic data noninvasively without exposure to ionizing radiation. Better techniques with fewer hazards are important advantages in the evaluation of patients who may require repeated studies through their lifetimes.

ACKNOWLEDGMENT

We wish to thank Dr. David M. Kramer for providing the gated images of the normal heart.

REFERENCES

1. Ackerman JJH, Grove TH, Wong GG, et al: Mapping of metabolites in whole animals by ^{31}P NMR using surface coils. Nature, *283*:167–170, 1980.
2. Alfidi RJ, Haaga JR, El Yousef SJ.: Preliminary experimental results in humans and animals with a superconducting whole-body nuclear magnetic resonance scanner. Radiology, *143*:175–181, 1982.
3. Battocletti JH, Salles-Cunha S, Halbach RE, et al: Exposure of rhesus monkeys to 20,000G steady magnetic field: Effect on blood parameters. Med Phys, *8*:115–118, 1981.
4. Beischer DE, Knepton JC: Influence of strong magnetic fields on the electrocardiogram of squirrel monkeys. Aerospace Med, *35*:939–944, 1964.
5. Bendel P, Lai CM, Lauterbur PC: ^{31}P spectroscopic zeugmatography of phosphorus metabolites. J Mag Res, *38*:343–356, 1980.
6. Budinger TF: Potential medical effects and hazards with NMR human studies. *In* Kaufman L, Crooks LE, Margulis AR (eds): Nuclear Magnetic Resonance Imaging in Medicine. Tokyo, Igaku-Shoin, 1981, pp. 207–231.
7. Crooks L, Arakawa M, Hoenninger J, et al: Nuclear magnetic resonance whole-body imager operating at 3.5K gauss. Radiology, *143*:169–174, 1982.
8. Crooks L, Hoenninger J, Arakawa M, et al: Tomography of hydrogen with nuclear magnetic resonance. Radiology, *136*:701–706, 1980.
9. Damadian R, Goldsmith M, Minkoff, L: NMR in cancer: XVI FONAR image of the live human body. Physiol Chem Phys, *9*:97–100, 108, 1980.
10. Davis PL, Crooks L, Arakawa M, et al: Potential hazards in NMR imaging: Heating effects of changing magnetic fields and RF fields on small metallic implants. AJR, *137*:857–860, 1981.
11. Edelstein WA, Hutchinson JMS, Smith FW, et al: Human whole-body NMR tomographic imaging: Normal sections. Br J Radiol, *54*:149–151, 1981.
12. Flaherty JT, Weisfeldt ML, Buckley BH, et al: Mechanisms of ischemic myocardial cell damage assessed by phosphorus-31 nuclear magnetic resonance. Circulation, *65*:561–571, 1982.
13. Gaffey CT, Tenforde TS, Dean EE: Alterations in the electrocardiogram of baboons exposed to DC magnetic fields. Bioelectromagnetics, *1*:209, 1980.
14. Garlik PB, Radda GK, Seeley PJ, et al: Phosphorus NMR studies on perfused heart. Biochem Biophys Res Comm, *74*:1256–1262, 1977.
15. Godwin JD, Herfuens RL, Skioldebrand CG et al: Evaluation of dissections and aneurysms of the thoracic aorta by conventional and dynamic CT scanning. Radiology, *136*:125–133, 1980.
16. Gordon RE, Hanley PE, Shaw D, et al: Localization of metabolites in animals using ^{31}P topical magnetic resonance. Nature, *287*:736–738, 1980.
17. Hansen G, Crooks LE, Davis P, et al: In vivo imaging of the rat anatomy with nuclear magnetic resonance. Radiology, *136*:695–700, 1980.
18. Heneghan MA, Biancaniello TM, Heidelberger E, et al: Nuclear magnetic resonance zeugmatographic imaging of the heart: Application to the study of ventricular septal defect. Radiology, *143*:183–186, 1982.
19. Hinshaw WS: Imaging formation by NMR: The sensitive point method. J Appl Phys, *47*:3709–3721, 1976.
20. Hinshaw WS, Andrew ER, Bottomley PA, et al: Display of cross-sectional anatomy by nuclear magnetic resonance imaging. Br J Radiol, *51*:273–280, 1978.
21. Hinshaw WS, Bottomley PA, Holland EN: Radiographic thin-section image of the human wrist by nuclear magnetic resonance. Nature, *270*:722–723, 1977.
22. Holland GN, Bottomley PA, Hinshaw WS: ^{19}F magnetic resonance imaging. J Mag Res, *28*:133–136, 1977.
23. Hollis DP, Nunnally RL, Jacobus WE, et al: Detection of regional ischemia in perfused beating hearts by phosphorus nuclear magnetic resonance. Biochem Biophys Res Comm, *75*:1086–1091, 1977.
24. Kaufman L, Crooks LE, Margulis AR (eds): Nuclear Magnetic Resonance in Medicine. New York, Igaku-Shoin, 1981.
25. Kramer DM, Schneider JS, Rudin AM, et al: True three-dimensional nuclear magnetic resonance zeugmatographic images of a human brain. Neuroradiology, *21*:239–244, 1981.
26. Lai CM, Lauterbur PC: True three-dimensional image reconstruction by nuclear magnetic resonance zeugmatography. Phys Med Biol, *26*:851–856, 1981.
27. Lauterbur PC: Image formation by induced local interactions: Examples employing nuclear magnetic resonance. Nature, *242*:190–191, 1973.
28. Lauterbur PC, Dias MHM, Rudin AM: Augmentation of tissue water proton spin–lattice relaxation rates by in vivo addition of paramagnetic ions. *In* Dutton PL, Leigh JS, Scarpa A (eds): International Symposium of Frontiers of Biological Energetics: Electrons to

Tissues, Vol. 1. New York, Academic Press, 1978, pp. 752–759.

29. Leigh, JS.: Nuclear magnetic resonance. *In* Jones DW (ed): Introduction to the Spectroscopy of Biologic Polymers. New York, Academic Press, 1976.
30. Mansfield P, Pykett IL, Morris PG, et al: Human whole body line-scan imaging by NMR. Br J Radiol, *51*:921–922, 1978.
31. Muramaya M: Orientation of sickled erythrocytes in a magnetic field. Nature, *206*:420–422, 1965.
32. Pykett IL: NMR imaging in medicine. Scientific American, *246*:78–88, 1982.
33. Pykett IL, Newhouse JH, Buonanno FS, et al: Principles of nuclear magnetic resonance imaging. Radiology, *143*:157–168, 1982.
34. Ross RJ, Thompson JS, Kim K, et al: Nuclear magnetic resonance imaging and evaluation of human breast tissue: Preliminary clinical trials. Radiology, *143*: 195–205, 1982.
35. Roy OZ: Technical note: Summary of cardiac fibrillation thresholds for 60 Hz currents and voltages applied directly to the heart. Med Biol Eng Comput, *18*:657–659, 1980.
36. Togawa T, Okai O, Oshima M: Observation of blood flow EMF in externally applied strong magnetic field by surface electrodes. Med Biol Eng, *5*:169–170, 1967.
37. Ross BD, Radda GK, Gadian G, et al: Examination of a case of suspected McArdle's syndrome by ^{31}P nuclear magnetic resonance. N Engl J Med, *304*:1338–1342, 1981.
38. Watson AB, Wright JS, Loughman J: Electrical thresholds for ventricular fibrillation in man. Med J Aust, *1*:1179–1182, 1973.
39. Williams ES, Kaplan JI, Thatcher F, et al: Prolongation of proton spin relaxation times in regionally ischemic tissue from dog hearts. J Nucl Med, *21*:449–453, 1980.
40. Wolff S, Crooks LE, Brown P, et al: Tests for DNA and chromosomal damage induced by nuclear magnetic resonance imaging. Radiology, *136*;707–710, 1980.

INDEX